HEAD AND NECK CANCER

Management of the Difficult Case

Paul J. Donald, M.D., F.R.C.S.
Associate Professor and Vice Chairman
Department of Otorhinolaryngology
University of California, Davis

1984
W.B. Saunders Company
Philadelphia • London • Toronto • Mexico City • Rio de Janeiro • Sydney • Tokyo

W. B. Saunders Company: West Washington Square
Philadelphia, PA 19105

1 St. Anne's Road
Eastbourne, East Sussex BN21 3UN, England

1 Goldthorne Avenue
Toronto, Ontario M8Z 5T9, Canada

Apartado 26370—Cedro 512
Mexico 4, D.F., Mexico

Rua Coronel Cabrita, 8
Sao Cristovao Caixa Postal 21176
Rio de Janeiro, Brazil

9 Waltham Street
Artarmon, N.S.W. 2064, Australia

Ichibancho, Central Bldg., 22-1 Ichibancho
Chiyoda-Ku, Tokyo 102, Japan

Library of Congress Cataloging in Publication Data

Donald, Paul J.

Head and neck cancer.

1. Head—Cancer—Treatment. 2. Neck—Cancer—Treatment. I. Title.

RC280.H4D66 1984 616.99′49106 83–3364

ISBN 0–7216–3141–X

Head and Neck Cancer: Management of the Difficult Case ISBN 0-7216-3141-X

Last digit is the print number: 9 8 7 6 5 4 3 2 1

This volume is dedicated to the interest, patience, enthusiasm, continued encouragement, and sacrifice that my wife, Roz, and my children, Scott, Allison, Heather, and Andy, showed during its production.

CONTRIBUTORS

DAVID A. DEER, M.D.

Medical Director, Radiation Oncology Department, Bethany Medical Center, Kansas City, Kansas

Radiotherapy

ROBERT E. GILLIS, Jr, D.M.D., M.S.D.

Clinical Associate Professor, Department of Otorhinolaryngology, University of California at Davis School of Medicine; Staff appointments at University of California, at Davis Medical Center, Mercy Hospitals of Sacramento, and Sutter Community Hospital, Sacramento, California

Maxillofacial Prosthetics

BERNARD R. GREENBERG, M.D.

Associate Professor of Medicine, University of Arizona College of Medicine; Chief, Section of Hematology/Oncology, Veterans Administration Medical Center, Tucson, Arizona

Chemotherapy

REBECCA J. LEONARD, Ph.D.

Assistant Professor, University of California at Davis School of Medicine; Chief, Division of Speech Pathology, University of California at Davis Medical Center, Sacramento, California

Speech Rehabilitation

BRUCE W. PEARSON, M.D., F.R.C.S.(C)

Associate Professor of Otorhinolaryngology, Mayo Medical School, Mayo Clinic; Consultant in Otorhinolaryngology, St. Mary's Hospital, Rochester, Minnesota

Larynx

ANN E. FURIEL SIEVERS, R.N., M.A.

E.N.T. Clinical Nursing Specialist, E.N.T. Clinic, University of California at Davis Medical Center, Sacramento, California.

Nursing Aspects; Nutrition

PREFACE

In recent times, surgeons have been privileged to have readily available a number of outstanding textbooks covering the basic principles on the management of head and neck cancer. Heretofore, there has not been a text specifically devoted to describing approaches to the difficult and problematic cases. Most of the patients who fall into this category suffer from tumors that are either massive in extent or that extend beyond the cervicofacial area to encroach upon adjacent anatomic regions such as the brain or thorax. Their management often requires a unique set of intricate surgical steps, both for ablation of the tumor and for the eventual reconstruction. Some of the tumors in this category exhibit unusual histologic and biologic behavior. Because of the debilitation resulting from the tumor and the extensiveness of the surgery, many of these patients are difficult to manage postoperatively. Later, they often require the assistance of both a maxillofacial prosthetist and a speech therapist in their rehabilitation.

The surgeon faced with the enigmas inherent in these lesions is often forced to conduct an exhaustive search of the literature in order to extract the information that may provide a solution to his particular problem. The purpose of this book is to provide a concise and comprehensive reference source in those cases in which complete excision is difficult or complex, and reconstruction to restore function and cosmesis is problematic. The book is not intended for the beginning resident or the practitioner who does occasional head and neck tumor surgery. It is directed at the senior resident level, and is specifically intended to aid those surgeons who are regularly engaged in head and neck tumor exenterative surgery and from time to time are faced with the difficulties encountered in those problem cases.

The format of this monograph in each chapter is to initially briefly outline the pertinent points of pathology, etiology, and presentation of the lesions in each major anatomic area of the head and neck. Concentration is directed toward the natural history of the disease, the peculiar anatomic details, the pathophysiology of the tumors, and most especially the surgical management of the area involved. There is some variation in emphasis among chapters. Those on malignant melanoma and pediatric tumors, for instance, are a little more general in nature, because these diseases are very uncommon, exhaustive treatises on them are wanting, and their management is highly controversial. On the other hand, chapters such as the one on the oral cavity provide detailed discussions of conservation surgery, the management of lesions in specific areas of the region, and the excision of massive tumors with the subsequent reconstruction. Procedures such as wedge resection of the tongue and the composite resection are not covered because they are so well described in the standard textbooks on head and neck surgery.

There is bound to be some overlap of material, such as the application of mediastinal resection both in thyroid cancer and in malignancy of the cervical esophagus. The details of mediastinal resection are carefully outlined in the chapter on surgery of the hypopharynx and cervical esophagus, and only the modifications peculiar to thyroid cancer with mediastinal involvement will be described in the chapter on the thyroid. The thyroid chapter also presents a guide to attempt the differentiation of benign from malignant tumors, as well as details on how to avoid injury to the recurrent laryngeal nerve.

The management of tumors in some areas (such as the base of the tongue, the anterior pharyngeal wall and the cervical esophagus) remains somewhat controversial, with solid statistical information on the best choice of procedure as yet unavailable. The author's usual methods of handling these difficult lesions are outlined as well as the appropriate techniques to reconstruct the gullet.

The chapter on the nose and paranasal sinuses concentrates on the management of two major problem areas: lesions of the nasal dorsum and vestibule, and those large paranasal sinus tumors that require craniofacial resection. Not only are the combined procedures detailed but the anesthetic and postoperative management are thoroughly discussed as well. Particular attention is paid to the physiologic considerations of altered intracranial homeostasis and its necessary restoration during and after these operations. This problem is dealt with in even greater detail in the chapter on the skull base. This latter chapter presents a number of avant-garde procedures to successfully exenterate neoplasms that invade the base of the skull from a host of cervicofacial areas such as the deep lobe of the parotid gland, the nasopharynx, and the neurovascular structures under the temporal and sphenoid bones.

A detailed account of the author's approach to the excision of lesions at the various levels in the temporal bone is found in the chapter on the ear and temporal bone. A meticulous recounting of each step in resection of the temporal bone is an amalgamation of the best features of a number of contributions by many of the giants in the field of head and neck surgery.

The chapter on the salivary glands initially attempts to clarify the confusion that surrounds the classification of the tumors arising in these structures. The surgical approach concentrates on the more unusual problems: dealing with recurrent pleomorphic adenoma, the excision of large extensive malignancies that invade the infratemporal fossa or temporal bone, and the management of adenoid cystic cancers. The management of tumors of the minor salivary glands is detailed as well.

The chapter on the larynx deals mainly with conservation surgery and voice-preserving techniques. The excellent contribution of Dr. Bruce Pearson of the Mayo Clinic is an outstanding embellishment to this book. His description of the voice-conserving procedure he developed is easy to follow and, with some practice, easy to duplicate.

The final chapters concern those specialized fields that are integral to the management of these difficult cases. In many anatomic areas, the ultimate resection has been achieved and become established. Irradiation and antitumor drug therapy are often vital adjuncts to the surgical management and represent the only hope to improve both local control and patient survival.

Increasing evidence is accumulating showing that tumor eradication and reasonable patient survival can be hoped for only when a judicious combination of these three modalities is employed.

The main focus of both the chapters on chemotherapy and irradiation is their utilization in combination with surgery. The basic principles of antitumor activity are clearly and briefly outlined in the beginning of each chapter. The utility of the modalities in each site is reviewed, but the main thrust is the discussion of various formats of combined therapy and their success rates.

A smooth postoperative course and ultimate recovery of the patient is often heavily dependent upon the quality of the nursing care. The prevention of complications and their diligent management by the bedside nurse is of paramount importance. A detailed account of the treatments involved in the "control of the wound," as aptly coined by Conley, and the management of the often difficult and complex psychosocial problems of these patients is covered in the chapter on Nursing Aspects. Organization of the flow of nursing care both pre- and post-treatment, as well as in the home following discharge, is also included. Good nutritional care is essential to the healing of the wound and the rapid recovery of the patient. The use of parenteral hyperalimentation and the various high-protein, high-caloric food substitutes has broadened the armamentarium of the nutritionist who previously had to rely solely on intravenous glucose and varying combinations of regular food to administer the badly needed calories. The chapter on nutrition provides detailed information on the composition, caloric content, and even cost of many of the available commercially prepared formulas. Types of parenteral and enteral procedures are detailed.

Maxillofacial prosthodontics is one of the most rapidly advancing fields in dentistry. Almost unheard of twenty years ago, it has become an integral part of the rehabilitation of the problem head and neck cancer patient. The chapter on Maxillofacial Prosthetics concentrates more on the application of prosthetic rehabilitation in the difficult case than on the basic principles of the specialty, with considerable attention given to the surgical details that will facilitate the fitting and retention of the prosthesis.

Saving "the best for last" is aptly applied to the final chapter in this book. The chapter on speech rehabilitation is one of the best, most orderly approaches to an understanding of the effects of head and neck surgery on speech production and its possible remediation that I have encountered. Dr. Leonard has done an exceptional job in reviewing the pertinent literature, then clearly and succinctly coalescing the facts in a lucid and meaningful way. The effects of the various surgical procedures in the oral cavity on speech are discussed in great detail, and rehabilitative measures for the pharyngectomized as well as the laryngectomized patient are beautifully described.

An important caveat is essential at this juncture. The nature and extent of these lesions dictate that the surgery, in order to be successful, must be radical. Problem surgery is not for the faint of heart. Armed with the knowledge that with extensive exenteration of the tumor, the patient has a good chance of being rid of the malignancy, and that most can be surgically and prosthetically rehabilitated, the surgeon is able to approach these lesions with considerable optimism.

Lastly, the patient himself must not be forgotten. Often during the deliberations of the complexities of the preoperative work-up, the intricacies of the surgery, and the coordination of the specialists involved in the patient's care, there is a tendency to concentrate on the tumor rather than on the unfortunate person who possesses it. The patient is in pain, suffers not only the compromises of disturbed function, but also the agony of an often grossly altered physiognomy and its devastating social consequences. Eclipsing these adversities is the pervasive fear of possible impending death and the helplessness of being the victim of a complex surgical procedure, the comprehension of the nature and consequences of which defy the surgeons's detailed explanation. Compassion, empathy, and patience are vital tools in the management of these severely afflicted individuals.

It is hoped that this book will fill a need relevant to the practice of the head and neck surgeon who is engaged in the treatment of these challenging patients.

PAUL J. DONALD

ACKNOWLEDGMENTS

I would like to acknowledge the contributions and support of a number of individuals who were of inestimable assistance in the production of this work. Dr. A. Edward Percy, now deceased, was a big supporter of this project, and without his help it would not have been brought to fruition. Dr. Percy's unlimited generosity and warm encouragement were greatly appreciated. His sage counsel and ready wit are sorely missed by students, residents, and faculty alike.

The magnificent artwork of Nelva Richardson is easily one of the most important contributions to this book. Mrs. Richardson was a joy to work with and had the uncanny ability to conceptualize the many procedural details and unusual approaches that were completely unfamiliar to her. With some crude line drawings of my own and a few verbal instructions as a guide, she produced precisely what was needed, and always in a timely fashion. It was pure pleasure to work with an artist of her outstanding ability and good humor.

Finally, I wish to thank the typists who worked so diligently on the manuscript. Connie Van Amstel and Irene Ross began with the first two chapters. However, the bulk of the work fell on the capable shoulders of Amy Barbeau, whose effort on behalf of this work was herculean to say the least. She happily worked overtime to complete the typing and proofing at the earliest time possible. Her hard work and diligence are greatly appreciated.

P.J.D.

CONTENTS

1

ORAL CAVITY

Paul J. Donald, M.D.

Carcinoma of the oral cavity accounts for approximately 55 per cent of all human malignancies in the United States.[1] The lesion is histologically squamous cell carcinoma in 95 per cent of cases.[2,3] The worldwide variation of incidence of oral cancer is striking; the oral cavity is the site of 1 per cent of all cancers in West Germany, strongly contrasting with a 45 per cent incidence in Bombay, India. Male predominance is characteristic in the United States; however, some notable exceptions are seen elsewhere in the world. In the state of Andra Pradesh in India, on the island of Singapore, and in the city of Durban, South Africa, the female incidence is considerably higher than the male.[2] This is also true in Scandinavia, where the Plummer-Vinsòn syndrome is common.

PATHOLOGY

Etiology. Oral lesions commonly occur in the so-called salivary puddle,[4] a horseshoe-shaped area that encompasses the lateral regions of the tongue, the floor of the mouth, the retromolar trigone, and the anterior tonsillar pillar. Figure 1–1 shows the distribution of a series of oral cavity carcinomas seen at the Memorial Hospital in New York.[5] It is interesting to note that 80 per cent of the lesions are confined to only 20 per cent of the oral cavity surface. Thus Lederman's conception of the etiologic implication of these mucosal areas being continuously bathed in saliva in which carcinogens are suspended has considerable relevance.

The precise etiology of these neoplasms remains obscure, but a number of factors have been elucidated. A common association has been noted between the interstitial glossitis of tertiary syphilis and lingual cancer. The predilection of syphilis-induced malignancy for the dorsum of the tongue (Fig. 1–2), in contrast to the usual site of origin of these cancers, is distinctive. Trieger et al[6] reported an 18 per cent incidence of serologically positive syphilis in their series of patients. Gorlin and Vickers[7] state that carcinoma of the tongue is four times more common in patients afflicted with syphilis. Trauma, sepsis, alcohol, tobacco, and dietary deficiencies have all been implicated. The presence of broken and carious teeth and infected gingivae has long been thought to be etiologically significant, and although no consistent statistical proof of a link with cancer has been forthcoming, the association appears to be common. The importance of chronic irritation in the genesis of cancer at any site is frequently noted. The fact that one half of all patients with oral cancer are edentulous, and are therefore usually denture wearers, lends some credence to this opinion. In fact, oftentimes the "denture sore" produced by the irritation of a denture is indistinguishable on gross examination from a carcinoma (Fig. 1–3).

Heavy tobacco use and alcohol consumption are undoubtedly implicated in the genesis of oral cancer. Whether these substances act directly on the mucosa or as a trigger mechanism on a predisposed cellular situation is not yet clear. There is substantial evidence showing that the cellular immunocompetence of an individual is markedly diminished with heavy cigarette smoking[8] and high alcohol intake.[9,10]

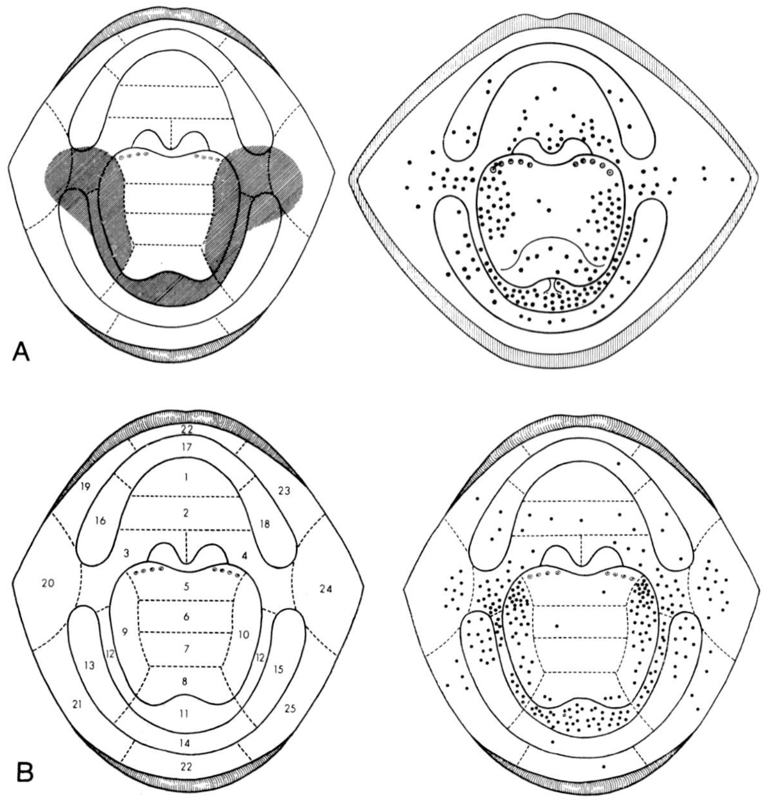

Figure 1–1. *A, Left,* Segmental distribution of the incidence of oral cavity cancer in 252 cases. Each segment occupies an approximate equivalent area of mucosa. *Right,* A scattergram indicating the distribution of 256 cases of oral carcinoma.
B, Left, Preferred site of predilection for squamous cell carcinoma of the oral cavity. *Right,* Scattergram of 209 consecutive cases of oral cavity cancer. (Adapted from Moore C, Catlin D: Anatomical origins and locations of oral cancer. Am. J. Surg. 114:511, 1967.)

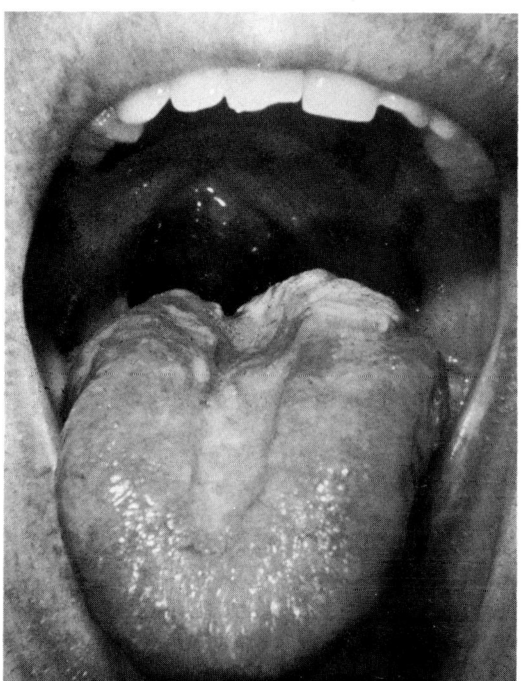

Figure 1–2. Carcinoma on the dorsum of the tongue.

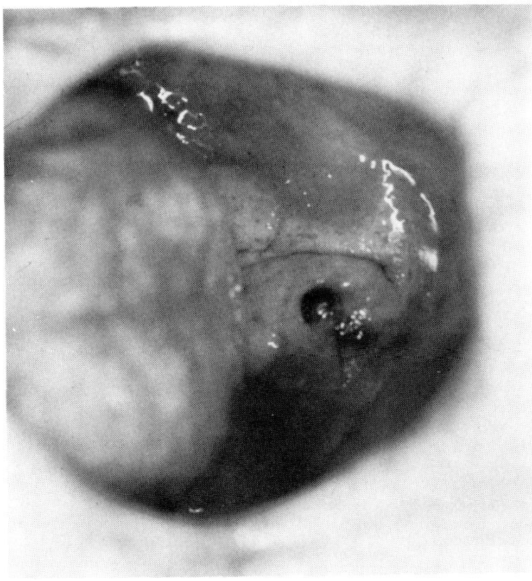

Figure 1–3. Denture sore on hard palate, closely resembling an exophytic carcinoma.

A number of lesions that are thought to be the precursors of malignancy have been identified in the mouth. The importance of leukoplakia (Fig. 1–4) as a progenitor of carcinoma has been debated. The fact that carcinomas are commonly found in leukoplakic areas, including some previously proved histologically benign, lends some support to their importance. A study by Waldren and Shafer[11] showed that between 14 and 18 per cent of leukoplakias are dysplastic or malignant on the first biopsy. Subsequent sampling of the benign ones showed that a further 5 per cent eventually became carcinomatous. Queyrat's erythroplasia is seen most commonly in the region of the soft palate and the anterior tonsillar pillar, but it has also been observed on the buccal mucosa. Its premalignant potential is well established. The condition of so-called erythroplakia, an ostensible hybrid of leukoplakia and erythroplasia, is considered to be more malignant still.[12] In most instances of erythroplakia, there is histologic evidence of at least severe dysplasia and often carcinoma in situ or microinvasive carcinoma.

A further complexity in the management of patients with oral cavity cancer is the problem of multicentric carcinoma. There is a tendency in some individuals to develop multiple foci of squamous cell carcinoma. These may be either in situ or frankly invasive. These patients have a mucosa often predisposed to cancer formation by chronic heavy tobacco abuse and alcohol consumption. This so-called field cancerization[4] renders the definitive treatment of these lesions most difficult.

Metastasis. The local aggressiveness, the regional metastatic potential, and even the distant metastatic rate increase as distal progression of tumor location is made from the tongue tip to the oropharynx. Lesions of the tongue base generally have a dismal prognosis compared with those of the oral tongue. Unilateral cervical metastases are usually present, and bilateral disease is common. Throughout the tongue, but especially in the posterior one third, the musculature acts like a "muscular pump," disseminating tumor cells in the interstices between muscle fibers that are a considerable distance from the primary tumor.

The incidence of regional metastases varies

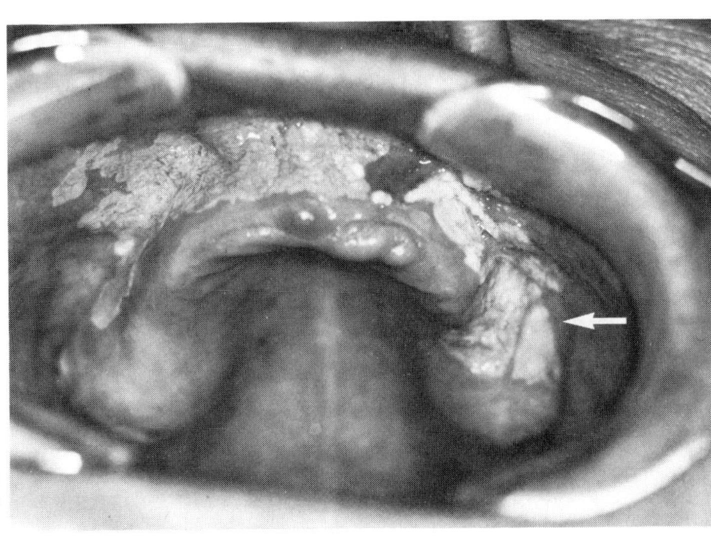

Figure 1–4. Extensive leukoplakia on upper alveolar ridge. Arrow denotes verrucous carcinoma.

Table 1–1. REGIONAL LYMPH NODE INVOLVEMENT BY SITE*

	Tongue (2751)	*Floor of Mouth (1013)*	*Gingiva (423)*	*Buccal Mucosa (654)*
Nodes present at admission	36%	38%	33%	32%
Nodes involved later (occult)	29%	18%	17%	13%
Total lymph node involvement	65%	56%	50%	45%

*From DiTroia JF: Nodal metastases and prognosis in carcinoma of the oral cavity. Otolaryngol Clin North Am 5:335, 1972, Table 1.

among series. Strong[13] reported on 314 patients with carcinoma of the anterior two thirds of the tongue gathered in a 5-year period between 1957 and 1963. The number of patients with palpable lymph node metastasis on presentation was 98, an incidence of 31.2 per cent. Only 4 patients had contralateral or bilateral nodal involvement. Table 1–1 illustrates the incidence of regional lymph node metastases in a large composite group of 4841 patients with oral cavity carcinoma from different sources. In this group, a total of 59.1 per cent had either manifest or occult metastases. In approximately one third of each anatomic group, the metastasis was occult in nature. However, the incidence of occult metastases is highly variable among series, which is evidence of the general unreliability of clinical palpation. Batsakis[15] depicts this variability with a table reproduced here as Table 1–2.

Metastasis varies with both size and site of the tumor. T_3 and T_4 lesions are much more commonly seen with metastases than are smaller lesions. Cancers on the tongue tip have a much lower metastatic rate than those in the middle third, and these in turn have a lower rate than those of the posterior third of the oral tongue.[21] This also holds true for the bilaterality of the nodal metastases. Fries et al,[22] in a combined study of oral cavity tumors from Germany, Switzerland, and Austria, found that cancer of the buccal mucosa had the highest metastatic rate: 75 per cent. The mandibular alveolar ridge was next highest at 61.2 per cent, followed by the floor of the mouth at 59.9 per cent. The tongue itself had metastases in 40 per cent of cases. In the smaller series of buccal mucosal carcinomas quoted by Batsakis, the metastatic rate was lower, varying from 37 to 50 per cent.[15] There was, however, some concurrence in the rates cited for the alveolar ridge, which ranged from 30 to 80 per cent in both his and the European group.

Table 1–2. INCIDENCE OF CLINICALLY OCCULT CERVICAL METASTASES*

Authors	*Incidence*
Lyall and Shetlin[16]	60%
Kremen[17]	50%
Southwick et al[18]	40%
Sako et al[19]	27.6%
Ward et al[20]	25%

*From Batsakis JG: Tumors of the Head and Neck: Clinical and Pathological considerations. Baltimore, Williams and Wilkins, 1974 pp 86–111.

Sites of Predilection. The oral cavity is generally divided into the lips, buccal mucosa, tongue, floor of the mouth, hard palate, and alveolar ridges. However, the area of the distal oral cavity—the retromolar trigone, adjacent floor of the mouth, anterior tonsillar pillar, and soft palate—is a unit (Fig. 1–5) that anatomically and biologically forms a kind of transition zone.[23] Tumors in this region are managed in a similar fashion to those involving the oropharynx and often extend into it. Malignancies remain asymptomatic in this region for a considerable time before becoming manifest as localized pain, trismus, or cervical adenopathy. Lesions of the distal floor of the mouth adjacent to the retromolar trigone of the mandible are particularly pernicious. This area has been dubbed the "coffin corner" because of the ability of tumors therein to remain occult until they obtain substantial size. The examining physician must move the tongue well to the side and illuminate this area adequately to pick up these lesions while they are still small.

The buccal mucosa is not nearly as common a site for primary carcinoma as the other regions in the oral cavity. Batsakis[15] classifies these lesions according to their presentation on gross examination as ulcer-infiltrative, exophytic, or verrucous. The verrucous variety is the most benign in its natural course, almost never metastasizes, and can most easily be adequately encompassed by a local resection. The ulcer-infiltrative type is the most locally aggressive, has the highest metastatic rate, and requires the most radical excision. The anatomic composition of the area predisposes it to rapid through-and-

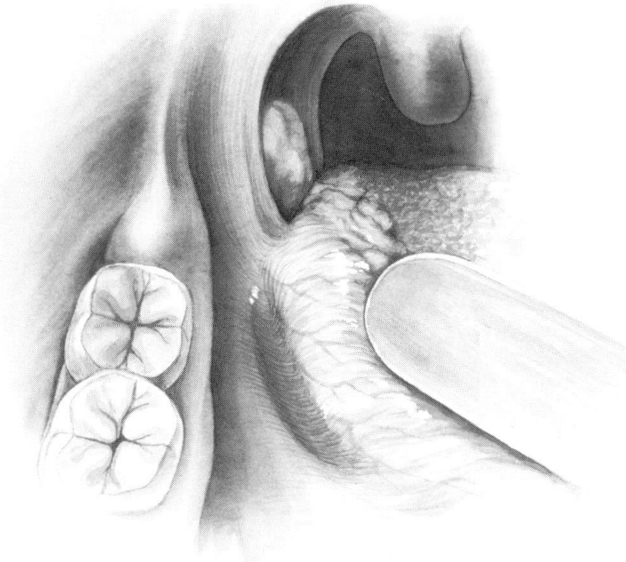

Figure 1–5. The distal oral cavity. Note the retromolar trigone area behind the third molar tooth and the posterior extreme of the floor of the mouth, the so-called "coffin corner."

through penetration by aggressive tumors. The buccal mucosa lies against the buccinator muscle, which is sheathed in the buccopharyngeal fascia. Superficial to this lies subcutaneous fat and skin.

The alveolar ridge is an area in which the diagnosis of cancer may be mistaken for some time. In the upper jaw and palate, the appearance of an exophytic mass must raise the suspicion of the maxillary sinus as the site of origin. It is important to note in this regard that expansion of the maxillary sinus into the alveolar process occurs in 50 per cent of persons.[24] Carcinoma is 2 to 3 times more common in the lower jaw than in the upper.[25] The exophytic and ulcerative character of the neoplasm in its early stages is grossly indistinguishable from the infected granulation tissue accompanying pyorrhea. A high index of suspicion in susceptible individuals is mandatory. Following extraction of a carious tooth, a failure of the site to heal—the so-called dry socket—must be equally suspiciously viewed in the same population. However, according to Thoma[26] most alveolar ridge lesions occur in the edentulous patient. Sharp and Wood[27] stated that 50 per cent of the tumors in their series arose in previously leukoplakic areas.

MANAGEMENT PRINCIPLES

In keeping with the philosophy of this monograph, the basic principles of management of oral cavity lesions will be merely overviewed, with detailed discussion reserved for specialized areas. Generally speaking, T_1 lesions (less than 2 cm in size) may be treated equally well with irradiation or surgery. This decision depends on a number of factors. For example, the proximity of the tumor to bone tends to favor the choice of surgery because of concern that irradiation therapy may lead to the development of osteoradionecrosis of the mandible (Fig. 1–6). The presence of mandibular tori (Fig. 1–7) is similarly a deterrent. Often the final decision as to modality of therapy is primarily the patient's.

The treatment of T_2 lesions (between 2 and 4 cm) is a little more controversial. Lesions that are 2 to 2½ cm, or occasionally even 3 cm, in size, are superficial in type, and are not accompanied by cervical lymphadenopathy generally do fairly well with irradiation therapy alone. All T_2 lesions that are larger or deeply infiltrative, especially when accompanied by cervical lymph node metastasis, are resected en bloc. The so-called suprahyoid neck dissection should not be done except to establish an adequate soft tissue margin around the tumor. The fact that metastatic tumor may bypass the submandibular nodes and lodge in the jugular chain militates against use of this procedure as a definitive attempt at nodal clearance.[28]

Gilbert et al[29] reported a local control rate of 77 per cent in T_1N_0 but only 21 per cent in T_2N_0 lesions of the anterior floor of the mouth treated with radiotherapy. The inci-

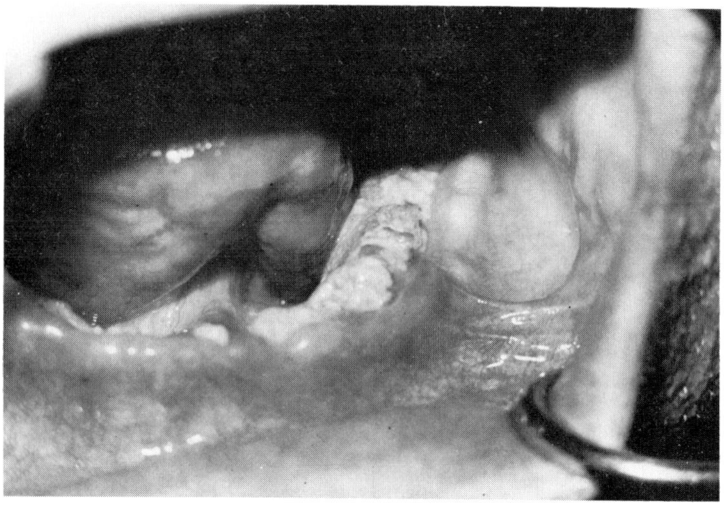

Figure 1–6. Extensive osteoradionecrosis of the mandible.

dence of osteoradionecrosis in his patients was 22 per cent. Berthelsen et al[30] found a 79 per cent control rate with T_1 lesions and a 76 per cent rate in T_2 carcinomas similarly treated by radiation. These patients were all N_0 at the time of first examination. Pierguin et al[13] noted an astoundingly high local control rate of 95 per cent in 153 patients with lesions 4 cm and less in diameter treated with interstitial irradiation. The telling statistic, however, is that at 4 years the actual survival rate was only 40 per cent. Those who succumbed did so to metastatic disease. Fu et al[32] recorded optimistic results with irradiation therapy for neoplasms less than 4 cm in size. In 50 patients, a 76 per cent control rate was experienced. Similarly, Delclos et al[33] reported an 82 per cent local control rate in 34 patients with tumors less than 4 cm.

Table 1–3 illustrates the collective experience of a number of surgeons in their management of small lesions by conservation-type surgery. It is important to note that many of the patients had cervical metastases. In a further series of 26 patients published by Schramm et al,[35] a 100 per cent control rate was observed with surgical resection of this type. This was a series of anterior oral cavity tumors, 5 cm or less in diameter, and only 15 per cent of the entire group eventually developed metastases to the neck. With one exception, all the patients followed for longer than 2 years, and all patients who had cervical metastases developed them within 18 months.

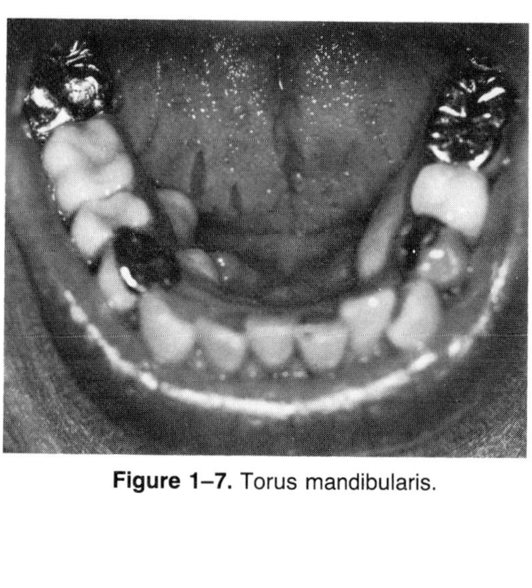

Figure 1–7. Torus mandibularis.

Large lesions are frequently accompanied by cervical metastases, either manifest or occult. Surgical excision combined with irradiation has provided the best survival rates. This was dramatically illustrated by the review of Krause et al[36] on the University of Iowa study of 472 patients. The determinant 5-year survival after surgical excision alone was 45 per cent, and that following primary irradiation therapy alone was 35 per cent. A regimen combining 4500 rads of irradiation to the lesion and both necks followed 4 weeks later by excision improved the determinant 5-year survival to 76 per cent. A similar combined therapy program utilized by La Ferrier et al[37] produced comparable results. Postoperative combined therapy, popularized by the M. D. Anderson group, allows the surgeon the luxury of operating in an unirradiated field, thus lowering the postoperative complication rate while at the same time making it possible to use a higher total irradiation dose.[38]

An ambitious cooperative study directed by Snow et al[39] has produced some revealing

Table 1–3. FIVE-YEAR LOCAL CONTROL AND SURVIVAL RATE WITH CONSERVATION THERAPY FOR ORAL CAVITY CARCINOMA*

	5-Year Survival		*Local Control*	
Author	*(No.)*	*(Per Cent)*	*(No.)*	*(Per Cent)*
King	38/65	59%	53/65	82%
DeSanto	32/46	70%	36/46	73%
Keim and Lowenberg	27/34	79%	27/34	79%
Flynn and Moore	Not stated		19/23	82.6%
Marchetta	14/23	61%	17/23	76%
Som and Nussbaum	8/18†	44%	Not stated	
TOTALS	119/186	64%	182/229	80%

*From Donald PJ: Conservation therapy for oral cavity carcinoma. Trans Pacific Coast Oto-Ophthalmological Soc 58:111, 1977.

†Two years or more.

statistics regarding combined therapy. The patient population is composed of those with Stage III and Stage IV lesions, with the patients randomly assigned to one of three treatment groups: a preoperative combined therapy group, a postoperative combined therapy group, and a radical radiation group. Although the Snow paper is a preliminary report, it showed no statistically significant difference in 18-month survival rates between the preoperative and postoperative combined therapy group. Interestingly, the radical radiation group, which had a comparable patient mix with regard to lesion site and size, had a respectable 18-month survival compared to the combined group. Sixteen of the original group of 38 who received radiation only are alive and free of disease, but at 18 months, 2 in the surviving group had required surgery for local recurrence. Surgical salvage was attempted in 9 failures of the original 38, but only one third of those survived free of disease: 2 for 18 months and 1 for a shorter follow-up period. The problems of high complication rates and poor survival of patients in their surgical salvage group is a common finding in our own experience.

Composite resection of the tongue, floor of mouth, and mandible is a standard procedure found in a number of surgical atlases.[40–43] Some modifications of this time-honored method that produce superior functional and cosmetic results without compromising survival have been recently described by La Ferrier et al.[37] Instead of using a lip-splitting incision, they use a horizontal curvilinear neck incision that extends from the mastoid tip to the level of the midbody of the opposing side of the mandible, remaining 4 cm below the mandible through its course (Fig. 1–8). Although a McFee incision can be constructed using a parallel incision 2 cm above the clavicle, we do not recommend it in cases that have been irradiated (Fig. 1–9). The watershed area of cutaneous blood supply, the area that is nourished by opposing vertically disposed blood vessels responsible for the nutrition of the skin of the head and neck, is isolated by this incision. Rather, a curvilinear or lazy S–shaped vertical incision

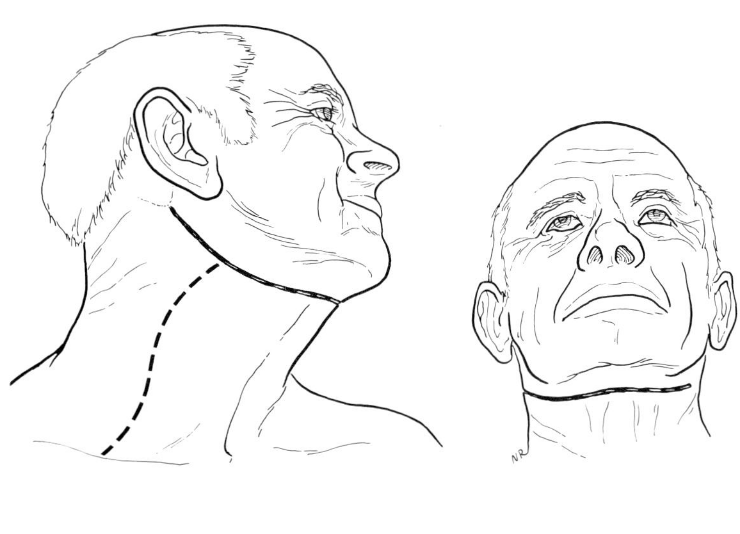

Figure 1–8. Incision for visor flap. Dotted line represents extension if radical neck dissection is necessary.

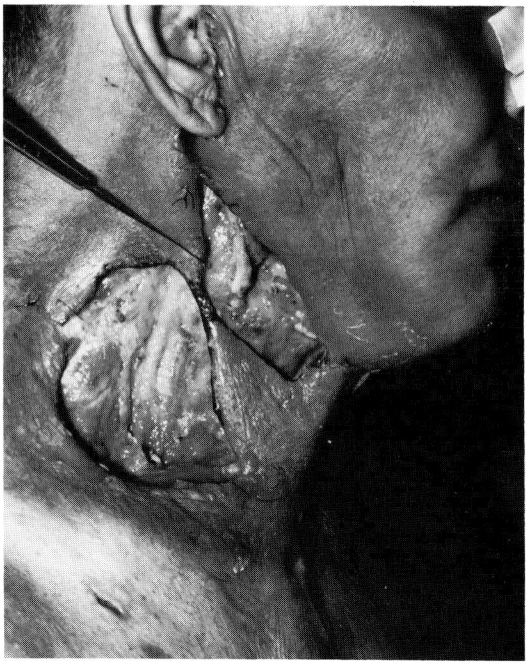

Figure 1–9. Patient treated with preoperative irradiation. The McFee incision was employed and a large area of cervical skin flap necrosis resulted.

should be dropped from the submandibular cut. The intersection should be at right angles and located posteriorly to the carotid artery (Fig. 1–8). La Ferrier makes intraoral incisions in the gingival-labial and gingival-buccal sulci that communicate with the neck incision so that the soft tissue of the lip and chin can be retracted superiorly like a knight's visor (Fig. 1–10). Care must be taken to avoid damage to the mental nerve on the side of the mandible opposite the lesion. A totally insensible lower lip will not register the presence of saliva or food, and is a serious social incapacity. Gentle retraction of the flap using Penrose drains produces little flap damage and permits excellent visualization for performing the definitive resection.

Once the tumor extirpation has been done, postoperative lingual mobility is made possible by skin-grafting the defect. A split-thickness skin graft is sutured medially to the lingual and, if the oropharynx is involved, pharyngeal and palatal resection edges, and laterally to the buccal and labial mucosa (Fig. 1–11). The authors stress that a substantial pouch of skin must be created that actually descends a short distance into the upper neck. The pouch is then packed firmly with antibiotic-soaked cotton balls. This bolster is firmly anchored with tie-over sutures. The bolster is removed at 10 days and lingual mobility encouraged.

A remarkable improvement in postoperative occlusion can be achieved by a 4-week period of intermaxillary fixation. This obviates much of the lateral mandibular swing during chewing that is otherwise so commonly seen following partial mandibulectomy. The unopposed pull of the pterygoid muscles of the intact side is partially neutralized by the fibrosis that occurs on the operated side during the period of fixation.

In the past two decades, intraoral soft tissue reconstructive demands have been primarily met by the use of regional flaps. The forehead flap (Fig. 1–12), although somewhat cosmetically disfiguring, provides an excellent lining. Not only does it permit excellent tongue mobility but it also provides a source of well-vascularized soft tissue, encouraging healing in a recipient bed often damaged by irradiation. Sufficient bulk is applied to efface the defect commonly left by the hemimandibulectomy. The cosmetic deformity of the flap can be reduced by attention to some details of surgical technique. Superiorly, the incision should, when possible, hug the hairline. Inferiorly, the incision is best made through the superior edge of the eyebrows. The knife edge should be beveled to avoid amputating the hair follicles here. A dip in the region of the glabella corresponds to a normal crease-line of this area. The horizontal incisions at the distal end of the flap should terminate at the lateral extent of the eyebrow. Similarly, when the flap's pedicle is returned, it should be amputated so that it abuts the opposite lateral brow margin, thus creating a symmetrical defect in the forehead (Fig. 1–13). One of the principal disfiguring features of the forehead defect is the sharp drop-off between the normal forehead skin and the skin graft lining the donor site. This may be reduced by beveling the incision toward the defect. A further improvement can be achieved by allowing the donor site to granulate in for 14 to 21 days following resection and then applying a skin graft to the granulating bed.[44, 45] Although some shrinkage of this tissue occurs with time, the transition from the forehead to the graft is not nearly so obvious when this method is utilized. A marked discrepancy in color between the donor site and the surrounding skin is encountered in those individuals who have considerable sun exposure to the graft site. Strict avoidance of direct sunlight must be practiced to avoid this unsightly complication.

The problem of the cosmetic defect consequent to this procedure coupled with the

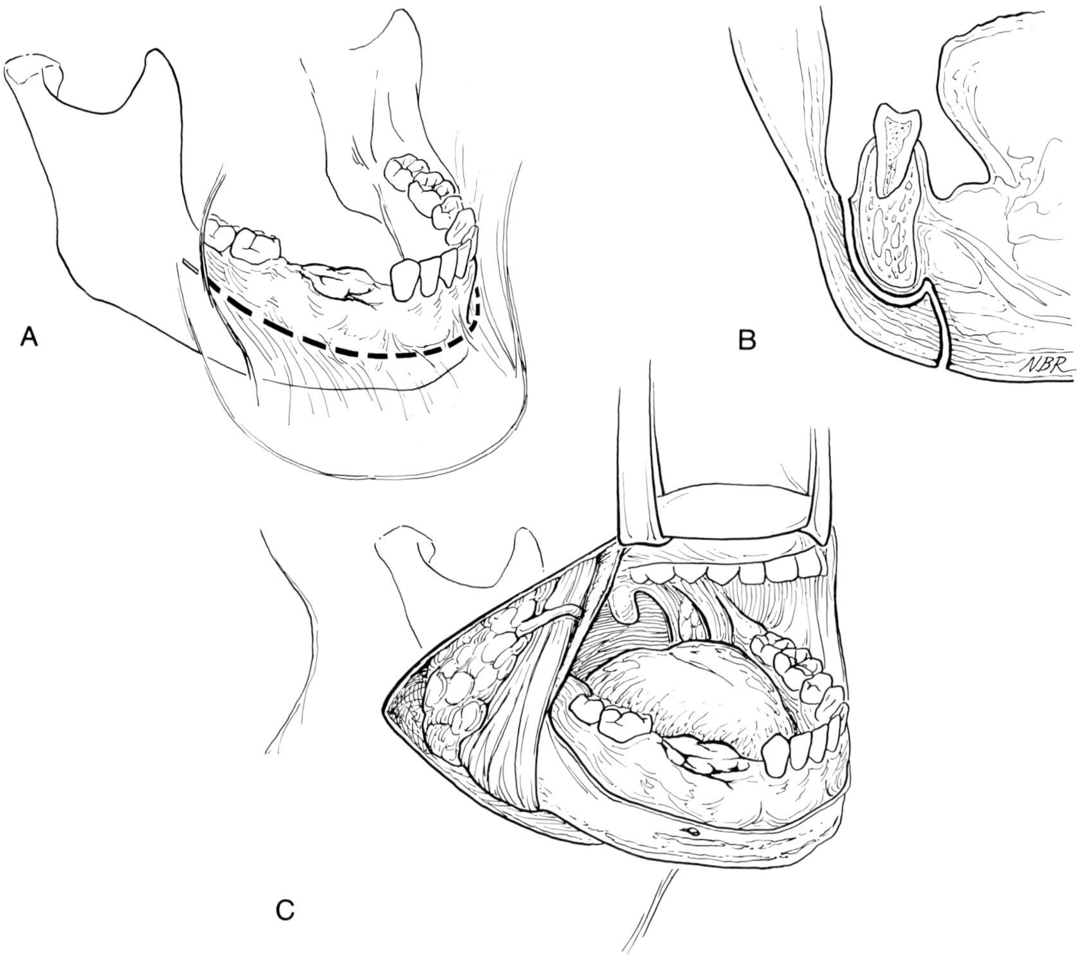

Figure 1–10. *A,* Vestibular incision in oral cavity. *B,* Connection between intra- and extraoral incisions. *C,* Lip retraction with soft rubber Penrose drains gives excellent tumor exposure.

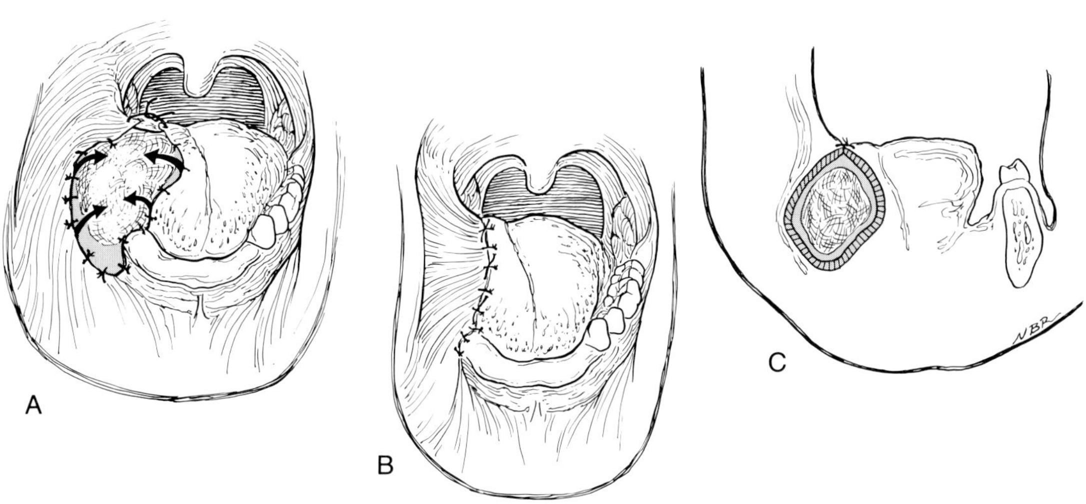

Figure 1–11. *A,* Split-thickness skin graft used to line defect. This is inserted like a pouch and held in place by a pad of medicated gauze or cotton balls. *B,* Cheek to tongue approximated to oversew the bolster on skin graft. *C,* Coronal view showing bolster in place.

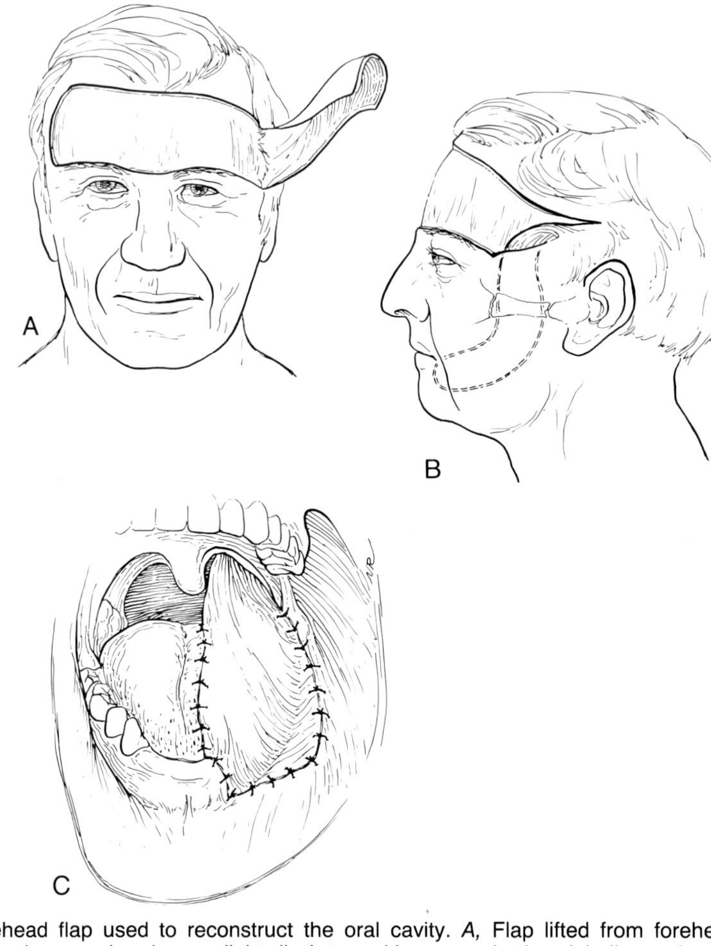

Figure 1–12. Forehead flap used to reconstruct the oral cavity. *A,* Flap lifted from forehead. Note how inferior incision hugs the eyebrow and makes a slight dip into a skin crease in the glabellar region. The distal end of the flap extends to the limit of the eyebrow. *B,* Flap is folded on itself and tucked under the zygomatic arch. The arch is fractured at two sites in order to provide additional room so as not to compromise the blood supply to the flap. Note that the upper incision is horizontal, in order to incorporate the blood supply from the occipital and postauricular arteries. *C,* The intraoral view showing flap reconstruction of a lateral tongue and the buccolingual sulcus.

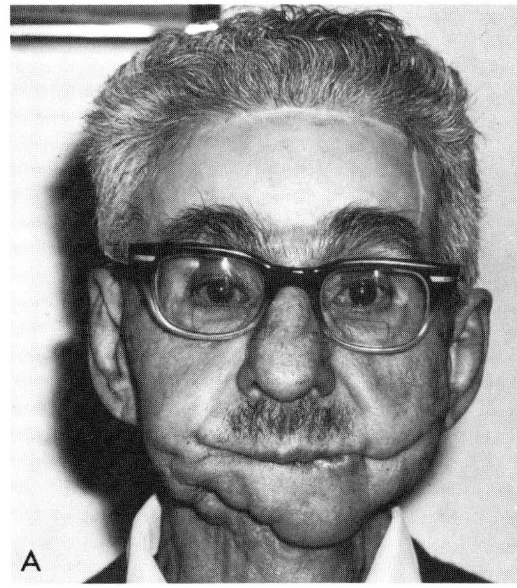

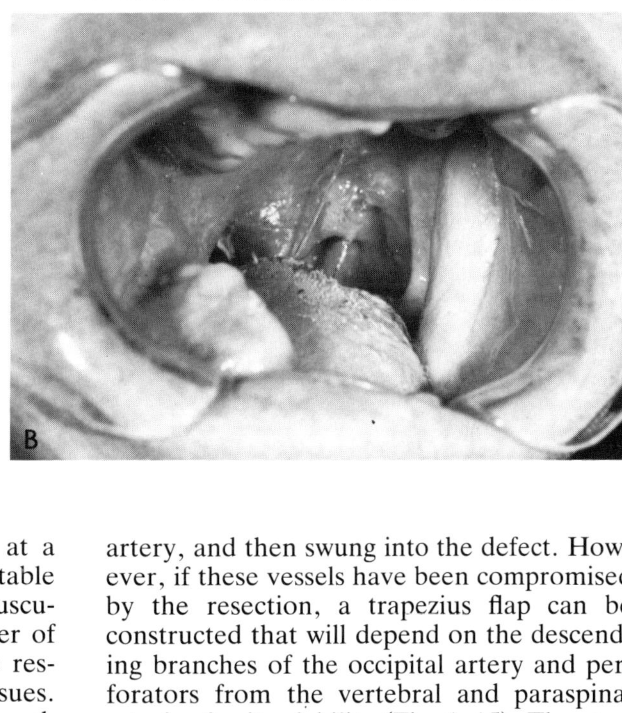

Figure 1–13. *A,* A 65-year-old white male patient following extensive resection of anterior oral cavity carcinoma. Forehead flap used for reconstruction. Note the line of the flap incision as it abuts the hairline. It extends only to the lateral aspect of each brow and inferiorly is obscured in the eyebrow. *B,* Forehead flap lining intraoral defect.

necessity of returning the flap pedicle at a second sitting prompted a search for suitable alternatives. The introduction of the musculocutaneous flaps has provided a number of successful one-stage procedures for the restoration of resected oral cavity soft tissues. Islands of skin from the neck and upper trunk receiving their blood supply through blood vessels perforating underlying attached muscle are pedicled on axial vessels and swung into the defect. The skin provides the lining while the muscle provides bulk (Fig. 1–14). For most resections, the trapezius and sternomastoid flaps are ideally suited. The trapezius flap was developed by Demergasse in Argentina and is eloquently described by Bertotti.[46] He notes that it works best when it is pedicled on the transverse cervical artery, or as a second choice the posterior scapular artery, and then swung into the defect. However, if these vessels have been compromised by the resection, a trapezius flap can be constructed that will depend on the descending branches of the occipital artery and perforators from the vertebral and paraspinal arteries for its viability (Fig. 1–15). The sternomastoid flap, despite its supply from three sources at three levels,[47] is probably the least dependable of the musculocutaneous flaps. In this flap even more than the others, the principle of loosely suturing the subcutis to the underlying muscle is absolutely essential because the skin is so loosely attached to the underlying muscle. The shearing action of skin over muscle during this flap's dissection has great potential for damaging the perforating vessels. It is a common experience to witness some degree of epithelial necrosis in

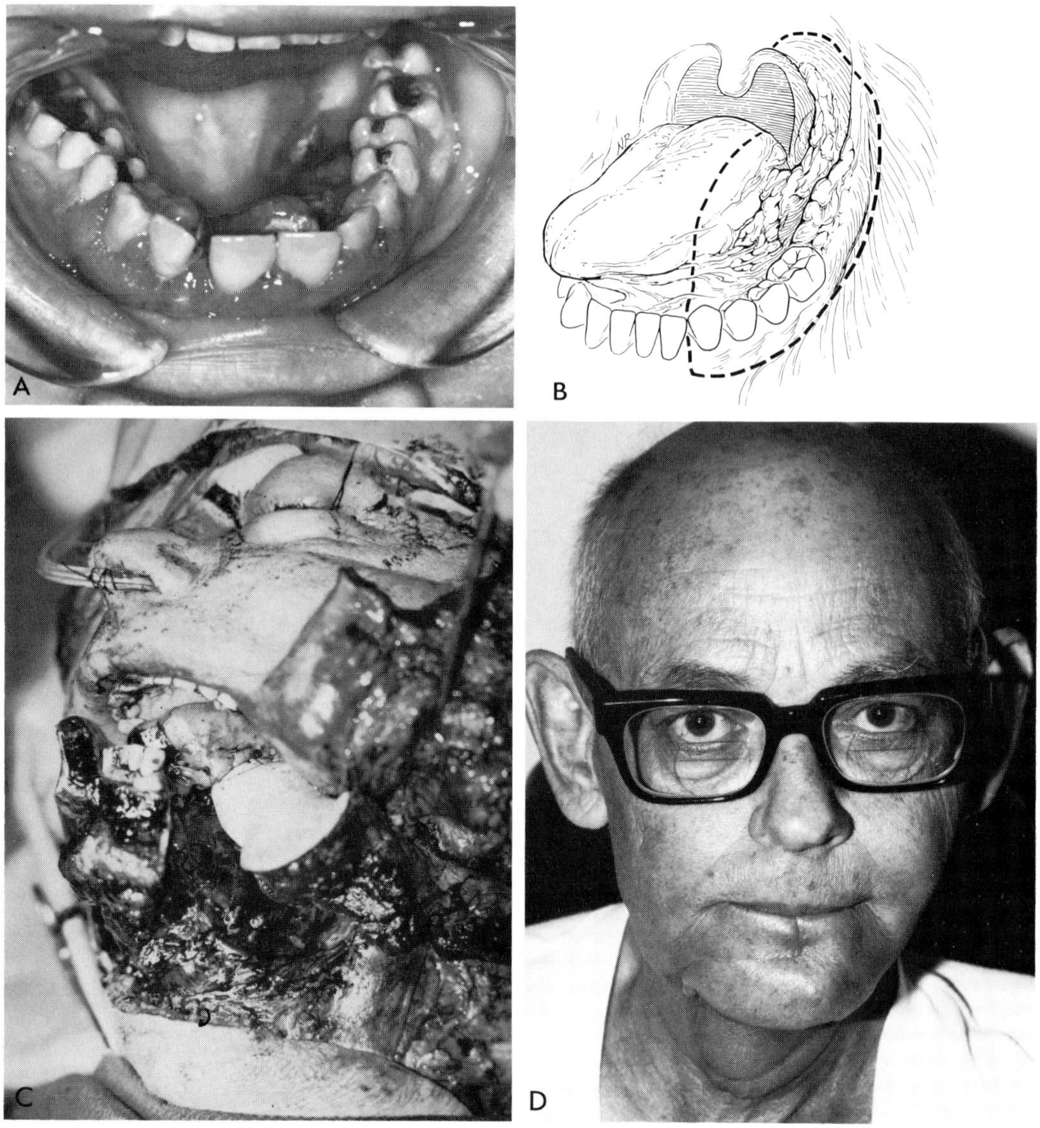

Figure 1–14. *A,* Large oral cavity tumor extending into the oropharynx. Tumor begins just opposite the canine tooth and extends onto the soft palate of the same side. *B,* Resection margin outlined. *C,* Following composite resection of jaw, tongue, lateral pharyngeal wall, soft palate, and radical neck dissection, the defect is replaced with a trapezius-musculocutaneous flap. *D,* Postoperative result.

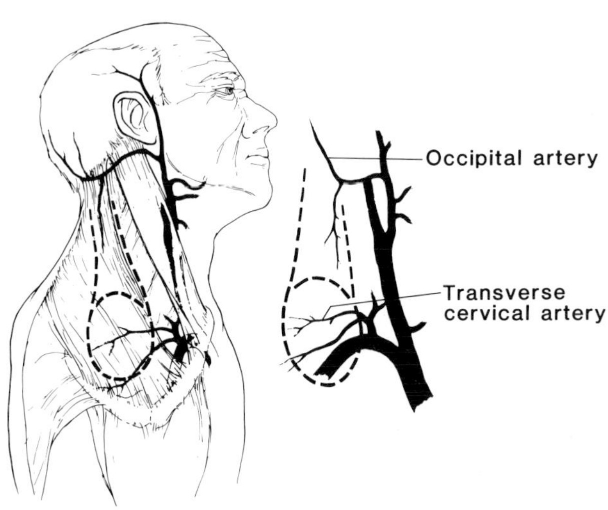

Figure 1–15. Superiorly based trapezius-musculocutaneous flap.

this flap. Fortunately, re-epithelialization is the rule and fistulization is rare.[47, 48] In both the sternocleidomastoid and trapezius flaps, the donor site can often be closed primarily. Occasionally, especially with the trapezius flap taken from the back, a split-thickness skin graft is needed to complete the closure of the donor site.

CONSERVATION SURGERY

Conservation surgery for carcinoma of the larynx has become highly developed over the past 10 to 15 years. The increased awareness of medical and dental practitioners with regard to oral cavity carcinoma has made its early diagnosis more commonplace. Although irradiation and surgery result in roughly equivalent survival rates in patients with these small neoplasms, often the complications, expense, and time lost from gainful employment favor the latter over the former modality. This is especially true when the principles of conservation surgery are applied.

Although function-preserving procedures for the larynx are found in most standard texts, similar procedures for the oral cavity are difficult to find. A corollary between the narrow tissue margin of resection necessary to ensure adequate tumor extirpation relative to the true vocal cord is also found in the mandibular periosteum. The work of Marchetta et al[49, 50] indicates that the lymphatics that drain the floor of mouth and tongue do not circle the mandible but pass directly into the upper cervical lymph nodes. In general, the sparse lymphatics that drain the meager lymph from osseous tissue encircle the bone they drain between the two layers of investing periosteum. Contrary to the earlier notions of Polya,[51] there is presently no evidence to indicate that continuity exists between these lymphatics of the mandible and those in the floor of the mouth or in the tongue. In a review of 80 cases of oral cavity carcinoma, Marchetta and his associates found no evidence of tumor in bone, periosteal lymphatics, or periosteum when a tumor of the floor of the mouth was up to 1 mm away from mandibular periosteum.[49, 50] In the 15 patients in whom periosteum was involved, the incidence of lymph nodal metastases was 27 per cent. In the remaining 65 patients without periosteal involvement, the metastatic rate was 65 per cent, implying an extraperiosteal route of metastatic srpead.

The work of Marchetta and coworkers prompted the development of procedures that split the mandible in a horizontal or vertical plane, permitting adequate tumor excision and the preservation of mandibular continuity. Such "face-saving" operations[52] eliminate the need for extensive reconstructive efforts in areas that are particularly difficult to rebuild. This is especially true of the anterior regions of the oral cavity. Fortunately, mandibular bone invasion by squamous cell cancer is a slow process. Byars[53] has shown that this remains true until the medullary cavity or the major neurovascular foramina have been invaded, at which time tumor spread becomes more rapid.

Although these procedures have withstood the test of time, some doubt as to their safety has been cast by the work of Ossoff and colleagues.[54, 55] By injecting lymph vessels in the floor of the mouth of dogs, they found that some of the efferent lymphatics were tightly adherent to the mandibular periosteum. As yet, no studies have been done to establish a human corollary.

Marginal Mandibulectomy

This procedure is indicated for the excision of tumors of the attached gingiva (Fig. 1–16) that extend no more than 2 to 3 mm into the immediate gingival, labial, buccal, or lingual mucosa. There must be no evidence of bone erosion radiographically or on radionuclide scanning. The tumors generally are of the superficially invasive and exophytic varieties, and will seldom be larger than 4 cm in size. Tumors that are more extensive or that are accompanied by cervical lymphadenopathy

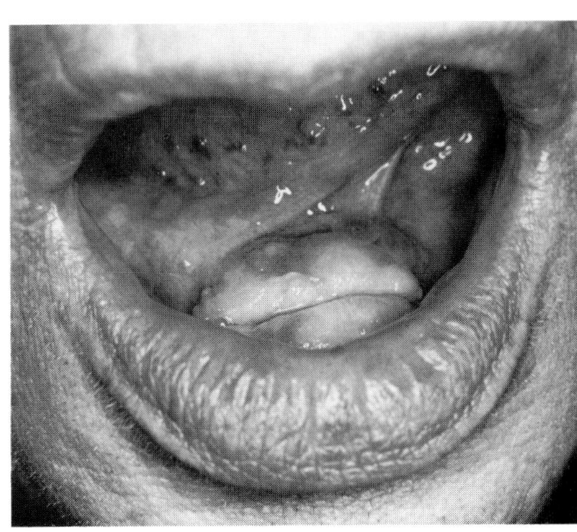

Figure 1–16. Alveolar ridge carcinoma.

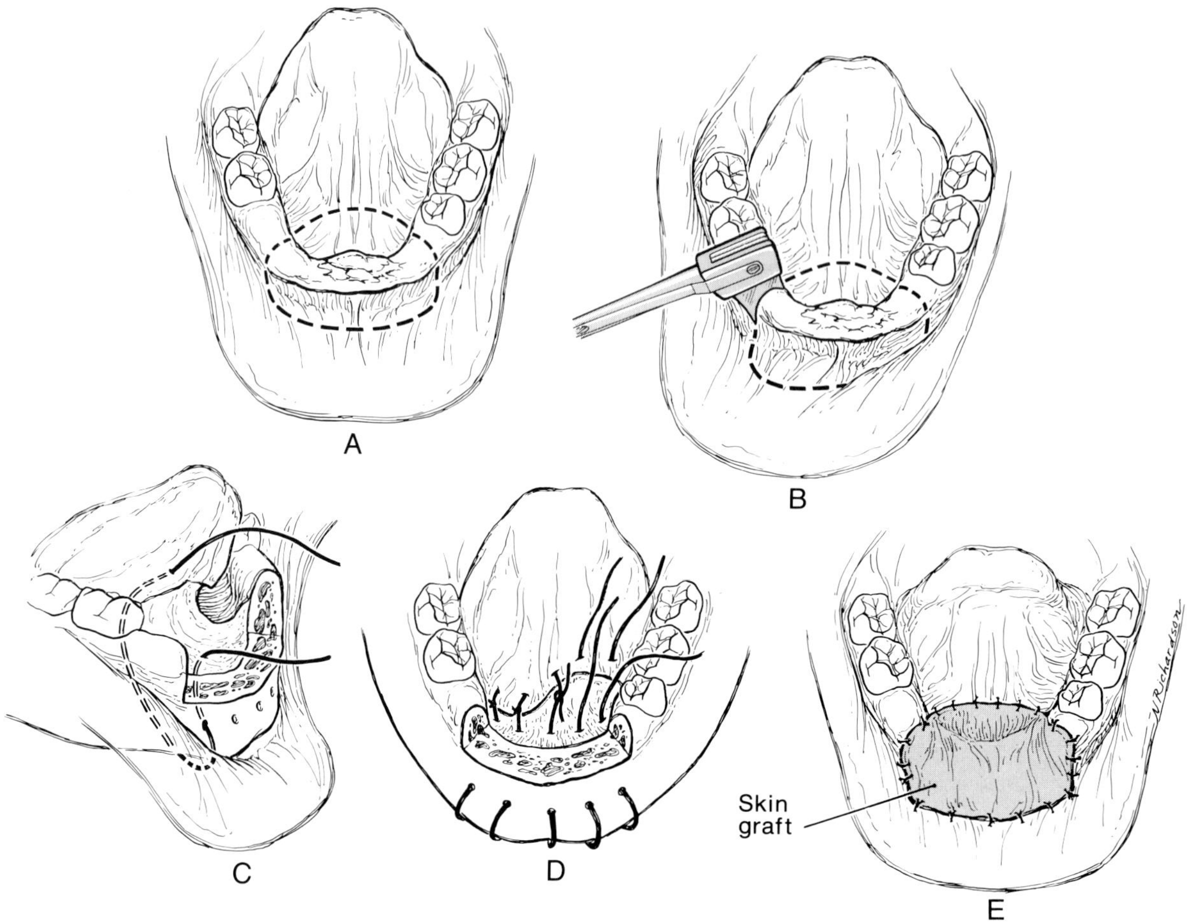

Figure 1–17. Marginal mandibulectomy. *A,* Tumor of fixed gingiva outlined with a 2-cm margin. *B,* Stryker saw used to make bony cuts. *C,* Chronic sutures through drill holes in mandible used to close dead space. *D,* Dead space effaced. *E,* Skin graft placed to cover remaining defect.

require either a full-thickness excision of mandibular bone or a combination of a marginal mandibulectomy and a lingual or buccal split.

The excision is done entirely intraorally. The area of resection, allowing a 2-cm margin of healthy tissue around the tumor, is outlined with methylene blue, using a nonsiliconized needle. The cutting cautery is used to make the incision down to the bone and into the adjacent soft tissues to the estimated depth of the bony resection. Care must be taken to keep the soft tissue cuts vertical, avoiding the natural tendency to slant the incisions toward the tumor (Fig. 1–17). A bone saw is used to make vertical cuts through the mandible a distance of 1½ to 2 cm. Shallower cuts are made in the edentulous mandible in which alveolar bone is lost and only basal bone remains. In the atrophic mandible, the marginal resection must be abandoned and full-thickness bone must be excised.

Horizontal incisions in the soft tissue now extend from the vertical incisions on the labial-buccal and lingual aspects of the resection. Once these deep incisions abut the mandible, a sagittal saw is used to complete the bony cuts, and the bloc is removed. Alternatively, the bone incision can be done by making multiple penetrating bur holes and then connecting them with an osteotome.

The raw area is usually readily covered by a dermis graft or split-thickness skin graft. It is essential to stent these grafts in position. Numerous quilting sutures may be inserted as suggested by McGregor,[57] but the surest means of anchoring the graft in place is with some form of bolster or stent. Larger areas may be covered with a forehead flap or bilateral nasal labial flaps as suggested by Freund.[56] A preformed acrylic stent (Fig. 1–18) can be fixed to the dentition by prosthetic clips or anchored to the lower jaw by circummandibular wires. Any necessary reshaping of the splint to accommodate the graft is

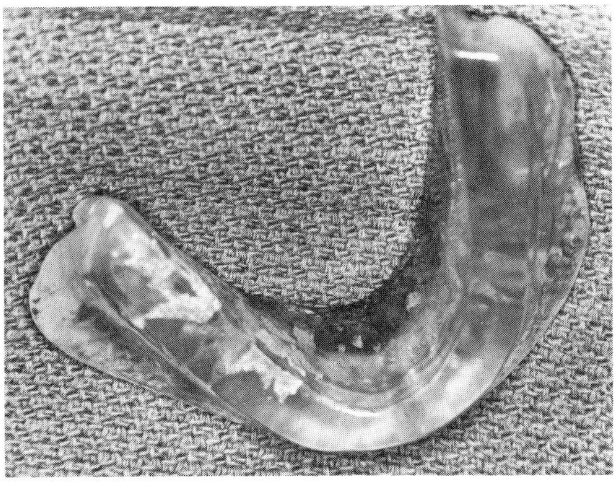

Figure 1–18. Preformed acrylic stent.

done at the operating table prior to fixing it in place. If insufficient acrylic is present to adequately obturate the graft, additional cold cure acrylic may be added. The splint is left in place for 10 to 14 days. Some means of continuous splinting is essential until a permanent denture is fashioned. This splinting will reduce the graft shrinkage that invariably ensues during the subsequent weeks of healing. If a prosthetist is not available to provide a splint, bolstering of the graft can be accomplished with cotton dental rolls. However, keeping the bolster in place is often difficult because of the considerable movement of the tongue.

Lingual and Buccal Plate Excisions

Vertical excisions of manidbular bone are indicated in oral cavity tumors that extend to the proximity of the buccolabial or lingual portions of the mandible (Fig. 1–19). An adequate margin of resection necessitates the excision of partial-thickness bone in the vertical plane. Primary tumors of the lip or buccal mucosa uncommonly extend to the depths of their reflection onto the mandibular gingiva. On the other hand, lingual and floor-of-mouth tumors often extend onto the gingiva or close to it. According to Marchetta's studies, a slim margin of 1 mm of uninvolved tissue between mandibular periosteum and the tumor ensures the safety of a conservation procedure.

Similar to the marginal mandibulectomy, vertical plane excisions can only occasionally be done entirely intraorally. Usually the lesions are more extensive and the excision must extend through the mylohyoid muscle. In these instances a cervical incision should be added. It is placed horizontally about two finger-breadths below the body of the mandible (Fig. 1–20). Flaps are elevated over an area that enables sufficient exposure of the submandibular and submental triangles. In the absence of cervical lymph node involvement, a so-called suprahyoid dissection is performed. This is not in lieu of a neck dissection but simply a means of getting an adequate tissue margin around the lesion. The excision often entails the removal of one submandibular salivary gland and occasionally both. Although care should be exercised to preserve the ramus mandibularis, no compromise of the tumor resections should be made in order to achieve this. A simple, rapid means of preserving the nerve is to incise the fascia overlying the submandibular salivary gland at the inferior pole. As the fascia is dissected from the gland in a superior

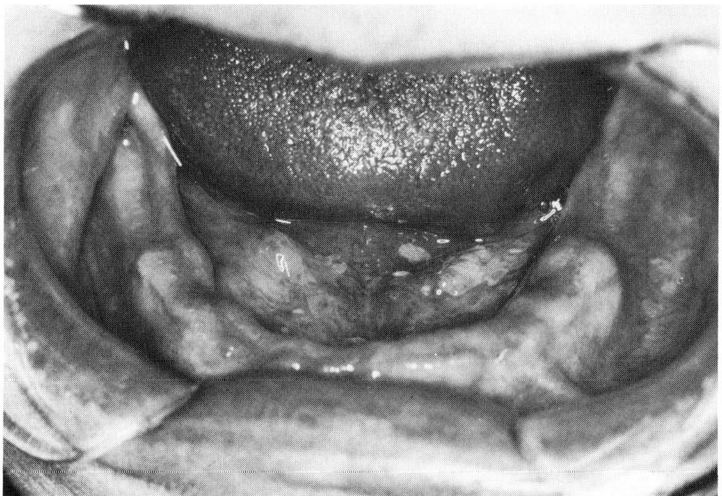

Figure 1–19. Carcinoma of the anterior floor of the mouth, and associated leukoplakia. Malignancy approximates the lingual plate of mandible on the left.

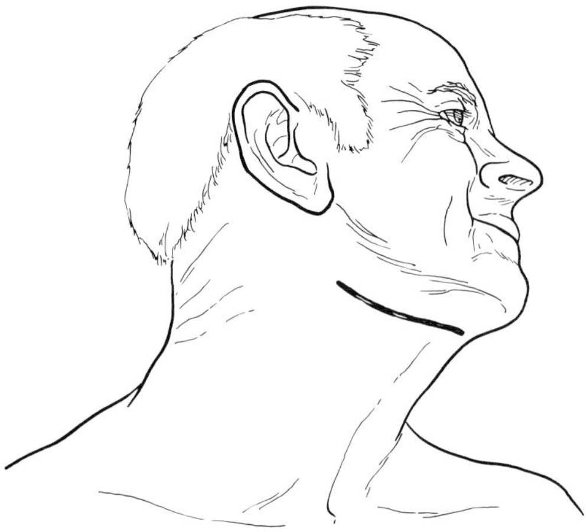

Figure 1–20. Cervical excision for inferior exposure in lingual or buccal plate excision.

direction, the nerve is carried with it. The dissection is carried to the body of the mandible, and the nerve's safety is ensured. The inadequacy of the suprahyoid dissection in removing lymphadenopathy needs re-emphasis. If the site or size of the primary lesion carries a 25 per cent or greater incidence of occult nodal involvement, then prophylactic irradiation therapy to the neck is mandatory. If palpable adenopathy is detected, radical neck dissection is done in continuity. The incision is outlined in Fig. 1–8.

The intraoral part of the excision is marked out using multiple punctures with a nonsiliconized needle dipped in methylene blue. A lip split is seldom, if ever, necessary for adequate exposure. The soft tissue excision usually extends through the mylohyoid muscle. The adequacy of the excision width is best controlled from below. The necessity of making the soft tissue cuts precisely vertical must be re-emphasized, and the natural tendency to slant the incision toward the tumor as the deeper planes are reached must be firmly resisted.

Any teeth in the line of excision are now extracted. Care must be taken to leave an adequate shell of alveolar bone surrounding the teeth adjacent to the resection margin. An exposed tooth root may lead to infection, poor healing, and eventual tooth loss. The vertical incision through the bone is made with a sagittal cutting saw (Fig. 1–21). It is important to remember that the buccal plate of the mandible is much thicker than the lingual, and the inferior aspect of the mandible is much broader than the alveolar portion. The vertical bone cut is directed as nearly perpendicular to the inferior plane of the mandible as possible. It can also be accomplished with multiple closely spaced bur holes that are then connected with an osteotome. This cut in the sagittal plane of the mandible is now connected by vertical cuts at right angles to, and at the extremities of, the sagittal cut. Once the specimen is free, all soft tissue attachments are severed and it can be "pulled through" the floor of the mouth.

Reconstruction is similar to that of the marginal mandibulectomy. However, especially in buccal plate excisions, care is taken to reconstruct a sulcus. An effaced gingival-buccal sulcus may thwart even the best attempts at prosthetic rehabilitation.

Combined Excisions

Probably the most commonly performed conservation procedure is the combination of a vertical and horizontal mandibulectomy (Fig. 1–22). This is used for tumors that originate in the tongue or floor of the mouth on the lingual side, or for those on the lip or

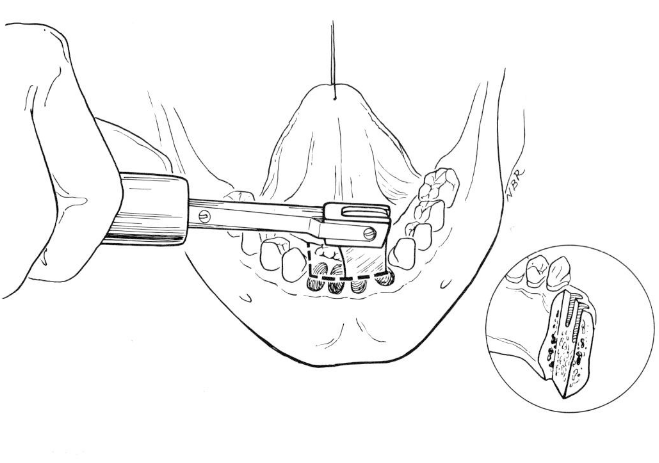

Figure 1–21. Bony cuts for lingual plate excision. Notice how the plane of the incision is at right angles to the mandible.

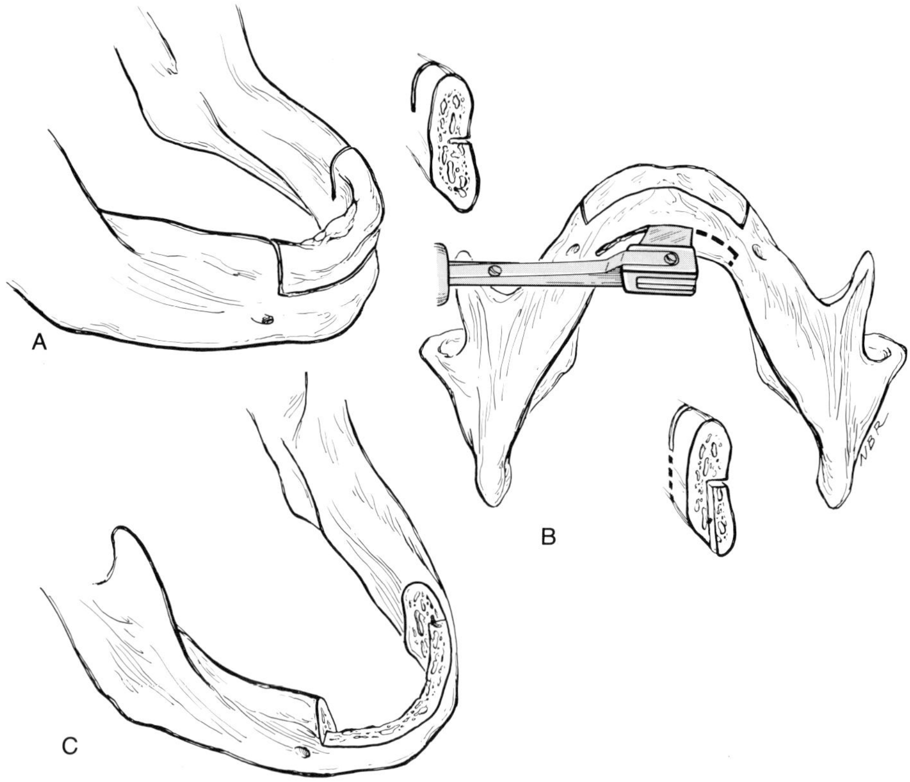

Figure 1–22. Combined marginal mandibulectomy and lingual split. *A,* Marginal incisions made through alveolar ridge. Horizontal cut made on buccal but not lingual surface. *B,* Lingual plate incision made with sagittal saw connects with the horizontal cut of the marginal mandibulectomy. *C,* Resection completed with residual buccal-inferior bone strut remaining to connect both mandibular bodies, thus retaining mandibular arch configuration.

buccal mucosa on the buccolabial side that encroach on the alveolar gingiva.

Once the mucosal cuts are completed, the marginal mandibulectomy incisions are made in the usual way, with the exception of the horizontal portion. This cut is carried through only half the thickness of the mandible, from the plate on the side opposite the tumor to the midportion of the medullary cavity. For example, in a floor-of-mouth tumor encroaching on the gingiva, the horizontal bony incision would be from the buccal plate to the midportion of the medullary cavity. The sagittal cut is begun at the inferior aspect of the jaw and carried superiorly to meet the horizontal cut of the marginal portion of the operation (Fig. 1–22*B*). The residual bar of bone is often thin and fragile, especially if the buccal plate is excised. Since this procedure is most applicable in the anterior aspect of the mandible, this bony strut is usually sufficiently strong, except in the markedly atrophic mandible.

Reconstruction of the area is the same as in the previously mentioned conservation procedures. If an accidental fracture occurs through the residual bone in the operative defect, interosseous wires are placed and the patient is put into intermaxillary fixation. In the three patients in which this has occurred, in our experience, all had successful healing despite postoperative irradiation.

A number of authorities feel that these tumors merit a full-thickness bony excision. Som and Nussbaum[60] state strongly that periosteal involvement mandates a full-thickness resection. On the other hand, Keim and Lowenberg[58] showed no bone invasion in 22 consecutive cases of oral cavity tumors that invaded the gingiva. King[59] had excellent local control in 65 patients of whom many had periosteal involvement; however, none of the tumors were greater than 4 cm in size and all were superficial in type. Whereas the arch area in the anterior region is notoriously difficult to reconstruct, in the lateral aspect of the mandible, a segmental resection and replacement with a rib or hip graft (Fig. 1–23) is probably technically easier than the conservation procedure.

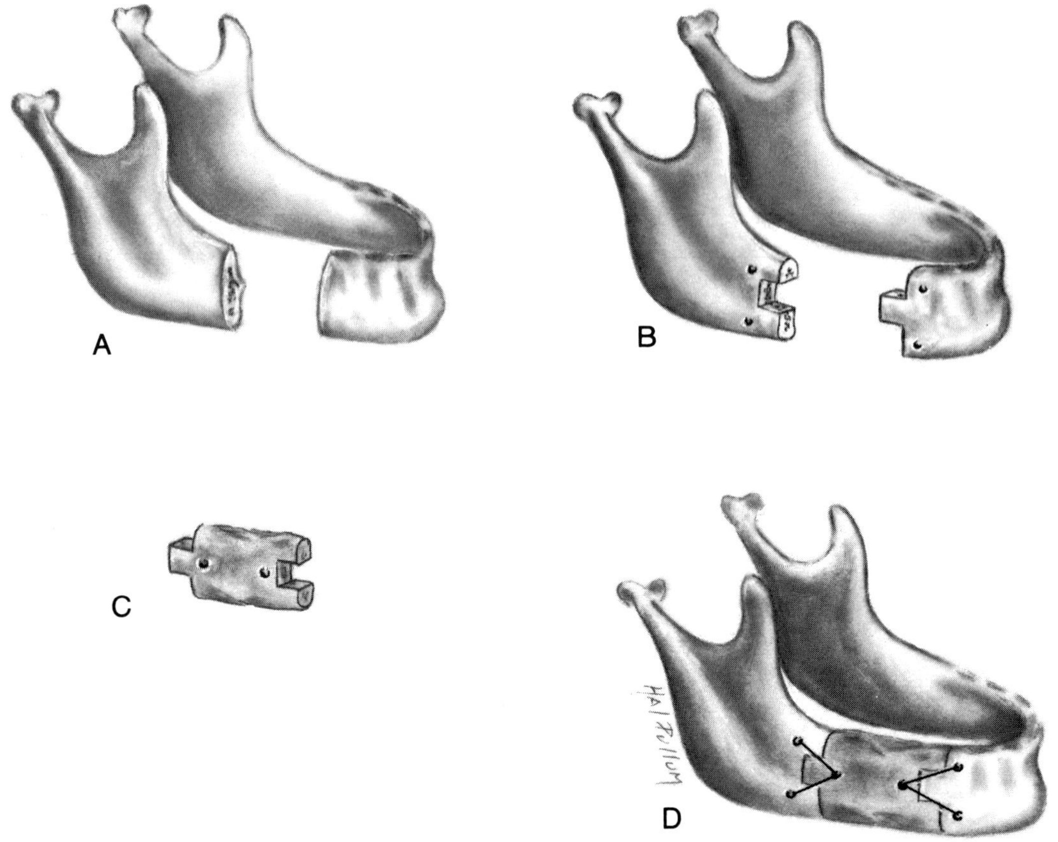

Figure 1–23. Segmental mandibular excision for oral cavity carcinoma of limited extent. *A,* Area of excision. *B,* Mortising of joint with drill holes fashioned. *C,* Rib graft with reciprocal mortising. *D,* Graft in place.

REHABILITATION FOLLOWING ANTERIOR RESECTIONS

Most standard texts of head and neck surgery adequately describe the procedure of composite resection of the anterior aspects of the oral cavity. Little attention is paid to either the details of the incapacity inflicted by this surgery on these patients or the rectification of these disabilities. Unfortunately, surgical resections, especially of extensive lesions, often leave patients severely handicapped. Oral incompetence with drooling, problems with alimentation, and severe articulation defects, in addition to an often hideous appearance, frequently make the patient an anathema to family and friends (Fig. 1–24). These problems are so grave that a number of head and neck surgeons elect irradiation therapy for these tumors, accepting a reduced survival, and reserve surgery for salvage of those who fail this modality, despite the increased morbidity that results from salvage surgery.

Surgical reconstruction and rehabilitation of patients who have had extensive resections of the anterior aspects of the oral cavity provides one of the greatest challenges in head and neck surgery. A detailed consideration of each anatomic area reveals a unique group of specific functional contributions to each facet of normal oral physiology. In managing the defects consequent to extirpative surgery, a clear plan of action must be formulated based upon the restoration of function of these structures and utilizing a host of surgical, prosthetic, and physiotherapeutic measures.

Although each anatomic area of involvement will be dealt with individually in a sequential manner, reconstruction of a number of contiguous areas is usually demanded in many commonly encountered resections.

Lips

The lips are the guardians of the oral cavity. Their ability to approximate prevents drooling during rest or speech, and during mastication they are responsible for maintain-

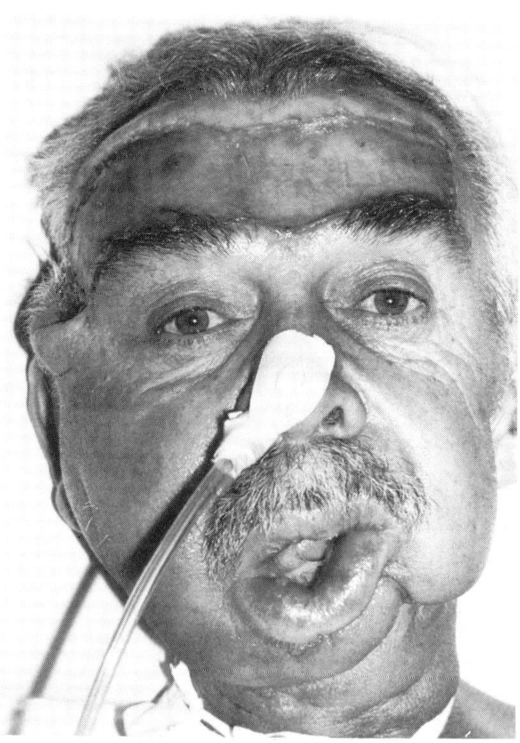

Figure 1–24. A flaccid, inactive lower lip secondary to denervation resulting from tumor excision.

ing the food in the mouth. Although the orbicularis oris is often thought to be solely responsible for these functions, important contributions are made by a number of other facial muscles. The deepest muscular layer lying adjacent to the labial mucosa is made up principally of the buccinator and the deepest fibers of the orbicularis oris. At this level, the middle portions of the buccinator muscle decussate at the angle of the mouth, with the lower fibers seeking and then traversing the upper lip, and the upper fibers, the lower lip. The buccinator fibers that lie superior and inferior to the decussating ones course straight across the upper and lower lips respectively. These fibers blend with those of the orbicularis oris muscle, which are similarly disposed, and the two muscles together are responsible for drawing the lips together and against the adjacent surface of the teeth and alveolar gingivae (Fig. 1–25).

The more superficial layer of the lip musculature is made up principally of the depressor and levator anguli oris muscles and their interdigitation with the orbicularis oris, whose fibers are now oriented in an oblique direction. This enables the lips to be pursed and pouted. The levator anguli oris alaeque nasi, the zygomaticus major and minor, and the mentalis muscles are all integrated at this level. They insert into the decussating fibers of the levator and depressors, the oblique fibers of the orbicularis oris, and the skin of the lips.[61]

The lower lip is functionally more important than the upper, in part owing to the action of the lower jaw. Even though the upper lip may hang like a curtain, the active lower lip will perform all of the activities essential to normal functioning.[62] On the other hand, even if the upper lip is fully innervated and operative, oral continence will be lost if the lower lip is flaccid and inactive (Fig. 1–24). In reconstructing the lip, whenever possible, replacement of lost labial tissue is done with adjacent labial tissue; hence the success of the Abbe and Estlander flaps. Reconstruction of the lower lip from adjacent nonlabial tissue is far less successful than that of the upper.

Often following anterior resection of the oral cavity for large tumors, the lower lip is partially or completely denervated. Despite heroic attempts to restore the integrity of the mandible and mobility of the tongue, rehabilitation will be thwarted if oral continence is not ensured. Often the lower lip is quite large, usually as the result of edema secondary to the effects of either the surgery alone or in combination with irradiation. This is especially frequent in cases in which bilateral neck dissection has been done. A reduction in bulk by wedge resection of the lip will usually restore continence, especially if some semblance of muscle activity remains.

The more severe condition of the prolapsed, totally denervated lip can be rehabilitated by a wedge resection followed by the use of a fascial sling.[64] A small incision is made just above the zygomatic arch and about 6 mm of arch is divested of soft tissue covering. The fascial strip is fed around the arch with an aneurysm needle. This sling of fascia lata is then tied around one zygomatic arch, knitted through one half of the lower lip, and brought out in the midline. A second fascial strip is similarly placed on the opposite side, the lip is cinched into position (Fig. 1–26), and the two strips are sutured together. Once the lower lip approximates the upper lip, oral continence is greatly improved. When motor function is lost to the lip secondary to trauma or surgical excision for tumor, sensation is often also lost. This precludes the patient's appreciation of the presence of saliva or oral contents on the lip. Occasionally, some return of tactile sense will

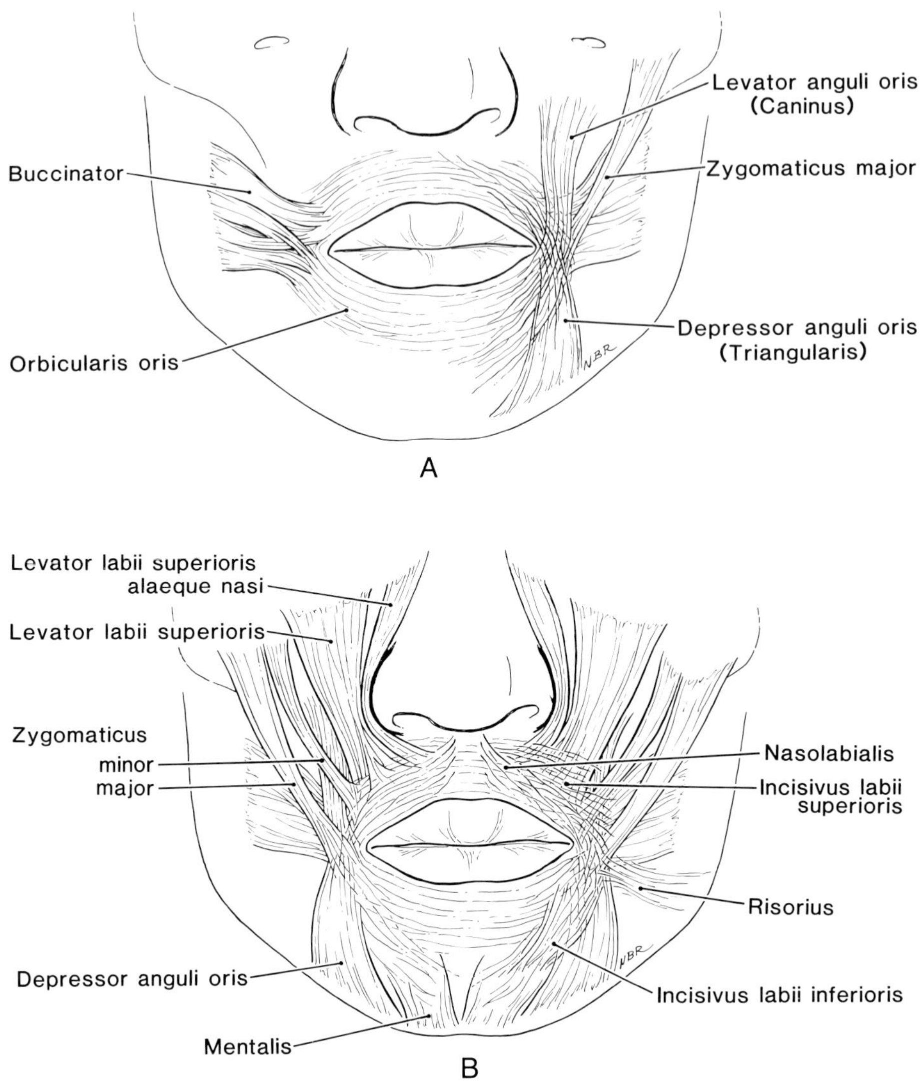

Figure 1–25. Muscle layers of the lip. *A,* Deep layer, composed principally of the buccinator and obicularis oris muscles. Note how the central slips of the buccinator decussate at the corners of the mouth (*right*), then interdigitate with the obicularis oris. *B,* Superficial layer, composed of more obliquely oriented obicularis fibers, showing their interdigitation with the muscles of facial expression that act on the mouth.

occur by regrowth of the sensory nerves from the least involved side; however, it is often incomplete and continues to be a vexing problem.

Mandible

The key to retention of both oral functioning and aesthetics is the preservation or the adequate reconstruction of the mandibular arch. The arch has a unique configuration that is extremely difficult to reproduce. Moreover, it forms an anchor for one of the major tongue muscles, the genioglossus; serves as a point of stabilization for the hyoid bone through the geniohyoid and the anterior belly of the digastric; and is the origin of the diaphragm of the floor of the mouth, the mylohyoid. Loss of this arch results in collapse of the anterior aspect of the oral cavity, resulting in total oral incompetence, dysphagia, severely distorted speech, and aesthetic deformity.

Numerous methods have been described to reconstruct this keystone of the oral cavity. Immediate bone grafting in a tumor patient who is often an elderly chronic alcoholic, protein depleted, and with grossly carious dentition is usually doomed to failure. If the

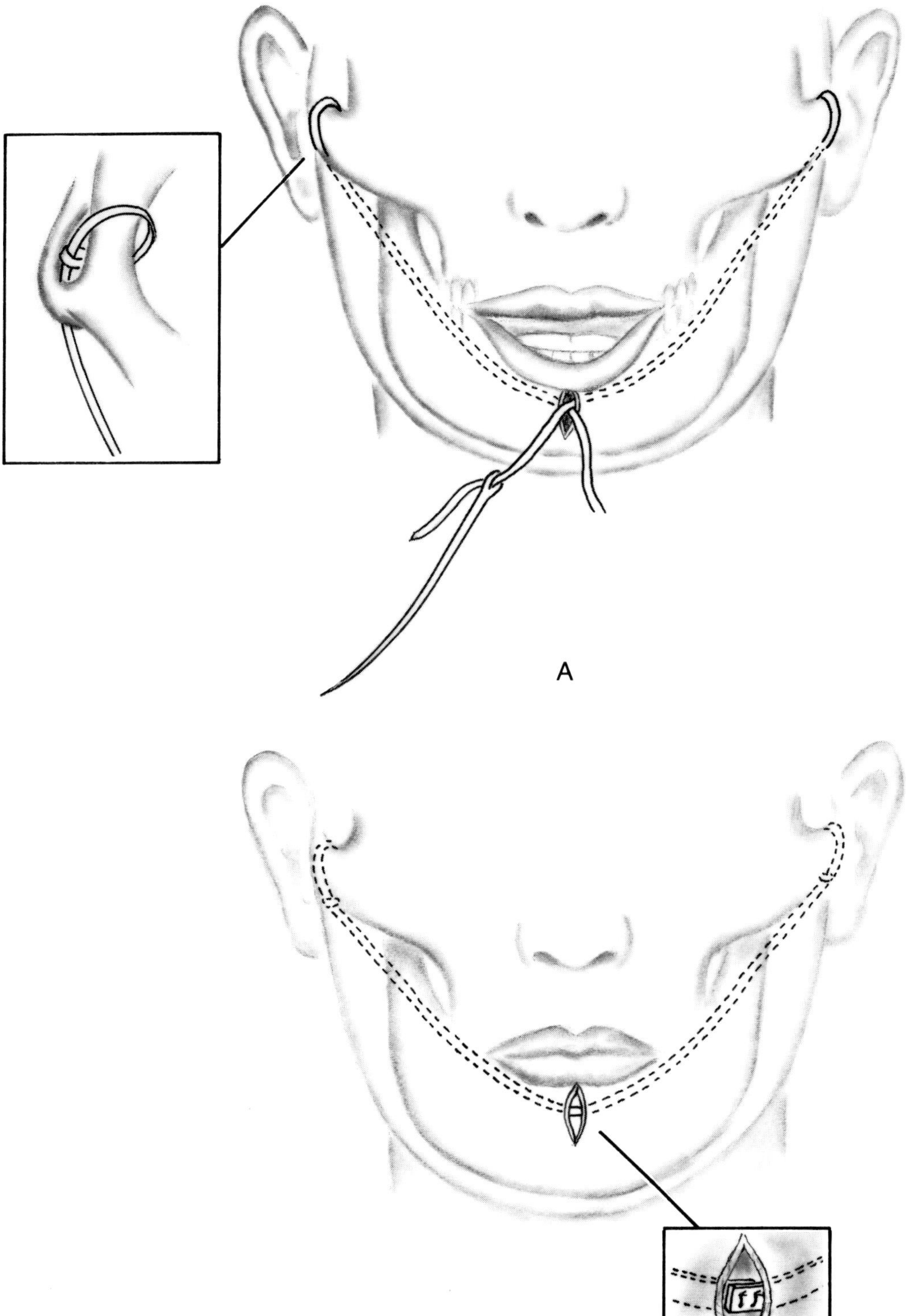

Figure 1–26. Fascial sling used to cinch inactive functionless lower lip into position. *A,* Fascia lata loop is slung over zygomatic arch and brought out through a central midline incision just below the lower lip. *B,* Lip clinched shut and fascia strips approximated in midline. Wound is then closed.

patient has had prior irradiation, an even higher extrusion rate can be anticipated. In most patients at our institution large tumor resections are usually followed by a full course of radiotherapy. This impedes the growth of osteoblasts, thereby retarding or precluding bone healing. In the majority of these patients, grafting is left until the wound is completely healed and 4 to 6 weeks have elapsed from the completion of postoperative radiation therapy.

The problem with this plan of attack is that of maintaining the gap between the mandibular fragments during the interlude between irradiation and reconstruction. The biphase appliance has been most efficacious in opposing the strong pull of the pterygoid muscles that tends to collapse these fragments (Fig. 1–27). During radiotherapy, the minor amount of deflection of the gamma rays by the screws of the appliance has a negligible effect on the adjacent bone or on therapeutic efficacy. If salvageable teeth are present, eyelet wires are applied in addition, to maintain occlusion and eliminate the torque on the screws that results from repetitive jaw opening. Continuous stress of this sort eventually results in loosening of the screws and loss of fixation. Care must be taken to place at least two screws in each fragment for stability.

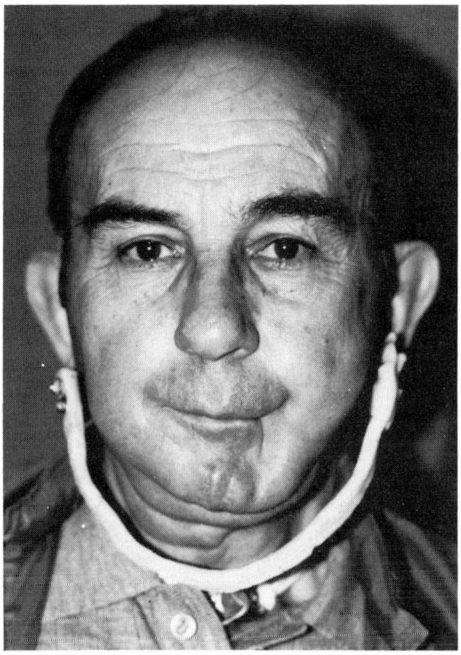

Figure 1–27. Middle-aged man following extensive excision of an anterolateral carcinoma of the tongue and floor of the mouth. Mandibular segments are maintained with a biphase appliance.

Allografts are entirely unsuitable for tissue replacement in this area. Tantalum and Vitallium trays filled with cancellous bone chips have met with limited success, especially when done as a primary reconstructive effort, probably because of the combination of the aforementioned adverse factors present in most of these patients.[65] Freeze-dried cadaver mandible[66] has been tried by Cantrell and Boyne[67] with similarly dismal results. Recently, Cummings[68] has attempted removing the mandibular arch, excising the attached cancer, freezing the bone twice in liquid nitrogen, and then reimplanting it. He expresses guarded optimism regarding the efficacy of this procedure, as he found local persistence of tumor in adjacent soft tissue. Popescu and Spirescu[69] described four cases done in the same way: two patients with squamous cell tumors and two others with benign lesions invading the mandible. Although they had no instances of local recurrence, they had a high rate of serious local complications. Panje[70] attempted this procedure three times without success, reporting that the bone became septic and extruded. Haymaker[71] has had short-term success with gross excision of tumor from the resected jaw, after which the bone is exposed to 10,000 rads of gamma irradiation and then reinserted as a free graft. However, subsequent irradiation of the patient as part of a combined therapy program often results in transformation of the graft to fibrous tissue.[72]

Bone grafting still remains the most commonly used method of reconstruction. The most suitable graft material is the patient's own bone. Although iliac crest is strong and bulky, it is extremely difficult to fashion into the form of an arch and is also limited in length. The 7th, 8th, and 9th ribs have a natural curvature that greatly aids in this reproduction. The rib can be further bent by excising a series of small wedges from the posterior cortical surface using a Stryker saw. The rib is then skewered with a Kirschner wire and bent into the desired configuration (Fig. 1–28).[73] Countersinking the ends of the Kirschner wire into holes drilled into the medullary cavity of the mandible increases graft stability. Mortising the joint not only adds to its stability but also increases the area of medullary contact, enhancing healing.

Maintaining fixation of the graft in these patients is often extremely difficult. If enough

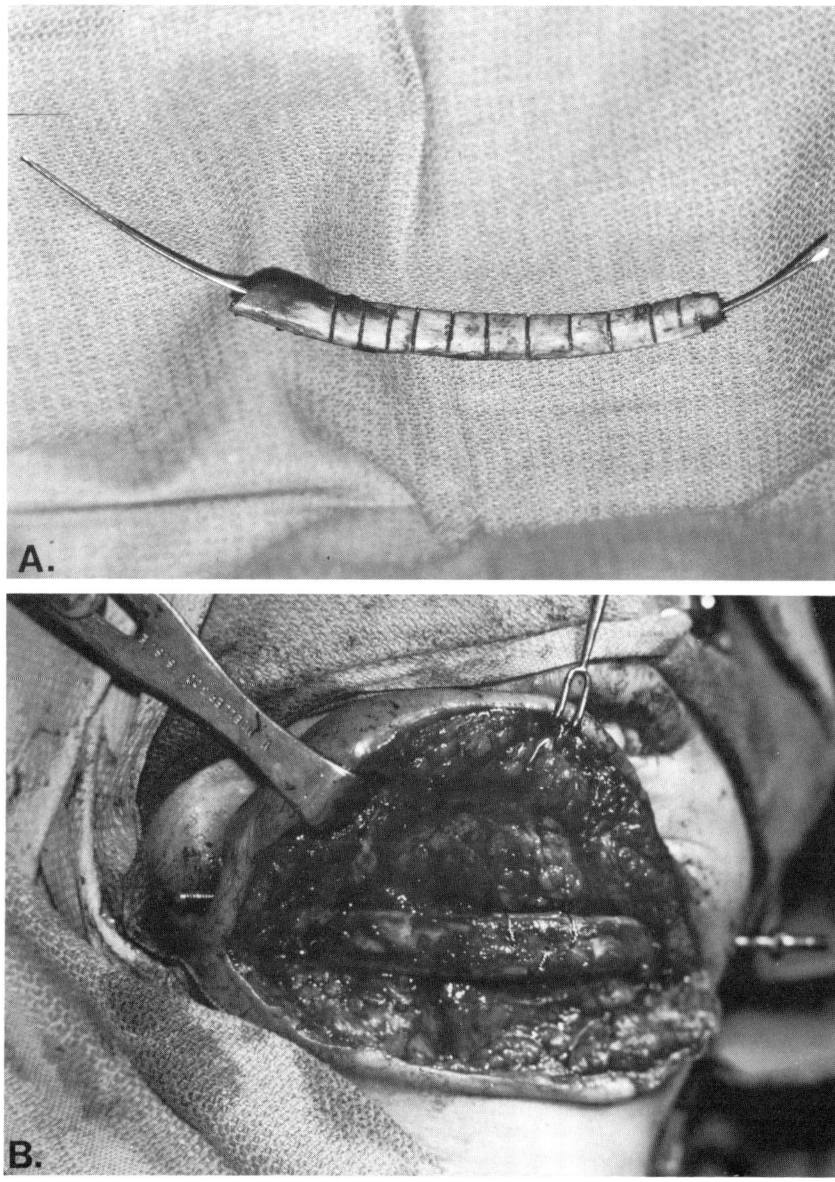

Figure 1–28. Anterior mandibular arch reconstruction with rib graft. *A,* Rib graft is sectioned through the posterior cortex, then skewered with Kirschner wire. Rib is bent into the desired configuration. *B,* Graft is in place by means of a mortise joint and a triangular wire. Additional rib is wired over the anterior aspect to improve chin projection.

stable bone remains, the biphase system is utilized. However, screws are not placed in the graft itself. Avoidance of mobility at the graft sites is important in preventing nonunion; therefore even the biphase appliance should be complemented with additional immobilization. Because most of these patients are edentulous, no anchor sites are available for the placement of arch bars or eyelet wires. Interosseous intermaxillary wires should be avoided because they may provide a route for the passage of microorganisms, thereby infecting the grafts. Fixation is maintained for 12 to 14 weeks. If no mobility or tenderness is elicited at the graft sites at this time, the biphase appliance is removed.

Occasionally, insufficient bone is available for secure biphase fixation. In such cases a simple Barton bandage provides adequate immobilization, so long as it is tightened every 2 to 3 days. A more elaborate type of head gear can be constructed with nylon straps, felt supports, and a Velcro fastening system (Fig. 1–29). The Barton bandage type

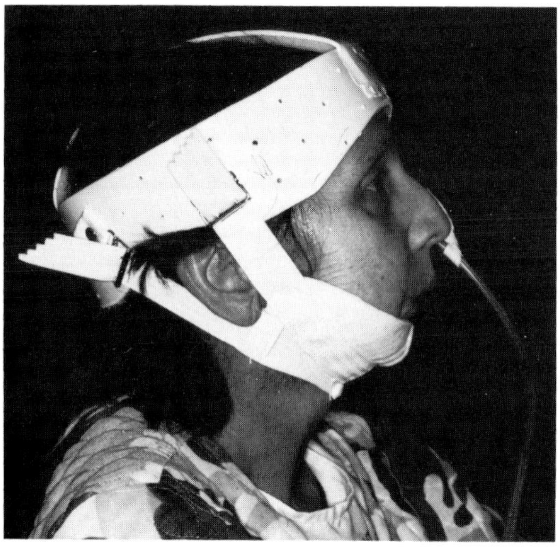

Figure 1–29. Nylon strap mandibular fixation sling based on the principle of the Barton bandage. Use of this sling was necessitated by inadequate residual bone for the biphase fixation of the mandibular graft. The suspension system was used for 3 months and resulted in excellent osseous healing.

of immobilization was adequate to permit healing in three of our patients in whom it had to be relied upon exclusively.

Chin

One of the most disfiguring consequences of anterior resection is the markedly receding chin or "Andy Gump" deformity. This is often brought about by a deficiency in the bony component, but in its severest forms results from the loss of both bone and overlying soft tissue.

Before a bone graft can be inserted to reestablish the continuity of the mandible, it must have adequate soft tissue coverage. When the malignancy is so extensive that a through-and-through excision is necessary, reconstruction requires a flap often of substantial size. The introduction of musculocutaneous flaps into the reconstructive surgical armamentarium has vastly improved the potential for coverage of very large defects. The mastery of microvascular surgical techniques also opens up the possibility for the use of osteocutaneous free flaps. However, in instances where previous surgery and irradiation have failed, it is often wise to suture the skin to the oral mucosa, delaying the reconstruction to a time when healing is complete and the danger of local recurrence has passed (Fig. 1–30).

The deltopectoral flap, formerly the workhorse in chin reconstruction, is being rapidly supplanted by the pectoralis major musculocutaneous flap. The bulk supplied by the muscle, the wide expanse of skin available, and the persistently intact blood supply are its principal advantages. The rich blood supply from the thoracoacromial artery will help to nourish future bone grafts. The deltopectoral flap still has its place, however, and should be considered when the addition of pectoralis major muscle to the chin may result in excessive projection.

Conley[74-76] has used a number of osteocutaneous composite flaps to reconstruct these defects in a few patients with some success. He has used both attached rib and clavicle as the osseous components, but frequent bone extrusion and absorption were encountered and the results were little better than with immediate bone grafting. The reason for this is the nature of the blood supply to the bones in these flaps. In their usual anatomic site, they are supplied from two sources: the small periosteal arteries and the nutrient artery. The nutrient artery piercing the head of the bone is responsible for the supply of the medullary and most of the compact bone of the diaphysis.[77, 78] The periosteal supply, which is that part which is preserved in chest flaps that include either rib or the shaft por-

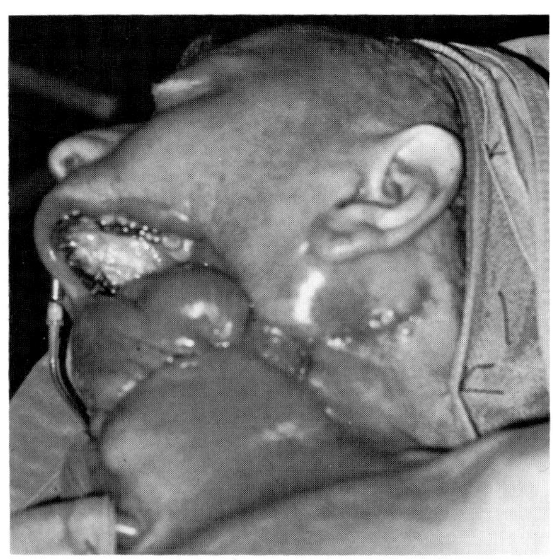

Figure 1–30. Skin-to-mucosa closure performed and reconstruction delayed because of extensive tumor resection done on a previously irradiated patient who is markedly malnourished. Tumor had eroded through the skin, causing fistulization, and a pathologic fracture eventuated because of extensive tumor involvement and osteoradionecrosis of the mandible.

tion of the clavicle, nourishes the outer portion of the compact bone. The principal periosteal artery in the rib is the anterior intercostal branch of the internal mammary artery, and unfortunately this is sacrificed in most composite flap transfers. Therefore, the only blood supply to the bone in these flaps is through collaterals from overlying muscle.

Using the goat as an experimental model, Medgyesi[79] showed an extensive and rich capillary blood supply from the overlying muscle and soft tissue to the periosteum of bone in a number of osteomyocutaneous flaps. Snyder et al[80] found some evidence of actively growing bone in a number of tubed flaps in humans. The cases of Conley and associates, with the exception of one temporal flap, showed either necrosis or creeping substitution on microscopic examination.[76] However, Cuono and Ariyan[81] showed evidence of viable medullary bone in a rib graft taken with a pectoralis major myocutaneous flap. Ostrup and Fredrickson[82] state that an intact medullary blood supply is required for bone transfer, in order to avoid the creeping substitution seen in free bone grafts and commonly experienced in composite flaps.

Panje[83] has used a trapezius musculocutaneous flap with attached scapular spine with excellent functional and cosmetic results in four patients. He fractures the bony fragment in the middle in order to achieve a semblance of the arch configuration. Fluorescein studies at the operating table and bone scans done later in the postoperative period reveal the maintenance of an excellent blood supply. The main disadvantages of this procedure are the difficulty in maintaining an intact blood supply to the flap from the transverse cervical artery during the neck dissection, the uncomfortable position of the patient's shoulder during the early postoperative weeks, and the difficulty in creating a satisfactory arch configuration from the graft.

Free flaps of cutaneous, muscular, and osseous tissue are excellent replacements for full-thickness loss. The bony component restores mandibular continuity, the cutaneous part replaces missing oral tissue or overlying skin, and the intervening flap muscle provides the soft tissue responsible for adequate chin projection and lateral contouring. Ariyan[84] found that composite free flaps of skin muscle and rib grafted to mandible by microvascular anastomoses survived and were adequately maintained on the anterior intercostal artery. This is fortunate, because primary medullary circulation can be established only by an anastomosis between the recipient artery and the nutrient artery piercing the head of the rib. The dissection necessary to preserve this nutrient vessel is exceedingly difficult. An important artery to the lumbar spine, the artery of Adamkiewicz, is in jeopardy during the maneuvers necessary to free up this vessel. Obtaining sufficient vessel length to provide an adequate cuff for anastomosis to the recipient artery is also very difficult.

Problems that face the use of compound free flaps for reconstruction of the chin area include the nature of the vessels in the recipient bed if the procedure is of a delayed nature, the danger of imminent irradiation if the reconstruction is done primarily, and finally, the enigma of reproducing the arch form. If the anterior intercostal artery is chosen as the main nutrient vessel to the rib in the graft, serial wedge cuts in the posterior rib surface and a series of greenstick fractures on the anterior surface further endanger the periosteal supply. The survival of the microvascular anastomosis in a previously irradiated bed was dramatically illustrated by Ostrup and Fredrickson in dogs.[82] The ability of these anastomoses to withstand a full course of irradiation, however, has yet to be proved. Irradiation tends to wreak most of its vascular damage on medium-sized arterioles. The dependency of a periosteal type of supply on the early establishment and maintenance of small-diameter collaterals between the vessels of the compacta and those of the medullary cavity[77, 78, 82] creates considerable doubt of graft success when postoperative irradiation is used.

The difficulty in arch reproduction and the problem of obtaining a medullary blood supply may have been answered by the work of Man and Fredrickson.[85, 86] They utilized the inner surface of the iliac crest with attached muscle and accompanying deep circumflex vessels. An outline of the required mandibular arch graft is inscribed on the inner cortex and it and the underlying medullary bone are taken. A generous cuff of overlying muscle must be included to protect the nutrient vessels that branch from the deep circumflex artery. Although their reported clinical experience is with only one patient, the procedure shows much promise.

Once the epithelial coverings of the lower third of the face have been restored, the mandibular graft inserted, and the continuity of the jaw re-established, the chin promi-

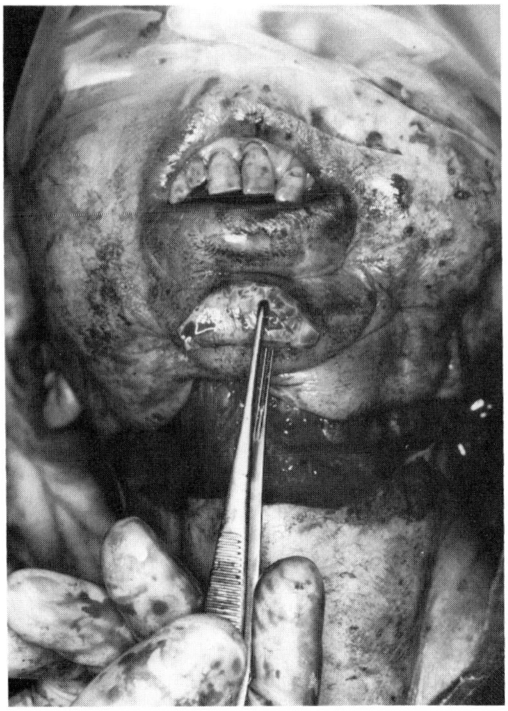

Figure 1–31. Instillation of irradiated cartilage graft to improve projection of the chin in a patient whose mandibular replacement graft rib was inadequate to produce sufficient mental projection.

nence is occasionally deficient. The insertion of an irradiated cartilage graft in a small pocket over the mentum restores a more normal appearing profile (Fig. 1–31).

In selecting from this extensive list of methods for lower face reconstruction, the author presently prefers the following: (1) a rib graft for mandibular reconstruction; (2) a pectoralis major flap for soft tissue and cutaneous coverage; and (3) an irradiated cartilage implant for mental augmentation.

Tongue

The fine, precise movements of the tongue result from the delicate coordination of its intrinsic muscles, which are oriented in longitudinal, vertical, and transverse planes. The verticalis linguae fibers are located only in the margins of the anterior tongue and are responsible for some of the delicate movements of the tongue tip. This may explain why, in cases in which tumor resection in the anterior oral cavity involved the removal of only relatively small portions of anterior tongue, the residual impairment of function is markedly out of proportion to the amount of resected tissue.

Clearly enunciated speech requires not only precise muscular coordination but adequate tongue length to contact the other oral articulators, as well as intact sensation to maintain the necessary kinesthetic sense. Often following extensive resections of large tumors, a longitudinal hemisection of the oral tongue is performed. Excellent function is commonly retained because of sufficient residual length and sensation, despite the fact that half of the bulk has been removed.

Marked improvement in speech can be achieved by reconstruction of the anterior tongue with a flap, but the loss of normal lingual sensation and fine movement markedly diminish the potential for perfectly articulated discourse. The success of this reconstruction also depends on the degree of fibrosis incurred during subsequent healing. The forehead flap is excellent for reconstructing both the anterior tongue and the floor of the mouth. However, the residual cosmetic deformity of the donor site has largely precluded its use. The deltopectoral flap has the principal drawback of excessive bulkiness. It is often much larger than required and is being largely supplanted by the sternocleidomastoid and trapezius myocutaneous flaps. Bulk again is a problem with these flaps but is occasionally an asset in disguise, especially in lateral defects (Fig. 1–14*D*). One vexing problem with these flaps is the frequent incidence of epidermolysis.[47] Although re-epithelialization is the rule, often with oral mucosa rather than skin, the patient is troubled in the first 2 or 3 postoperative weeks with delayed oral alimentation and fetor oris.

Often the principal limitation to good oral functioning is tethering of the anterior tongue in the floor of the mouth. Lingual release by sharp dissection, followed by lining of the defect with split-skin or dermis is a simple procedure with excellent results. The graft must be initially splinted with either dental rolls or some kind of dental stent for immobilization. When the restriction is more in the form of a band, a simple Z-plasty is all that is required as long as sufficient mobile tissue is present in the lateral oral gutters (Fig. 1–32).

Despite vigorous surgical efforts, the ultimate goal of acceptable speech is often not realized. Concentrated speech therapy usually improves the quality of articulation immensely. The surgeon's encouragement of

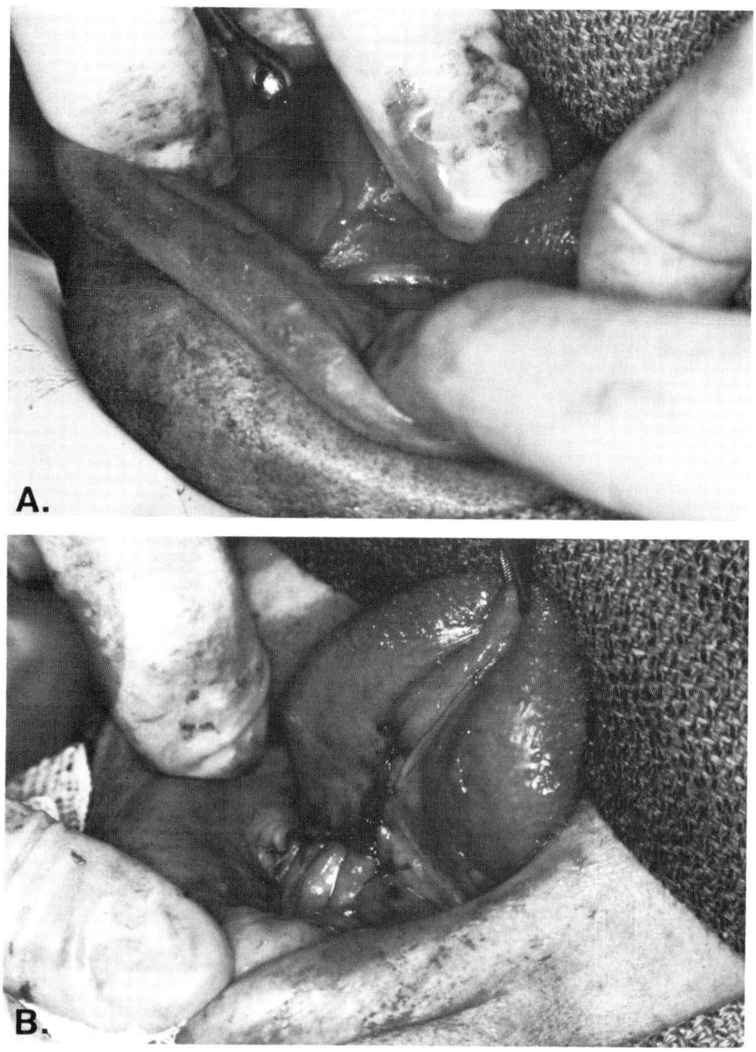

Figure 1–32. *A,* Tongue bound to the floor of the mouth by scarring following lingual plate excision of mandible and partial glossectomy. *B,* Z-plasty completed.

both patient and therapist in their strenuous participation is often rewarded with a surprising degree of success.

Alveolar Ridge and Gutters

Although adequate oral alimentation can be readily accomplished without dentition or even an alveolar ridge, precise articulation is virtually impossible without teeth. In addition, most patients desire dentition in order to return to a more normal diet and achieve a pleasing aesthetic appearance. Most often anterior oral cavity resections require the removal of partial or full-thickness mandible. The patient is often difficult, if not impossible, to rehabilitate prosthetically unless an alveolar ridge can be reconstructed. Moreover, this reconstructive effort will be doomed to failure unless the importance of the gingival-buccal and gingival-labial sulci is recognized.

Reconstruction of the alveolar ridge is fraught with difficulties, not the least of which is the provision of an adequately tough covering that will withstand the rigors of denture wearing. Once teeth have been extracted, the residual gingival tissue is thick and durable. When gingiva is resected as part of a tumor extirpation, it is commonly replaced by skin or dermal grafts. Unfortunately, the lack of toughness and durability, especially of the dermal graft, may make denture wearing painful and retention difficult. Moreover, denture retention is dependent not only on the character of the underlying epithelium but on the contour of the alveolar ridge as well. A smooth, conical ridge of sufficient height with minimal undercuts is necessary for denture retention.

The failure of onlay bone grafts to maintain adequate alveolar ridge height in the atrophic mandible has stimulated a number of fascinating innovations in the past decade. The early promise of Proplast and Proplast-coated metal implants has met with bitter disappointment and disastrous consequences. Harle,[87] in 1979, presented an excellent overview of the latest techniques of augmentation of the atrophic ridge. Although the various sandwich graft techniques have had some success, his visor osteotomy and its modification by De Koomen and coworkers[88] offer the greatest promise (Fig. 1–33). Their techniques, which involve a coronal split of the mandible followed by a superior sliding of the inner fragment upon the outer, have been applied successfully in mandibles with as little vertical height as 11 mm. However, none of the patients had undergone tumor resection or had received irradiation; thus, the suitability of these techniques for tumor patients remains to be seen. This author has had limited experience with augmentation, utilizing onlay grafts of irradiated cartilage with moderate success. Most patients undergoing an alveoloplasty require a vestibuloplasty at a later date in order to accommodate the denture flanges.

The area of mandibular resection itself may not need to actually have to withstand the pressure of the denture. If the arch is intact and sufficient denture-bearing surface is present outside the resected area, the prosthesis will be retained. The provision of adequate sulci is the measure most frequently required to ensure this retention. This is accomplished by an incision in the depths of the gingival-buccal or gingival-lingual sulcus, followed by supraperiosteal dissection as inferiorly as possible on the lingual or buccal plates of the mandible. Great care must be taken to avoid cutting the mental nerves; in some very atrophic ridges, these nerves may even present on the occlusal surface. A split-thickness skin graft is placed over the raw surface and sutured into position with absorbent material. Quilting sutures in the depths of the newly created sulcus are a great help in retaining the graft, but the keystone in graft immobilization is the stent. Although the graft immobilization technique of Esser[89] is as relevant today as it was 60 years ago, it has largely been supplanted by dental stents. The splint is held in place by circum-mandibular wires that are removed in 7 to 14 days. Once the wires are removed, the splint must be worn until a permanent denture is made.

In the last few years, the use of dermis for intraoral grafts has been supplanted by split-thickness skin grafts. The degree of take of split-skin is higher, and its durability under a prosthesis is much superior to that of dermis. Some shrinkage of both of these grafts takes place despite continuous splinting; however, it is rarely enough to preclude denture retention. It must be reiterated, though, that the patient's own gingiva, as long as it is firmly fixed and not redundant in amount, should be retained as much as possible on the occlusal surface of the ridge, because of its superior durability. Skin grafts on the retaining and occlusal surfaces of the mandible should be placed as close to the bone as possible. Dissection of the existing overlying soft tissue should keep adjacent to the periosteum, and the skin graft should be applied tightly to the

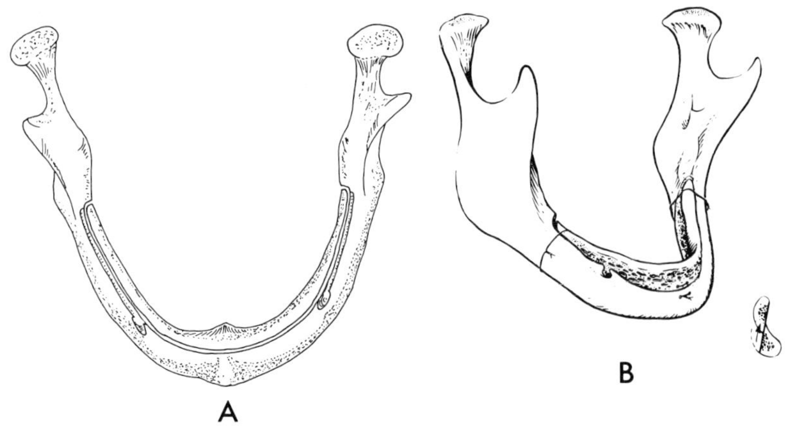

Figure 1–33. Visor osteotomy (after Harle). Mandible is vertically split. The inner plate is slid superiorly. *A,* View from below. Note how inferior alveolar nerve is spared. *B,* Inner plate slid into position and fixed with wire.

surface. The resultant tightly adherent graft will hold the denture well.

MANAGEMENT OF MASSIVE LESIONS

The massive T_4 lesion that invades bone, erupts through skin (Fig. 1–34) and extends beyond the confines of the oral cavity often presents with distant metastases or a metabolism that is too fragile to permit a potentially curable resection. Lesions of this magnitude often present with bilateral cervical adenopathy as well, and as a group, their prognosis is generally poor. However, a defeatist philosophy in the face of such horrendous tumors should be tempered with the knowledge that a significant number of patients can be cured if an approach of an appropriately radical nature is undertaken.

The surgeon who is courageous and skilled enough to undertake these heroic procedures must have a thorough knowledge of head and neck anatomy and physiology, as well as an understanding of the biology of these aggressive lesions. The techniques of radical tumor ablation must also be accompanied by considerable skills in reconstructive surgery in order to achieve a satisfactory result.

Adequate excision in these cases often requires removal of most of the mandible. Many of the patients represent failures of previous resections, and winning in these cases can be equated to "playing catch-up football." An extra-wide resection margin is essential to get ahead of a rapidly advancing tumor that has already eluded at least one previous therapist. Postoperative irradiation is of great help in the management of these patients, but can never be considered a method of shrinking the surgical margins. In general, surgical salvage of radiation failure is a poor concept as a therapeutic plan and should be heartily discouraged because of low survival and high complication rates.

Possibly the best way to illustrate the basic principles involved in the ablation of these large neoplasms, and especially the reconstruction of the extensive residual defects, is with a number of case examples.

CASE I. The patient depicted in the radiograph (Fig. 1–35*A*) had a metastasis from an unknown primary tumor. This massive tumor, measuring about 15 cm in diameter, deeply invaded the bone and penetrated the skin. A generous excision of mandible and overlying skin with a bilateral neck dissection was required for adequate excision (Fig. 1–35*B*).

Resections in these cases usually require a full-thickness excision from skin to mucosa, including intervening bone. Cutaneous excision in penetrating lesions should include a 3- to 4-cm margin of uninvolved skin. This is because of the frequent tendency of rapid tumor spread in the subepithelial plane once skin involvement occurs.

As previously mentioned, tumor spread through cortical bone is slow but progresses rapidly once the medullary cavity of the mandible is reached. In this patient, the tumor had extensive medullary involvement, and resection from one condyle to the opposing ramus was necessary. The tongue and floor of the mouth could be spared because of their lack of involvement. The resected tissue was reconstructed with a deltopectoral flap (Fig. 1–35*C*).

The patient became lost to follow-up for 2 years. When he was finally located, his hideous counte-

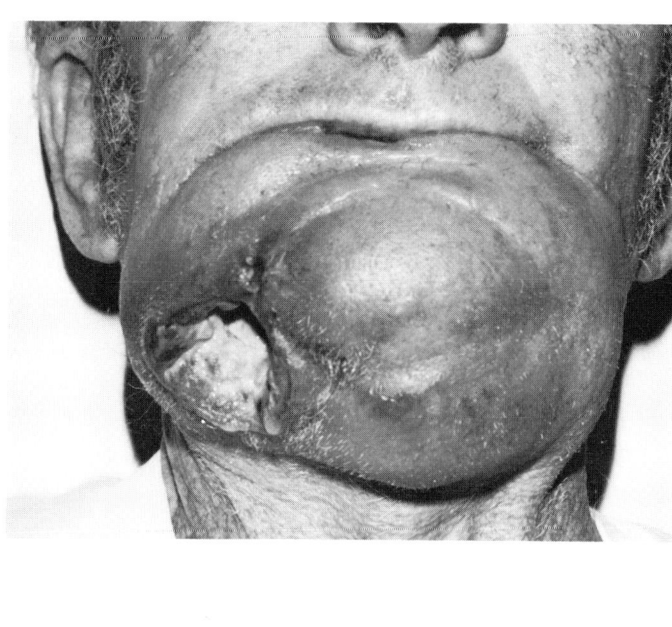

Figure 1–34. Massive oral cavity carcinoma beginning as a primary tumor in the lip that has extended through bone and fistulized through skin.

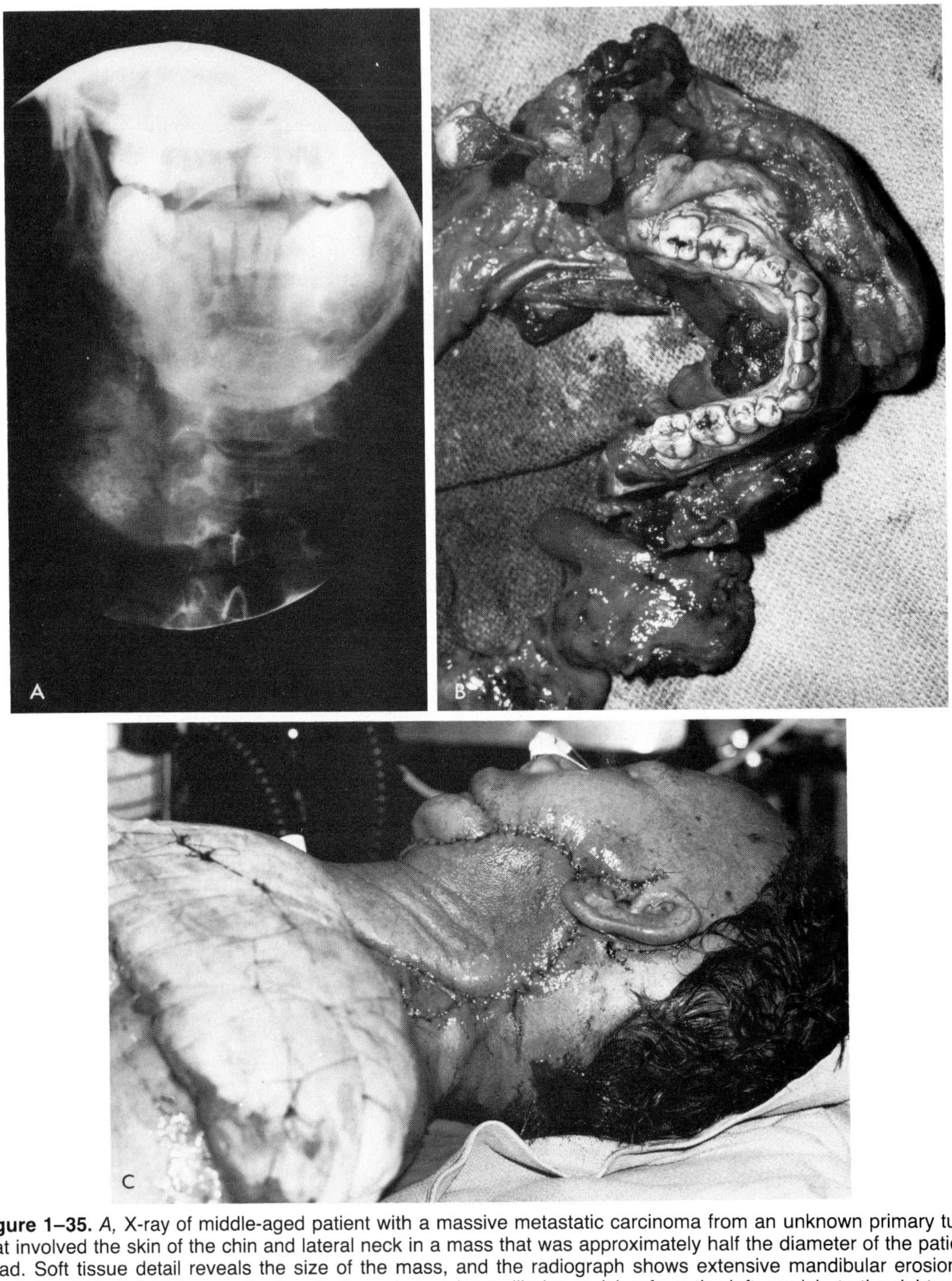

Figure 1–35. *A,* X-ray of middle-aged patient with a massive metastatic carcinoma from an unknown primary tumor that involved the skin of the chin and lateral neck in a mass that was approximately half the diameter of the patient's head. Soft tissue detail reveals the size of the mass, and the radiograph shows extensive mandibular erosion. *B,* Resection included bilateral radical neck dissection and mandibular excision from the left condyle to the right angle. The tongue was spared, but the skin of the left chin and neck was included in the specimen. *C,* Deltopectoral flap used to cover the defect.

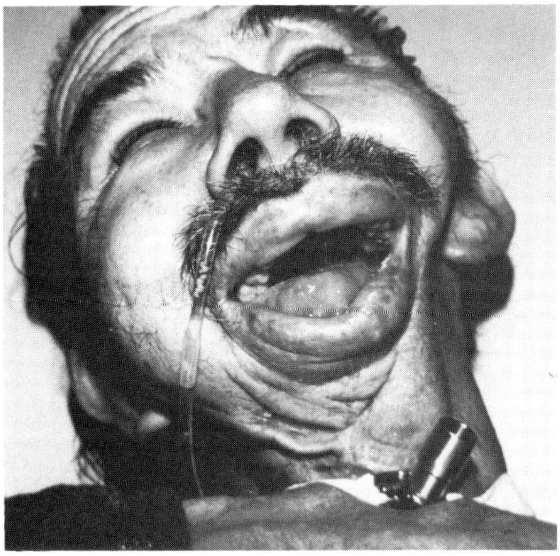

Figure 1–36. Grotesque visage results from inadequate soft tissue replacement and lack of bony support.

nance, oral incompetence (Fig. 1–36), and unintelligible speech had made him a socially unacceptable recluse. His own self-image was so severely affected that he tucked his head into his chest and hid the lower third of his face from view by a Styrofoam coffee cup fastened in place by an attached elastic band that was slung around his head. This posture combined with soft tissue contractures of his neck resulted in a permanent cervical flexion deformity.

His rehabilitation began with correction of the flexion contracture in his neck. This was accomplished by effacing the cervical webs, using multiple Z-plasties, and then manipulating his cervical spine under general anesthesia, once bone ankylosis had been ruled out. He was immobilized in the upright position with a halo brace (Fig. 1–37). The next stage was to supply a large flap of soft tissue to provide a bed for the installation of a bone graft. A pectoralis major musculocutaneous flap was selected because it would not only supply more than adequate skin coverage but it would also provide the necessary muscle bulk to augment the deficient chin and anterior neck (Fig. 1–38*A*, *B* & *C*).

An incision was made at the junction of the previously transposed deltopectoral flap and the residual chin skin. Skin flaps were developed so that a raw area of sufficient dimension was created to accept the flap. An important principle in reconstructing these cases, and one absolutely vital to their success, is to provide an excess of tissue in the flap. Touch-up trimming of superfluous flap can always be done once all the reconstructive steps have been completed. The disaster of being caught short of tissue in the middle of reconstruction thwarts any hope of a successful functional or cosmetic result. In this particular instance, concern regarding pressure on the flap pedicle precluded its subcutaneous placement. The hollowed supraclavicular aspect of the previously dissected neck posed such an acute angulation with the clavicle that the thoracoacromial artery would likely be severely compromised. The flap was rotated into position extracutaneously and the pedicle tubed. The pedicle was returned 3 weeks later.

Mandibular reconstruction posed a number of serious problems. The amount of graft material necessary eliminated the possibility of an osseous-musculocutaneous flap or an osseous or osteocutaneous free flap. Resections that stretch from one mandibular condyle to the opposite angle leave little hope for functional restoration; however, bone grafting can give some projection to the chin and, by supporting the tongue and floor of the mouth, assist in oral continence. It was elected to use two ribs, notch their posterior cortical surfaces to make them malleable, and skewer them with Kirschner wires. The Kirschner wires, in addition to skewering the two grafts together, lent them some stability, and helped to anchor one end into the mandibular ramus. They were bent into a horseshoe shape to reproduce the arch configuration of the mandible. Although the temporomandibular joint, mandibular ramus, and body of the mandible have been adequately restored by Obwegeser[90] in congenital abnormalities, such attempts in cancer patients are generally futile. Reconstruction of a temporomandibular joint in this patient was not attempted. The distal end of

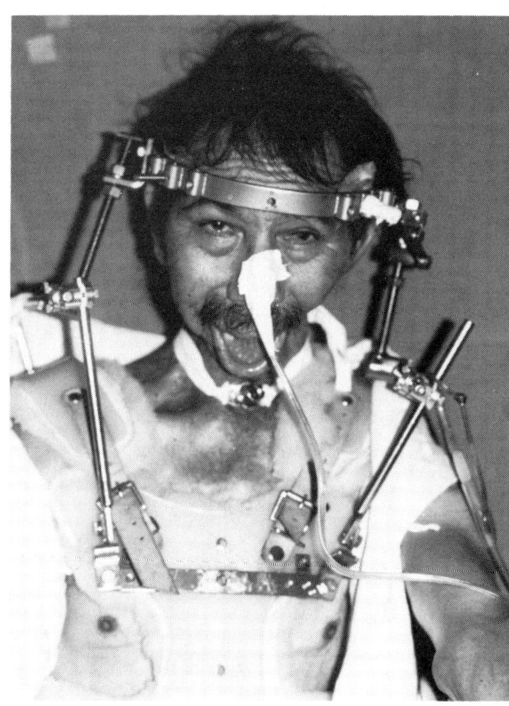

Figure 1–37. Initial step in rehabilitation is the straightening of the patient's spine following multiple Z-plasties in the neck to alleviate soft tissue contracture. Halo brace maintains head position.

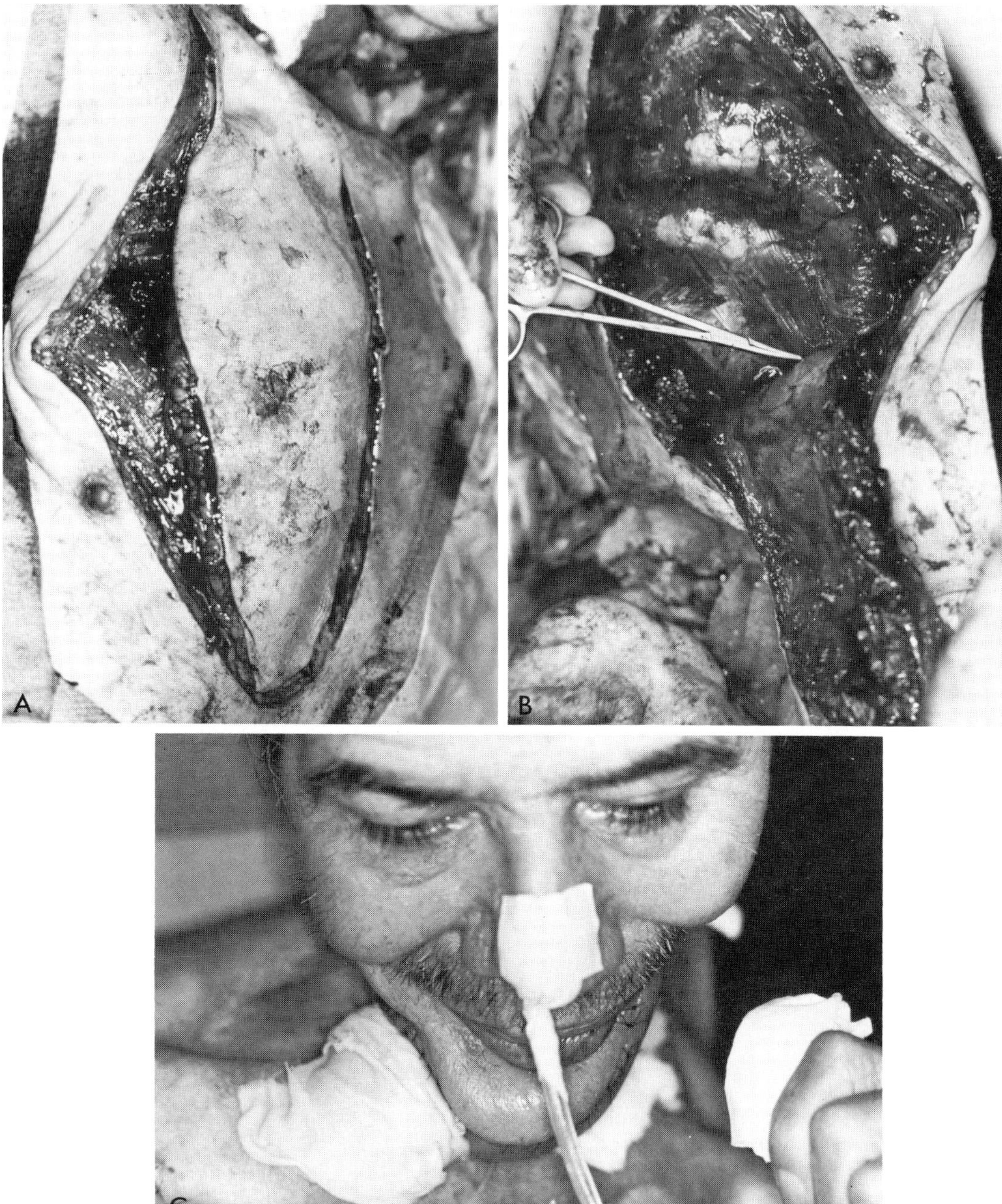

Figure 1–38. Reconstruction of the chin and anterior neck is begun by the use of a pectoralis major myocutaneous flap. *A,* Flap incised. *B,* Flap raised; hemostat points to vascular pedicle. *C,* Flap is rotated into position and placed outside the usual skin bridge, because of concern of compromising the pedicle of this massive flap by its compression between the lower cervical skin and the underlying clavicle.

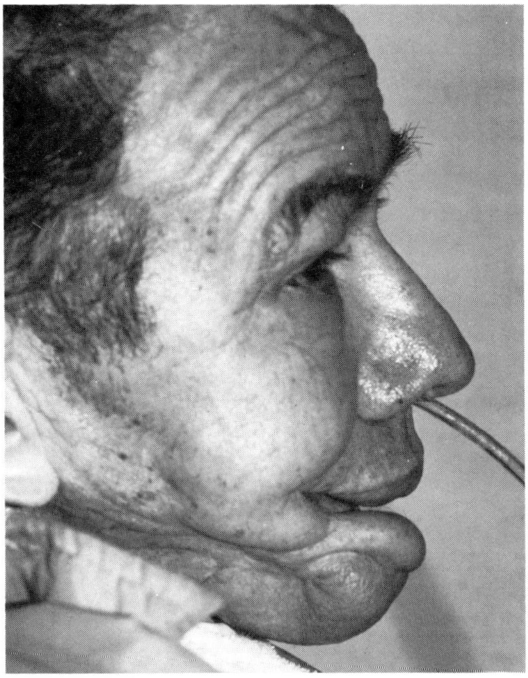

Figure 1–39. Patient shown 6 months after instillation of two tandem rib grafts extending from right to left mandibular angles. Nasogastric and tracheostomy tubes were eventually discontinued.

the graft was inserted into a fibrous tissue pocket, which was tunneled into the area roughly corresponding to the site of the opposing mandibular angle.

The patient has now been tumor-free for 5 years, has oral continence, is free of his nasogastric and tracheostomy tubes, and has understandable speech (Fig. 1–39).

CASE II. In the female, deltopectoral and pectoralis major flaps severely distort the breast. In an already deforming surgical procedure, the addition of a further aesthetic defilement of a socially and psychologically significant area of the body should be avoided. The nape of neck flap developed by Zovickian[91] provides excellent coverage and is a good match of texture and color.

The patient in Figure 1–40 had had a mandibular splitting procedure done at another institution for a lingual carcinoma that extended onto the floor of the mouth and was fixed to the periosteum of the lingual plate. An attempt to compensate for an inadequate surgical procedure with postoperative irradiation—a principle to be severely decried—had met with failure.

On presentation, her locally persistent disease extended through the skin. Resection included skin, mandible, tongue, and lateral oropharyngeal wall. Despite frozen-section confirmation of tumor-free margins, permanent section revealed the presence of malignant tissue. At a further operation additional tumor was resected from the tongue and the edges of closure (Fig. 1–41*A*). The resultant defect was not closed primarily, and skin was approximated to the mucosa (Fig. 1–41*B*).

Once complete healing had taken place, the staged construction of the flap was begun (Fig. 1–42). The delay of the flap should be done in at least three stages. Initially, the elevation of a bipedicled flap is followed by a 3-week rest. At 10-day intervals, successive progression is made around the distal end of the flap under local anesthesia, at two or three separate sittings. The lidocaine for injection should not be mixed with epinephrine in these stages, as there is experimental evidence showing the danger of flap necrosis secondary to sympathetic denervation hypersensitivity of the vessels.[92] As a result of the initial flap elevation, the nutrient vessels have been sympathectomized, rendering them exquisitely sensitive to exogenous epinephrine. Catecholamines induce vasospasm, resulting in severe hypoxia to the flap. In the definitive reconstruction, once the mucosa had been closed, the flap was wrapped around the neck like a scarf, eliminating the step of pedicle return (Fig. 1–43). An inner lining was created by elevating oral and oropharyngeal mucosa and filleting the tongue. Care must be taken in the mucosal closure to elevate flaps with broad bases and short lengths. Tissues suffering the ravages of past radiation and repetitive surgery do not tolerate further surgical manipulation well.

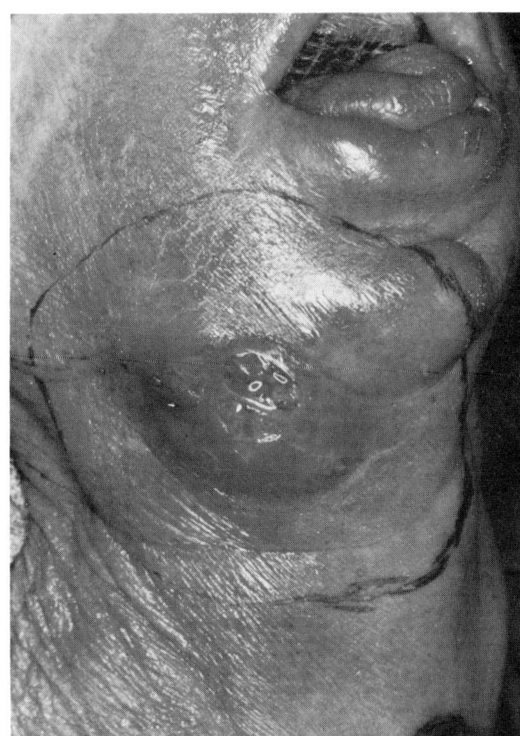

Figure 1–40. Recurrent carcinoma of the floor of the mouth and tongue following inadequate excision and full course irradiation. Note tumor burgeoning through the skin. Margin of excision is outlined.

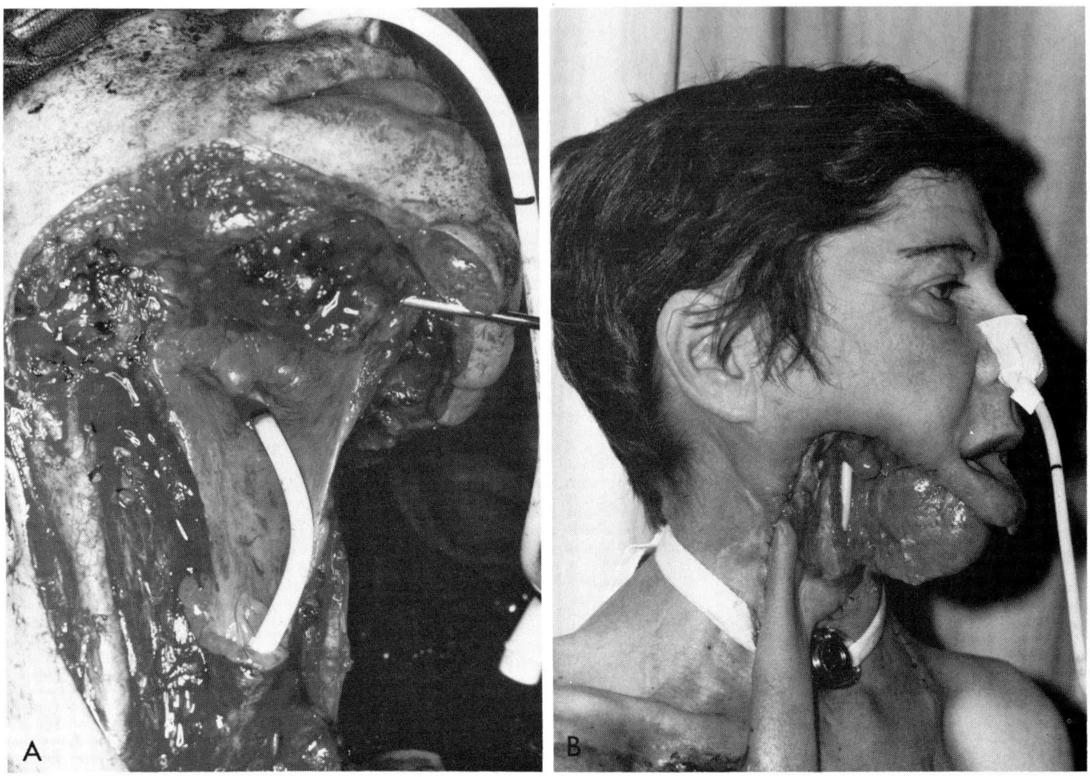

Figure 1–41. A second resection was necessary on the patient in Figure 1–40 because of evidence of persistent disease at the wound margins on histologic examination. *A,* Defect following reoperation. *B,* Defect ready for secondary closure.

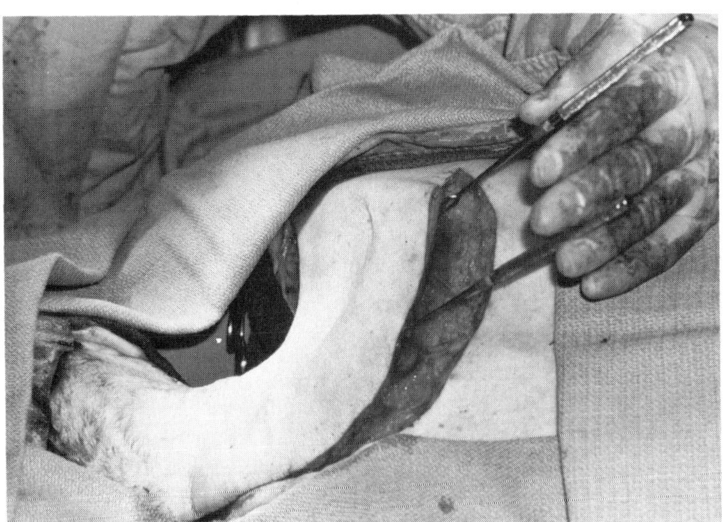

Figure 1–42. Initial stage in delayed elevation of Zovickian or scarf flap for reconstruction of oral cavity and oropharynx of patient in Figure 1–40. A large bipedicled flap is elevated initially, and then the distal end is severed in two successive stages.

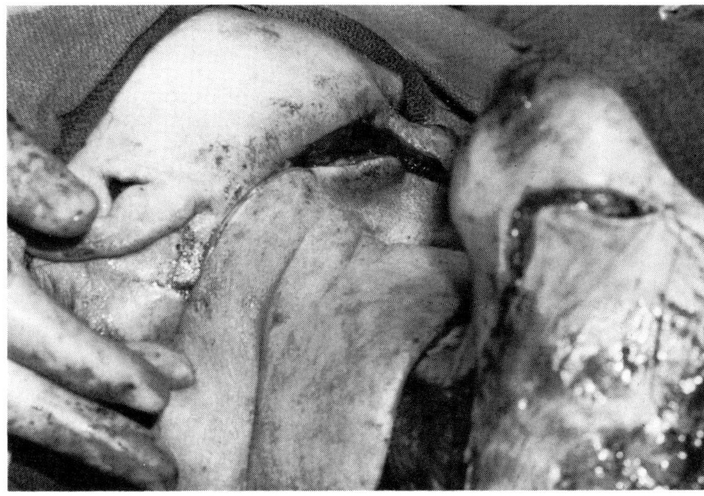

Figure 1–43. Final closure of cutaneous defect after mucosal continuity has been restored with lingual, pharyngeal, and buccal mucosal flaps. The scarf flap is wound around the neck and primarily approximated to the skin of the face and neck.

CASE III. Primary tumors of the buccal mucosa (Fig. 1–44) often require through-and-through excision. When internal and external linings are required for closure, the use of a musculocutaneous flap with a de-epithelialized bridge can be employed. The young woman in Figure 1–45 had a resection for an adenocarcinoma of the buccal mucosa that was fixed to skin and close to the anterior maxillary periosteum. The excision included the anterior wall of the maxillary sinus with preservation of the sinus mucoperiosteum. In addition, the oral commissure and lateral upper lip were removed in order to achieve a satisfactory margin. The upper lip was reconstructed with an Estlander flap.[93] A sternocleidomastoid musculocutaneous flap was constructed with its skin paddle bifurcated by a narrow, transverse de-epithelialized bridge (Fig. 1–45). A wider margin of muscle than skin is included in the flap in an attempt to compensate for the soft tissue resection extending under the facial skin. The flap is tunneled under the skin and the donor defect closed primarily. The distal end of the flap is folded into the mouth to replace the excised mucosa. Muscle is sutured under the skin to the soft tissue, and cutaneous closure is done.

CASE IV. It is wise to remember that not all reconstructive efforts are successful. The patient in Figure 1–44 required a bilateral radical neck dissection, an angle-to-angle mandibular resection, and a skin excision that involved the removal of a third of the upper lip, the entire lower lip, the skin of the lower third of the face, the inferior third of the tongue, and the larynx. The defect was covered with a pectoralis major musculocutaneous flap containing an area of approximately 400 square centimeters of skin. The flap was inserted through a wide subcutaneous tunnel. It remained healthy for approximately 26 hours, then

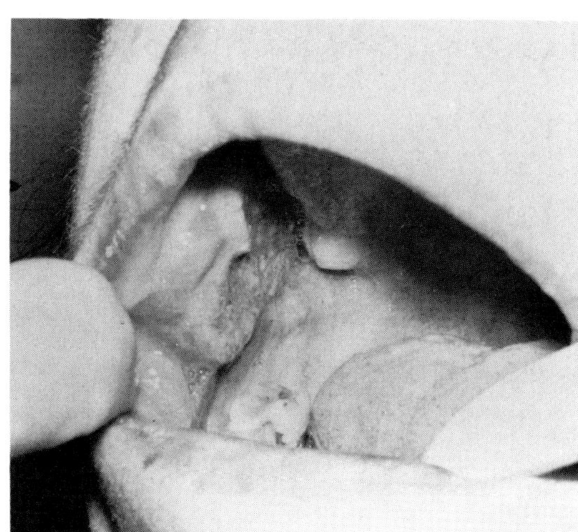

Figure 1–44. Extensive carcinoma of the buccal mucosa.

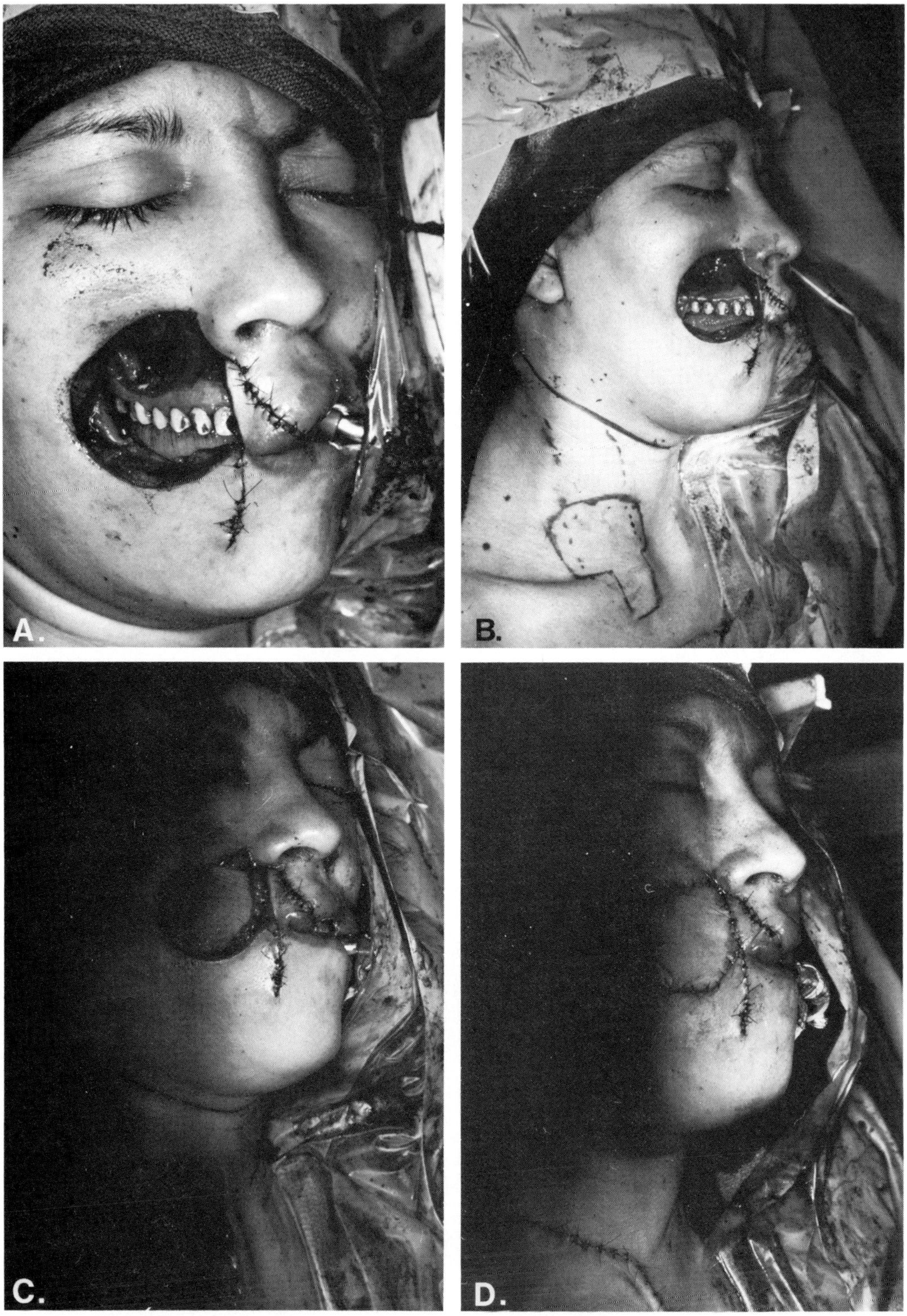

Figure 1–45. Young woman with an adenocarcinoma of the buccal mucosa requiring through-and-through excision. *A,* Surgical defect following Abbe-Estlander reconstruction of the right lateral mouth and commissure. *B,* Sternocleidomastoid island flap marked out on skin. Note the inferior paddle extending over the clavicle. A thin strip of epithelium is excised between the paddle and the flap proper. *C,* Flap is tunneled under a skin bridge and inserted into defect. The paddle is turned into the oral cavity to provide lining.

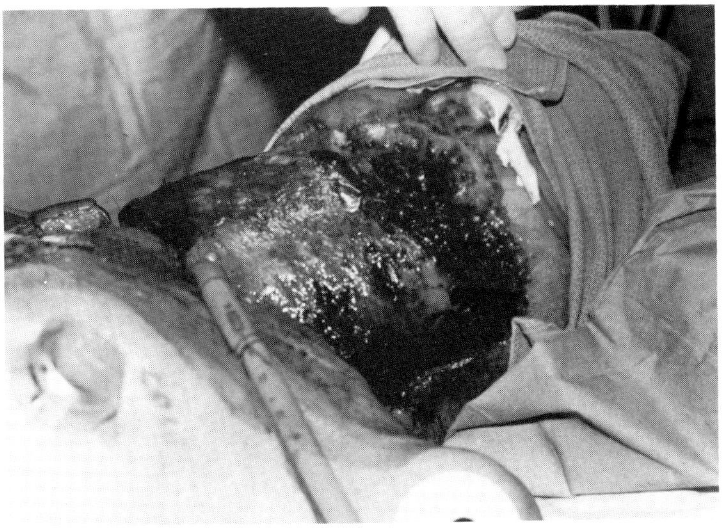

Figure 1–46. Slough of the major portion of a large (400 cm^2) pectoralis major myocutaneous flap used to cover defect from the oral commissures to the skin of the clavicles. Patient subsequently healed and had postoperative radiation therapy but died in his home of a myocardial infarction 6 months later.

it became dusky in color. By the time the neck skin bridging the pedicle was incised, most of the flap's circulation was lost, and about 70 per cent of the skin and muscle sloughed (Fig. 1–46). The marked edema of the face and neck skin resulted from ligation of both jugular veins as well as the extensive dissection and had squeezed off the circulation in the flap's nutritional supply. The flap may have been saved by extracutaneous positioning of the pedicle at the time of surgery or by vigilance in the early morning hours of the second postoperative day. The patient subsequently underwent debridement and had a skin graft performed. He underwent postoperative irradiation but died, tumor-free, 6 months later of a myocardial infarction.

References

1. Kornblut AD, DeFries HO: Forward. Otolaryngol Clin North Am 12(1), 1979.
2. Sellars SL: Epidemiology of oral cancer. Otolaryngol Clin North Am *12*(1):45, 1979.
3. Conley J (ed): Concepts in Head and Neck Surgery. New York, Grune & Stratton, 1970, p 99.
4. Lederman M: The anatomy of cancer. J Laryngol Otol *78*:1819, 1964.
5. Moore C, Catlin D: Anatomical origins and locations of oral cancer. Am J Surg *114*:510, 1967.
6. Trieger N, Shipp II, Taylor GW, et al: Cirrhosis and other predisposing factors in carcinoma of the tongue. Cancer *11*:357, 1958.
7. Gorlin RJ, Vickers RA: *In* Anderson WAD (ed): Pathology, 6th ed. St. Louis, CV Mosby, 1971, p 1084.
8. Cretien PJ: The effects of smoking on immunocompetence. Laryngoscope Supplement *8*:88, pp 11–13, 1976.
9. Palmer DL: Alcohol consumption and cellular incompetence. Laryngoscope Supplement *8*:88, pp 13–17, 1976.
10. Lundy J, Raaf JH, Deakins S, et al: The acute and chronic effects of alcohol in the human immune system. Surg Gynecol Obstet *141*:212, 1975.
11. Waldron CA, Shafer WG: Leukoplakia revisited. Cancer *36*:1386, 1975.
12. Shafer WG, Waldron CA: Erythroplakia of the oral cavity. Cancer *36*:1021, 1975.
13. Strong EW: Carcinoma of the tongue. Otolaryngol Clin North Am *12*:107, 1979.
14. DiTroia J: Nodal metastases in carcinoma of the oral cavity. Otolaryngol Clin North Am *5*:333, 1972.
15. Batsakis JG: Tumors of the Head and Neck: Clinical and Pathological Considerations. Baltimore, Williams & Wilkins, 1974, pp 86–111.
16. Lyall D, Shetlin CF: Cancer of the tongue. Ann Surg *135*:489, 1952.
17. Kreinen AJ: The case for elective (prophylactic) neck dissection. *In* Conley J (ed): Cancer of the Head and Neck. Washington DC, Butterworths, 1967, pp 183–185.
18. Southwick HW, Slaughter DP, Trevino ET: Elective neck dissection for intraoral cancer. Arch Surg *80*:905, 1960.
19. Sako K, Pradier RN, Marchetta FC, et al: Fallibility of palpation in the diagnosis of metastases to cervical nodes. Surg Gynecol Obstet *118*:989, 1964.
20. Ward GE, Edgerton MT, Chambers RG, et al: Cancer of the oral cavity and pharynx and results of treatment by means of the composite operation (in continuity with radical neck dissection). Ann Surg *150*:202, 1959.
21. Skolnik EM, Saberman MN: Cancer of the tongue. Otolaryngol Clin North Am *2*:603, Oct 1969.
22. Fries R, Platz H, Wagner RR, et al: Carcinoma of the oral cavity: on the prognostic significance of the primary tumor site (by organs) in the oral cavity. J Maxillofac Surg *8*:25, 1980.
23. Litton WB, Krause CJ: Surgical management of carcinoma of the oral cavity. Otolaryngol Clin North Am *5*:303, 1972.
24. Vidic B, Melloni BJ. Applied anatomy of the oral cavity and related structures. Otolaryngol Clin North Am *12*:3, 1979.
25. Cady B, Catlin D: Epidermoid carcinoma of the gum. Cancer *23*:551, 1969.
26. Waldron CA: Oral epithelial tumors. *In* Gorlin RI, Goldman HM (eds): Thoma's Oral Pathology, 6th ed, Vol 2. St. Louis, CV Mosby, 1970, p 834.
27. Sharp GS, Wood RC: Treatment of cancer of the gums. J Oral Surg *8*:185, 1950.

28. Schuller DE: Cancer of the oral cavity. SIPac, published by the American Academy of Otolaryngology, 1980.
29. Gibert ED, Goffinet DR, Bayshaw MA: Carcinoma of the oral tongue and floor of the mouth: 15 years' experience with linear accelerator treatment. Cancer *35*:1517, 1975.
30. Berthelsen A, Hansen HS, Rygard J: Radiation therapy of squamous carcinoma of the floor of. the mouth and the lower ridge. J Laryngol Otol, *91*:489, 1977.
31. Pierguin B, Chassagne D, Cox JD: Toward consistent local control of certain malignant tumors. Radiology *99*:661, 1971.
32. Fu KK, Chan EK, Phillips TL, et al: Time, dose, and volume factors in carcinoma of the oral tongue. Radiology *119*:209, 1976.
33. Delclos L, Lindberg R, Fletcher GH: Squamous cell carcinoma of the oral tongue and floor of the mouth. Am J Roentgenol, *126*:223, 1976.
34. Donald PJ: Conservation therapy for oral cavity carcinoma. Trans Pacific Coast Oto-Ophthalmol Soc *58*:111, 1977.
35. Schramm VL, Myers EN, Sigler BA: Surgical management of early epidermoid carcinoma of the anterior floor of the mouth. Laryngoscope *90*:207, 1980.
36. Krause CJ, Lee JG, McCabe BF: Carcinoma of the oral cavity—a comparison of therapeutic modalities. Arch Otolaryngol *97*:354, 1973.
37. La Ferrier KA, Sessions DG, Thawley SE, et al: Composite resection for oral cavity and oropharyngeal cancer. Arch Otolaryngol *106*:103, 1980.
38. Donald, PJ: Complications of combined therapy in head and neck carcinoma. Arch Otolaryngol *104*:329, 1978.
39. Snow JB, Gelber RD, Kramer S: Randomized preoperative and postoperative radiation therapy for patients with carcinoma of the head and neck: preliminary report. Laryngoscope *90*:930, 1980.
40. Lore JM: An Atlas of Head and Neck Surgery, 2nd ed, Vol 2, Philadelphia, WB Saunders, 1973, pp 506–509.
41. Spiessl B, Tschopp HM: Surgery of the jaws in head and neck surgery, face, and facial skull. *In* Naumann HH (ed): Head and Neck Surgery, Vol 2. Philadelphia, WB Saunders, 1980, pp 149–154.
42. Barbosa JF: Surgical Treatment of Head and Neck Tumors. San Francisco, Grune & Stratton, 1974, pp 93–104.
43. Freund HR: Principles of Head and Neck Surgery, 2nd ed. New York, Appleton-Century-Crofts, 1979, pp 152–175.
44. Calnan J, Innes FL: Exposed delayed primary skin grafts: A clinical investigation. Br J Plast Surg *24*:129, 1971.
45. O'Neill JV, Snyder GG: Delayed grafting of forehead flap defects. Laryngoscope *88*:1871, 1978.
46. Bertotti JA: Trapezius-musculocutaneous island flap in the repair of major head and neck cancer. Plast Reconstr Surg *65*:16–21, 1980.
47. Ariyan S: One-stage reconstruction for defects of the mouth using a sternomastoid myocutaneous flap. Plast Reconstr Surg *63*:618, 1979.
48. Sasaki CT: The sternocleidomastoid myocutaneous flap. Arch Otolaryngol *106*:74, 1980.
49. Marchetta FC, Sako K, Babillo J: Periosteal lymphatics of the mandible and intraoral carcinoma. Am J Surg *105*:505, 1964.
50. Marchetta FC, Sako K, Murphy JB: The periosteum of the mandible and intraoral carcinoma. Am J Surg *122*:711, 1971.
51. Polya SJ, Narratel D: Experiments on lymph ducts of the buccal mucous membranes. Orvostud ertek gyujt magy orz. Arch Budapest v.f. III:485, 1902.
52. Cunningham MP, Slaughter DP: A face-saving procedure: marginal resection of the mandible for anterior oral cavity cancer. Ill Med J *133*:166, 1968.
53. Byars LT: Extent of mandibular resection required for treatment of oral cancer. Arch Surg *70*:914, 1955.
54. Ossoff RH, Bytell DE, Hast MH, et al: Lymphatics of the floor of the mouth and periosteum. Presented at Research Forum, American Academy of Otolaryngology, 1978.
55. Ossoff RH, Sisson GA: Lymphatics of the floor of the mouth and periosteum. Otolaryngol Head Neck Surg *88*:652, 1980.
56. Freund HR: Principles of Head and Neck Surgery, 2nd ed. New York, Appleton-Century-Crofts, 1970, p 150.
57. McGregor IA: "Quilted" skin grafting in the mouth. Br J Plast Surg *28*:100, 1975.
58. Keim FW, Lowenberg S: Marginal mandibulectomy in the treatment of carcinoma of the floor of the mouth. Laryngoscope *80*:1566, 1970.
59. King GD: Transoral resections for carcinoma of the oral cavity. Otolaryngol Clin North Am *5*:321, 1972.
60. Som ML, Nussbaum M: Marginal resection of the mandible with reconstruction by tongue flap for carcinoma of the floor of the mouth. Am J Surg *121*:679, 1971.
61. Goss CM (ed): Gray's Anatomy of the Human Body, 29th ed. Philadelphia, Lea & Febiger, 1976, pp 383–386.
62. Bratcher GO: Personal communication, 1979.
63. Karapandzic M: Innervated myocutaneous arterial flap in lip reconstruction. Transactions of the Third International Symposium on Plastic and Reconstructive Surgery, New Orleans, 1980.
64. Norante JD, McCabe BF: Fascial sling suspension of the chin following resection of the anterior mandible. Laryngoscope *83*:336, 1973.
65. Lawson W, Lascalzo L, Baek S, et al: Experience with immediate and delayed mandibular reconstruction. Laryngoscope *92*:5, 1982.
66. DeFries HO, Marble HB, Sell KW: Reconstruction of the mandible: use of a homograft combined with autogenous bone and marrow. Arch Otolaryngol *93*:426, 1971.
67. Cantrell RW: Personal communication, 1976.
68. Cummings CW, Leipzig B: Replacement of tumor-involved mandible by cryosurgically devitalized autograft. Arch Otolaryngol *106*:252, 1980.
69. Popescu V, Spirescu IE: Bone resection, extracorporeal cryotherapy and immediate re-implantation in the treatment of mandibular tumors. J Maxillofac Surg *8*:8, 1980.
70. Panje WJ: Personal communication, 1980.
71. Haymaker R: Symposium on Head and Neck Cancer: Principles of Reconstruction. Cincinnati, June 17–19, 1982.
72. Haymaker R: Personal communication, 1982.
73. Millard DR, Garst WP, Campbell RC, et al: Composite lower jaw reconstruction. Plast Reconstr Surg *46*:22, 1970.
74. Conley J: Regional Flaps of the Head and Neck. Stuttgart, Georg Thieme Publications, 1976, pp 247–266.
75. Conley J: Use of composite flaps containing bone

for major repairs in the head and neck. Plast Reconstr Surg *49*:522, 1972.
76. Conley J, Cinelli PB, Johnson PM, et al: Investigation of bone changes in composite flaps after transfer to the head and neck region. Plast Reconstr Surg *51*:658, 1973.
77. Brookes M, Elkin AC, Harrison RG, et al: A new concept of capillary circulation in bone cortex: some clinical applications. Lancet *1*:1078, 1961.
78. Brookes M, Harrison RG: The vascularization of the rabbit femur and tibiofibula. J Anat *19*:61, 1957.
79. Medgyesi S: Observations on pedicle grafts in goats. Scand J Plast Reconstr Surg *7*:110, 1973.
80. Snyder CC, Bateman JM, Davis CW, et al: Mandibulo-facial restoration with live osteocutaneous flaps. Plast Reconstr Surg *45*:14, 1970.
81. Cuono CB, Ariyan S: Immediate reconstruction of a composite mandibular defect with a regional osteomusculocutaneous flap. Plast Reconstr Surg *65*:477, 1980.
82. Ostrup LT, Fredrickson JM: Reconstruction of mandibular defects after radiation using a free living bone graft transferred by microvascular anastomosis. Plast Reconst Surg *55*:563, 1975.
83. Panje WJ: Trapezius osteomyocutaneous island flap for reconstruction of the anterior floor of the mouth and mandible. Head Neck Surg *3*:66, 1980.
84. Ariyan S: The viability of rib grafts transplanted with the periosteal blood supply. Plast Reconstr Surg *65*:140, 1980.
85. Fredrickson JM: Free flap reconstruction of the mandible. Otolaryngol Head Neck Surg (in press).
86. Man C, Fredrickson JM: Mandibular reconstruction using free revascularized iliac crest. Anatomical investigation of bone-blood supply. J Otolaryngol (in press).
87. Harle F: Follow-up investigation of surgical correction of the atrophic alveolar ridge by visor osteotomy. J Maxillofac Surg *7*:283, 1979.
88. DeKoomen HA, Stoelinga PJ, Tideman H, et al: Interposed bone-graft augmentation of the atrophic mandible (a progress report). J Maxillofac Surg *7*:129, 1979.
89. Esser JF: Studies in plastic surgery of the face. Ann Surg *65*:297, 1917.
90. Obwegeser HL: Advances in reconstructive maxillofacial surgery. Presented at the Third International Symposium of Facial Plastic Surgeons, New Orleans, 1979.
91. Zovickian A: Pharyngeal fistula; repair and prevention using mastoid occipital based shoulder flaps. Plast Reconstr Surg *19*:335, 1957.
92. Klingenstrom P, Nylen B, Westermark L: Vasoconstrictors and experimental flaps. Acta Clin Scand *131*:187, 1966.
93. Estlander JA: Méthode de l'autoplastie de la jove ou d'une lèvre par un lambeau emprunté à l'autre lèvre. Rev Mens Med Chir *1*:344, 1877.

2

OROPHARYNX AND TONGUE BASE

Paul J. Donald, M.D.

In the decades prior to modern surgical and radiotherapeutic techniques, tumors of the oropharynx and tongue base had a dismal prognosis, the only exceptions being small tonsillar or tongue lesions that were usually picked up incidentally on examination. The patient was usually doomed to early recurrence. Today, however, newer, more radical surgical procedures, especially when combined with radiation therapy, have vastly improved the situation, making many of these patients surgically salvageable.

ANATOMY

The inferior anatomic boundary of the oropharynx is somewhat obscure. Gray's Anatomy[1] describes this limit to be the hyoid bone, which is about level with the depths of the valleculae. Some clinical textbooks[4-6] agree with this definition, while others[2, 3] place the inferior border at the tip of the epiglottis. This leaves uncertain the locale of the base of the tongue. By one definition, only that area adjacent to the circumvallate papillae would be included, whereas by the other, the entire tongue base would be oropharyngeal in location. This problem frequently makes unclear survival statistics quoted for patients with tumors in this region. Discussions of oropharyngeal tumors often refer only to tumors of the tonsil, soft palate, and pharyngeal walls. The base of the tongue is frequently an orphan.

In this chapter, the areas of surgical management will include not only the aforementioned areas and the tongue base but the retromolar trigone area as well. The *retromolar trigone* (Fig. 1–5, p. 5) in a strict anatomic sense resides in the oral cavity. However, because of its proximity to the mandibular ramus and anterior tonsillar pillar, as well as the biologic similarity of its tumors to those of the tonsillar region, it is included in the discussion of the management of oropharyngeal cancer. Retromolar tumors (Fig. 2–1) are particularly aggressive locally and have high metastatic rates similar to those of the anterior tonsillar pillar and soft palate. Skolnik et al[7] report that cervical metastases to the ipsilateral lymph nodes occur in 40 to 60 per cent of cases, and to the contralateral nodes in 5 per cent of cases. Wang[8] lumps retromolar trigone lesions and anterior faucial pillar lesions together. He found an overall cervical metastatic rate of 33 per cent and emphasized the locally aggressive nature of these lesions. Infiltration into the adjacent tongue is common with these lesions and caused a precipitous drop in survival rate in his series when radiation was used as the principal therapeutic modality.

The *pharynx* is a muscular tube suspended from the skull base. It opens anteriorly to the nose in its superior or nasopharyngeal portion and to the oral cavity in its middle or oropharyngeal part. The inferior border of the nasopharynx—thus the superior limit

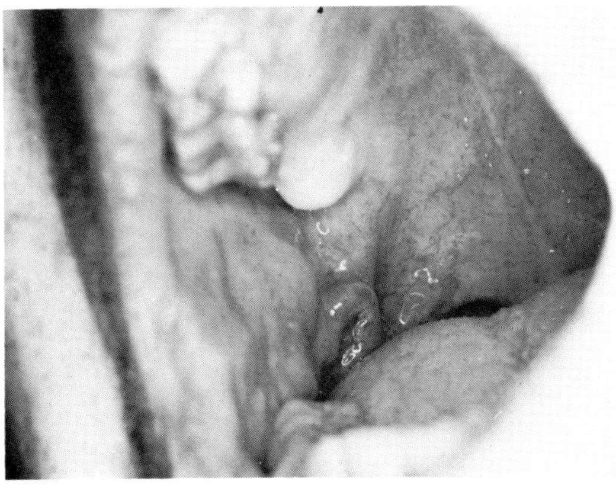

Figure 2–1. Squamous cell carcinoma of the retromolar trigone. Despite combined therapy with preoperative irradiation, this man died of local recurrence in the pterygoid muscles and distant metastatic disease.

of the oropharynx—is clearly established at the level of the soft palate.

The *tonsillar fossa* is separated from the medial surface of the mandibular ramus by a thin sheet of superior constrictor muscle and some scant fat and areolar tissue of the lateral pharyngeal space (Fig. 2–2). Tumors of the fossa are frequently endophytic. Invasion and attachment to bone can occur early in the course of the disease. Early detection of this phenomenon radiographically is difficult. Standard plane films and tomography demonstrate only lesions that are far advanced. Some evidence that triphasic bone scans are capable of more accurately assessing early invasion has recently come to light. The work of Baker, Krause, and Saxon[9] in the evaluation of subclinical bony involvement of the mandible in oral cavity cancer supports our own findings[10] that bone scanning is a far more sensitive indicator of early bone invasion than standard radiographic evaluation. Unfortunately the scan is also highly sensitive to inflammatory changes and thus produces occasional false-positive results. Because of the problems of tumor proximity to mandible and the difficulty in detecting subclinical invasion, bony resection in all but very early lesions is mandatory.

As progression is made around the lateral aspect of the oropharynx, the *posterior pharyngeal wall* appears to be a simple structure composed of mucosa, submucosa, pharyngobasilar fascia, underlying superior constrictor muscle, and overlying buccopharyngeal fascia.[11] Loose areolar tissue is contained in a potential space between the buccopharyngeal fascia and the thick prevertebral fascia. This loose connective tissue permits the easy gliding movement of the pharynx and cervical viscera over the cervical spine required by normal activity. It is a common experience to see extensive mucosal, submucosal, and muscular involvement of the posterior oropharyngeal wall with cancer, but no penetration of the buccopharyngeal fascia. The hardiness of this layer in resisting the penetration of malignant cells allows for an exception to the 2-cm resection rule. Although a minimum margin of 2 cm of healthy tissue is required for adequate resection of mucosal disease in the pharynx, a free dissection plane between the prevertebral and buccopharyngeal fascial layers almost always ensures a tumor-free plane. This is seen even in tumors with deep muscular penetration. However, once the tumor has transgressed the prevertebral space, it becomes fixed to the bodies of the cervical vertebrae and becomes unresectable. Con-

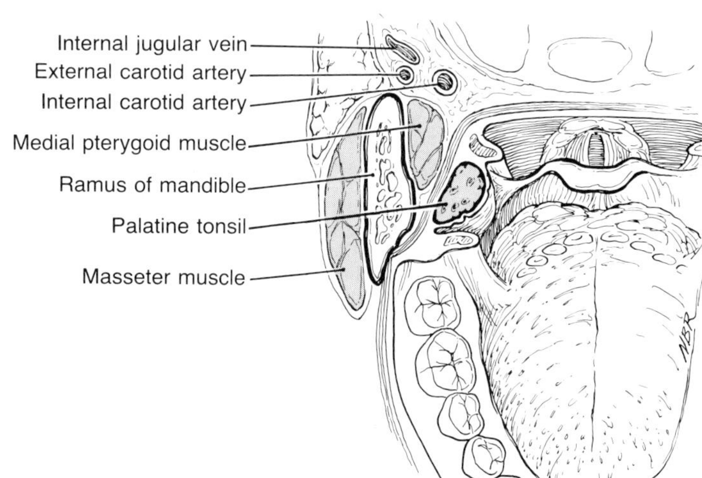

Figure 2–2. Proximity of the tonsil to the inner surface of the mandibular ramus.

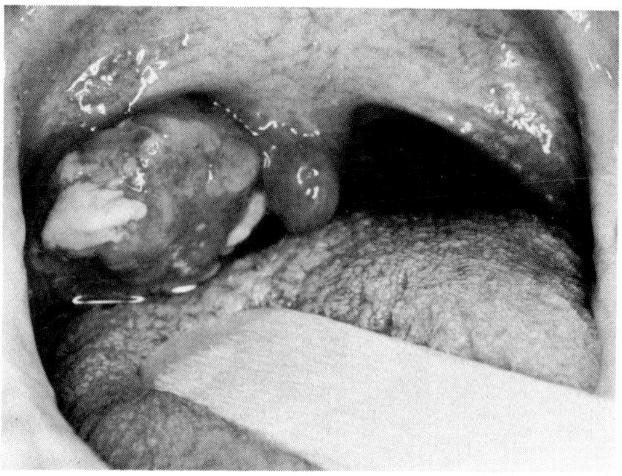

Figure 2–3. Large, bulky squamous cell carcinoma of the tonsil.

ceptually, a margin of bone could be excised from the vertebral bodies and if spinal instability resulted, cervical fusion could be done. However, usually the patient's general physical condition will not permit this, and those few whose health was adequate and to whom we offered this approach have declined. Furthermore, the proximity of the paraspinal musculature and the intervertebral foramina provides a ready means of local tumor extension and an inoperable situation. At the present state of knowledge, vertebral fixation is a sign of unresectability.

PATHOLOGY

By far the most common malignancy in the oropharyngeal region is squamous cell carcinoma.[12] These tumors may be exophytic and bulky (Fig. 2–3) or deeply infiltrating and ulcerating (Fig. 2–4). Occasionally, we see a tumor described as "superficially invasive" (Fig. 2–5). The grossly innocuous appearance of these sinister lesions must not tempt the surgeon to tailor a more conservative approach. The frequent finding of deeply extending chords of tumor cells in these cases dooms conservative measures to certain failure.

Many of these lesions in the faucial-palatine arch are surrounded by an area of Queyrat's erythroplasia (Fig. 2–6). As mentioned in the preceding chapter, these regions harbor numerous foci of carcinoma in situ and microinvasive cancer. The problem of multifocal cancer and "field cancerization" seen in the oral cavity continues to be a problem in the oropharynx.

The lymphocytic aggregations of the ring of Waldeyer may become a source of lymphoma (Fig. 2–7). In a compendium of a number of series reported by Parkhill,[12] an analysis of 416 malignancies of the palatine tonsil revealed 47, or 11.3 per cent, to be malignant lymphoma. If the unusual Mayo

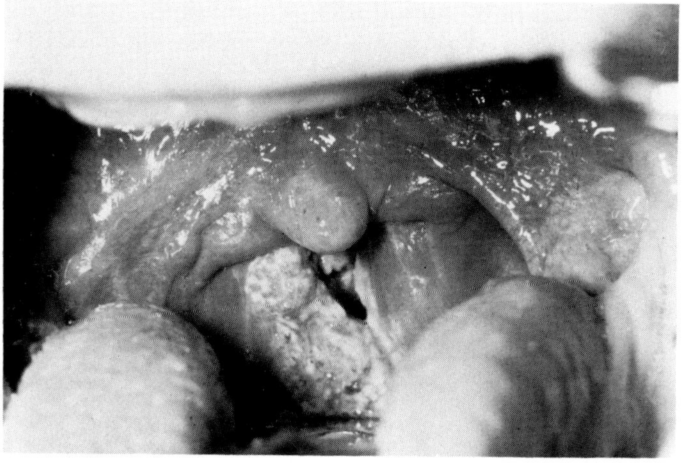

Figure 2–4. Endophytic ulcerative cancer of the posterior pharyngeal wall eroding into the cervical spine.

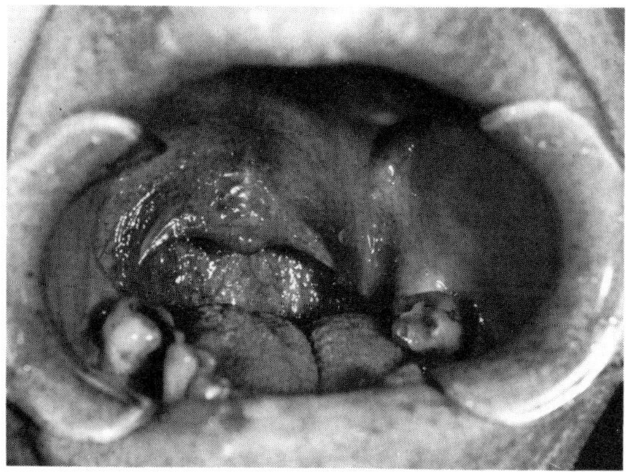

Figure 2–5. Carcinoma of the left tonsillar fossa of the "superficial invasive" variety.

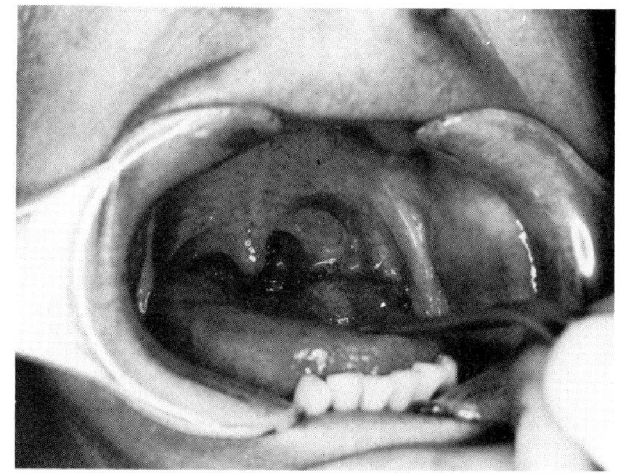

Figure 2–7. Lymphoma of the left lateral pharyngeal wall.

Clinic experience is extracted from this data (27 out of 64 of their cases being lymphoma), the incidence of lymphoma in the remaining 352 is 5.7 per cent. In general, the male incidence slightly exceeded that of the female, and the average age at diagnosis was 59 years. Following the palatine tonsil, the nasopharynx is the next most common site, with the lingual tonsil and the pharyngeal lymphoid aggregations being the least frequently involved. Accompanying cervical lymph nodal disease is common. In a large series of lymphomas involving Waldeyer's ring, Banfi et al[13] reported 62.3 per cent with cervical lymph node involvement. Only 22.5 per cent of the entire group of patients had lymphoma limited exclusively to the pharyngeal arch. In 74 of the 225 patients, lower limb angiography was done, and 44.6 per cent were found to have lymph node involvement outside the cervical area. Lymphoid malignancy in the head and neck is usually a manifestation of a systemic disease. This is especially true in Hodgkin's disease.[14] Surgery is rarely ever the method of choice for control in these disorders. Occasionally considerable difficulty is experienced by the pathologist in differentiating between a so-called anaplastic carcinoma and lymphoma. A high index of suspicion must be maintained in such patients, and further studies, such as the identification of cell surface markers and even electron microscopy, may be required to establish the diagnosis (Fig. 2–8).

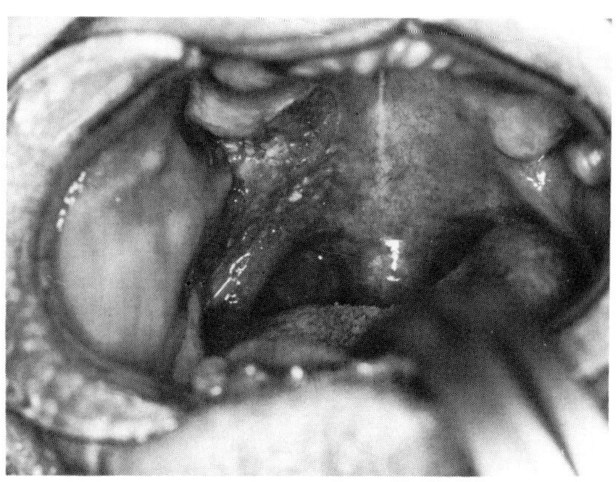

Figure 2–6. Epidermoid cancer of the tonsillar fossa and anterior pillar extending onto the soft palate and maxillary tuberosity. Lesion is surrounded by a brilliant scarlet-colored arc of Queyrat's erythroplasia.

The incidence of cervical lymph node metastases is high in oropharyngeal cancer. Toomey[15] quotes an overall figure of 50 to 75 per cent, and Lindberg[16] cites 60 to 80 per cent for cervical metastases from oropharyngeal carcinoma. Truluck and Putney[17] in 1971 reported on 168 cases of tumors in the tonsil, tongue base, and hypopharynx. Of the patients with tongue base lesions, 66 per cent had cervical metastases, while 56.3 per cent of those with tonsillar lesions had cervical spread. Wang[8] quotes a 33 per cent incidence of secondary tumors in 124 patients with anterior tonsillar pillar and retromolar trigone lesions. In T_3 lesions of the area, the metastatic rate rose to 43 per cent in his series. Quenelle et al[18] reported a 55 per cent metastatic rate in tonsillar fossa carcinoma in a series of 58 patients, while Edström et al[19] found cervical metastases in 27 of 37 patients (73 per cent) with tonsil tumors. When the tumor crosses the palatine arch or invades the tongue, contralateral metastases are seen in 10 to 20 per cent of cases.[16, 20]

Cancers involving the base of the tongue

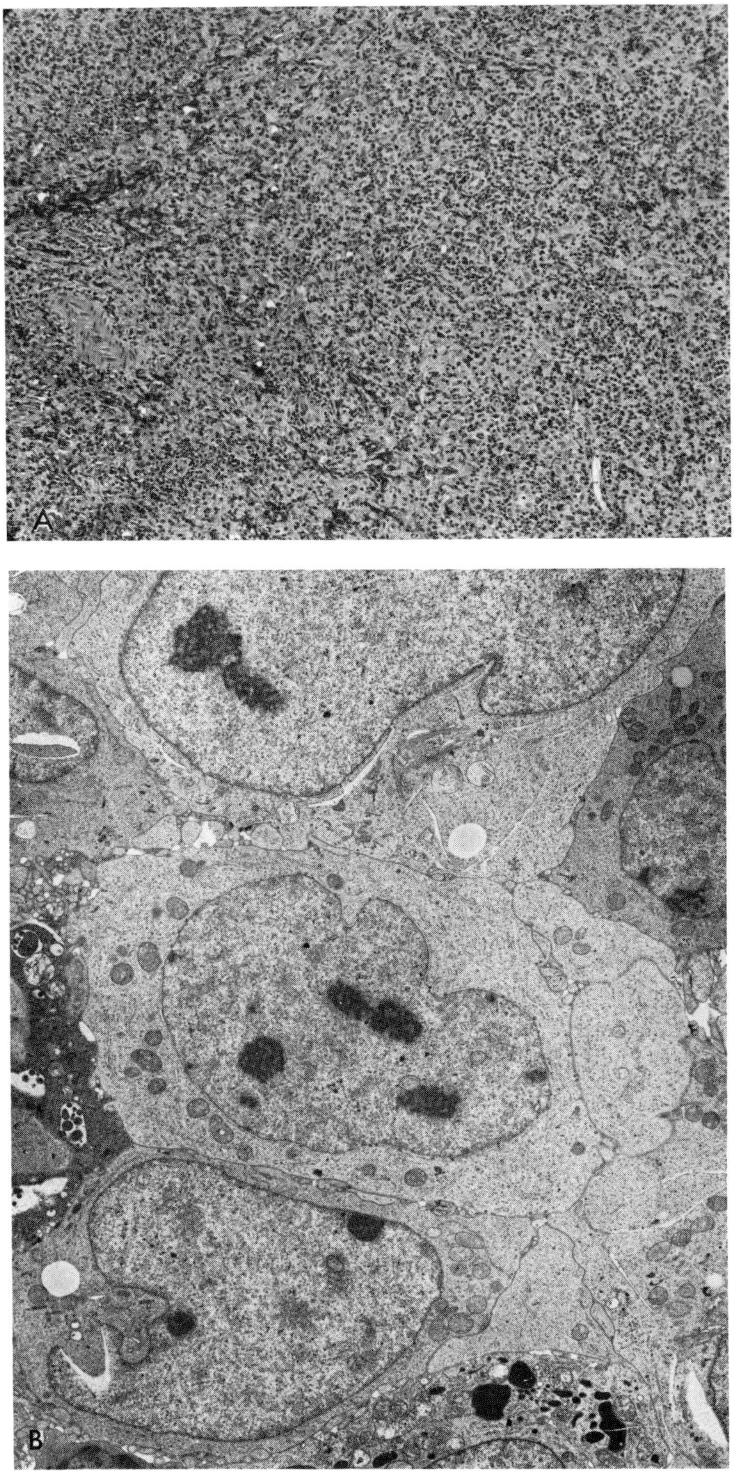

Figure 2–8. *A,* Photomicrograph of lymphoma of the tonsil that was initially diagnosed as anaplastic carcinoma. (H & E × 110) *B,* Electron micrograph showing three adjacent lymphocytic cells. There is a very primitive, diffusely distributed chromatin pattern with prominent nucleoli. The cytoplasm contains only scattered endoplasmic reticulum. (× 8250) (Courtesy of Dr. R. D. Cardiff, Department of Pathology, University of California, Davis.)

Illustration continued on opposite page

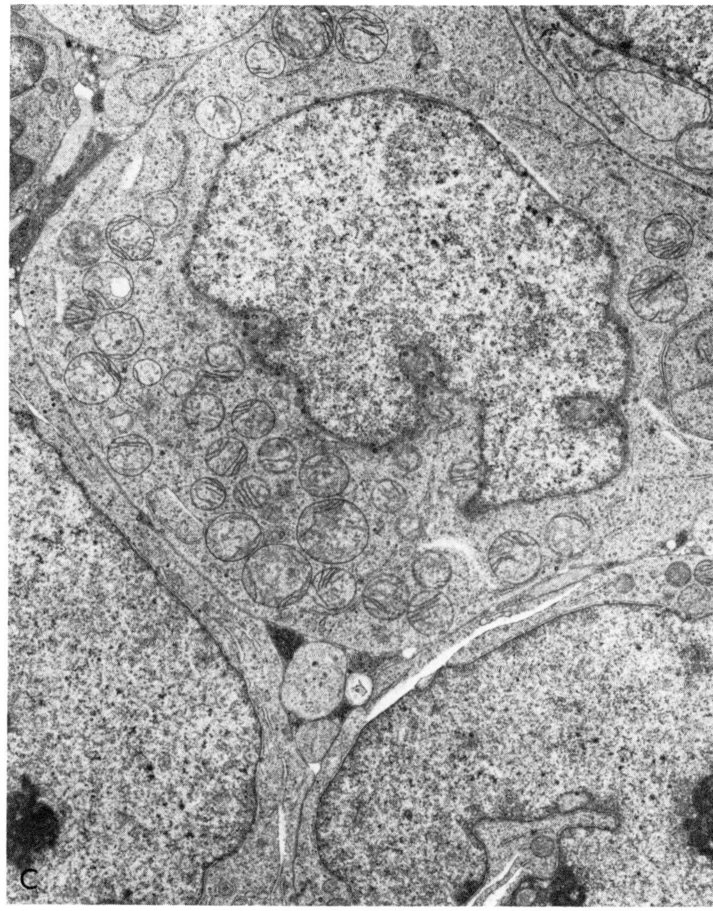

Figure 2–8. *Continued C,* Higher power magnification electron micrograph showing a single cell possessing very primitive cytoplasm and nucleus. Some nuclear pores are seen adjacent to the nucleus. There are no modifications of the cytoplasmic membranes such as desmosomes that would characterize squamous cells. (× 13,800) (Courtesy of Dr. R. D. Cardiff, Department of Pathology, University of California, Davis.)

are frequently anaplastic, extend rapidly among the muscle bundles of the structure, and often remain occult until a substantial size is reached. Cervical metastases are common. In an article by Ogura et al,[21] discussing the utility of elective neck dissection, it was reported that of 42 patients with cancer of the base of the tongue, 25 (59 per cent) had lymph node metastases. Bilateral disease was present in 8 of 42 patients, or 19.1 per cent. Out of a group of 102 patients with base-of-tongue carcinoma described by Whicker et al,[22] 78, or 21.6 per cent, had bilateral disease. Strong[23] reported a 76.5 per cent incidence of unilateral cervical involvement and a 22.8 per cent incidence of bilateral disease in his series of 136 patients.

TREATMENT

The management of oropharyngeal lesions, including those of the soft palate and tongue base, has been a source of controversy for many years. Up to 20 years ago, the primary mode of therapy was irradiation. Following this, surgery had its heyday, with some improvement seen in survival statistics.[22, 24] More recently, combined therapy has been used with greater frequency, showing further improvement in survivorship in most series. The pros and cons of timing of irradiation in relation to surgery are widely debated. The advocates of preoperative irradiation argue that there will be dissemination of malignant cells if a tumor nest at the surgical margin is cut through. In addition, the operative site will suffer from relative hypoxemia because of blood vessel interruption. They conclude that this will render irradiation relatively ineffective during the postoperative period. The proponents of postoperative therapy contend that preoperative irradiation reduces the tumor size so that the resection margins at the time of tumor extirpation are difficult to delineate. This point is especially well taken concerning tumors of the pyriform sinus and may, in fact, be the main reason of the superiority of results when postoperative radiotherapy is used in these cases.[25, 26]

Over the past 8 years we have switched from preoperative to postoperative irradiation as the primary form of combined therapy. This was based on our impression of at least equivalent survival results and the findings of marked diminution in the incidence of complications when the postoperative modality is used.[27]

Tonsillar Carcinoma. Survival rates in carcinoma of the tonsil are, as expected, relative to the size of the tumor and the extent of metastatic disease. One of the larger series of tonsillar tumors treated by radiotherapy has been published by Wang.[8] He followed 124 patients with lesions of the anterior pillar and retromolar trigone, one third of whom had metastases to cervical lymph nodes. His 3-year disease-free survival rate was 36 per cent. In those patients who had T_3 lesions, the survival rate dropped to 20 per cent. Furthermore, in any tumor that encroached on the tongue, the survival was only 28 per cent. There were no survivors among the patients who had bilateral lymph node metastases or in those whose nodes were fixed. Of the 79 failures, 30 were eligible for surgical salvage, and 21 (70 per cent) of these survived disease-free for 3 years. It is important to note that since only 38 per cent of the patients were eligible for surgical salvage, the *overall* surgical salvage rate was only 27 per cent. There is little doubt that the T_1 lesion of the tonsil itself responds well to radiotherapy. In an analysis of 201 tonsillar fossa lesions by the same author, 85 per cent of patients with T_1 lesions had a disease-free 3-year survival. A series of 125 tonsillar lesions at the University of Iowa reviewed by Krause[25] demonstrated a 5-year determinant survival rate of 75 per cent for T_1N_0 lesions when radiotherapy was the modality employed. However, the survival rate fell to 25 per cent when the lesion became T_1N_1. In the Iowa group, 94 patients with all varieties of T and N lesions had primary radiotherapy; 49 per cent were alive without disease at 3 years, and 39 per cent at 5 years.

There is general agreement that some form of combination therapy is best for management of lesions that extend beyond the confines of the tonsillar fossa, involve the base of the tongue, or present with cervical adenopathy. Wang[8] recommends this modality in all large oropharyngeal lesions, although he presents no results. In the Iowa series[28] there was a 67 per cent 2-year survival rate among 36 patients. The data of Snow and coworkers,[29] who compared the efficacy of preoperative and postoperative irradiation, are inconclusive and show survival rates for both at 18 months to be around 65 per cent. Our own experience using postoperative combined therapy shows about the same results.

Although Wang speaks optimistically about the surgical salvage of patients who fail to be cured with irradiation, others report grim statistics in their attempts at salvage surgery. In one study, of 21 patients who had failed to be cured by irradiation, 12 had tumors in the tonsillar fossa, 4 had disease of the anterior pillar, and 5 had tumors primarily in the base of the tongue. Following an attempt at salvage surgery, 48 per cent died of their disease and 43 per cent died of complications. More than 50 per cent of the original group died of locally recurrent disease. A similarly dismal experience is cited by Schleuning and Summers[30] in the management of tongue base carcinoma. Radiotherapy was employed in 79 such tumors, with only 10 cures. Surgical salvage was successful in only 13 (18.8 per cent) of the 69 patients with locally recurrent disease.

Carcinoma of the Base of the Tongue. Patients with tumors of the tongue base have a notoriously poor survival rate. Occult spread beyond the palpable limits of the tumor, frequent neck metastasis occurring often bilaterally, and a relatively high incidence of distant metastases combine to yield a poor prognosis. A large series of oral cavity lesions reported by Trible included 58 patients with tongue base cancer.[31] A number of different treatment modalities were used, and the overall 5-year survival was 27.6 per cent. Of the 16 survivors, 7 were treated with radiotherapy, 7 by surgery alone, and 2 with planned combined therapy. Unfortunately, no specific data were given representing how many total patients were treated by each specific modality.

Truluck and Putney[17] analyzed 36 patients with tongue base carcinoma. Combined therapy using preoperative irradiation was employed in 18 patients, with 6 (33 per cent) surviving 5 years. Strong[23] presented the results of treating 136 patients with carcinoma of the tongue base. The overall cure rate was 30 per cent, with Stage II disease having a 63.6 per cent and Stage IV a 21.7 per cent cure rate. Cure was not analyzed according to therapeutic regimen, but the recommendation for therapy is either combined irradiation and surgery, or triple therapy using *cis*-platinum and bleomycin in combination with the other two modalities.

Carcinoma of the Soft Palate. Carcinomas that involve primarily the soft palate produce cervical metastases in an average of one third of cases; with statistics varying from a high of 48.1 per cent reported by Ash[32] to a low of 27 per cent in the series of Russ et al,[34] with other studies yielding rates of 29.2 and 33 per cent.[33, 35] Small lesions less than 2 cm in size may be managed equally well by local resection or radiotherapy. Larger lesions are probably best managed by combined therapy.[33] In the series of 80 patients studied by Konrad et al,[35] it was curious to note that the survival results of irradiation, surgery, and combined therapy were almost the same (36, 50, and 44 per cent respectively). The 38 patients followed by Russ and coworkers[34] were treated primarily by radiation, with 33 per cent having a 5-year survival rate. It is astonishing that this should be their recommended modality of treatment when most of their patients succumbed to local recurrences.

Carcinoma of the Pharyngeal Wall. Little statistically significant information is available on the survival rate relative to management techniques in lateral and posterior pharyngeal wall malignancy. Rider in 1962 reported a 9 per cent success rate in controlling lesions of the oropharyngeal walls and 0 per cent when the disease was bilateral.[36] Fletcher et al[37] had a series of 145 patients treated by surgery, radiation, and combinations of the two. The overall 5-year actual survival rate was 41.3 per cent. In the Iowa series of 108 patients,[28] the 5-year determinant survival rate for those treated with irradiation therapy was 35 per cent, with surgery alone, 40 per cent, and with combined therapy using 4500 rads of preoperative irradiation, 67 per cent. The often-encountered pessimistic attitude regarding the prognosis for these patients is probably based on the early experience of individuals such as Rider. A great deal of concern regarding metastasis to retropharyngeal lymph nodes is unjustified. In our experience of well over 200 squamous cell cancers involving the lateral and posterior walls of the oropharynx, a metastasis in a retropharyngeal lymph node has never been encountered. The dissections of DeClercq and Chole,[38] who were investigating the pathophysiology of retropharyngeal abscesses, revealed no definitive lymph node material in this space in adults. This fact, and the resistance of the fascial envelopes of the pharyngeal musculature to tumor penetration, renders these lesions eminently resectable.

SURGICAL PRECEDURES

Total Glossectomy

Total glossectomy is a formidable procedure, but for a number of patients severely stricken with extensive malignancies of the tongue, it is the only hope for survival. The denial of this chance to a patient desperate for life, by a surgeon who fears the mutilation of such a procedure and then attempts to assuage his conscience by directing the unfortunate patient to other therapeutic modalities that give vain hope for survival, is to be condemned. The curious dichotomy in the minds of some surgeons who do not hesitate to perform a radical maxillectomy with orbital exenteration and extensive facial skin incision, but balk at total glossectomy, defies reason.

Recent advances in reconstructive surgery, prosthetics, and speech therapy have greatly improved the rehabilitative potential for these patients. The patient in Figure 2–9 had a total glossectomy for a massive lingual malignancy. The larynx was preserved and protection to the airway was afforded by the replacement of the excised tissue with a deltopectoral flap. Although oral alimentation is impossible without aspiration, the patient does not aspirate her saliva. She takes her meals by the periodic insertion of a nasogastric tube. Her speech is sufficiently articulate, especially with the use of an artifical tongue (see Chapter 14), to permit her to retain her employment as an office supervisor, which includes regular communication over the telephone.

Because of the frequency of cervical metastasis on presentation, the operation is done in continuity with a radical neck dissection. If bilateral nodal disease is present, a simultaneous bilateral neck dissection should be done. A staged neck dissection may be considered, but two factors militate against it. First, cutting the primary specimen from a region of known metastatic disease violates the principle of en bloc dissection and runs the risk of tumor spillage. Secondly, the delay

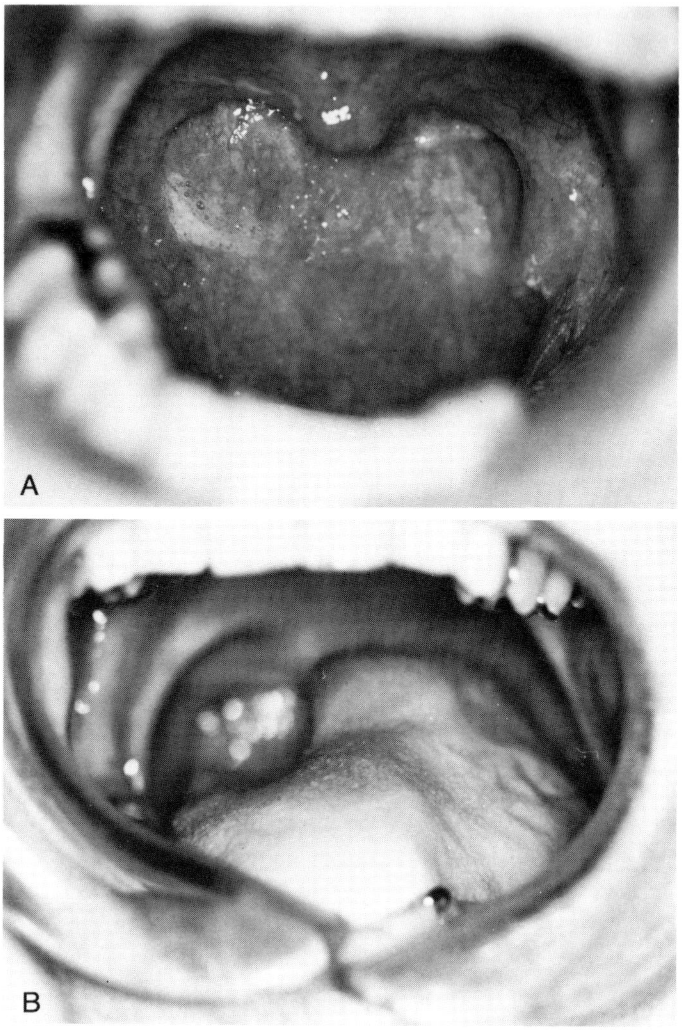

Figure 2–9. *A,* Patient with total glossectomy. *B,* Prosthetic tongue in place.

required between the first and second operations, in addition to the necessary time for healing of the staged neck, may take the patient beyond the "golden period" for postoperative irradiation. The morbidity of simultaneous bilateral neck dissection is considerable, and a good deal of judgment is essential in this situation.

A modified H incision or an apron flap is used in the skin. We prefer the former. On completion of the neck dissection the primary lesion is approached, with care taken to try to preserve the lymphatic drainage route to the neck. Unless at least a 2 cm margin of healthy tissue can be achieved by an incision in the vallecula, the larynx should be taken. However, a supraglottic laryngectomy has no place in a total glossectomy, as continuous aspiration is inevitable.

When the larynx can be spared, the lingual excision begins through an entrance in the vallecula or upper pyriform sinus with the least tumor involvement (Fig. 2–10). Care must be taken on entering the pharynx to avoid the superior laryngeal nerve and its sensory branch, the internal laryngeal nerve, which after piercing the thyrohyoid membrane courses submucosally through the anterior apex of the pyriform sinus. Its sensory innervation to the upper laryngeal mucosa is essential to airway protection. If a laryngectomy is indicated because of direct invasion of this structure or the spread of tumor to the pre-epiglottic space, a pharyngotomy through the pyriform sinus on the side of least involvement is done. The larynx is excised, separating it as high as possible from the remainder of the hypopharynx and pre-

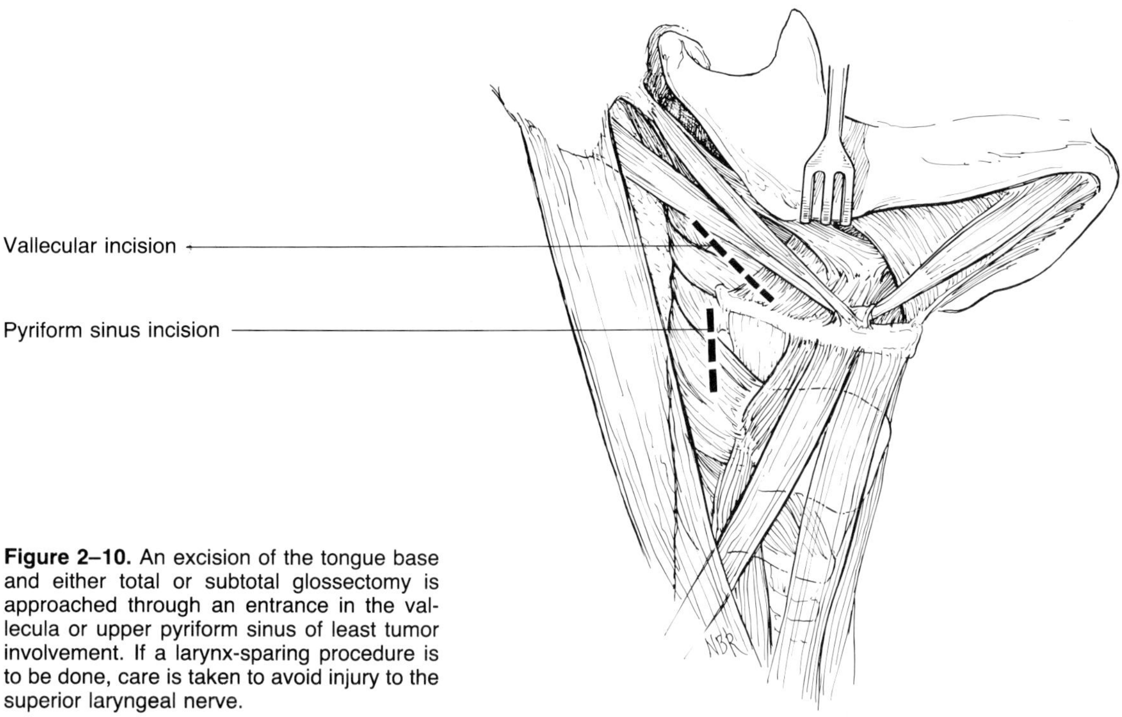

Figure 2–10. An excision of the tongue base and either total or subtotal glossectomy is approached through an entrance in the vallecula or upper pyriform sinus of least tumor involvement. If a larynx-sparing procedure is to be done, care is taken to avoid injury to the superior laryngeal nerve.

serving a maximal amount of pharyngeal mucosa. As the resection proceeds into the contralateral side of the pharynx, the entire tongue base is displayed and resection can proceed superiorly (Fig. 2–11). In the laryngeal preservation procedure, the tongue musculature is cut from its origins on the hyoid bone and resection proceeds along the lateral pharyngeal gutters (Fig. 2–12). In both resections, the line of incision continues from the pharyngeal gutters to the base of the tonsillar fossae. If either tonsillar area is involved with tumor, a partial mandibulectomy is performed on that side. Similarly, when tumor extends beyond the oral tongue and involves adjacent mandible, the bone must be sacrificed. If the malignancy spares the mucosa of the floor of the mouth, resection proceeds along the reflection of the mucosa onto the lingual aspect of the mandible (Fig. 2–13). Whenever possible, a small cuff of oral floor mucosa is preserved to aid in closure. As the

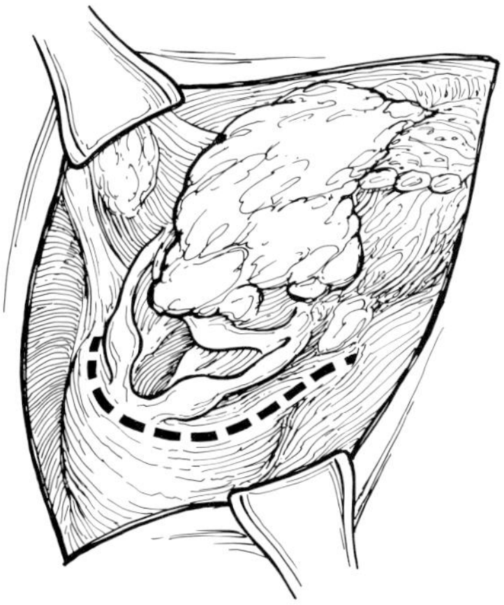

Figure 2–11. When the resection cannot spare the larynx, the hypopharyngeal mucosa is maximally preserved. The trachea is excised at the first ring and the procedure proceeds superiorly.

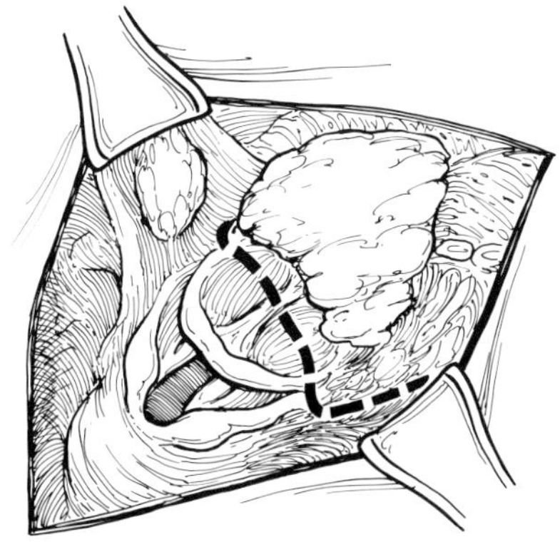

Figure 2–12. In the larynx-sparing procedure, an incision is made in the depths of the vallecula and along the superior border of the hyoid bone. The lesion is cleared by a 2- to 3-cm margin of healthy tissue.

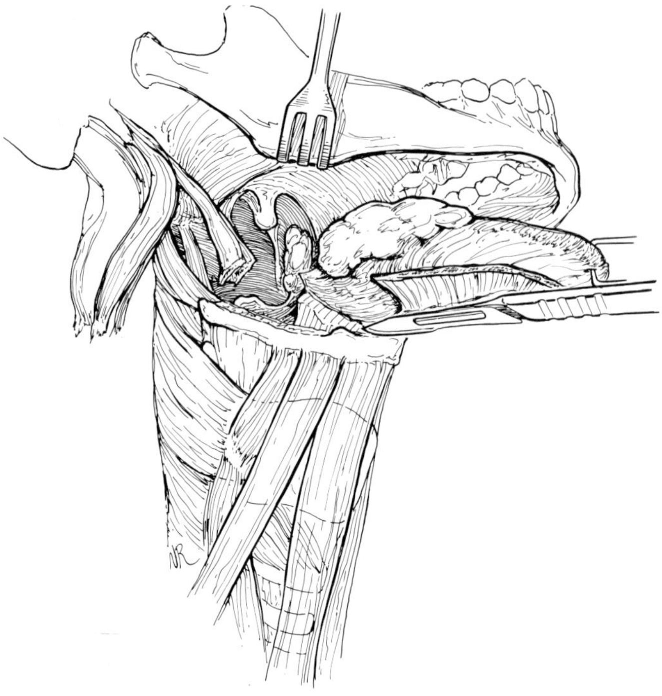

Figure 2–13. Outline of oral and tonsillar portion of resection of subtotal glossectomy when the tumor spares some anterior tongue.

oral incisions are made, great care must be taken to incise through the entire thickness of the mylohyoid, taking the underlying anterior bellies of the digastrics so that the superficial margin of excision here is the platysma (Fig. 2–14).

Once the tumor is cut, closure is often impossible without the use of a flap. The forehead flap, once the workhorse of oral cavity and oropharyngeal reconstruction, has almost entirely been supplanted by the myocutaneous flaps. A common objection to the use of myocutaneous flaps in the oral cavity—that of redundant tissue—is a tremendous asset in reconstruction following total glossectomy. One of the major problems in completing the oral phase of swallowing and in articulation during speech is the approximation of the tongue to the palate. If a bulky flap is used to replace lost lingual tissue, approximation of the jaws will permit this important palate-to-flap contact. The pectoralis major flap is most useful here, and inclusion of fat and muscle wide of the skin paddle will add to the flap's bulk. The deltopectoral flap is also suitable (Fig. 2–15). This latter, however, carries the major disadvantage of requiring a second procedure to return the pedicle. Pharyngeal approximation is done in the usual way, with the carotid arteries protected by dermis grafts and the neck wounds closed and drained. Oral closure is done with interrupted absorbable sutures supported by a second running suture of the same material.

Irradiation with a full dose of 5500 and 6000 rads to the primary area, and 4500 rads to both necks is given 4 to 6 weeks following surgery. Care is taken to keep the fields high enough on the side of the face, preferably to the zygomatic arches, in order to include the highest lateral pharyngeal lymph nodes. Bitter experience has taught us that these massive tumors with their proclivity for aggressive cervical metastasis do so even in a retrograde manner. We have seen a number of cases in which the uppermost part of the neck, containing the parotid gland, was spared from the radiation field for the sake of the patients' comfort, only to have them succumb to recurrent tumor in that high nodal region.

Rehabilitation of deglutition following surgery involves careful instruction by the surgeon and the clinical nurse specialist. It is hard to improve upon the excellent review by Meyers[39] describing the physiology of normal swallowing and the alterations incurred and adjustments required in the glossectomized patient. In the immediate postoperative period, all patients have a nasogastric tube and a tracheostomy in place. Once the wounds are healed, attempts at oral alimentation commence. The performance of a generous cricopharyngeal myotomy at the time

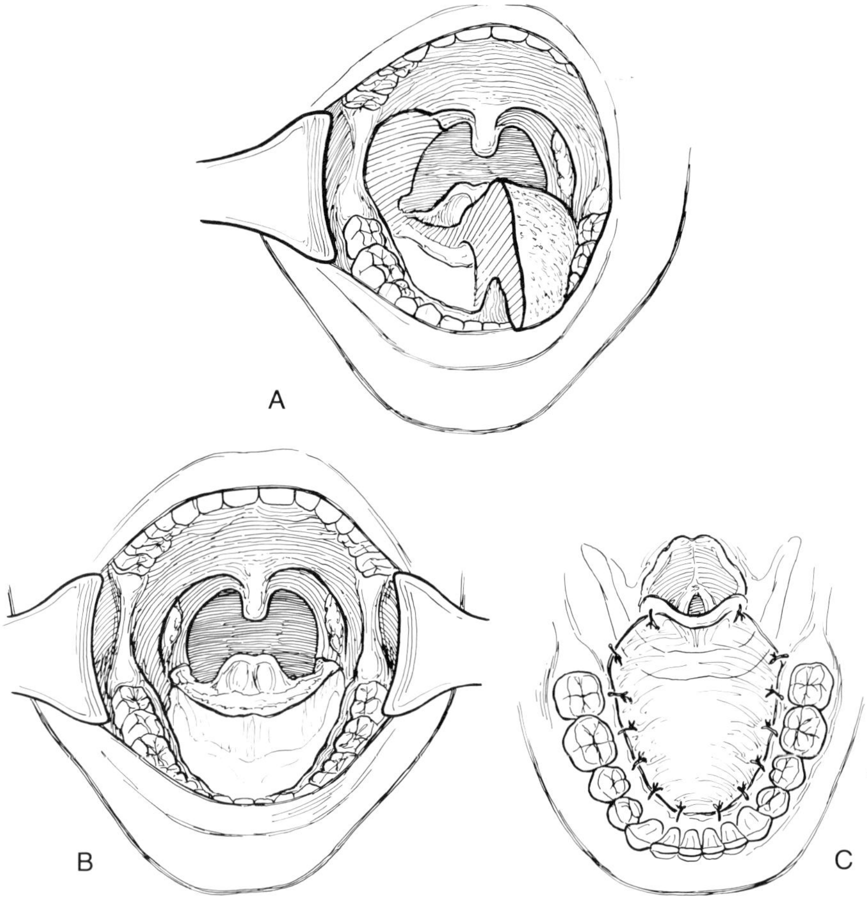

Figure 2–14. *A,* Resection completed. The deep margin is the platysma of the skin flap. All muscles deep to the tumor are resected. *B,* Total glossectomy completed in tumors with extensive posterior and anterior lingual involvement. *C,* Reconstruction with pectoralis major musculocutaneous flap or deltopectoral flap.

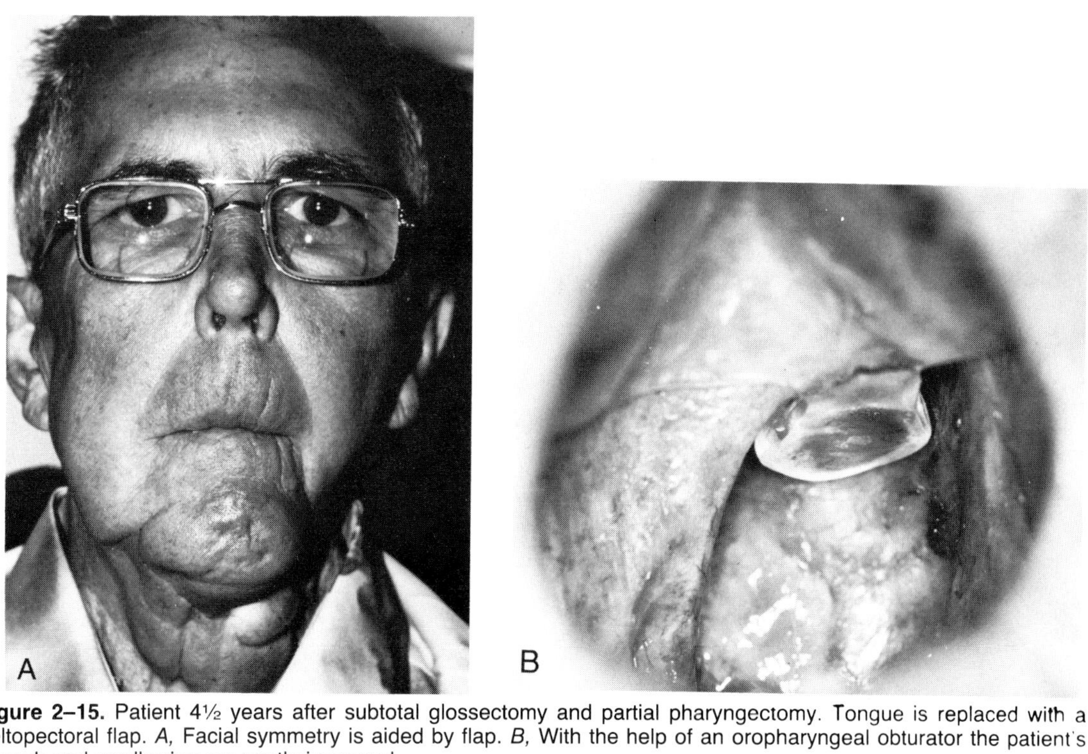

Figure 2–15. Patient 4½ years after subtotal glossectomy and partial pharyngectomy. Tongue is replaced with a deltopectoral flap. *A,* Facial symmetry is aided by flap. *B,* With the help of an oropharyngeal obturator the patient's speech and swallowing are vastly improved.

of surgery often prevents many of the difficulties encountered with pharyngeal pooling. As Meyers so aptly points out, the principal problem in the glossectomized patient is the absence of the "oral hold" phase of swallowing. Ingested material is immediately delivered to the oropharynx and proceeds directly to the hypopharynx. The material tends to pool in the pyriform recesses and spill into the larynx. A myotomy will prevent this "pharyngeal hold" phase of the swallowing sequence. Because effective delivery of ingested material to the pharynx has been precluded by the excision, gravity is the principal force that initiates the movement of the material to the digestive tract. The patient is instructed to "toss the material back" by extending the head back on the neck, which allows the upper digestive conduit to become a straight pipe with the funnel at the top. The patient uses small 10 to 15 cc boluses at first and works from liquids up to semisolids.

The cricopharyngeal myotomy is relatively easy to perform (Fig. 2–16). A dull tracheostomy hook is placed around the posterolateral border of the thyroid cartilage and the pharyngeal musculature exposed by retracting the larynx anteromedially. A strip of muscle 3 to 4 mm wide is removed from the posterolateral aspect of the cricopharyngeus and the inferior constrictor. Cutting against the index finger placed through the pharyngotomy will allow the surgeon to incise down to the submucosa without violating the mucosa. Care is taken to excise the muscular strip far enough posteriorly to avoid damage to the recurrent laryngeal nerve on that side.

The laryngectomized patient, of course, need not be concerned about aspiration during swallowing, but is similarly hampered by the loss of whatever lip anesthesia eventuates from the mandibulectomy.

The early introduction of vigorous speech therapy is essential (see Chapter 17). It is surprising how good the speech of a totally glossectomized patient can be. If the larynx is taken, however, speech is unattainable.

Resection of Tumors of the Lateral and Posterior Pharyngeal Walls

Tumors originating in the region of the lateral and posterior pharyngeal walls have a remarkable inability to penetrate the fascial envelope that encircles the constituent musculature. This factor permits successful resection of tumors in which a 2-cm deep margin cannot be obtained. On the other hand, because of the tendency of these tumors to spread submucosally, a mucosal margin of 2½ to 3 cm is advised when encircling the

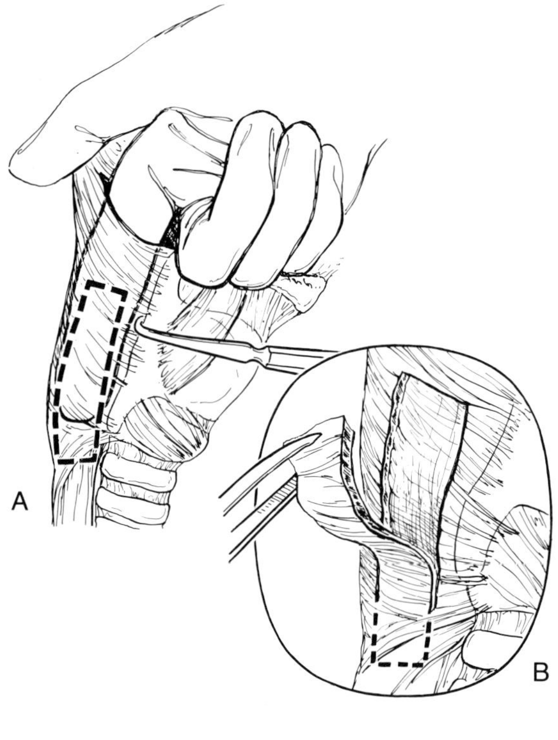

Figure 2–16. Cricopharyngeal myotomy. *A,* Finger in place facilitating muscle exposure and palpating depth of cut. *B,* A generous strip of cricopharyngeus and inferior constrictor muscle is excised.

neoplasm. Small lesions less than 2 cm in diameter are curable by radiotherapy or local excision. Closure in these T_1 tumors is obtained by either primary approximation or skin grafting. The defect may even be allowed to granulate in, with epithelialization usually being complete in 3 weeks. This open method, which is also used in the pharyngeal flap operation for vellopharyngeal incompetence, is usually less painful than primary approximation.

The excision can be done with the patient's head in the Rose position, the tongue being retracted with a Dingman or other variety of self-retaining mouth gag (Fig. 2–17). Alternatively, exposure can be achieved through a median labial-mandibuloglossotomy (Fig. 2–18). The latter approach is discussed in Chapter 3.

There is usually extension of the larger tumors to the lateral pharyngeal wall and the tonsillar fossa. Once the fossa is reached, a hemimandibulectomy is usually necessary. Spread to the soft palate in these cases is common, as is involvement of the nasopharyngeal wall mucosa. Involvement of the eustachian tube torus used to be an absolute contraindication to surgery. At our present stage of knowledge and technical development, however, it is now possible to excise the pharyngeal end of the eustachian tube, drilling away the bone at the apex of the petrous temporal bone and a portion of the clivus in order to get a satisfactory margin. It is important to note that the internal carotid artery is at risk because of its exit at the petrous apex and its subsequent course through the superior half of the foramen lacerum. Therefore, as the surgeon approaches this artery, careful control from below and above is essential.

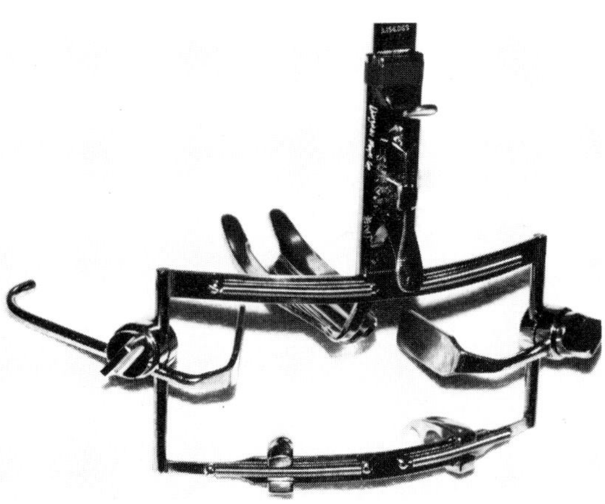

Figure 2–17. Dingman mouth gag.

In most instances, however, control of the tumor margins can be achieved at a level below the eustachian tube. The first step in the procedure must be an exploration of the retropharyngeal space in order to verify lack of tumor fixation to the anterior longitudinal ligament. The neck dissection is carried out and the primary approached through a lateral pharyngotomy incision. This provides excellent access to the tumor, and the resection proceeds, with maintenance of a wide margin of healthy tissue around the neoplasm. Excision is relatively bloodless provided that careful control of the ascending pharyngeal arteries is maintained. Because of the proximity of the carotids, vigilance is necessary throughout the excision as each successive cut is made.

The forehead flap is ideal for reconstruction of this defect (see Chapter 1, Fig. 1–12). (The bulkiness of myocutaneous flaps makes them unsuitable for this site.) The forehead flap with its excellent blood supply is relatively thin, but it is wide enough to resurface the entire pharynx and long enough to reach into the hypopharynx. Maximal length can be achieved by passing it through the infratemporal fossa, deep to the zygomatic arch. Excision of the temporalis muscle above its insertion into the coronoid process allows the residual muscle to retract partially out of the infratemporal fossa to make room for the passage of the flap. Further space may be achieved by creating two osteotomy cuts on the zygomatic arch and outfracturing the arch. The flap is passed into the upper end of the pharynx and is sutured in place with interrupted absorbable sutures. No sutures are placed along the upper aspect of the flap.

The pedicle is returned to the forehead 3 weeks postoperatively, but a word of warning is appropriate at this point. This task is unfortunately often relegated to a junior houseofficer. This is a grievous error, as the incision of the flap from its pedicle often must be done high in the oropharynx or even in the nasopharynx. Considerable blood loss may ensue, requiring considerable expertise to control. In withdrawing the flap from the infratemporal fossa, care must be taken to remove all the epithelium from its buried portion. Residual epithelial strips along the path of the flap have been responsible for recurrent abscesses in three patients in our own experience who eventually required reopening of the lateral aspect of the forehead

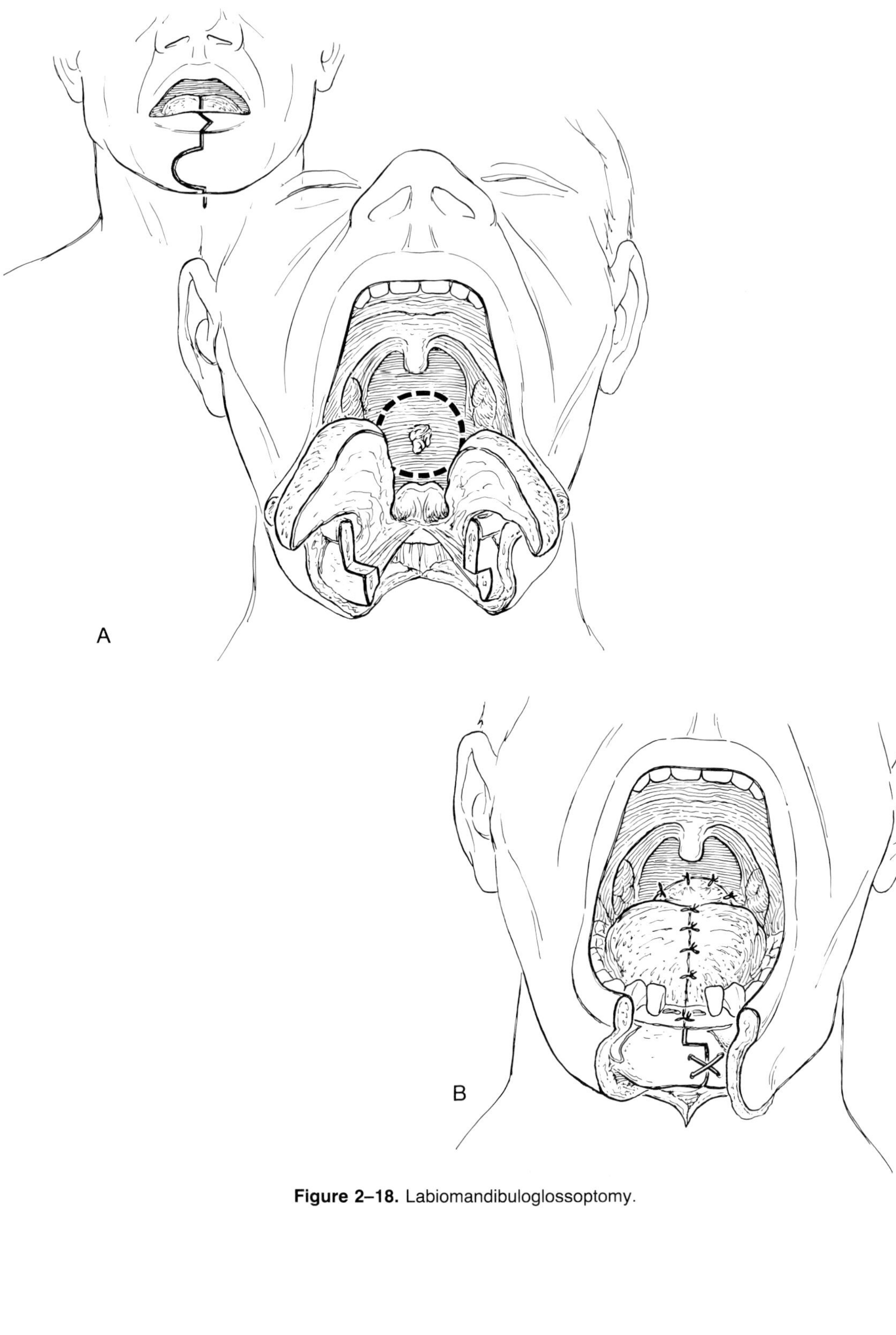
A

B

Figure 2–18. Labiomandibuloglossoptomy.

wound and exploration of the tract through which the flap was placed.

Small to moderate defects of the posterior and lateral pharyngeal walls can be closed primarily with generous undermining. Because of the significant cosmetic defect left by the forehead flap, it has been largely discontinued despite its marvelous suitability in replacing oropharyngeal defects. The trapezius musculocutaneous flap, especially that which is superiorly based, has supplanted the forehead flap in most cases. A one-stage reconstruction can be done that will leave a minimal cosmetic defect (Fig. 2–19). In addition, if the tumor extends into the oral cavity and the mandibulectomy extends beyond the angle of the jaw, the muscle bulk now helps to restore the esthetics of the area.

With loss of the posterior and lateral walls of the oropharynx, there is no stripping action of this part of the tube to propel a bolus of food into the hypopharynx. In these patients this early stage of swallowing is a passive phenomenon, but passage of ingesta can be

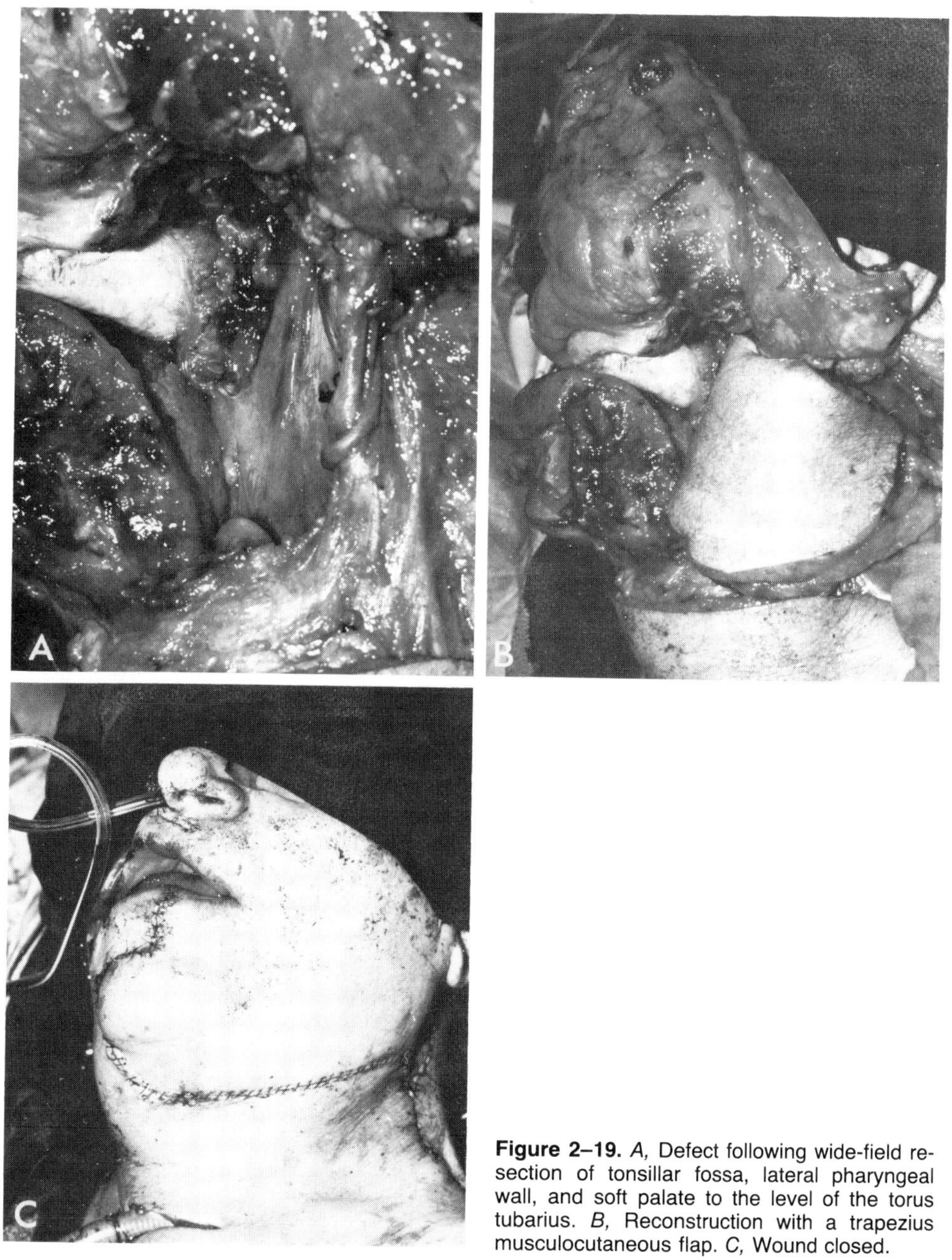

Figure 2–19. *A,* Defect following wide-field resection of tonsillar fossa, lateral pharyngeal wall, and soft palate to the level of the torus tubarius. *B,* Reconstruction with a trapezius musculocutaneous flap. *C,* Wound closed.

aided by a cricopharyngeal myotomy. When the soft palate is also excised, the problem of initiating deglutition is further compounded by the lack of closure of the vellopharyngeal port, and nasal regurgitation becomes an annoying problem. Much of this can be avoided by the use of a nasopharyngeal obturator, which is most effective when used intraoperatively. A more complete discussion of this is found in Chapter 3.

Surgery for Extensive Malignancies

Each extensive neoplasm in the oropharynx presents with its own unique set of problems. The basic principle of the composite resection for large pharyngeal neoplasms is similar to that for distal oral cavity resections. With few exceptions, a radical neck dissection is done in continuity. The mandible is resected from the coronoid notch to just beyond the angle, depending on the oral extent of the tumor. All mucosal disease is skirted by a 2-cm margin of healthy tissue, but as the hypopharynx is approached, this margin is widened to 2½ to 3 cm. All or part of the soft palate often needs to be resected, and it must be kept in mind that areas of Queyrat's erythroplasia should be included in the specimen. When the maxillary tuberosity or the hard palate is involved, a partial maxillectomy must be done.

The deep aspect of resection in tonsillar fossa and lateral pharyngeal wall neoplasms includes the medial pterygoid muscle. A generous margin of muscle should be resected, even though bleeding from this area—usually from the pterygoid venous plexus—is often profuse. Once the specimen has been removed, hemostasis is initially attempted with pressure. This must be augmented with stick ties and even pledgets of hemostatic gauze or cotton. Reconstruction is done either with simple approximation of pharyngeal wall mucosa to buccal mucosa or the interposition of a flap.

Various problems arise that are peculiar to each case. The following case histories will serve to illustrate the basic principles as well as offer some possible solutions to a number of troublesome problems.

CASE I. A 37-year-old woman was first seen with a $T_2N_0M_0$ lesion of the right tonsillar fossa and anterior pillar. She elected not to have conventional therapy and after a year of attempting quack cures re-presented herself for definitive therapy. The lesion was as depicted in Figure 2–20. A photo could not be obtained because of the severity of her trismus. She had a 1.5-cm hard mass in the right posterior triangle of the neck.

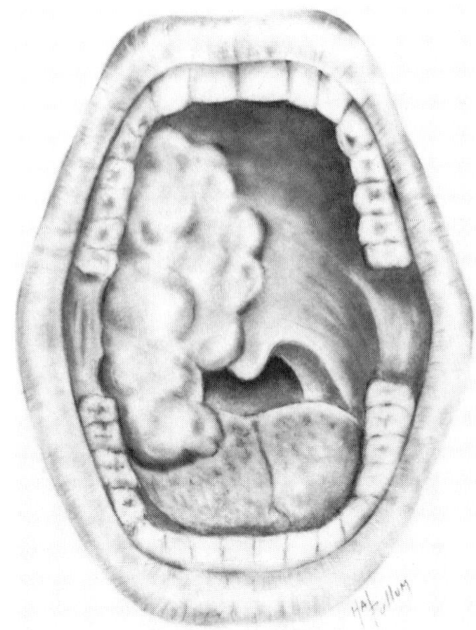

Figure 2–20. (Case I) Large oropharyngeal carcinoma originating in the tonsillar fossa.

A composite resection of the right side was done that included lateral tongue, lateral pharyngeal wall, tonsillar fossa, soft palate, hemimandible, maxilla, some buccal mucosa, and a right radical neck dissection (Fig. 2–21). The mandibulectomy and massive oropharyngeal resection gave excellent access to the skull base. The osteotome could then be placed against the basisphenoid and the pterygoid plates excised at their origin (Fig. 2–22). The excision of the posterior and posteroinferior maxilla along with the distal upper alveolus encompassed the palatal extent of the tumor and that invading the posteroinferior maxillary sinus, and completed the excision of the pterygoid muscles in their entirety (Fig. 2–23). No flaps were turned, and reconstruction was by primary approximation of the wound edges. A course of postoperative irradiation completed the therapy.

Discussion. At the time the patient presented with trismus, the generally accepted dictum was that this symptom indicated a hopeless prognosis. Pterygoid plate erosion and involvement of the pterygoid muscles with tumor had been considered an unresectable situation. Because of the patient's youth and her willingness to try anything for a potential cure, the pterygoid resection was advised.

Speech has been remarkably enhanced by a nasopharyngeal obturator. Swallowing was greatly improved by a cricopharyngeal myotomy done

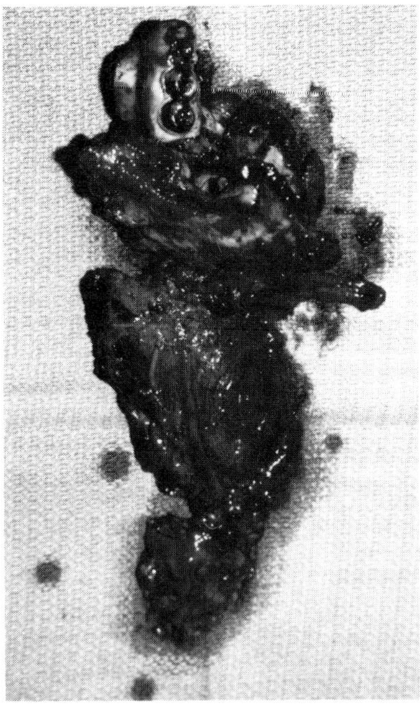

Figure 2–21. (Case I) Composite resection includes posterior maxillectomy, hemimandibulectomy, buccal mucosa, pharynx, tongue, pterygoid muscles, and an incontinuity radical neck dissection.

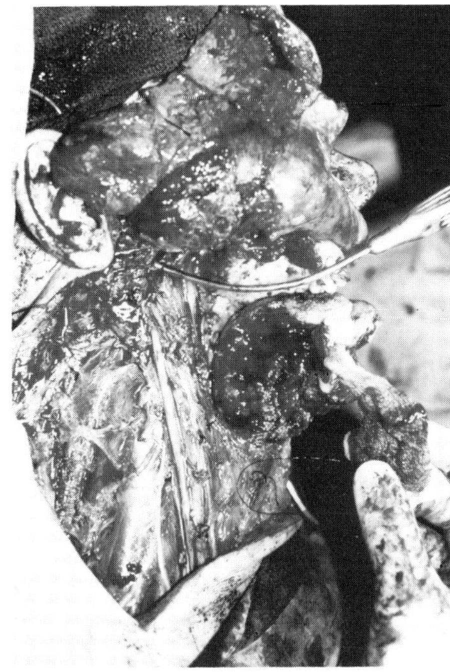

Figure 2–23. (Case I) Resection completed. Suction tip is at the skull base.

some months later. The patient is alive and well 5 years following treatment (Fig. 2–24).

CASE II. A 69-year-old man presented with a persistent sore throat and mild dysphagia. He had had a full course of radiotherapy for a pyriform sinus carcinoma 3 years previously that was augmented 2 years later by the implantation of radon seeds. His oropharynx and hypopharynx had been exposed to 10,000 rads. Because of persistent neck disease he had a radical neck dissection, all done at another institution. On presentation, he had a massive carcinoma of the base of the tongue that involved the vallecula and extended into the oral cavity (Fig. 2–25).

A total laryngectomy, partial pharyngectomy, radical neck dissection, and subtotal glossectomy were done. All of the tongue was excised except for about one quarter of the oral portion. The folly of primary approximation of the cutaneous wound edges was apparent when, 2 weeks post-

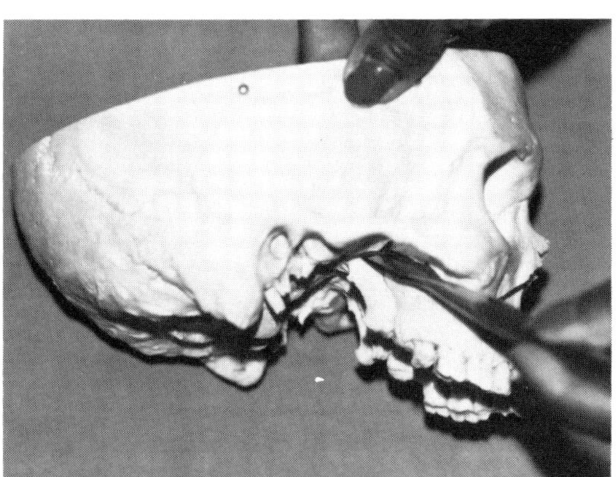

Figure 2–22. (Case I) Osteotome placed against the base of the pterygoid plates to ensure complete excision of the pterygoid muscles.

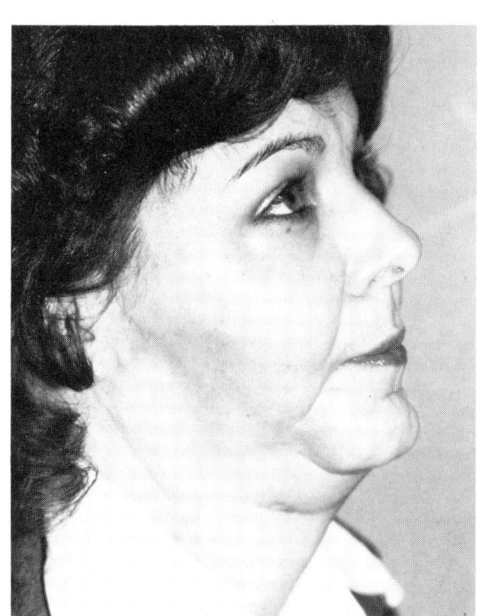

Figure 2–24. (Case I) Patient is alive and well 5 years after resection, with acceptable cosmetic appearance.

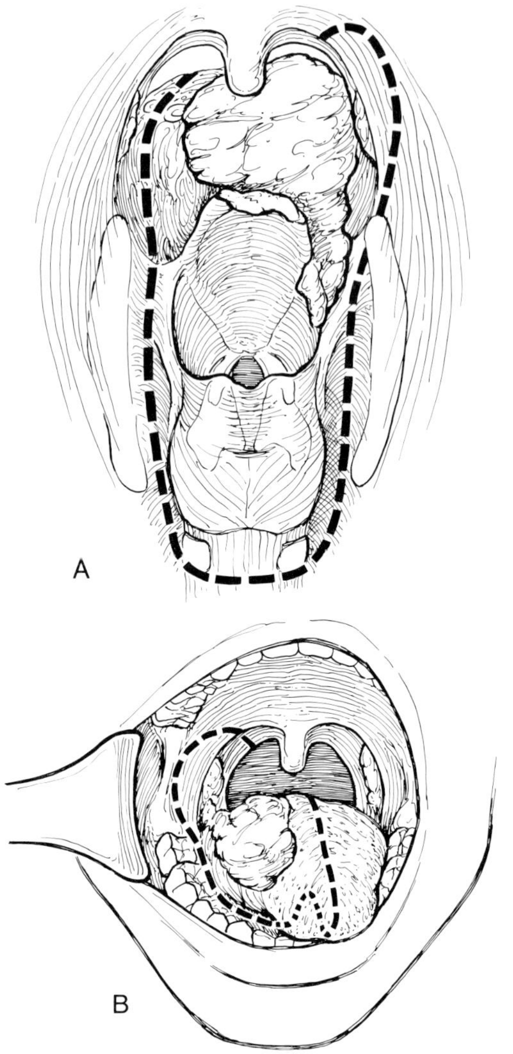

Figure 2–25. (Case II) Outline of resection for large base-of-tongue lesion with extension into pyriform sinus. *A,* Pharyngeal view. *B,* Oral view.

operatively, a gargantuan fistula opened. It extended from just under the mentum of the mandible to the manubrium, exposing both common carotid arteries from the root of the neck to their bifurcation (Fig. 2–26). Fortunately, the dermis grafts placed over both of these arteries at the time of surgery rapidly epithelialized, saving the patient from a carotid blow-out. Once the wound had matured (Fig. 2–27), the floor of the mouth and the anterior and lateral pharyngeal walls were reconstructed with a lined deltopectoral flap. During the delay stage of the flap, the undersurface of its dorsal end and the deltoid muscle of the donor site were lined with a split-thickness skin graft. At the time of the definitive procedure, the skin graft had not only taken, but had become tough enough to hold a suture well (Fig. 2–28). The skin graft was then trimmed to size as the flap

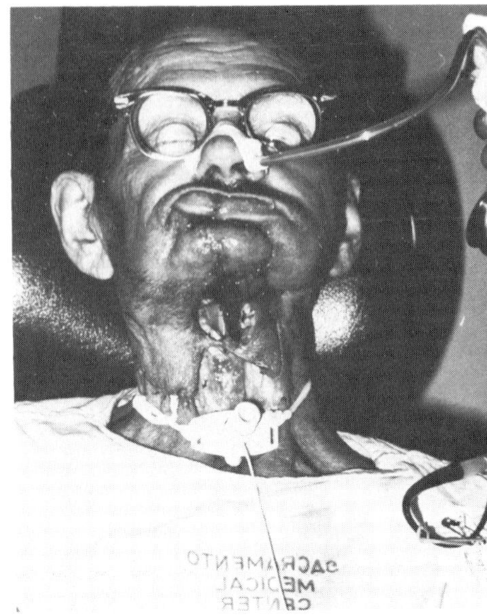

Figure 2–26. (Case II) Massive wound dehiscence from under the chin to the sternum, exposing both common carotid arteries that fortunately epithelialized from their overlying dermis grafts.

was turned to close the defect; the skin graft replaced lost mucosa, and the chest skin, the lost skin of the neck (Fig. 2–29).

The patient did well until 2 years later, when he developed another primary tumor in the nasopharynx to which he eventually succumbed.

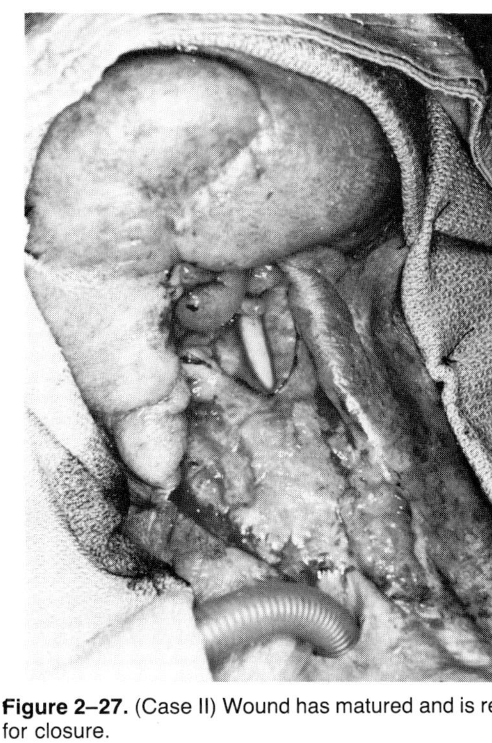

Figure 2–27. (Case II) Wound has matured and is ready for closure.

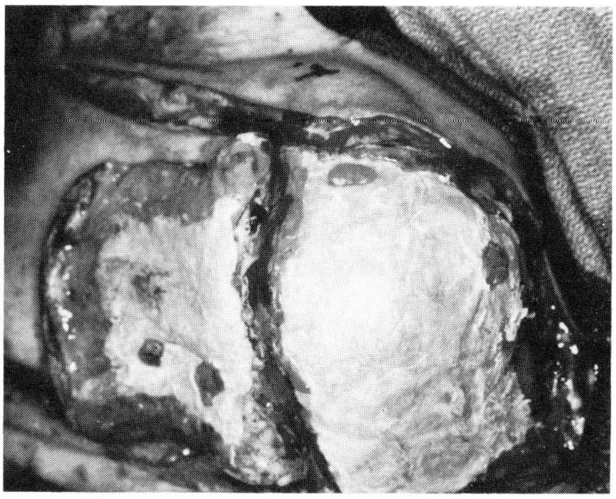

Figure 2–28. (Case II) Deltopectoral flap lined with a thick split-thickness skin graft. The skin graft is sutured to the oral and pharyngeal mucosa. The flap skin supplies the outer surfacing.

Discussion. The wisdom of primary closure of a large excision site in the upper aerodigestive tract of a patient who has undergone previous irradiation in addition to prior surgery is very much in question. Primary reconstruction using richly vascularized flaps has a lot to recommend it. However, the establishment of an adequate control fistula, probably best described by Novack,[40, 41] is in many cases the best choice. A simple method of closing a huge defect such as that depicted in this case is the use of a lined flap. Although Bakanjian, who has popularized the deltopectoral flap, recommends the use of it without a staged delay in most cases,[42] we feel more comfortable with delaying the flap for 10 days to 3 weeks before the planned reconstruction. At the stage of the delay, the split-skin graft is placed against the raw surface of the deltoid end of the flap as well as against the underlying muscle. Quilting sutures

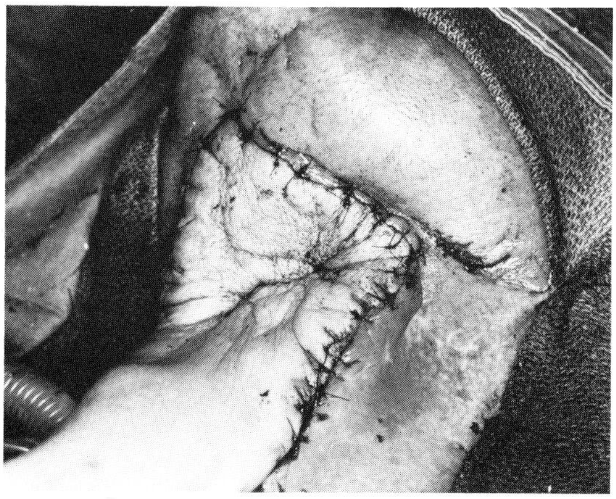

Figure 2–29. (Case III) Flap in situ sutured to the bed by quilting sutures, which are placed in the direction of the flap's axial vessels.

similar to those recommended by McGregor[43] are placed to hold the graft in place, and the two grafts are separated by medicated gauze and a split-open rubber glove. The edges of the flap are then sutured in place until the primary reconstruction takes place.

When the flap is turned, the skin graft is exceptionally strong and holds the suture well. Care must be taken to ensure adequate contact of the remaining raw surface of the flap to a similar raw surface on the neck, so that a blood supply sufficient to nourish the flap will be present once the pedicle is severed.

The value of the dermis graft in carotid artery protection cannot be overemphasized. In well over 400 dermis grafts we have had no local complications from their use. On the other hand, the number of carotid artery blow-outs has been few, thanks to the rapid re-epithelialization of these grafts.

CASE III. A 44-year-old woman presented with a massive T_4 lesion of the oral cavity and oropharynx that was stuck to the skin of the cheek. The tumor began at the right oral commissure and extended to the right side of the posterior pharyngeal wall. The lateral third of the anterior tongue and tongue base were infiltrated with the neoplasm, as was the soft palate and a generous portion of the right hard palate.

The patient had been initially treated with a full course of irradiation for a tonsillar carcinoma. When this failed to achieve cure, a limited composite resection was done, but tumor persisted. A course of chemotherapy was ineffectual. Fortunately the cancer, although it continued to enlarge, had not become fixed to the spine or skull base, and there was no evidence of distant spread. Because of the patient's relative youth, her excellent general health, and her desire for a desperate attempt at salvage, surgery was undertaken.

The first step in the resection was to make a small incision that would allow access to the retropharyngeal area, to verify lack of penetration of the buccopharyngeal fascia and the absence of tumor fixation to the carotid artery (Fig. 2–30). The resection included the area from the mandible to the midline and the inferior half of the maxilla. The tongue was excised to just beyond the midline in its oral portion and into the base almost to the vallecula. Portions of the right upper and lower lip were resected, as was the mucosa and skin of the cheek and upper neck. The pharynx was removed to the midline, and the soft palate was resected as well. The extensive skin excision was necessary because of tumor fixation (Fig. 2–31).

The upper and lower lips were approximated in an attempt to recreate the oral commissure. Oral continuity was re-established by using a forehead flap for the inner lining and a deltopectoral flap for the outer (Fig. 2–32).

The patient developed widespread metastases a few months later and died.

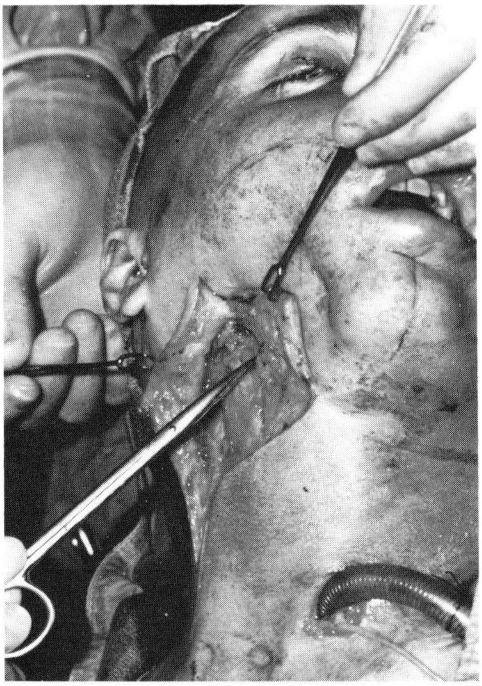

Figure 2–30. (Case III) Small cervical incision ensures lack of fixation of tumor to carotid or cervical spine.

Discussion. In this desperate situation, a wide-field resection was done in the face of an exceptionally aggressive cancer. The huge defect could have been left open with skin sutured to mucosa and skin grafts to cover the remaining raw areas, as was done in the patient depicted in Figure 1–30. The exposure of the carotid artery was extremely problematic because of the impossibility

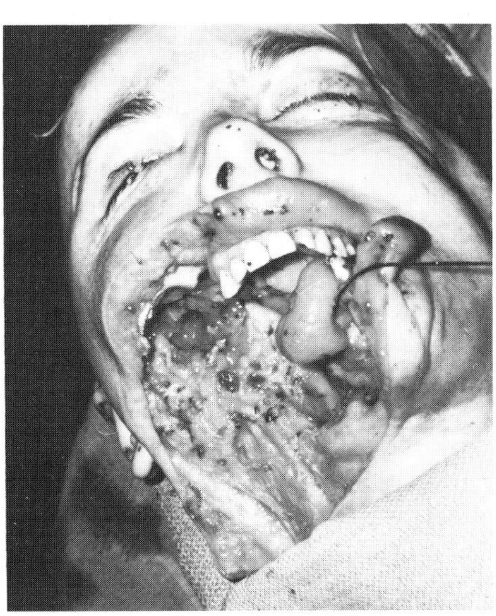

Figure 2–31. (Case III) Completed partial resection of pharynx, mandible, maxilla, 2nd pharynx. Extensive skin excision was required because of cutaneous involvement with cancer.

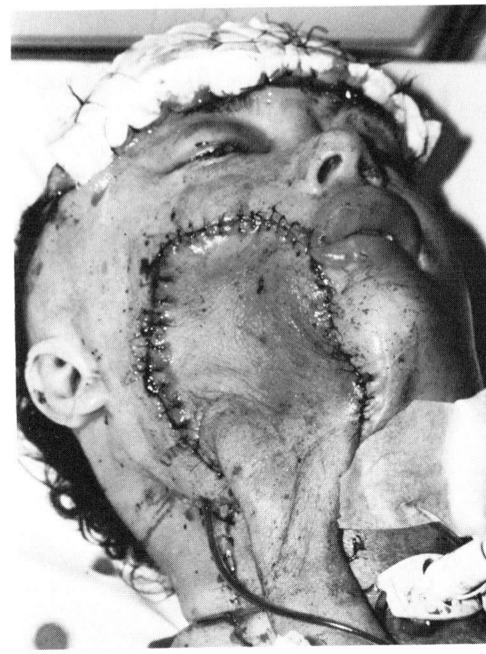

Figure 2–32. (Case III) Oral cavity closed with a forehead flap to line the inner surface and a deltopectoral flap to line the outer.

of approximating the pharyngeal mucosa to the residual skin or the neck. Using one flap back-to-back with another provided an oral and pharyngeal lining and re-established cervicofacial skin continuity. Alternatively, an undelayed split-thickness skin-graft–lined pectoralis major flap could be used. This would provide not only inner and outer epithelium but also the tissue bulk so badly needed to provide fullness to this side of the face.

The inclusion in this portion of the dissertation of two patients who eventually succumbed to their disease or to a second primary tumor is deliberate. It is essential to recognize that in patients with such extensive malignancies even the most vigorous efforts are successful in totally ablating the disease in only 25 to 30 per cent of cases. Furthermore, these patients may develop a second primary in the head and neck or in another organ system entirely. The more aged patient may die of ongoing systemic problems aggravated by the stress of the surgery. However, each individual patient represents a throw of the dice. If the indications are that he has a reasonable chance of surviving the treatment and that the surgeon has a good chance of surgically encompassing the disease, he deserves our "best shot." Finally, the role of palliation must never be forgotten. Although a resection may be extensive, the relief of pain and the ablation of a putrifying, bleeding, odorous mass may improve the patient's comfort immensely. Let us not be accused of hating cancer more than we like people, but let us shun the fear of operating on a desperate patient because it may spoil our track record.

References

1. Goss CM (ed): Gray's Anatomy, 29th ed. Philadelphia, Lea & Febiger, 1973, p 1197.
2. Davies J: Embryology and anatomy of the head and neck, face, palate, nose and paranasal sinuses. *In* Paparella MM, Shumrick DA (eds): Otolaryngology, Vol I, 2nd ed. Philadelphia, WB Saunders, 1980, p 116.
3. English GM: Otolaryngology. Hagerstown, MD, Harper & Row, 1976, p 414.
4. Fletcher GH, Jesse RH, Healey JE, et al: Oropharynx. *In* MacComb WS, Fletcher GH (eds): Cancer of the Head and Neck. Baltimore, Williams & Wilkins, 1968, p 180.
5. Ballenger JJ: Diseases of the Nose, Throat, and Ear, 12th ed. Philadelphia, Lea & Febiger, 1977, p 237.
6. DeWeese DD, Saunders WH: Textbook of Otolaryngology. 2nd ed. St. Louis, CV Mosby, 1964, p 69.
7. Skolnik EM, Campbell JM, Meyers RM: Carcinoma of the buccal mucosa and retromolar area. Otolaryngol Clin North Am 5:327, 1972.
8. Wang CC: Radiation therapy in the management of oral malignant disease. Otolaryngol Clin North Am 12:73, 1979.
9. Baker H, Krause CJ, Saxon KG: Evaluation of triphasic bone scan to detect subclinical invasion of the mandible by squamous cell carcinoma of the oral cavity. Otolaryngol Head Neck Surg 9:327, 1982.
10. Donald PJ: The use of Te^{99} bone scan in the detection of early mandibular invasion in oral cavity cancer. (In preparation.)
11. Romanes GJ: Cunningham's Manual of Practical Anatomy, Vol 3, 13th ed. New York, Oxford University Press, 1968, p 147.
12. Parkhill EM: Tumors of the palatine tonsil. *In* Dockerty MB, Parkhill EM, Dahlin DC (eds): Tumors of the Oral Cavity and Pharynx. Washington, DC, Armed Forces Institute of Pathology, 1964, p 243.
13. Banfi A, Bonadonna G, Carnevali G, et al: Lymphoreticular sarcoma with primary involvement in Waldeyer's ring. Cancer 26:341, 1970.
14. McNelis FL, Pai VT: Malignant lymphoma of the head and neck. Trans Am Soc Laryngol Rhinol Otol, 1969, p 253.
15. Toomey JM: Cysts and tumors of the pharynx. *In* Paparella MM, Shumrick DA (eds): Otolaryngology, Vol III, 2nd ed. Philadelphia, WB Saunders, 1980, p 2323.
16. Lindberg R: Distribution of cervical lymph node metastases from squamous cell carcinoma of the upper respiratory and digestive tracts. Cancer 29:1445, 1972.
17. Truluck CH, Putney FR: Survival rates in cancer of the tongue, tonsil, and hypopharynx. Arch Otolaryngol 93:271, 1971.
18. Quenelle DJ, Crissman JD, Shumrick DA: Tonsillar carcinoma: treatment results. Laryngoscope 89:1842, 1979.
19. Edström S, Jeppsson PH, Lindström J: Carcinoma of the tonsillar region. Aspects on treatment modalities with reference to a study on patients treated by radiation. Laryngoscope 88:1019, 1978.
20. Healy GB, Strong MS, Uchmaklic A, et al.: Carcinoma of the palatine arch. The rationale of treatment selection. Am J Surg 132:498, 1976.
21. Ogura JH, Biller HG, Wette R: Elective neck dissection for pharyngeal and laryngeal cancers: an evaluation. Ann Otol Rhinol Laryngol 80:646, 1971.
22. Whicker JH, DeSanto LW, Devine KD: Surgical treatment of squamous cell carcinoma of the base of the tongue. Laryngoscope 82:1853, 1972.
23. Strong EW: Carcinoma of the tongue. Otolaryngol Clin North Am 12:107, 1979.
24. Freund HR: Posterior oral carcinoma. *In* Principles of Head and Neck Surgery, 2nd ed. New York, Appleton-Century-Crofts, 1979, p 193.
25. Krause CJ: Personal communications, 1980.
26. Donald PJ, Hayes, HR, Dhaliwa R: Combined therapy for pyriform sinus cancer using postoperative irradiation. Otolaryngol Head Neck Surg 88:738, 1980.
27. Donald PJ: Complications of combined therapy in head and neck carcinoma. Arch Otolaryngol 104:324, 1978.
28. Lee JG: Resection margins of carcinoma of the oral cavity, oropharynx, hypopharynx, and larynx: a clinical study. Master's thesis, University of Iowa, 1973.
29. Snow JB, Gelber RD, Kramer S: Randomized preoperative and postoperative radiation therapy for patients with carcinoma of the head and neck: preliminary report. Laryngoscope 90:930, 1980.
30. Schleuning AJ, Summers GW: Carcinoma of the tongue: review of 220 cases. Laryngoscope 82:1446, 1972.
31. Trible WM: Cancer of the oral cavity: five year end results in 237 patients. Ann Otol Rhinol Laryngol 78:716, 1969.
32. Ash CL: Oral cancer: a twenty-five year study. Am J Roentgenol Radium Ther Nucl Med 87:417, 1962.
33. Fee WE, Sonja LS, Rubenstein R, et al: Squamous cell carcinoma of the soft palate. Arch Otolaryngol 105:710, 1979.
34. Russ JW, Applebaum EL, Sesson GA: Squamous cell carcinoma of the soft palate. Laryngoscope 87:1151, 1977.
35. Konrad HR, Canalis RF, Calcaterra TC: Epidermoid carcinoma of the palate. Arch Otolaryngol 104:208, 1978.
36. Rider WD: Epithelial cancer of the tonsillar area. Radiology 78:760, 1962.
37. Fletcher GH, Jesse RH, Healey JE, et al: Oropharynx. *In* MacComb WS, Fletcher GH, (eds): Cancer of the Head and Neck. Baltimore, Williams & Wilkins, 1968, p 179.
38. DeClercq LD, Chole RA: Retropharyngeal abscess in the adult. Otolaryngol Head Neck Surg 88:684, 1980.
39. Myers EN: Total glossectomy in cancer of the oral cavity. Otolaryngol Clin North Am 5:343, 1972.
40. Novack AJ: Carcinoma of the anterior and lateral aspects of the floor of the mouth. Otolaryngol Clin North Am 12:97, 1979.
41. Novack AJ: The surgical management of malignant lesions of the floor of the mouth. Otolaryngol Clin North Am 12:97, 1979.
42. Bakanjian VY: The deltopectoral flap. *In* Grabb WC, Meyers MB (eds): Skin Flaps. Boston, Little, Brown, 1975, p 225.
43. McGregor IA: "Quilted" skin grafting in the mouth. Br J Plast Surg 28:100, 1975.

3

HYPOPHARYNX, CERVICAL ESOPHAGUS, AND MEDIASTINUM

Paul J. Donald, M.D.

Squamous cell cancer affecting the hypopharynx and the cervical esophagus carries with it one of the most ominous prognoses of any site in the upper aerodigestive tract. As location of malignancy progresses downward from the oral cavity to the stomach, the 5-year survival rate falls accordingly. From the tongue tip to the oropharynx the downswing of the survival curve is less steep; however, the curve plummets with progression through the hypopharynx and cervical esophagus. The aggressive biologic activity of the lesions and the minimal symptoms experienced by patients through the early course of this disease are jointly responsible for this unfortunate circumstance.

Biologically, these lesions have a propensity for rapid local mucosal and submucosal spread and a proclivity for regional and even distant metastasis. So-called "skip areas" and multifocal disease are not uncommon in the pyriform recesses and are almost the rule in cervical esophageal lesions. The rather localized nature of epidermoid tumors, so commonly observed in the rest of the head and neck region, is not a feature of hypopharyngeal and esophageal lesions.

The occult nature of the clinical presentation encountered in these neoplasms accounts for their large size when first seen. Often a cancerous cervical lymph node, indicating metastasis, is the only sign of trouble. The unfortunate stigma of a neck scar from a biopsy that should not have been done in a patient bearing the diagnosis of metastatic squamous cell carcinoma is a tragedy in the experience of most head and neck surgeons (Fig. 3–1). Most often a quick look with a laryngeal mirror reveals the source of the primary lesion. The symptom of mild dysphagia is commonly reported in a family practice setting, and fortunately hypopharyngeal and cervical esophageal tumors are rarely encountered in the experience of these practitioners. Only a chance pharyngoesophagogram will reveal the malignancy that may lurk there. Pain on swallowing, hoarseness, dyspnea, and hemoptysis are all late signs.

ANATOMY

Hypopharynx

For the purpose of consistency, the start of the hypopharynx will be demarcated at the level of the valleculae and the lateral pharyngoepiglottic folds. The termination of this area inferiorly is at the level of the cricopharyngeus muscle (Fig. 3–2). Contained within the hypopharynx is, of course, the larynx, malignancies of which have an altogether different biologic character from those of the pharynx. However, once a tumor has migrated outside the confines of the larynx and has transgressed the hypopharynx, it

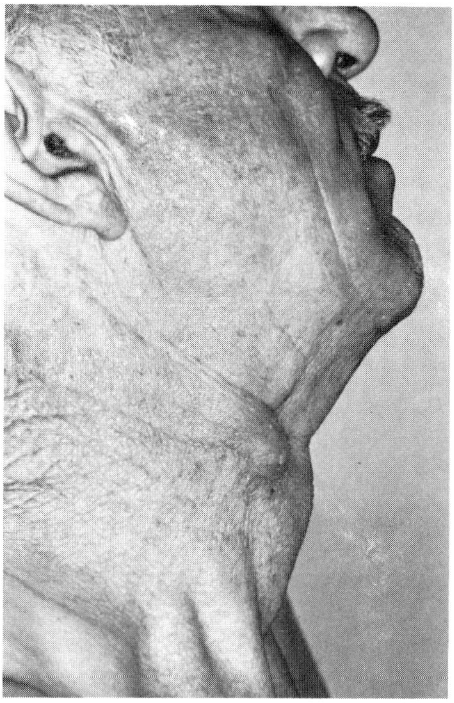

Figure 3–1. Neck scar with tumor growing through it following a biopsy of a cancerous cervical lymph node metastatic from a pyriform sinus carcinoma.

assumes the more aggressive behavior of this latter region.

The hypopharynx includes both pyriform fossae and an intervening area of pharynx directly posterior to the larynx; the anterior wall of this area is called the postcricoid area, and the posterior wall simply the posterior pharyngeal wall. Each pyriform fossa is rimmed by the aryepiglottic fold medially, the lateral pharyngoepiglottic fold anterolaterally, and the lateral hypopharyngeal wall lateroposteriorly. The aryepiglottic fold is considered to be the medial wall of the pyriform sinus. This fold is actually part of the larynx, but the medial wall of the pyriform sinus begins 1 cm below the fold's superiormost extremity. This medial wall pyriform mucosa is in continuity with that of its opposing side through the aforementioned postcricoid area. The lamina of the cricoid cartilage is the principal skeletal component supporting this latter region. The posterior cricoarytenoid muscles and a portion of the interarytenoid muscles intervene between the mucosa and the cartilage. The posterior surface of this—the posterior wall of the larynx—forms the postcricoid area, which also serves as the anterior wall of the posterior hypopharynx. At the inferior border of the cricoid the hypopharynx becomes the cervical esophagus.

The posterior wall of the pharyngeal area is continuous with that of the oropharynx above and the cervical esophagus below.

The hypopharynx is composed of the middle and inferior constrictor muscles of the pharynx and their investing fascial layers. The loose areolar fascia between the bucco-

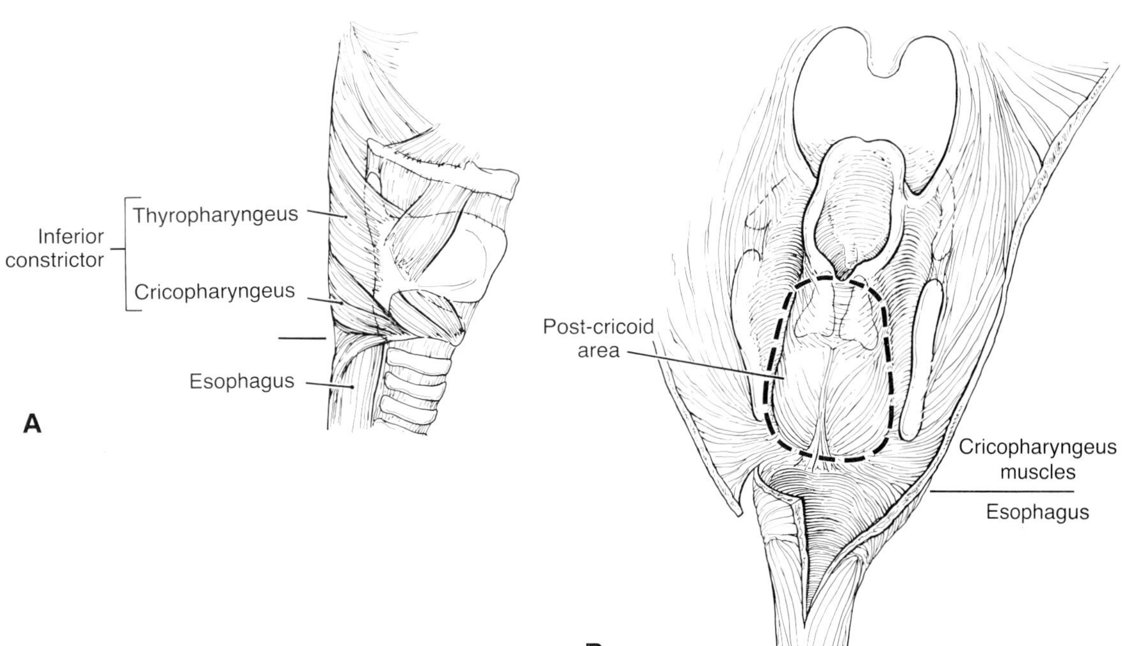

Figure 3–2. Anatomic boundaries of the hypopharynx. *A*, External view. *B*, Internal view.

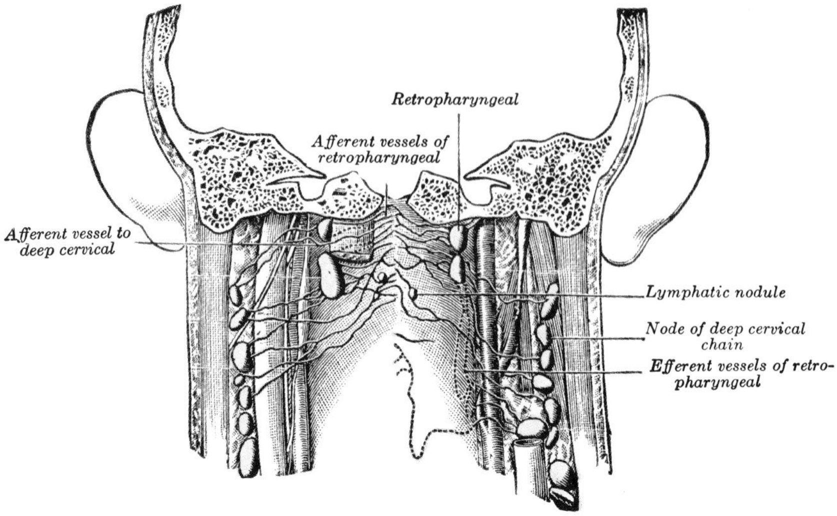

Figure 3–3. Illustration of the nodes draining the pharynx. Note the high retropharyngeal nodes of Rouvière, which are inaccessible to the palpating finger. (Poirier and Charpy; from Goss CM (ed): Gray's Anatomy of the Human Body, 29th ed. Philadelphia, Lea & Febiger, 1975.)

pharyngeal fascia investing the muscular coats and the stout fascia of the prevertebral area exists in the same way that it does in the oropharynx and is called by some the "alar fascia."

The pyriform fossae, except at their posterior extremities, are contained within the alae of the thyroid cartilage. Superiorly, the aryepiglottic and, slightly more inferiorly, the lateral cricoarytenoid muscles separate the fossae from the laryngeal lumen. The arytenoid cartilage composes part of this medial wall posteriorly. Inferiorly, the cricoid cartilage makes up this wall as the pyriform progresses toward the cervical esophagus.

The lymphatics of the hypopharynx penetrate the thyrohyoid membrane to terminate in the nodes of the middle jugular chain. The drainage of the postcricoid area is less profuse than that of the pyriform recesses, and the pattern of drainage is similar to that of the cervical esophagus.[1] The lymph nodes in which they terminate are grouped around the upper esophagus and trachea as well as in the supraclavicular fossa. The drainage from the posterior wall may ascend the lymphatic chain in the lateral and posterolateral neck, emptying into the midjugular chain, and may even reach the highest retropharyngeal node, the node of Rouvière (Fig. 3–3).[12]

Cervical Esophagus

The cervical esophagus is roughly the upper one third of that organ, but no precise demarcation exists. It begins at the level of the cricopharyngeus muscle opposite C_6 and ends at the thoracic inlet. As the esophagus descends into the chest, it proceeds in a posterior direction carried by the trachea, which fronts it. The cervical tracheal membranous wall lies anteriorly to the esophagus and is separated from it by a flimsy layer of connective tissue. While in the neck, the trachea and esophagus deviate approximately 0.5 cm from the midline of the spine. The cervical esophageal lumen measures about 2.3 cm by 1.7 cm and is somewhat flattened compared to its more rounded configuration in the chest. The relatively thin wall of the organ is responsible for its reputation as a delicate, poorly healing structure, and surgery to the esophagus has traditionally been fraught with misery because of its fragility. Compounding this problem is the extreme mobility of the esophagus. The prevertebral fascia that binds it to the prevertebral area is made up of loose areolar tissue which permits the repetitive gliding traverse of the organ during swallowing. An excursion the distance of a vertebral body is common during the swallowing act, and such a degree of movement inevitably adds to the risk of any surgical procedure.

The major contributors to the blood supply of the cervical esophagus are the inferior thyroid arteries. Their twigs pierce the muscular coat in the ascending and descending course of each artery as well as near its termination. Minor contributions are also made directly from the subclavian, common

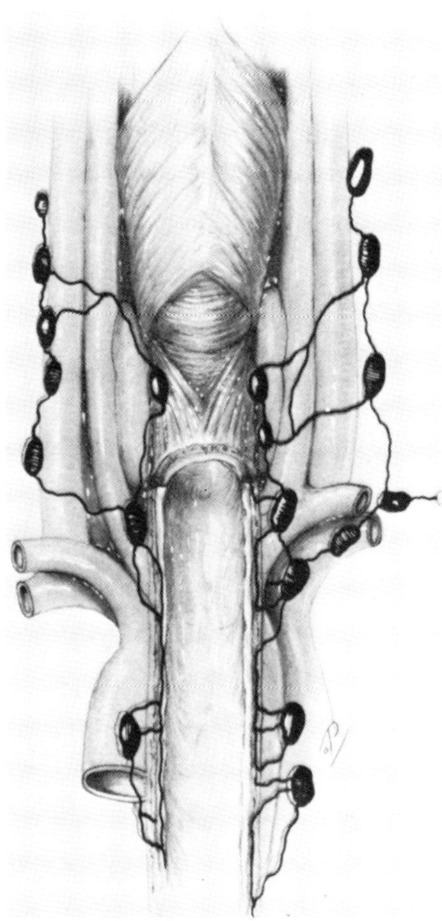

Figure 3–4. Lymphatic drainage of the cervical esophagus and its integration with those of the hypopharynx. (From Postlethwait PW: Surgery of the Esophagus. New York, Appleton-Century-Crofts, 1979.)

carotid, vertebral, costocervical, superficial cervical, and even the superior thyroid arteries. A richer supply emanates from the right inferior thyroid artery than from the left; however, the overall circulation and nutrition does not differ between the sides.[3]

The lymphatic drainage described in 1932 by Rouvière,[4] based to a large degree on the work of Sakata,[5] has been little improved upon by the work of later investigators. A rich lymphatic network drains the mucosa and submucosa, and to a lesser degree the muscularis. These vessels are disposed in a longitudinal and transverse manner with the longitudinal vessels outnumbering the transverse by a ratio of 6 to 1.[5] This, in part, probably accounts for the rapidity of submucosal spread that is characteristic of esophageal carcinoma. Connecting lymphatic vessels directly penetrate the muscular layer and terminate in adjacent thoracic nodes. The longitudinally disposed lymphatics of the thoracic esophagus run a particularly long course, with many of them reaching the neck, piercing the muscularis and entering the cervical nodes (Fig. 3–7*B*). Rouvière makes the point that the lymphatics of the upper two thirds of the esophagus have a great propensity to run superiorly and drain into these nodes. The lymph of the cervical esophagus drains directly into these nodes of the inferior neck (Fig. 3–4). These facts support the clinical findings that the inferior jugular aggregation of nodes are often involved in esophageal carcinoma in the neck and upper chest and that "skip areas," often of considerable separation from one another, are not uncommonly seen between cancers in the esophagus.

Mediastinum

The mediastinum is an extensive area located between the medial reflections of the pleurae; it houses the heart, great vessels, esophagus, trachea, and pulmonary hila. The portion of this region that principally concerns the head and neck surgeon is the superior compartment. The area is roofed anteriorly by the manubrium sterni and the clavicular heads. A markedly thickened periosteal layer underlies the manubrium and during surgical dissection affords protection to the great vessels that lie underneath. Directly adjacent to this heavy fibrous layer is the thymus gland. It occupies a variable volume of the immediate lower neck and upper mediastinum, extending as far inferiorly as the 4th rib. The gland is relatively large at birth, reaching its maximum size at about the age of 2 years, but at puberty it begins to regress. In the adult, the gland involutes and is largely replaced by fat; the remainder measures 5 cm by 4 cm and is approximately 6 mm thick.

Intimately related to the deep surface of the thymus is the mediastinal fat pad. Numerous lymphatic channels and the pretracheal lymph nodes are found in this layer. The investing fascia of this pad also sheaths the great vessels as they cross the trachea. Near the inferior limit of the superior mediastinum, the aorta crosses the trachea from right to left. As it crosses, it gives off the right brachiocephalic artery, which while crossing the trachea from left to right may ascend into the lower neck. The left subclavian and left common carotid arteries emerge from the aorta on the left side of the trachea (Fig. 3–5). The left innominate vein crosses

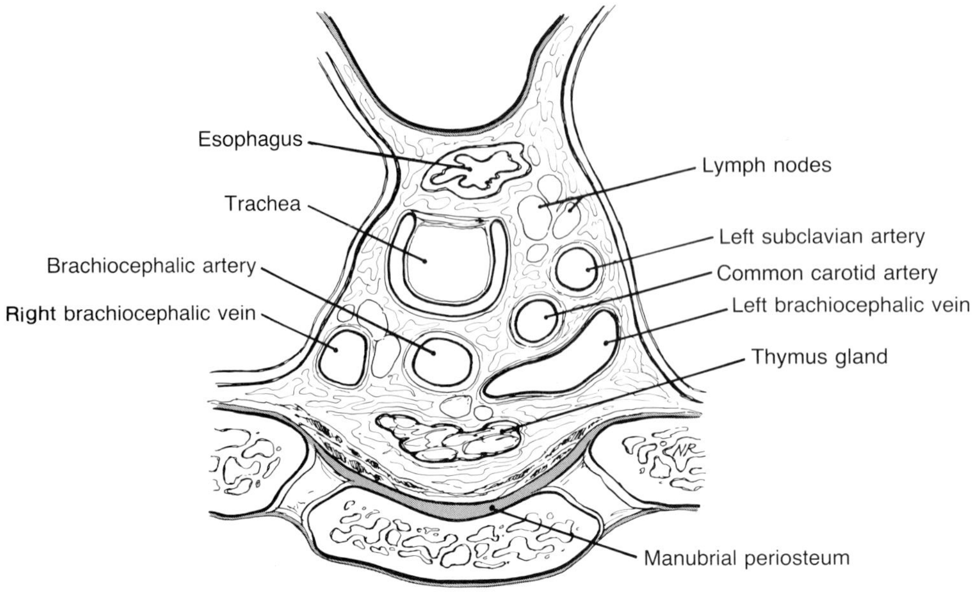

Figure 3–5. Horizontal sectional view of the upper mediastinum taken at approximately the upper third of the manubrium sterni.

the trachea more superiorly than the aorta, obscuring a clear view of the trachea and lateral lymphatics. Both vagi as well as the right recurrent nerve are lateral to the trachea and deep to the vascular compartment. The width of the upper mediastinum varies with the patient's weight, measuring on the average between 5.6 and 7.4 cm (Table 3–1).

The lymphatics of the mediastinum that are surgically accessible are located in the pretracheal and paratracheal areas. As Sisson[6] has pointed out, no clearly established anatomic relationship has been elucidated between the cervical and mediastinal lymphatics. There is, however, the common finding that carcinoma involving lymphatics at the root of the neck remain stationary for a time and then spread to the mediastinum. The presumptive link between the two systems seems to be supported not only by this clinical correlate but also by the survival data in this patient group.[6] Although the nodes are not too plentiful, they are indeed present. In 20 fresh cadaver dissections, Mast and Jafek[7] found an average of three nodes in the pretracheal area, six in the right paratracheal area, and eight in the left paratracheal area. The ranges of these values are 0 to 8, 2 to 13, and 2 to 15 respectively.

PATHOPHYSIOLOGY

Squamous cell carcinomas of the hypopharynx may begin de novo or may spread from adjacent structures, especially the larynx and tongue base. Tumors with a geographic center on the aryepiglottic fold, lateral pharyngoepiglottic fold, and vallecula often involve the pyriform sinus before they become symptomatic. However, these tumors are symptomatic much earlier than those that begin in the pyriform recesses per se. This is some indication of the insidious nature of these neoplasms.

Most series of patients with primary tumors in this locale contain very few T_1 lesions.[8] The symptoms of odynophagia, dysphagia, and voice change often do not appear until the lesion has attained massive proportions.

Table 3–1. CORRELATION OF CADAVER WEIGHT AND AVERAGE INTERPLEURAL DISTANCE*

Cadaver Weight (kg)	*No. of Cadavers*	*Average Distance Between Pleural Reflections (cm)*	*Range (cm)*
40–59	6	5.6	4.3–6.5
60–79	8	6.9	6.0–8.3
80–99	8	7.4	6.3–8.7

*Reprinted from Carter DR: The anatomy of the mediastinum. Ear Nose Throat J *60*:157, 1981.

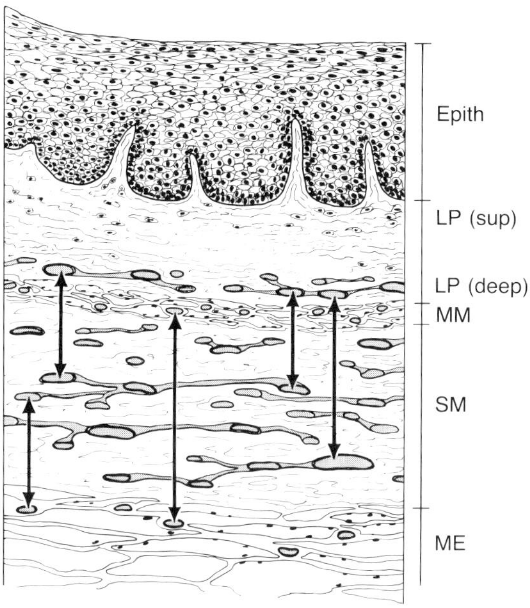

Figure 3–6. Drawing of idealized photomicrograph illustrating the rich lymphatic network in the lamina propria and submucosa of the esophageal epithelium and its numerous interconnections, providing a possible explanation of the frequent finding of multifocal cancer in the esophagus. *Epith* = epithelium; *LP* = lamina propria; *MM* = muscularis mucosae; *SM* = submucosa; *ME* = esophageal muscle.

Patients often present with weight loss and cervical adenopathy before developing symptoms referable to the hypopharynx. Moreover, hoarseness, hemoptysis, and airway obstruction generally do not ensue until there is laryngeal involvement. One patient in our own series did not seek attention until he developed intractable right heart failure secondary to upper airway obstruction caused by the large size of his tumor.

The rapid, aggressive spread of these carcinomas is in part due to the lack of restricting anatomic barriers in the hypopharynx.[9] The cervical esophagus harbors lesions that rapidly penetrate the mucosal walls to involve adjacent structures, and it has been postulated that this may be because of its lack of serosal covering.[10] The prevertebral fascia and the loose areolar fascia between it and the investing fascia of the muscular layers of the organ curiously provide a temporary but effective barrier to posterior spread of the cancer. The rich lymphatic network in the lamina propria and submucosa of the esophageal epithelium may explain the rapid longitudinal spread that is so commonplace with malignancies here (Fig. 3–6). The skip areas may be explained by the fact that the tumor cells embolize in the submucosal layer below the muscularis mucosae, travel a short distance longitudinally in this lamina, and then replicate and rupture through the epithelial surface at a point some centimeters away from the original tumor.

That the hypopharynx has a lesser tendency to develop multiple tumor foci with intervening skip areas may be due to histologic differences in its submucosal layer (Fig. 3–7). Instead of the thick submucosal layer and the well-developed muscularis mucosae characteristic of the esophagus, the pharynx possesses a dearth of the former and a replacement of the muscularis by a dense layer of elastic tissue. The pharyngeal mucosa is closely approximated to the longitudinal and circular muscle layers.[11] As the hypopharynx blends into the cervical esophagus, the thick elastic layer of the lamina propria becomes

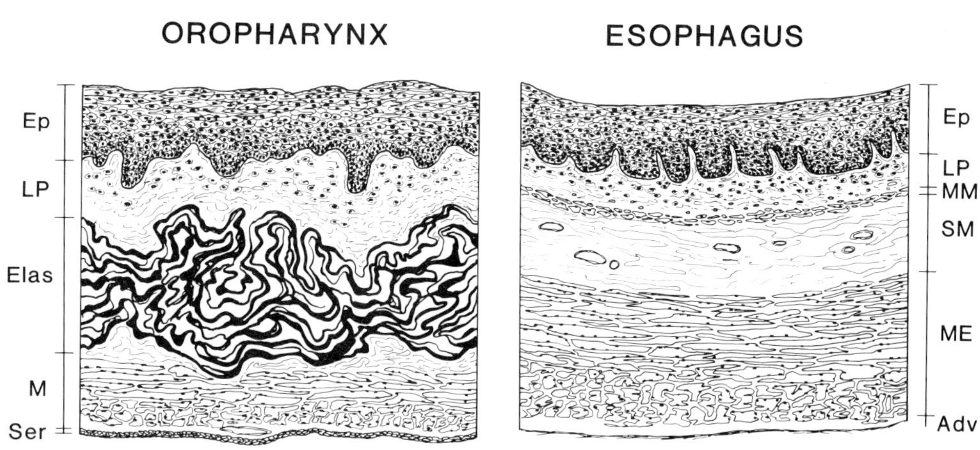

Figure 3–7. Comparison of the submucosal layers of the oropharynx and the esophagus. The thick elastic layer of the oropharynx may provide a barrier to tumor penetration. No such barrier exists in the esophagus, and the mucosa is applied directly to the muscularis. The hypopharynx is a transitional zone regarding the elastic layer. Here the elastic layer becomes attenuated, and the lamina propria possesses much loose connective tissue and is richly invested with lymphatics. *Ep* = epithelium; *LP* = lamina propria; *Elas* = elastic layer; *M* = muscularis; *Ser* = serosa; *MM* = muscularis mucosae; *SM* = submucosa; *ME* = esophageal muscle; *Adv* = adventitia.

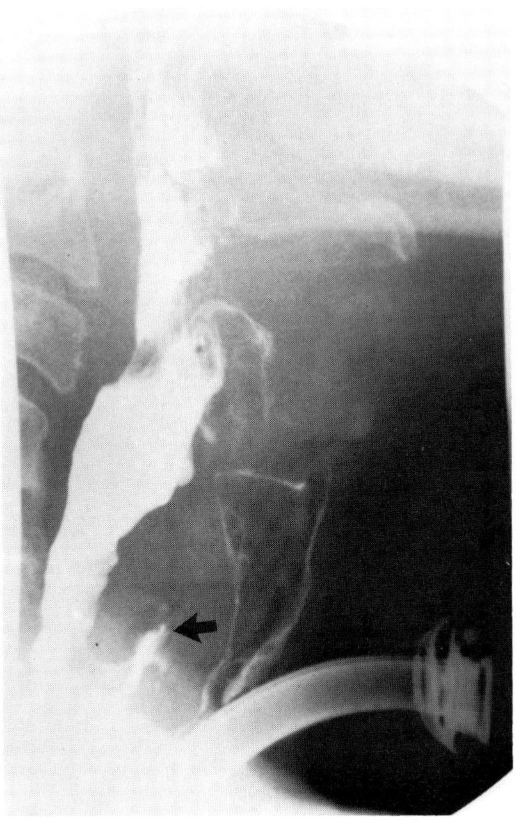

Figure 3–8. Barium swallow of an elderly man with cervical esophageal carcinoma that had eroded through the entire wall of the esophagus and developed a sinus tract into the neck (arrow).

plusher and more richly endowed with lymphatics. The frequency of "multiple hypopharyngeal primaries" in this area as a possible manifestation of the multifocal cancer from a single tumor, in contrast to the rarity of this phenomenon elsewhere in the pharynx, may be explained on this basis; however, this finding is far less commonly seen in the hypopharynx than in the esophagus.

Carcinomas of the cervical esophagus commonly remain occult until they have reached considerable size. Dysphagia and odynophagia are not uncommonly preceded by a period of weight loss, the presentation of a lump in the neck, or symptoms of invasion of adjacent structures such as the larynx, the vagus and recurrent laryngeal nerves, or the cervical sympathetic trunk (Fig. 3–8). Symptoms of swallowing disturbance may also include the regurgitation of bloody material.

Rarely, a carcinoma may develop in a Zenker's diverticulum (Fig. 3–9).[12] This alone is an excellent reason to perform esophagoscopy on every patient with this abnormality prior to its excision. The regurgitation characteristic of a pharyngoesophageal diverticulum is bloody only if a malignancy is present. Most patients with this cancer have prolonged histories of diverticula. Possibly the longstanding irritation of the mucosa secondary to stasis of food in the pouch may play a part in the initiation of such lesions.

DIAGNOSIS

A barium esophagogram followed by laryngoscopy and esophagoscopy is the standard diagnostic procedure for all of these lesions of the hypopharynx and cervical esophagus. The typical "apple core" appearance of esophageal cancers is infamous (Fig. 3–10) The new body scanners are showing promise in delineating the extraluminal extent of these lesions (Fig. 3–11).

One of the most common presenting symptoms of all of these tumors is a lump in the neck (Fig. 3–12). This finding may be the only sign or symptom until indirect laryngoscopy or esophagoscopy reveals its primary source. It is not unusual for a patient with a painless, slowly growing neck mass to be treated with a number of courses of different antibiotics and occasionally have the misfortune to have a nodal biopsy before more skilled consultation is sought.

By far the most common hypopharyngeal lesion is that found in the pyriform recesses. In Kirchner's series, 152 lesions were found in the pyriform sinus, whereas only 8 were seen in the postcricoid area and 7 in the posterior pharyngeal wall.[13] In a series from the Mayo Clinic, 20 lesions were found in the posterior pharyngeal wall and only 7 in the postcricoid area.[9] Som and Nussbaum[14] discuss the management of 61 large hypopharyngeal lesions that they described as postcricoid but which appear to have been large circumferential lesions whose precise geographic center was difficult to discern. The massive size of the lesions in their series is representative of most surgeons' experience. In our own series only 6 of 37 pyriform sinus tumors were T_1 or T_2 in size.[15]

Although Conley[8] states that over 50 per cent of patients with pyriform sinus cancer have regional metastases when first diagnosed, Ogura[16] noticed cervical secondaries in 90 per cent of his patients. Harwick[17] noted a 40 per cent incidence of contralateral nodal involvement in his patients. In our series,[15] 79 per cent of patients had lymph node me-

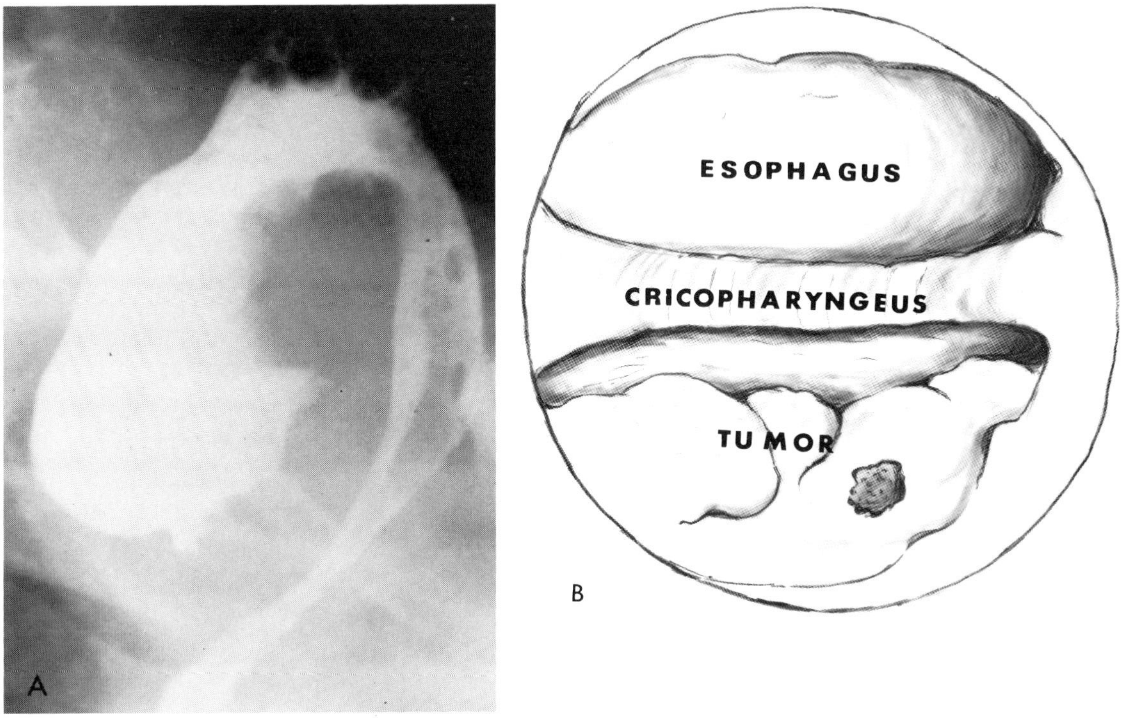

Figure 3–9. A squamous cell carcinoma in a Zenker's diverticulum. *A*, Barium swallow showing irregular space-occupying lesion in the diverticulum. *B*, Drawing of endoscopic view of tumor. (From Donald PJ, Huffman DI: Carcinoma in a Zenker's diverticulum. J Head Neck Surg 2:71, 1979.)

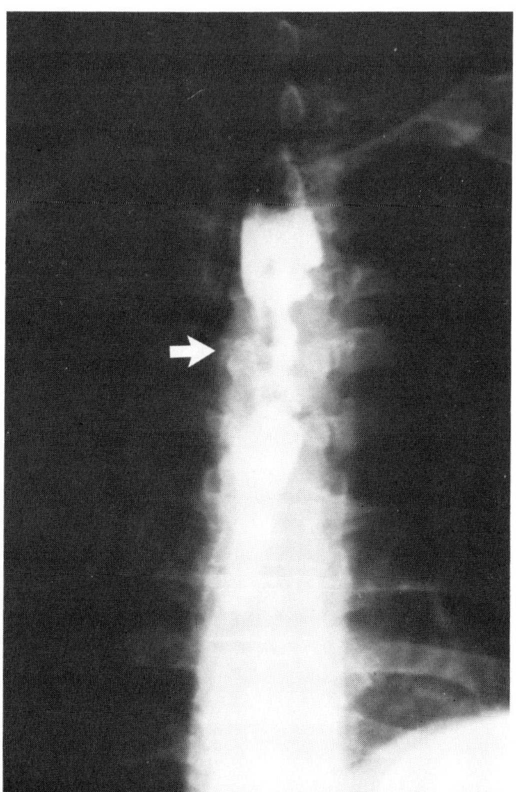

Figure 3–10. Barium swallow showing the typical "apple core" appearance (arrow) of esophageal cancer.

tastases, and in over half of these cases the secondary lesions were N_2 or N_3 in extent. Kirchner[13] reports finding palpable adenopathy in 71 per cent of his 116 cases, while Razack et al[18] note an incidence of 87.6 per cent.

In cervical esophageal cancer, nodal metastases are also common. Postlethwait,[10] citing a growing trend toward routine use of scalene fat-pad biopsy for esophageal carci-

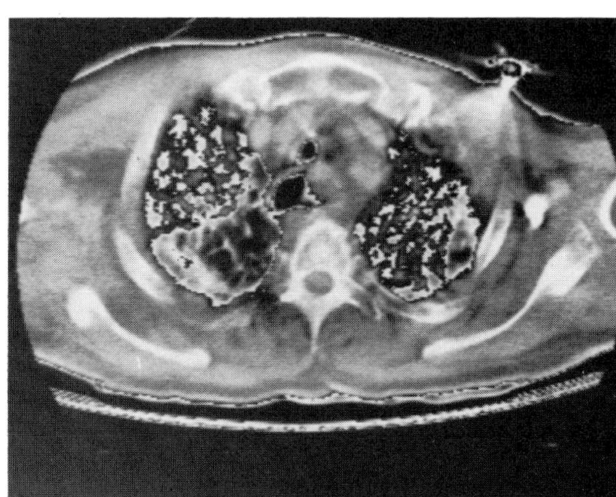

Figure 3–11. CAT scan of the neck in horizontal section, showing the extraesophageal extent of carcinoma of the esophagus.

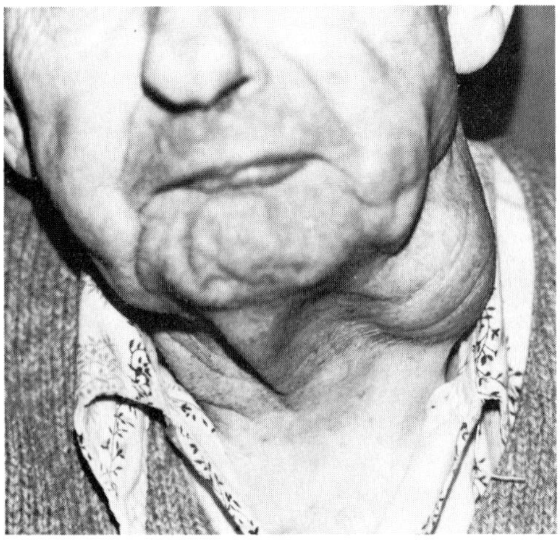

Figure 3–12. Mass in the neck was the only symptom in this elderly man with a large pyriform sinus carcinoma.

noma in general, describes his own experience with 78 such biopsies, which revealed metastatic cancer in 40 cases. In Mustard's series,[19] a similar pattern was seen.

TREATMENT

There is little argument that surgery is the most effective therapeutic modality for hypopharyngeal lesions. The experience of Som and Nussbaum[14] in which 1 patient out of 27 with hypopharyngeal cancer treated with primary irradiation therapy survived 5 years is echoed by others.[15, 19-22] A recent report by Million and Cassisi[23] indicates a favorable prognosis when radiotherapy is used for very small lesions, but these diminutive lesions are unfortunately rare.

As has been noted, most often the lesions encountered are of substantial size, and radical excision with in-continuity radical neck dissection is generally the rule. In addition, although this is still somewhat controversial, we believe that there is good evidence to show that use of postoperative irradiation therapy adds significantly to the survival rate.[15] In our own experience the survival rate has been better with postoperative rather than preoperative irradiation; this may be due to the fact that the shrinking effect on the tumor caused by preoperative irradiation makes it difficult to establish accurate resection margins at the time of surgery. In addition, the complication rate is much lower when the irradiation is used postoperatively.[21]

Wide extirpation of the lesion is the rule. Rarely, if ever, can the larynx be spared, because of the intimate relationship of the pyriform sinus mucosa to the laryngeal skeleton (Fig. 3–13). A radical neck dissection is always done even in the absence of adenopathy. Postoperative irradiation generally does a creditable job of eliminating occult cancer in lymphatics of the neck. However, it is not uncommon to have to operate on a protein-depleted, asthenic patient who has been imbibing alcohol heavily, neglecting his nutrition, and is in a state of negative nitrogen balance. These individuals are at a high risk of developing a major postoperative complication that will necessitate a delay in radiation therapy. Unfortunately, once the "golden period" of 4 to 6 weeks has elapsed between surgery and irradiation, the efficacy of the latter modality rapidly diminishes. We have seen a number of patients develop neck

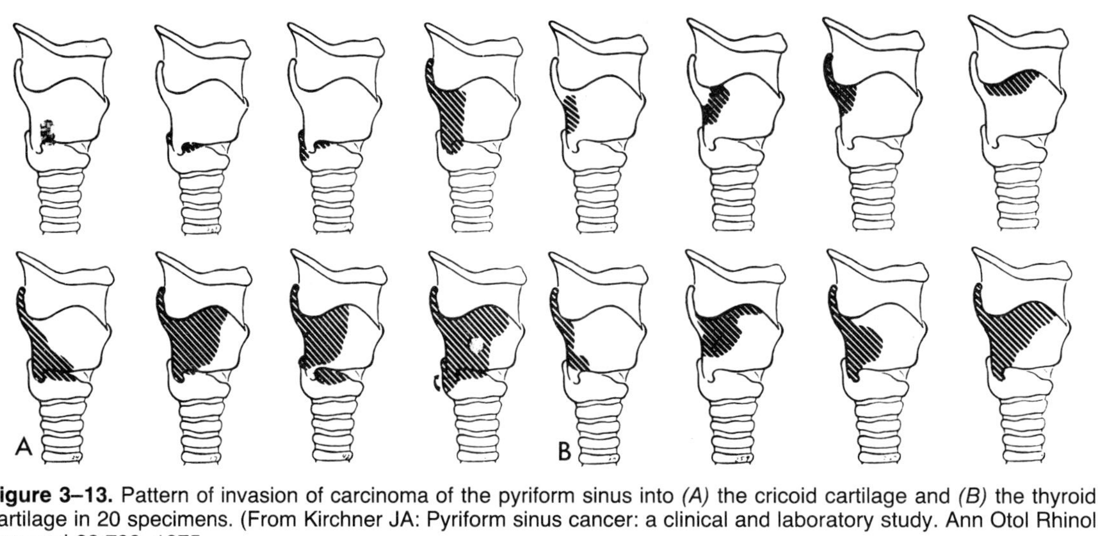

Figure 3–13. Pattern of invasion of carcinoma of the pyriform sinus into *(A)* the cricoid cartilage and *(B)* the thyroid cartilage in 20 specimens. (From Kirchner JA: Pyriform sinus cancer: a clinical and laboratory study. Ann Otol Rhinol Laryngol 83:793, 1975.

metastases in the interim between surgery and the start of irradiation when dissection of the neck ipsilateral to the tumor was not done.

The problem cases of hypopharyngeal carcinoma involve those patients who have massive lesions, those with bilateral lymph node involvement, and those with lesions extending into the cervical esophagus.

Bilateral Neck Dissection

Bilateral adenopathy may be handled with either a staged neck dissection or a simultaneous bilateral neck dissection. Whether one procedure is superior to the other is not clear, but our preference with palpable bilateral nodes is to do a simultaneous dissection. A radical neck dissection is performed on the side of greatest pharyngeal tumor involvement, but the dissection on the contralateral side spares the internal jugular vein if possible. If both veins are to be sacrificed, certain precautions must be observed. Facial swelling and edema can be reduced if the patient's head is tipped up at a 30-degree angle during the surgery. In fact, if the head is flat or slightly dependent, the swelling can be so pronounced that it will produce exorbitism. Even with the head elevated, it is wise to tape the eyes securely shut. Because of this

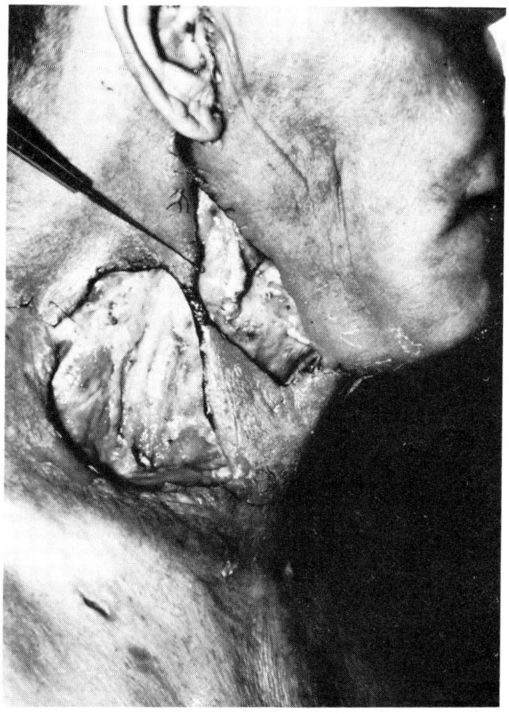

Figure 3–14. Exposed carotid artery following slough of neck flaps.

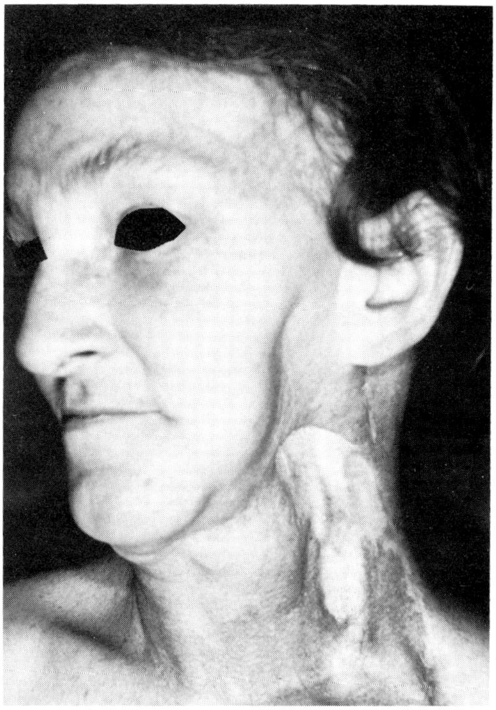

Figure 3–15. Re-epithelialization of large dehiscent area of neck by dermal graft on carotid artery.

slightly head-up position, the patient should have a CVP catheter placed preoperatively, so that in the event of an air embolism, the air may be easily withdrawn from the right atrium. A precordial Doppler scanner provides an excellent highly sensitive monitor in the event of this complication.

Once one jugular vein has been ligated, tremendous engorgement of the venous system on the contralateral side ensues. If the internal jugular vein must be taken on this side, blood loss will be reduced if its ligation is delayed until the end of the dissection of this neck. Careful hemostasis is essential as the dissection proceeds. Meticulous cross-clamping of veins prior to cutting them supersedes the advantage of rapid dissection and clamping of vessels as they bleed, since the increased venous pressure results in excessive blood loss with this latter method.

At the conclusion of the procedure the application of dermal grafts to the carotids provides excellent prophylaxis against the catastrophe of carotid blow-out if the artery should become exposed in the postoperative period. The graft when exposed to air rapidly epithelializes and will not only cover the exposed artery but will spread to cover large raw areas that have become devoid of epithelium (Figs. 3–14, 3–15).

Occipital Triangle Dissection

Metastases high in the neck should be resected with a generous cuff of parotid gland as well as the stylohyoid, stylopharyngeus, and posterior digastric muscles. If the disease is high and posterior in location, a generous portion of underlying trapezius muscle may need to be excised. Dissection of the occipital and suboccipital triangles may also need to be done, in order to encompass the occipital lymph nodes. These nodes are part of a controversial group of lymphatic aggregations described as the "nuchal nodes" (Fig. 3–16) that drain mainly into the upper internal jugular chain.[4, 24, 25]

The occipital triangle is that portion of the posterior triangle of the neck that is bounded superiorly by the junction of the posterior border of the sternomastoid and the anterior border of the trapezius muscle. The inferior border is the posterior belly of the omohyoid muscle. The floor of the triangle is formed by the splenius capitus superiorly and the levator scapulae inferiorly. The area of concern in this dissection is the superiormost aspect of the occipital triangle. Deep to both the trapezius and splenius capitus muscles is the semispinalis capitus, which roofs over the suboccipital triangle. Access to this region is facilitated by extending the mastoid portion of the incision in a superior and slightly posterior direction. In order to excise an adequate margin of surrounding healthy tissue, a substantial block of underlying trapezius, semispinalis capitus, and splenius capitus muscle tissue may need to be removed (Fig. 3–17). The floor of the dissection is made up of the suboccipital triangle, which is bordered by the superior oblique superiorly, the inferior oblique inferiorly, and the oblique capitus major and minor medially. The deep cervical vein emerges from the center of the triangle and must be controlled as the deep part of the dissection continues. The occipital artery is easily visualized in its superficial aspect, but seeks this surface from its course deep to the posterior belly of the digastric against the undersurface of the temporal bone. It arises between the superior oblique muscle and the posterior belly of the digastric to supply the occipital scalp. The so-called nuchal nodes are found in this region.[24] The contents of the suboccipital triangle can remain in continuity with the upper end of the sternomastoid muscle as the radical neck dissection proceeds.

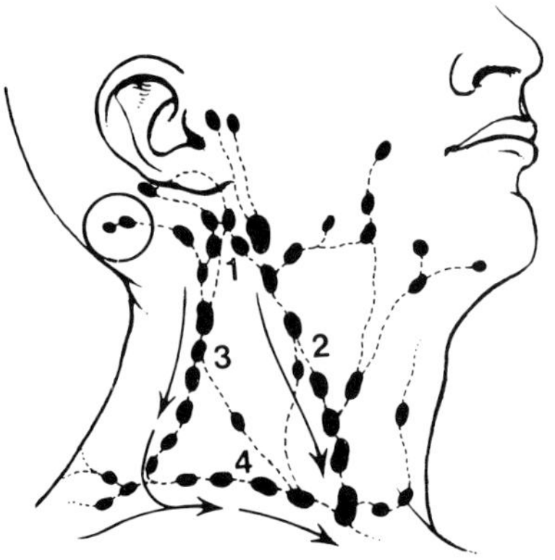

Figure 3–16. Lymph nodes of the neck: (1) the junctional nodes; (2) internal jugular chain; (3) the spinal chain; (4) the supraclavicular nodes. Encircled area represents the "nuchal nodes." (Modified from Fisch U: Lymphography of the Cervical Lymphatic System. Philadelphia, WB Saunders, 1968.)

Total Laryngopharyngectomy

Total exenteration of the larynx and pharynx is often necessary in patients with large hypopharyngeal lesions. Preservation of a small strip of mucosa that can be only tightly approximated over a nasogastric tube is to be discouraged. Not only is the patient frequently troubled later by severe dysphagia, but the cancer-excising potential of the operation is often compromised.

The surgery is approached through a modified H incision (Fig. 3–18). This provides optimal exposure and supplies ample opportunity for any necessary modification, should extension of the surgery be required. In addition, such exigencies as bilateral neck dissection or mediastinal resection can be easily provided for (Fig. 3–19).

With lesions involving the posterior wall, preliminary endoscopic assessment of pharyngeal mobility must be confirmed at surgery. If mobility is not present, posterior pharyngeal wall transgression of tumor with fixation to the spine is suspected. If resectability is in doubt, a small cutaneous incision in the line of the proposed neck dissection provides access to the normally easily dissectable retropharyngeal plane. Tumor penetration will be revealed by fixation of the pharyngeal wall to the prevertebral fascia. The pharynx in some instances may be separable from the spine, but firm dissection is required to do so. A whitish, plaquelike appearance of the muscular wall is usually

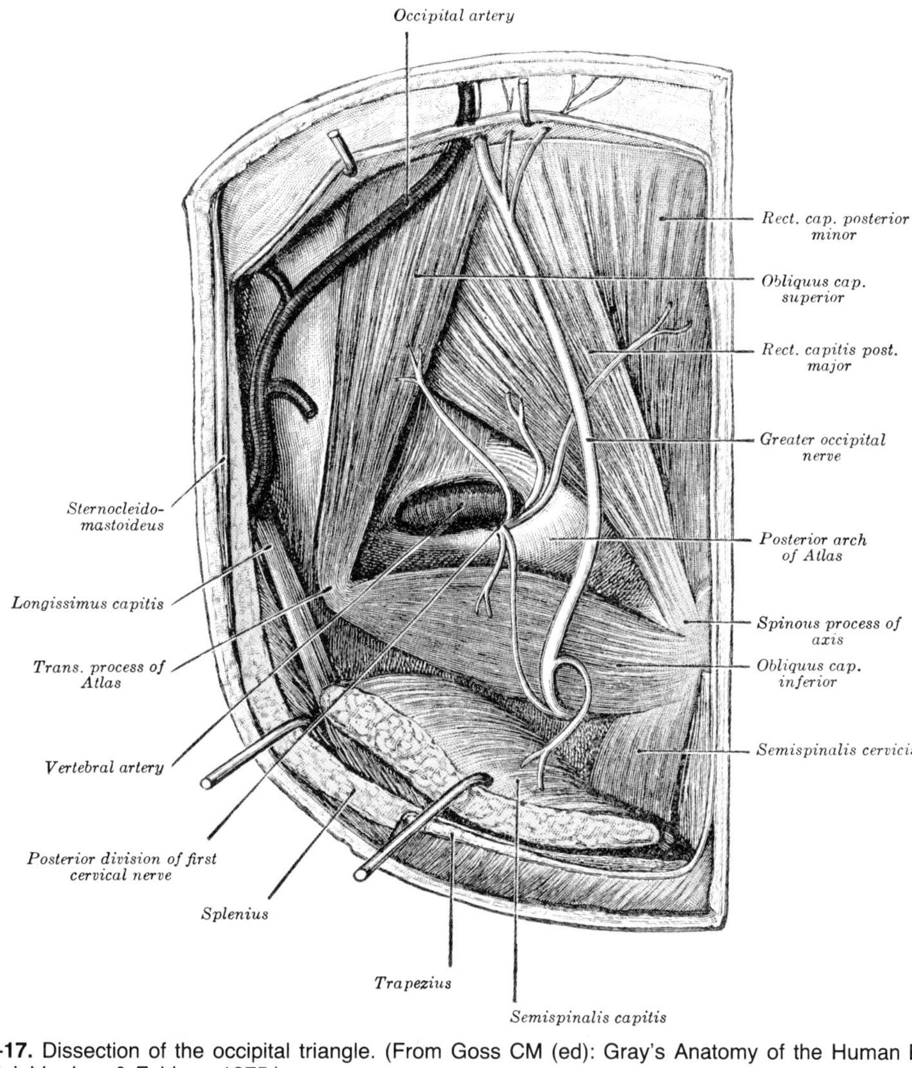

Figure 3–17. Dissection of the occipital triangle. (From Goss CM (ed): Gray's Anatomy of the Human Body, 29th ed. Philadelphia, Lea & Febiger, 1975.)

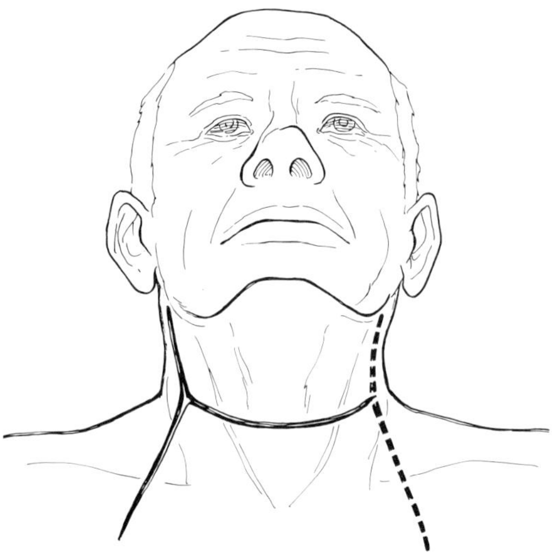

Figure 3–18. Modified H incision. Dotted line represents extension into full H incision for bilateral neck dissection.

encountered in this situation, indicating tumor penetration and therefore unresectability. Fixation of tumor to the common carotid artery similarly indicates a poor prognosis. The artery may be resected and grafted, but the eventual survival rate is poor. In one review, it was no better than 10 per cent.[26]

If the pharynx is free of fixation, the radical neck dissection is then executed. Care is taken to ensure that the radical neck bloc is pedicled on the fascia connecting it to the pharynx. It is through this layer that the lymph vessels traverse. If one remembers that the carotid artery should be located deep to this connection, the continuity will be maintained. Lifting the bloc superiorly and using finger dissection anterior to the artery helps to preserve the en bloc nature of the dissection (Fig. 3–20).

Management of the thyroid gland in laryngectomy and even radical neck dissection is somewhat controversial. Standard practice is to remove any lobe of the gland that has a palpable mass. Local extension of neoplasm into the thyroid is not uncommon, and our practice in large circumferential pharyngeal lesions is to take the entire gland. However, if the lobe on the side opposite the neck dissection is perfectly soft and that side of the neck is devoid of adenopathy, the lobe is saved.

The parathyroid glands are preserved when possible. When total thyroidectomy is done, postoperative vigilance for signs of hypocalcemia secondary to hypoparathyroidism is essential (Figs. 3–21 and 3–22). Even with preservation of one thyroid lobe, myxedema may occur because of diminished vascularity to the gland resulting from the neck dissection or from subsequent irradiation.[26]

As the superior margin of tumor resection is being delineated, the extent of involvement

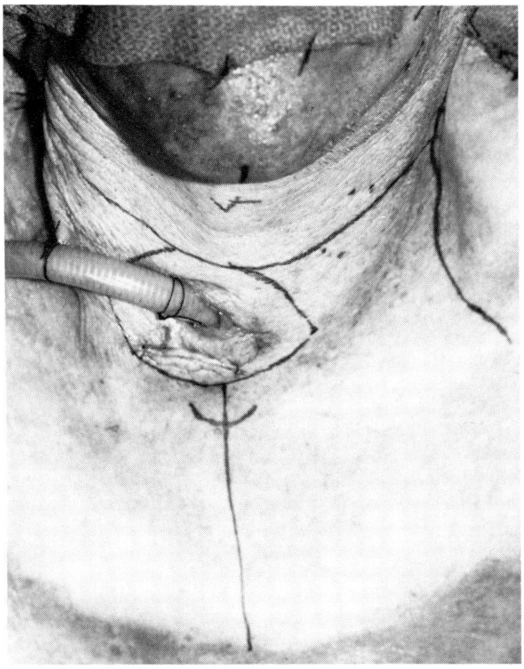

Figure 3–19. Extension for mediastinal dissection.

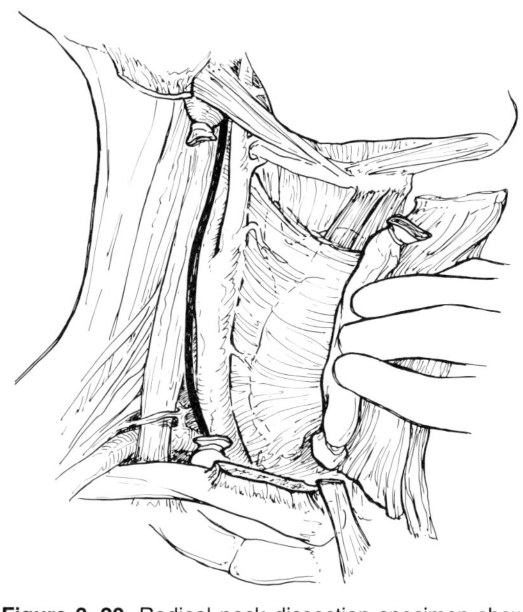

Figure 3–20. Radical neck dissection specimen showing continuity throughout its the length with the pharyngeal fascia, through which tumor may spread via the contained lymphatics.

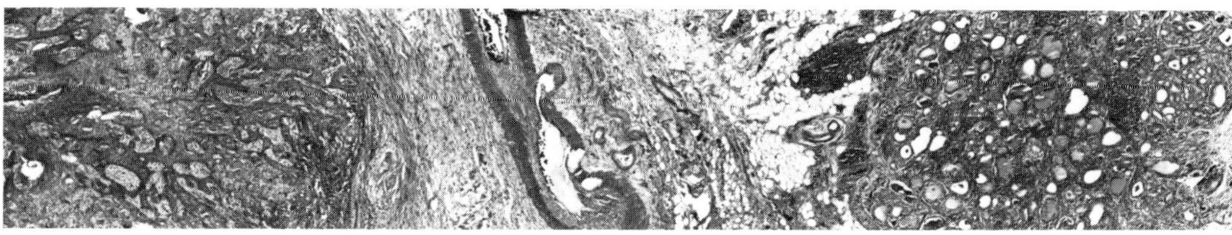

Figure 3–21. Photomicrograph illustrating microinvasion of the thyroid gland by a hypopharyngeal carcinoma. (H & E × 30)

of the tongue base must be accurately assessed. A wide margin is necessary in instances of lingual involvement because of the pernicious nature of cancer once it invades this organ. If at all possible, the hypoglossal nerves are spared (Fig. 3–23); however, this must not be at the expense of adequate tumor resection. Often the nerves can be dissected from the surface of the mylohyoid muscle and retracted superiorly. A generous margin of tongue can then be excised wtihout significantly compromising subsequent lingual function.

During the skeletonization of the larynx, the hypoglossal nerve on the side opposite the neck dissection is at risk because of its proximity to the greater cornu of the hyoid. The nerve can be protected by grasping this cornu with an Allis clamp, detaching the common tendon of the digastric muscle and the stylohyoid insertion, and then freeing up the cornu by dissection along its deep surface. The nerve may have to be taken as the subsequent excision proceeds, but this maneuver may prevent its needless sacrifice. The lower end of the laryngectomy is established on the basis of the inferior extent of the pharyngeal tumor and, if the cervical esophagus is involved, on whether or not it encroaches upon the anterior wall. Because the posterior wall of the trachea is so close to the anterior wall of the esophagus, it is necessary to take the trachea below the level of esophageal involvement. This is often a hard decision, for if the trachea must be taken low, excision of the manubrium is necessary for safe construction of the tracheostoma. In borderline situations in which the trachea is a bit short, but not so much as to mandate the excision of the manubrium, extra skin may be recruited by constructing an advancement flap of chest skin which is then slid into the upper mediastinum (Fig. 3–24).

Cervical esophageal involvement is usually an indication for mediastinal resection. Low hypopharyngeal malignancy involving the cricopharyngeus warrants an examination of the mediastinum. Mediastinoscopy will reveal evidence of nodal involvement of the anterior compartment. Large nodes usually bode ill, but microscopic adenopathy is potentially curable using a combination of resection and postoperative radiotherapy.

The oropharyngostoma is best constructed

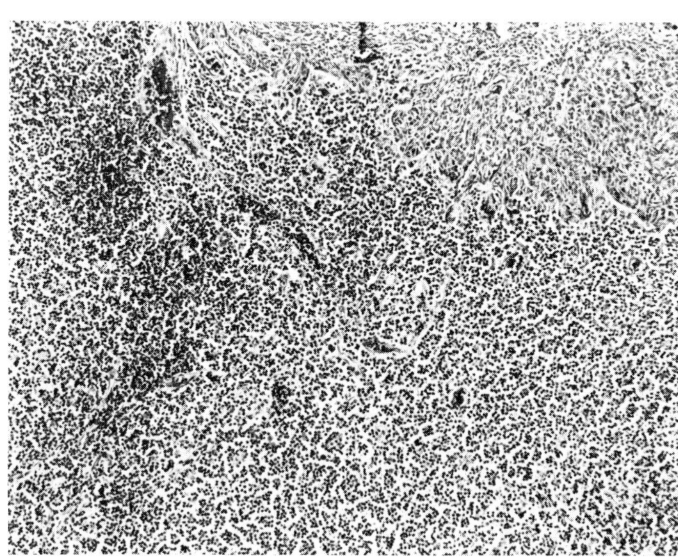

Figure 3–22. Photomicrograph showing microinvasion of a parathyroid gland by a squamous cell carcinoma of the pyriform fossa (H & E × 130).

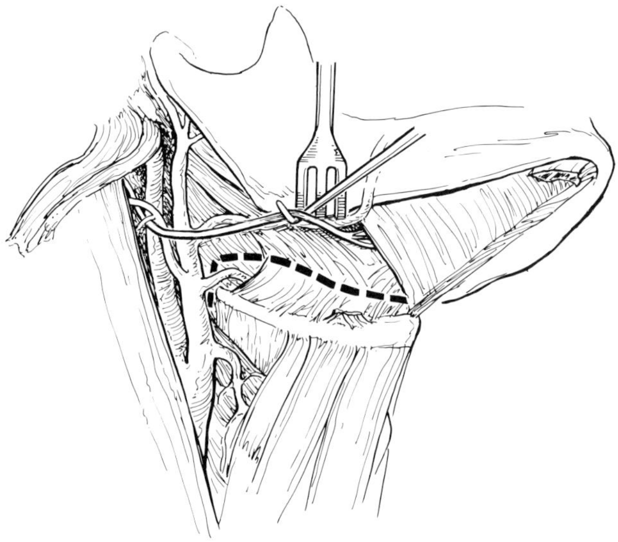

Figure 3–23. Hypoglossal nerve may be dissected from the fascia of the lateral aspect of the pharyngeal constrictors if no tumor penetration exists.

by pulling down the upper skin flap like a curtain and making a transverse incision in the middle of it. The slit opens and the anterior margin is sewn to the base of the tongue and the walls of the pharynx to the posterior skin edge (Fig. 3–25). If a substantial tongue resection is necessary, the tongue and lateral pharynx may need to be sewn to the inferior edge of the upper flap. In this instance, if the lower flap cannot be advanced to the posterior pharyngeal wall, the gap is bridged with a skin graft (Fig. 3–26).

A nasogastric tube is placed into the esophagostoma for feeding. The oropharyngostoma is packed with iodoform-soaked gauze, dressed with fluffed gauze, and held in place with a Barton-type bandage. A nasal tube attached to continuous suction is placed in the oropharynx to evacuate saliva and reduce contamination of the wound edges. The nurs-

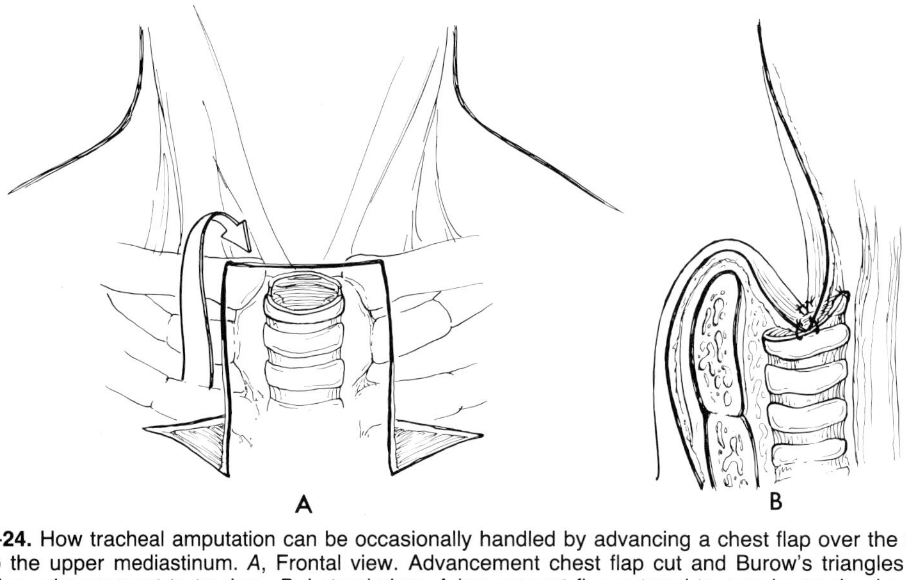

Figure 3–24. How tracheal amputation can be occasionally handled by advancing a chest flap over the manubrium sterni into the upper mediastinum. *A*, Frontal view. Advancement chest flap cut and Burow's triangles excised to facilitate flap advancement to trachea. *B*, Lateral view. Advancement flap sutured to anterior tracheal wall in upper mediastinum.

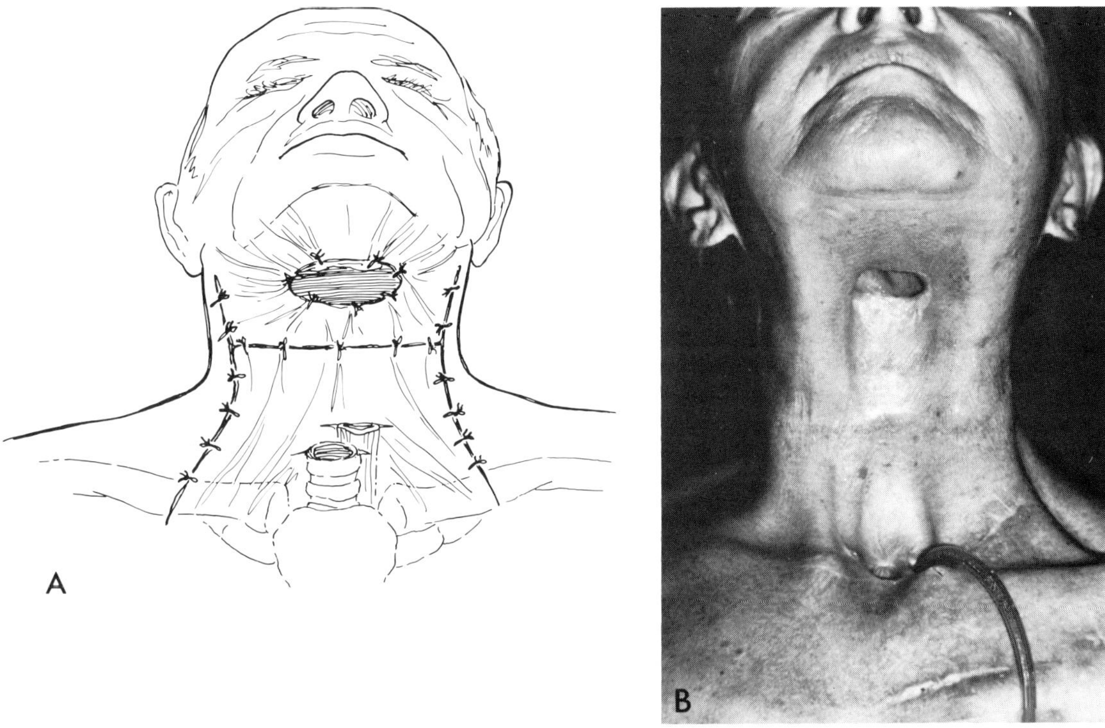

Figure 3–25. *A*, Pharyngostoma created by placing a slit in the upper flap of the modified H incision. *B*, Healed pharyngostoma ready for pharyngoesophageal reconstruction.

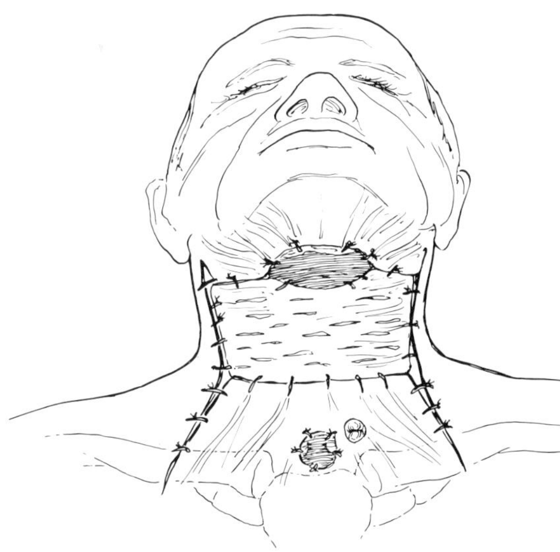

Figure 3–26. When the upper flap is of insufficient length, the gap between the posterior pharyngeal wall and the lower skin flap is bridged with a skin graft. The esophagostoma is positioned laterally and when possible superiorly to the tracheostoma.

ing staff needs to be aware of the requirement for frequent dressing changes. This is essential to avoid aspiration and subsequent pneumonia as well as to prevent local infection.

Reconstruction

Reconstruction may be either immediate or delayed. We tend to favor delay because the potential for wound complications in these debilitated patients is so great. A major wound breakdown may significantly delay the beginning of radiotherapy, and if longer than 6 weeks passes between the time of surgery and the onset of irradiation, there is doubt whether the radiotherapy will be of much value. In addition, there is considerable reluctance on the part of many radiotherapists to irradiate a dehiscent wound; however, an established pharyngocutaneous fistula or granulating wound, in the face of irradiation, will usually continue to heal, albeit more slowly. New fistulae, wound infection, or massive skin flap loss may force a delay that could result in the appearance of a tumor nodule in the wound site or a metastasis in the unoperated neck. Early reconstruction of the gullet, even with the institution of a "decompression" fistula, creates the potential for increased complications.

In the well-nourished, younger patient who has not received prior irradiation, immediate reconstruction can be done. We have found the most effective technique to be that described by Bakamjiam,[28] in which a medially pedicled chest flap based on the perforating branches of the internal mammary artery is used. There is preferably a delay of 3 weeks, although because of the exigencies of the tumor in many cases, this delay often cannot be done. If a delay is possible, it is necessary to raise only the deltoid portion of skin and incise the flap's outline (Fig. 3–27).[29] In most instances, especially in an otherwise healthy patient, an immediately rotated flap survives without major complication.

The flap is elevated and tubed on itself with the cutaneous surface facing inside (Fig. 3–28). Interrupted, everting, absorbable sutures are used to tube the skin. A second layer in the subcutis is done using a vertical mattress suture tied loosely enough to avoid vascular compromise at the wound edges. The distal end of the skin tube is anastomosed end-to-end to the oropharyngostoma. A double layer of sutures will ensure a watertight closure. The esophagus is sutured into the back surface of the flap as an end-to-side anastomosis, and the flap is tubed for a short distance beyond this. The bottom end of the deltopectoral flap is left open and serves for decompression. The cervical skin flaps are closed over the reconstructed gullet, and the feeding tube is maintained through the enclosed aspect of the chest flap. Any exposed raw area is skin-grafted.

In the delayed cases, it is very simple and convenient to employ the skin of the anterior neck for the inner lining. Despite the detrimental effects of radiation therapy, this skin stands up well to the demands of a pharyngoesophageal lining. The method used is based on the time-honored technique of Wookey.[30] The surgery is delayed until 4 to 6 weeks have passed from the time of cessation of radiotherapy. A flap is designed with

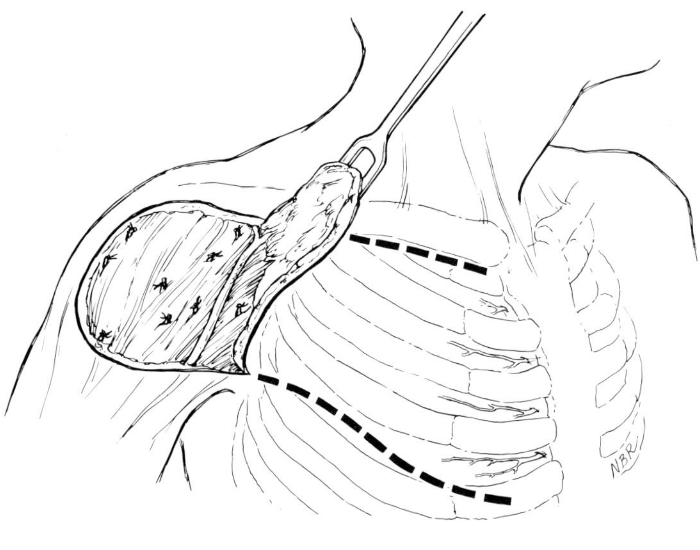

Figure 3–27. In delaying the deltopectoral flap, only the portion of the flap over the deltoid muscle—that part which is supplied by the musculocutaneous perforators—need be elevated. The rest of the flap, which is supplied in the main by the perforating branches of the internal mammary arteries in the 2nd, 3rd, and 4th intercostal spaces, is simply outlined.

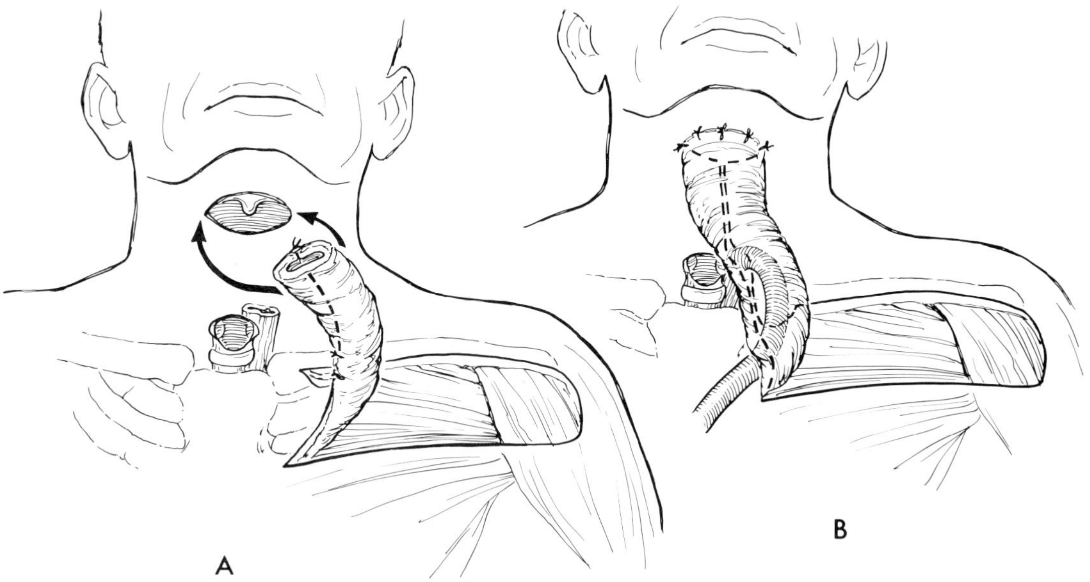

Figure 3–28. *A*, The deltopectoral flap is tubed using simple everting sutures. A watertight closure is accomplished with a second layer of loosely placed vertical mattress sutures in the subcutis. *B*, The deltoid end of the tube is sutured end-to-end to the pharynx. The medial portion of the tube is anastomosed end-to-side to the esophagus, with the esophageal anastomosis placed in the back surface of the flap. The flap is tubed for a short distance beyond this anastomosis. The nasogastric tube is placed through this site, which also serves for decompression.

its center in the midline of the neck (Fig. 3–29). It must be sufficiently wide when tubed so that it will give an internal diameter of adequate dimension. As the flap is elevated, greater length is generally taken on the side without the neck dissection. As the skin is peeled off the carotid artery on the neck-dissected side, the previously placed dermis graft will be seen to have become a layer of fibrous tissue. An easy dissection plane is generally found between this layer and the skin. Once the flaps have been elevated on either side, they are approximated one to the other. Special attention must be paid to the end near the tracheostoma where the skin edge must be elevated enough so that the skin flap providing the outside layer can be approximated to the cutaneous tissue adjacent to the tracheostoma (Fig. 3–29*B*).

The outside lining utilizes a regional skin flap: either deltopectoral or nape of the neck. The latter is preferred in women because it avoids deforming the breast (Fig. 3–30). The deltopectoral flap, being more reliable and less fraught with complications, is preferred in men. The nape-of-neck flap must be delayed in at least three stages (see Chapter 1, p. 33) because of the tenuous nature of its blood supply. The occipital arteries, the major nutrient vessels of this flap, can successfully supply a substantial flap of skin if the procedure is sufficiently delayed. An advantage of this flap is that there is no necessity to return a pedicle, since the flap slides around the neck like a scarf. On the other hand, the deltopectoral flap pedicle requires a return 3 weeks or more following the definitive procedure.

These reconstructed gullets serve as excellent food conduits and can be used for esophageal speech. The long-term complications include the occasional case of stricture and, in males, hirsutism (Fig. 3–31) of the flap lining. Hirsutism is a vexing problem and can be eventually eliminated by repeated mechanical epilation through a cervical esophagoscope and laser ablation of the hair follicles. A stricture is usually easily managed with bougienage and only rarely requires revision.

Management of Lesions of the Cervical Esophagus

A precise therapeutic approach to cervical esophageal carcinoma remains difficult to delineate. A large body of opinion concurs with that of Resano,[31] who believes that whereas malignancies of the lower third of the esophagus are amenable to surgical extirpation, those in the cervical part are best managed

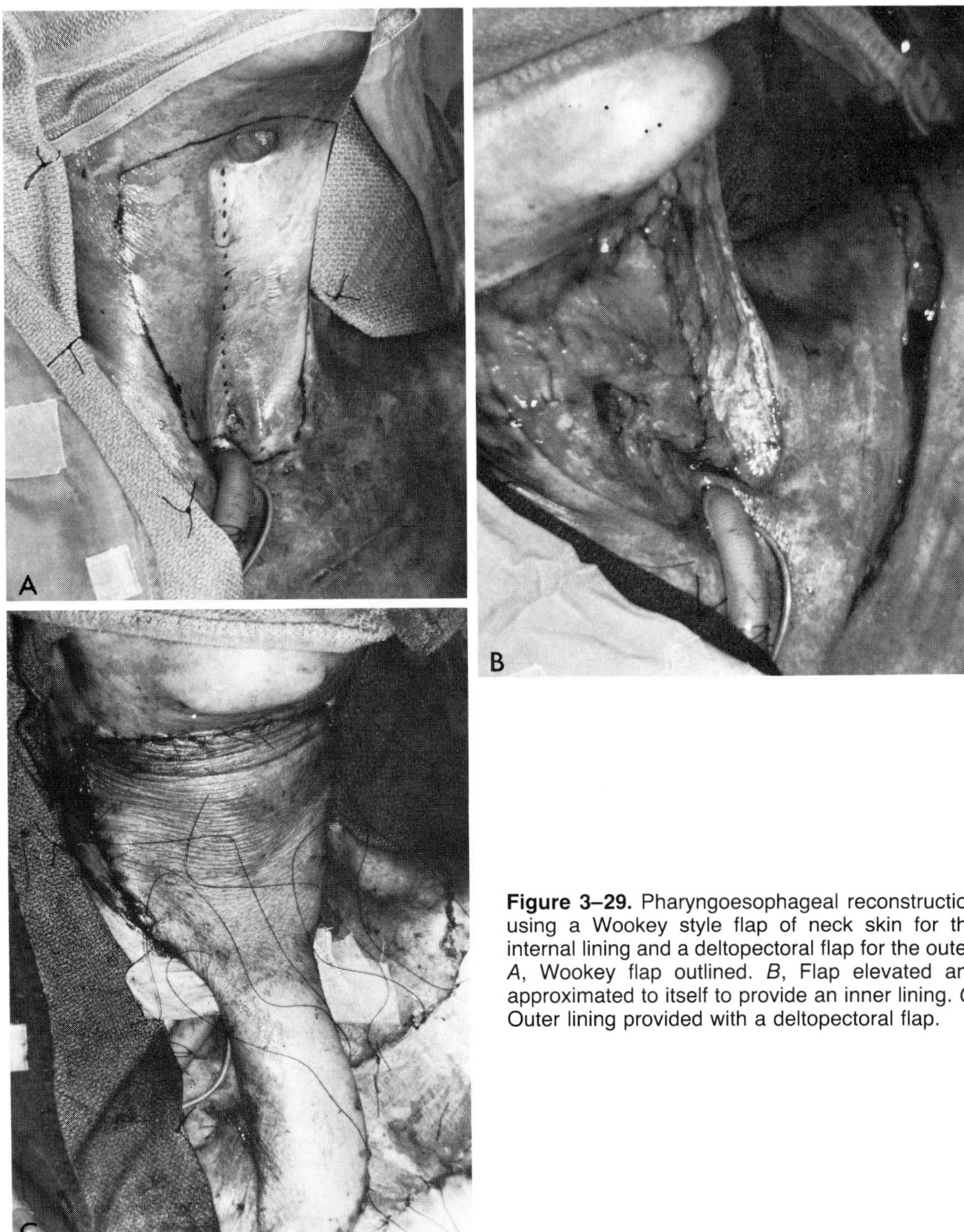

Figure 3–29. Pharyngoesophageal reconstruction using a Wookey style flap of neck skin for the internal lining and a deltopectoral flap for the outer. *A*, Wookey flap outlined. *B*, Flap elevated and approximated to itself to provide an inner lining. *C*, Outer lining provided with a deltopectoral flap.

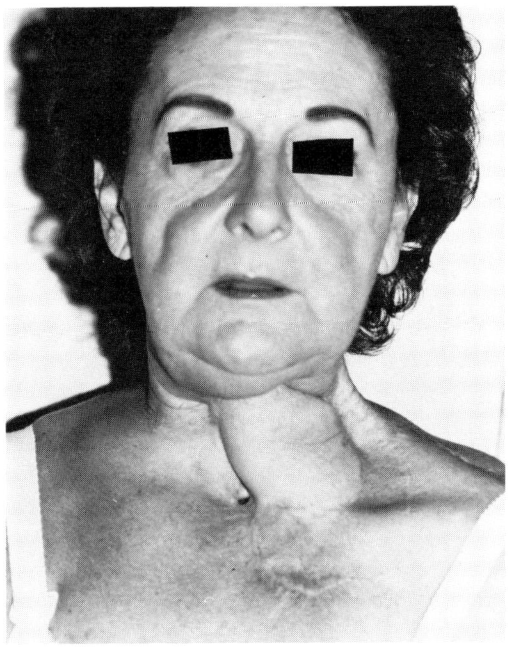

Figure 3–30. Zovikian flap used to resurface Wookey type reconstruction of the pharyngoesophagus. Although entailing a many-staged delay, this flap is cosmetically more acceptable in women.

by radiotherapy. The frequent problem of late diagnosis, with the tumor remaining undetected until there is transmural penetration and it is already invading the larynx, trachea, carotid arteries, or spinal column, leaves only a few patients presenting with potentially resectable lesions. Tracheal and laryngeal penetration complicate the surgical attack and lower the survival rate, but do not render the lesion unresectable. Exophytic lesions tend to have a more favorable prognosis than endophytic ones. We heartily agree with the comment of Parker[32] that a search for cure in those patients with potentially resectable lesions must not be abandoned because of the air of pessimism that commonly pervades the therapeutic considerations in these cases.

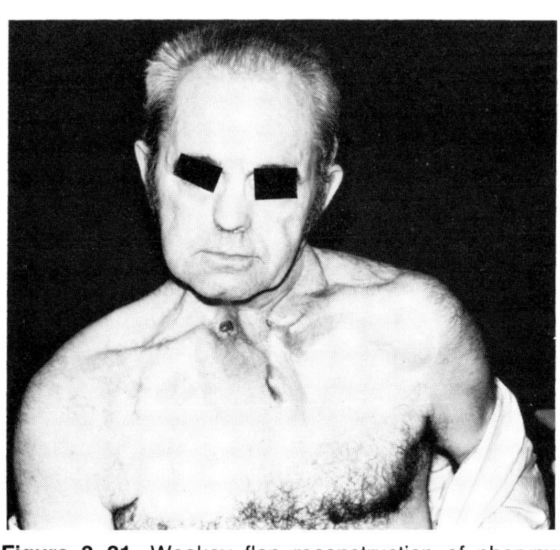

Figure 3–31. Wookey flap reconstruction of pharynx covered with Zovikian flap. This patient was exceedingly hirsute, and the reconstructed pharynx was occasionally obstructed by hair, requiring depilation through an esophagoscope.

The 5-year cure rate of 25 per cent following radical surgical extirpation is little improved since the report of Mustard[19] more than 20 years ago. Laryngopharyngocervical esophagectomy is the mainstay of treatment. The efficacy of postoperative irradiation has yet to stand the test of time. In the past, sporadic reports of a few random cases revealed no clear indication of its value.

When the cervical esophagus is involved with tumor, the resection should extend into the upper thorax. Often this cannot be adequately achieved without exposure of the mediastinum. Tumor extension near the junction with the thoracic esophagus and beyond is best treated by total esophagectomy.

Total esophagectomy is a procedure of substantial magnitude that carries a significant mortality rate. It probably should not be undertaken in the elderly or debilitated patient. Irradiation therapy in these individuals is probably the best choice despite the poor tumor control rate. However, the chronically starved, protein-depleted patient can be improved greatly when a high-calorie diet augmented by parenteral hyperalimentation is instituted.

Reconstruction often poses a problem because of the extensive distance a piece of gut must be transposed in order to achieve an upper anastomosis. The upper resection margin is often as high as the lower oropharynx. A piece of gut, either colon or jejunum, must stretch from there to the stomach. A common problem is sloughing of the cervical end, which can be prevented by tubing the cardiac end of the stomach and either anastomosing it directly to the pharynx or bringing it out onto the chest. If the latter course is chosen, the cervical portion of the gullet can be reconstructed with a tubed deltopectoral flap (Fig. 3–32*A*). At a second stage, the two tubes are hooked up and the patient is allowed to swallow when healing is complete, usually 10 days later (Fig. 3–32*B*).

Pharyngocervical esophageal reconstruction can also be accomplished by utilizing the pectoralis major musculocutaneous flap. The

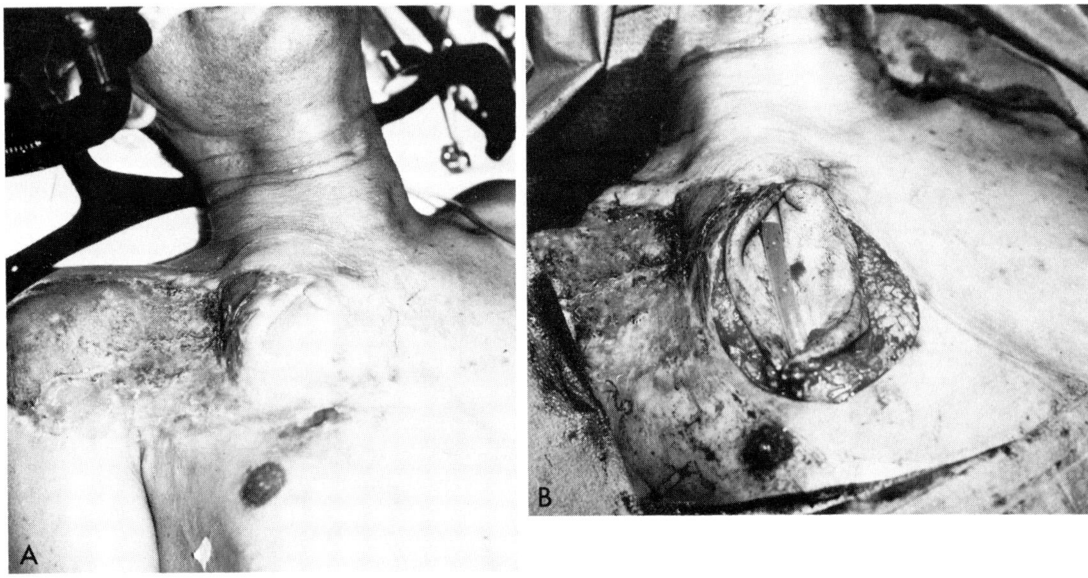

Figure 3–32. *A*, This patient had a deltopectoral flap anastomosed to the upper hypopharynx. Excision of the clavicular head avoids an acute angulation of the flap as it proceeds into the neck. The cardiac end of the stomach was tubed and brought subcutaneously into close approximation with the sternal end of the deltopectoral flap. *B*, In the final stage, the skin bridge between the lower end of the deltopectoral flap and the transposed gastric tube is tubed on itself and the defect covered with a local rotation flap.

disadvantage of this flap is its great bulk, which may be so extreme as to require additional skin to effect cervical cutaneous closure. However, the blood supply is excellent and it obviates the need for a second stage in most instances. For the sake of safety in a somewhat debilitated patient or if the integrity of the anastomosis is in doubt, a decompression fistula is advised. The use of this flap is not so problematic in slender males, in whom the amount of subcutaneous fat is scarce and the pectoralis major musculature spare.

The pectoralis major musculocutaneous flap is especially useful in patients who postoperatively developed a stricture. The stenotic area is transected and the gullet split in its longitudinal axis. The pectoralis major flap is then inserted in the form of a gusset, greatly widening the area of stenosis (Fig. 3–33).

The flap may be further used in cases of tracheoesophageal fistula. A fistulous tract may arise in a number of ways. It may have been placed deliberately as a tracheopharyngeal shunt for the establishment of voice, as in the Staffieri laryngectomy, or for the placement of a voice prosthesis such as the Singer-Blom valve or the Panje button. Less commonly it may result from traumatic perforation brought about by the swallowing of a sharp foreign body by a postlaryngectomy patient. These fistulae, if they cause aspiration, must be closed. This is usually the case in the situation of a traumatically induced fistula.

In tracheoesophageal fistulas the connection occurs between the membranous posterior trachea and the anterior wall of the pharyngoesophageal segment. Adequate, well-vascularized soft tissue should be interposed between the two. Because these patients have often undergone radiation therapy, fibrosis and lack of easy dissection planes are common findings. To obtain adequate exposure of the fistula and sufficient surgical control inferiorly often requires a modified mediastinal approach. The removal of the head of one clavicle and a limited sternal resection are usually all that is necessary to permit adequate exposure. The pectoralis major flap is sutured into the esophageal defect once its edges have been freshened. The epithelium faces the esophageal lumen, and the muscle side faces the trachea. Tracheal wall closure is accomplished either by primary approximation, if this can be done free of tension, or by application of a patch of split-thickness skin. The muscle bulk of the flap's pedicle fills in the dead space left

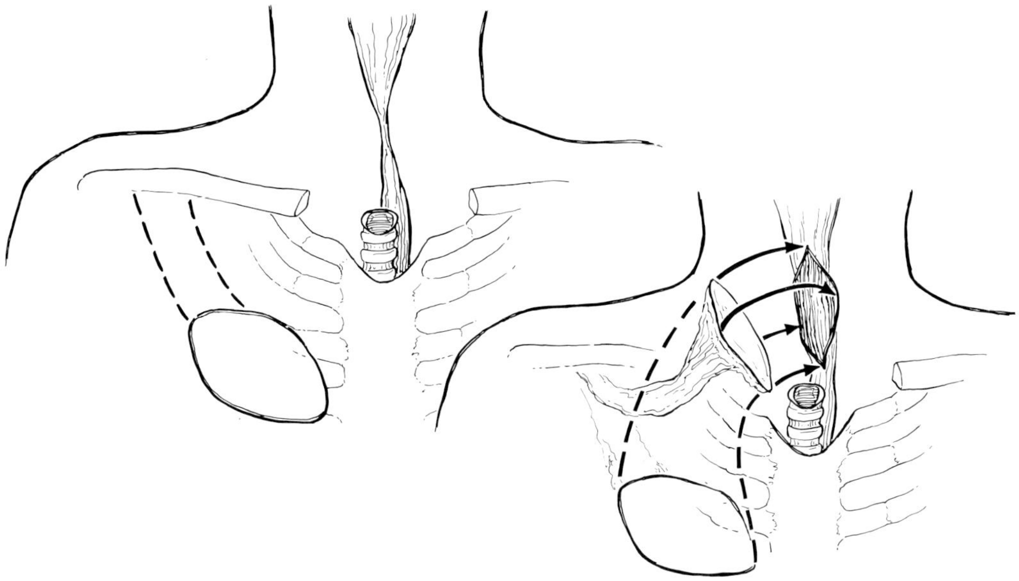

Figure 3–33. A pectoralis major flap is sewn into the longitudinally split stenotic area in the pharyngoesophagus like a gusset.

by the clavicular-sternal resection. The neck wound is closed, a nasogastric tube passed, and oral feeding begun in 2 weeks.

Mediastinal Resection

The extent of a mediastinal resection is predicated upon the degree of involvement of the trachea (Fig. 3–34). If a cervical esophageal malignancy invades the overlying trachea and subglottic larynx, the margin of resection necessitates a very low tracheostomy. In order for the amputated trachea to approximate the skin, a resection of a portion of manubrium is required. This resection differs from that used for a stomal recurrence following laryngectomy in that no skin is excised. The problem is that the trachea is too short to stretch over the manubrium in order to be sutured to the skin. An advancement flap on the chest can be made and slid into the uppermost mediastinum in the marginal case, but in most instances manubrial resection is necessary.

The problem with resecting the manubrium

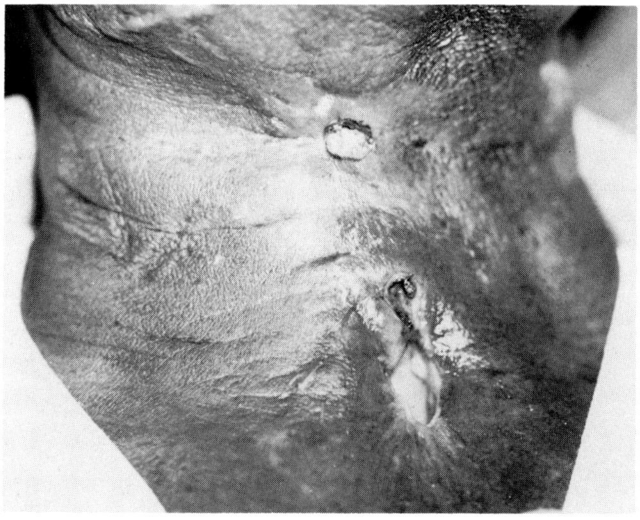

Figure 3–34. Patient with a stomal recurrence following laryngectomy. In this case the tumor invaded the underlying esophagus, necessitating pharyngocervical esophagectomy.

is the danger incurred by the subsequent proximity of the trachea to the innominate artery. The constant wearing away of the arterial wall by the trachea may result in tracheoinnominate fistula or rupture of the artery into the mediastinal space. The frequency of this complication stimulated Sisson[33] to develop protection for the artery by the interposition of pectoralis major muscle flaps, and adoption of this step resulted in a vastly improved survival rate.

The incision extends vertically from the inferior limb of an apron flap or from the horizontal part of a modified H incision (Fig. 3–18). The incision extends about 2 cm past the angle of Louis. Care is taken to identify and clamp the anterior jugular venous arch as it passes through Burn's space, because it forms a ready source of air emboli.

The area of tumor involvement of the stoma, if a stomal recurrence is present, or of overlying skin in the case of pharyngeal tumor, is encircled by a wide margin of healthy skin (Fig. 3–35). In most cervical esophageal or subglottic cancers, skin penetration is uncommon. The superior margin of resection of the pharynx (if it is involved) is established and the bloc dissected inferiorly. Residual thyroid gland, if any, is included as the dissection plane carries down along the plane of both carotid sheaths. Once dissection has proceeded as far into the root of the neck as possible, attention is turned to entering the mediastinum.

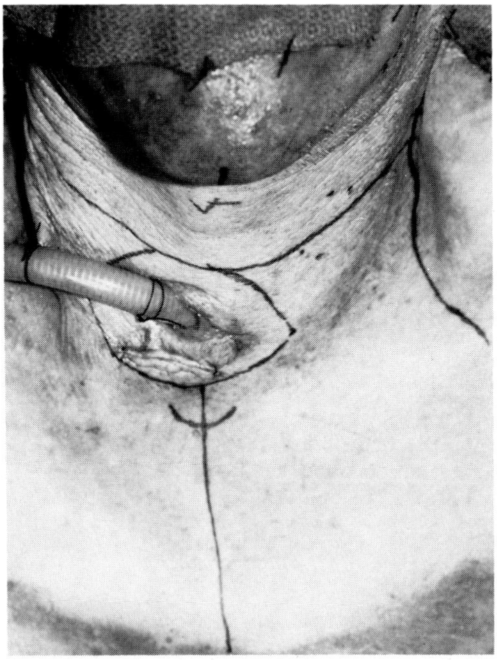

Figure 3–35. Area of proposed excision of skin involvement and mediastinal resection is marked out.

The periosteum is cut in the midsternal line to the required level of bony resection (Fig. 3–36*A*). Unlike the mediastinal resection for thyroid cancer, the manubrium is not simply split, but removed, in order to get the necessary prolapse of skin down to the trachea. The periosteal incision in the midline of the sternum is carried out laterally over the sternoclavicular joints across the clavicular heads and about a quarter of the way along the anterior surface of the medial aspect of the bone. The greatest hazard in the clavicular resection is inadvertent rupture of the subclavian vessels lying just deep to the bone. The most effective safeguard in preventing this is preservation of the clavicular periosteum. Some time should be spent in careful dissection of this layer on the bone's deep surface, creating a wide tunnel in order to insert a malleable retractor (Fig. 3–36*B*). An electric saw is used to sever the bone up to the last few millimeters of the deep cortical surface, which is then finished off with an osteotome. The cut surface is grasped with bone-holding forceps, the remaining deep periosteum stripped, and the sternoclavicular joint separated (Fig. 3–36*C*).

Once both clavicular heads have been removed, the heavy layer of periosteum on the deep surface of the manubrium is dissected. As previously mentioned, as the manubrium is being cut, this stout layer provides protection for the underlying great vessels. A malleable retractor is slid between this layer and the overlying bone while the electric saw is used to excise the manubrium from the first rib and the remaining sternum (Fig. 3–36*D*). Once the bone is removed, this fascial layer is excised en bloc with the underlying fat, thymus, and mediastinal lymphatics (Fig. 3–36*E*).

As the dissection proceeds more deeply, the left innominate vein is often seen crossing the field from left to right, obscuring the dissection. It is cross-clamped with Mixter clamps, divided, and suture ligated (Fig. 3–36*F*). Some postoperative swelling of the left arm is anticipated, but this dissipates somewhat with time. Soft tissue is stripped superiorly off the trachea, with care taken not to penetrate the pleurae on the lateral boundaries of the mediastinal space. Bleeding must be meticulously controlled by ligature or cautery, as a mediastinal collection of blood will

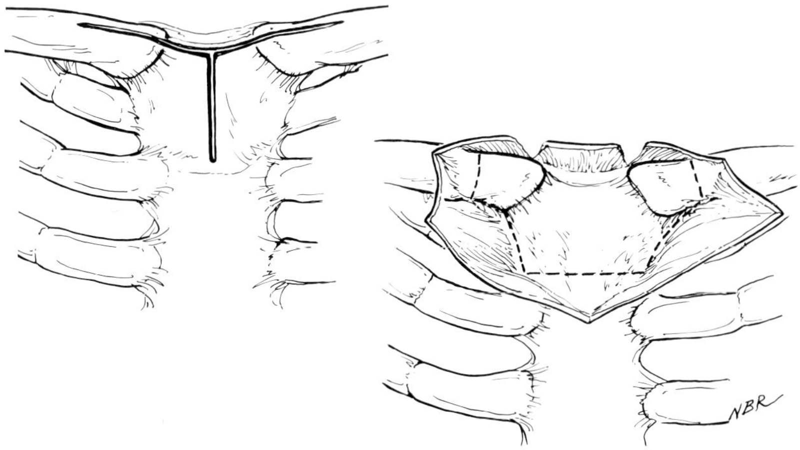

A

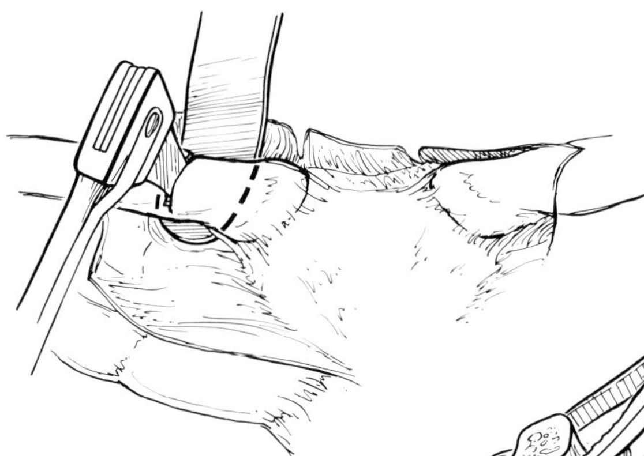

B

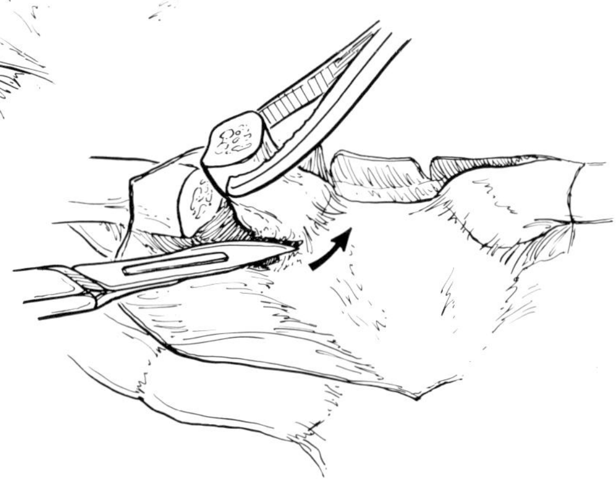

C

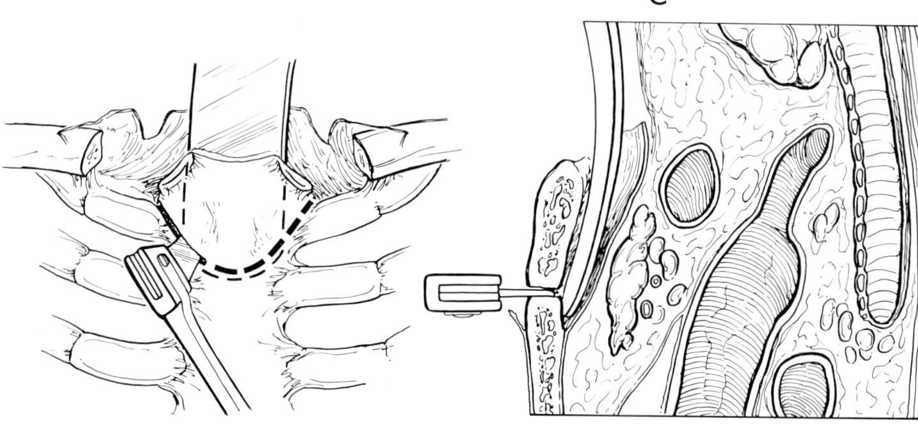

D

Figure 3–36. Mediastinal resection. *A*, The periosteum of the manubrium and clavicular heads is incised and dissected widely. Dashed line represents the proposed bony resection. *B*, A malleable retractor is inserted under the clavicular periosteum to prevent damage to the underlying vessels. *C*, The clavicle is grasped with bone-holding forceps and the sternoclavicular joint is separated by sharp dissection. *D*, A wide malleable retractor is inserted between the manubrium and its thick periosteum. A power saw or osteotome is used to remove the manubrium down to the level of the 2nd rib.

Illustration continued on following page

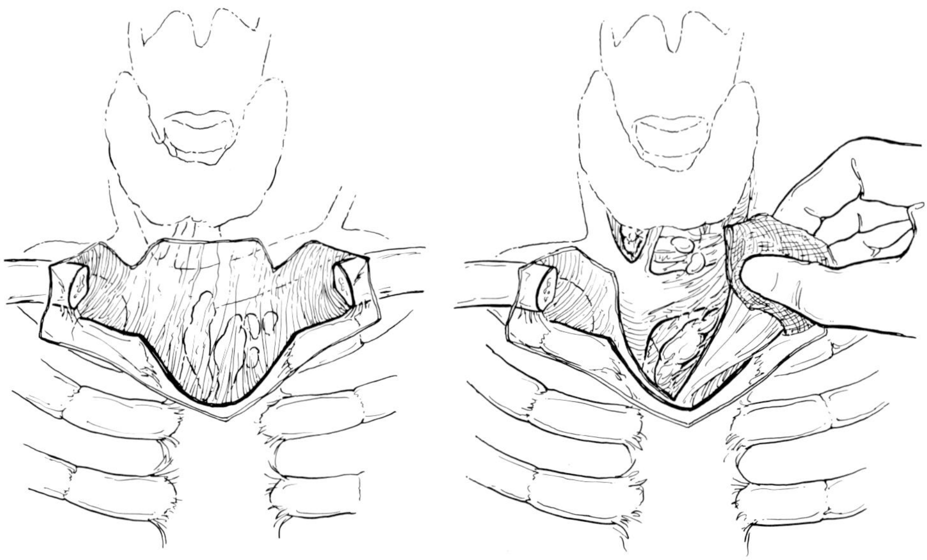

E

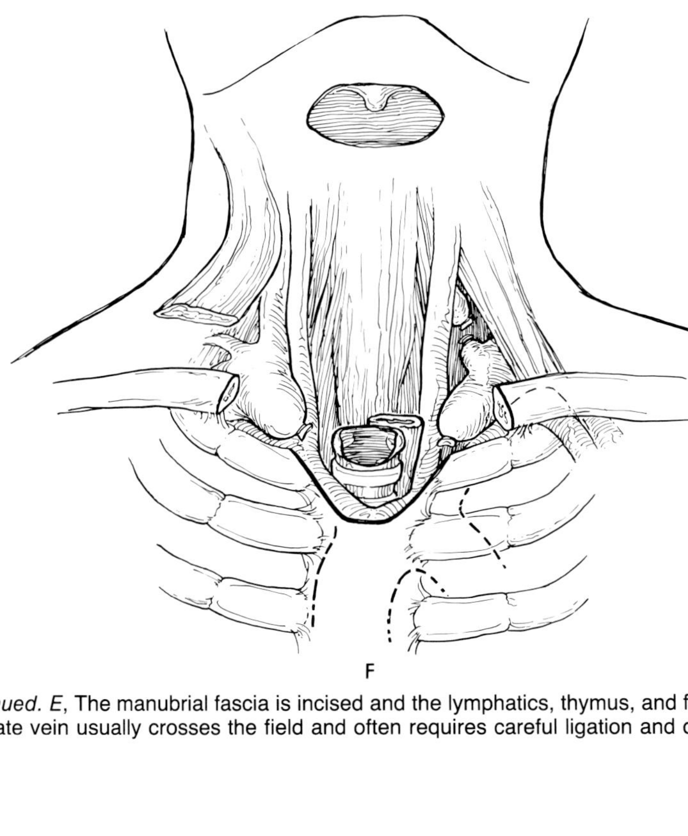

F

Figure 3–36 *Continued. E*, The manubrial fascia is incised and the lymphatics, thymus, and fatty tissue are removed. *F*, The left innominate vein usually crosses the field and often requires careful ligation and division.

often be substantial before it produces sufficient symptoms for detection. Subsequent infection of a mediastinal collection is disastrous.

The dissection continues until the site for the establishment of the inferior resection margin is delineated. The trachea and esophagus are then amputated, and the bloc is stripped superiorly and then removed (Fig. 3–37).

A substantial flap of pectoralis major muscle is now developed to interpose between the trachea and the innominate artery. The overlying skin is undermined, and a muscle flap pedicled on the internal mammary arterial perforators is fashioned. It is vital to preserve the superficial fascia of the muscle in order to safeguard the vascular supply. The muscle flap is elevated, usually with facility from the chest wall, and its distal end severed. Hemostasis with suture ligatures is the best method of stemming hemorrhage from the amputated muscle stump. The flap is turned 180 degrees into the mediastinal defect (Fig. 3–38*A*); this not only affords innominate arterial protection but also fills in the dead space in the mediastinum left by the resection. Absorbable sutures are used to approximate the muscle to the trachea and the sternal periosteum.

The trachea can now be approximated to the skin, keeping in mind that the skin must be brought in a long way to reach the tracheal

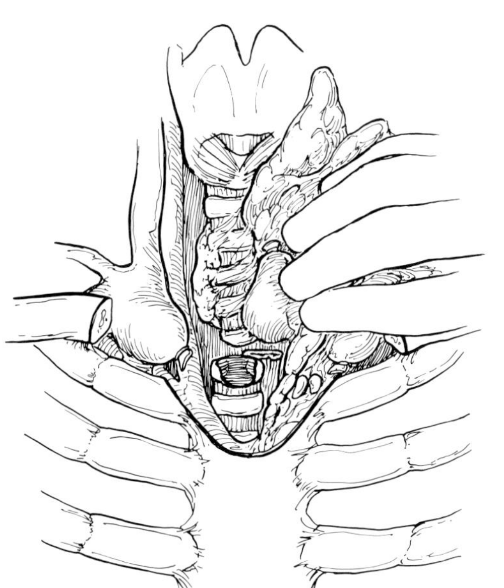

Figure 3–37. The trachea and esophagus are amputated and the mediastinal contents dissected superiorly.

stump. With the skin excision necessitated by tumor involvement, the closure requires the advancement of a skin flap. A bipedicled skin flap may be elevated and slid superiorly, while the raw area inferiorly is covered with a split-thickness skin graft; alternatively, a thoracoacromial flap (Fig. 3–38*B*) may be used. The stay sutures anchoring the trachea must be numerous and snugly cinched. When the skin is not involved with tumor, a short laryngectomy tube may be needed to keep the stoma open, especially in the early postoperative period, since in most cases of cervical esophageal cancer sufficient neck skin is usually present to achieve stomal closure.

The wound must be adequately drained, preferably with suction drainage. Suction tubes are placed under the neck flaps, the tunnel for the muscle flap, and the mediastinum.

When the skin is excised from the region of the tracheostoma, as in the operation for stomal recurrence, the skin deficit as well as innominate artery protection can be accomplished with a pectoralis major musculocutaneous flap. The muscle portion of the flap and the pedicle are interposed between the trachea and the innominate artery, filling in the dead space left by the resection. The stoma is made in the center or inferior third of the flap by placing a stab incision, taking care not to injure the flap's nutrient artery (Fig. 3–39*A*). The trachea is sutured to the skin in a circumferential fashion, but all the sutures are tagged and left untied until the last step. The endotracheal tube is then withdrawn, the trachea pulled through the stab incision in the flap, the tube reintroduced, and the sutures tied (Fig. 3–39*B*). The skin tends to pucker over the muscle down to the trachea. A laryngectomy tube often has to be worn permanently following this procedure.

For pharyngeal and cervical esophageal tumors, primary reconstruction should be done at this stage. If the pharyngeal excision is low, a stomach pull-up may be safely done. However, a deltopectoral flap is most commonly used. It is tubed and advanced to the pharynx, where an end-to-end anastomosis is done (Fig. 3–40). The thoracic esophagus is sutured end-to-side, with the anastomosis made on the deep surface of the tubed flap. A decompression fistula is created with the end of the flap onto the chest. This can be closed with local flaps about 3 to 6 weeks postoperatively.

Text continued on page 92

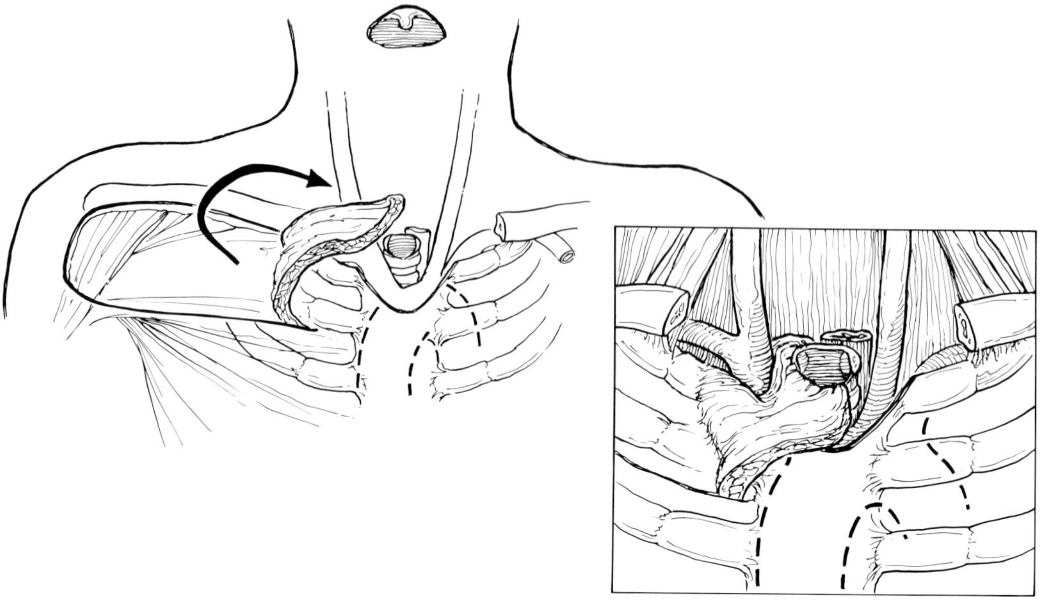

A

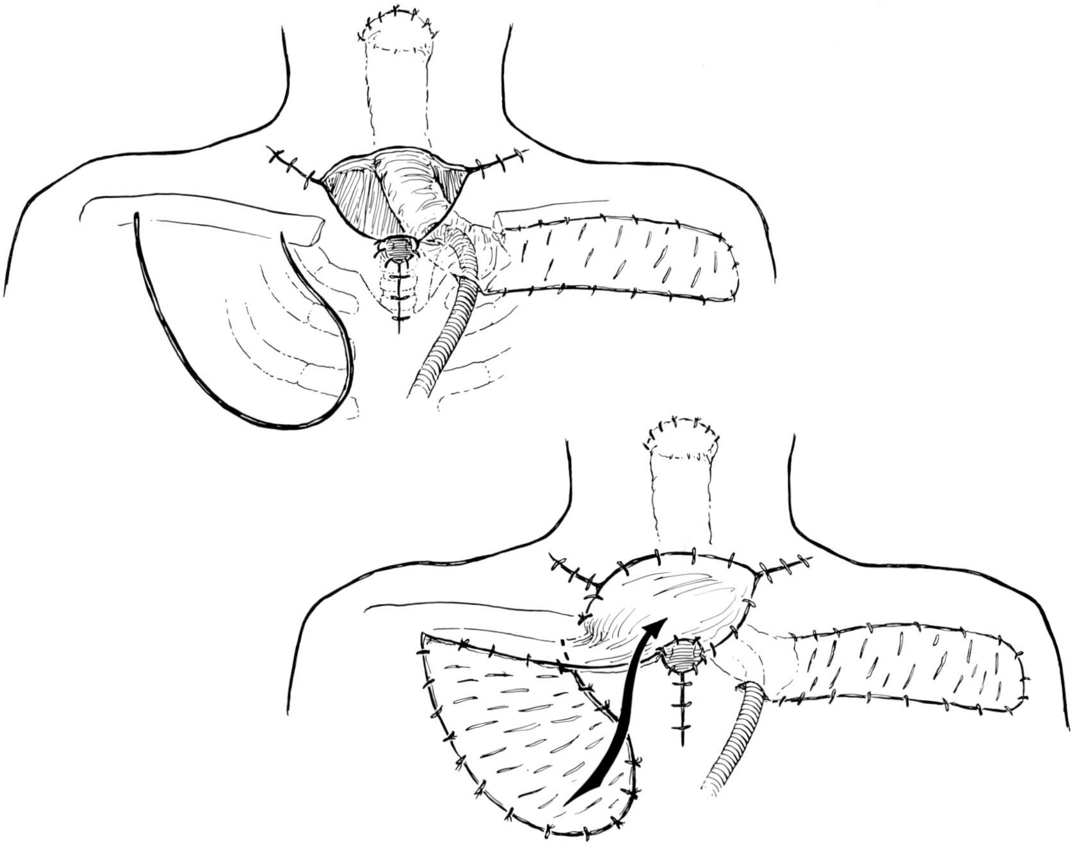

B

Figure 3–38. *A*, A medially based pectoralis major muscle flap is amputated laterally, hemostasis in the base secured with suture ligatures, and the flap turned 180 degrees into the wound. *B*, A thoracoacromial chest flap is transposed to achieve closure. The defect is covered with a split-thickness skin graft.

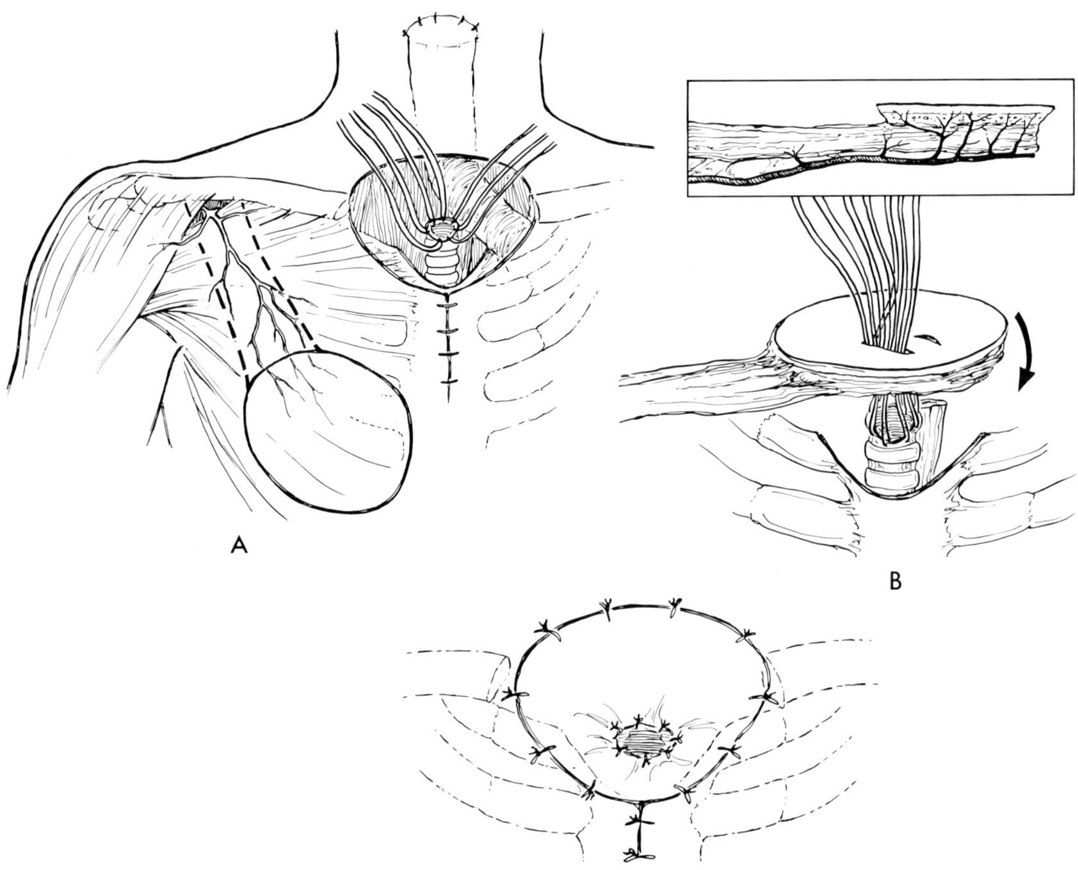

Figure 3–39. Pectoralis major musculocutaneous flap used to replace the skin deficit left by the resection and provide protection for the innominate artery. *A*, The flap is elevated and a stab incision is made in the axis of the flap's nutrient vessel. *B*, Muscle of the flap is interposed between the innominate artery and the trachea. The tracheal stump is pulled through the flap and approximated to the flap skin. *C*, Flap in place.

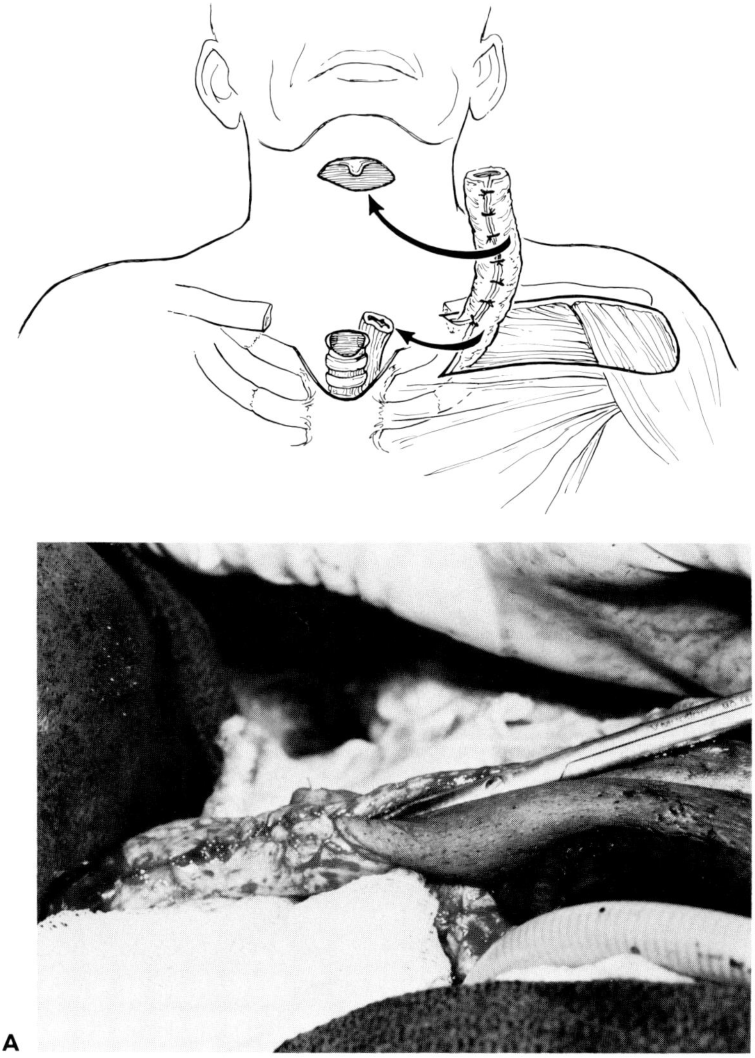

A

Figure 3–40. Pharyngoesophageal reconstruction in conjunction with mediastinal resection. *A*, A deltopectoral flap is tubed and approximated to the pharynx.

Illustration continued on opposite page

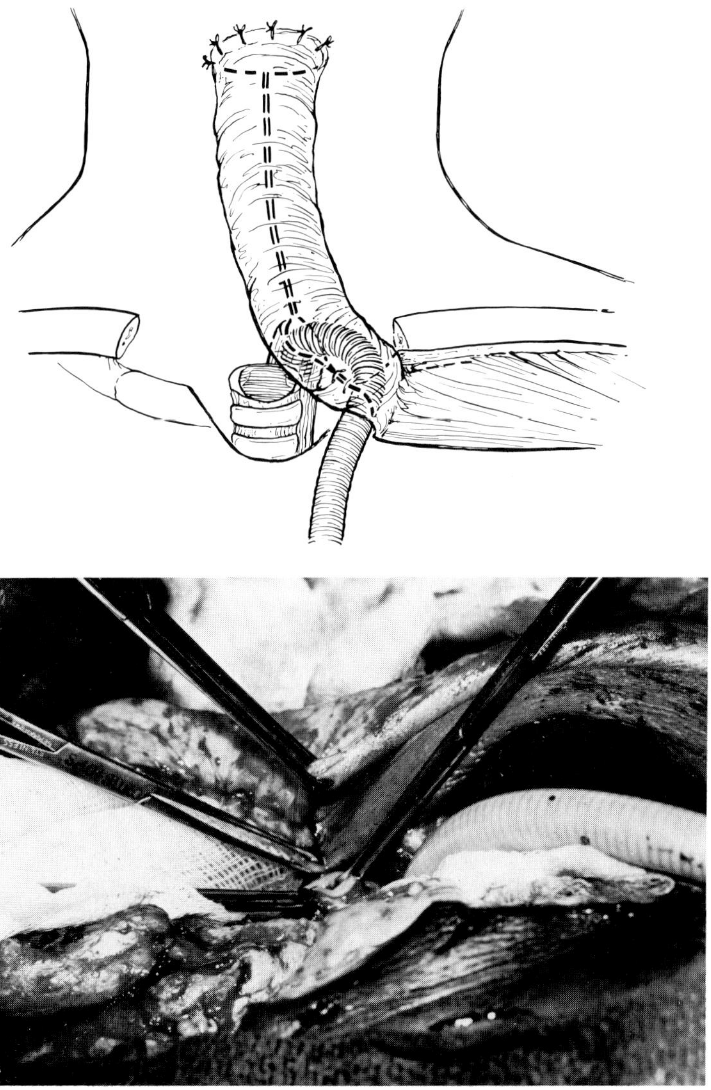

B

Figure 3–40 *Continued. B*, Anastomosis is completed in an end-to-side manner to the upper thoracic esophagus in the mediastinum. The nasogastric tube is brought out through the sternal end of the deltopectoral flap.

References

1. McComb WS, Healey JE, McGraw JP, et al: Hypopharynx and cervical esophagus. *In* McComb WS, Fletcher GH (eds): Cancer of the Head and Neck. Baltimore, Williams & Wilkins, 1967, pp 213–240.
2. Gray H: Anatomy of the human body. *In* Goss CM (ed): The Lymphatic System, 29th ed. Philadelphia, Lea & Febiger, 1975, pp 744–745.
3. Postlethwait PW: Surgery of the Esophagus. New York, Appleton-Century-Crofts, 1979, pp 554–580.
4. Rouvière H: Anatomie des lymphatiques de l'homme. Paris, Masson et Cie, 1932, 115.
5. Sakata K: On the lymphatics of the esophagus and on the regional lymph nodes with consideration of metastasis of the carcinoma. Mitt Grenzgeb Med Chir 11:634, 1903.
6. Sisson AA, Bytell DE, Becker SP: Mediastinal dissection—1976: indications and newer techniques. Laryngoscope 87:751, 1977.
7. Mast WR, Jafek BW: Mediastinal anatomy for the endoscopist. Arch Otolaryngol 101:596, 1975.
8. Conley J: Cancer of the pharynx. *In* Concepts in Head and Neck Surgery. New York, Grune & Stratton, 1970, pp 112–114.
9. Soule HE: Tumors of the hypopharynx and parapharyngeal area. *In* Dockerty MB, Parkhill EM, Dahlin DC, et al (eds): Tumors of the Oral Cavity and Pharynx. Washington, DC, Armed Forces Institute of Pathology, 1968, pp 167–242.
10. Postlethwait PW: Surgery of the Esophagus. New York, Appleton-Century-Crofts, 1979, pp 341–414.
11. Bloom W, Fawcett DW: Oral cavity and associated glands. *In* A Textbook of Histology, 10th ed. Philadelphia, WB Saunders, 1975, pp 617–618.
12. Donald PJ, Huffman DI: Carcinoma in a Zenker's diverticulum. J Head Neck Surg 2:71, 1979.
13. Kirchner JA: Pyriform sinus cancer: a clinical and laboratory study. Ann Otol Rhinol Laryngol 84:793, 1975.
14. Som ML, Nussbaum M: Surgical therapy of carcinoma of the hypopharynx and cervical esophagus. Otolaryngol Clin North Am 2:631, 1969.
15. Donald PJ, Hayes RH, Dhaliwal R: Combined Rx for pyriform sinus cancer using postoperative irradiation. Otolaryngol Head Neck Surg 88:738, 1980.
16. Ogura JH, Saltzstein SL, Spjut HJ: Experiences with conservation surgery in laryngeal and pharyngeal carcinoma. Laryngoscope 71:258, 1961.
17. Harwick RD: Carcinoma of the pyriform sinus. Am J Surg 130:493, 1975.
18. Razack MS, Sako K, Kalnis I: Squamous cell carcinoma of the pyriform sinus. Head Neck Surg 1:31, 1978.
19. Mustard RA: The use of the Wookey operation for carcinoma of the hypopharynx and cervical esophagus. Surg Gynecol Obstet 111:577, 1960.
20. Silver CE: Surgical management of neoplasms of the larynx, hypopharynx and cervical esophagus. Curr Probl Surg 14:2, 1977.
21. Donald PJ: Complications of combined therapy in head and neck carcinomas. Arch Otolaryngol 104:329, 1978.
22. Goepfert H: Carcinoma of the hypopharynx and cervical esophagus. *In* Suen JY, Meyers, EN, (eds): Cancer of the Head and Neck. New York, Churchill Livingstone, 1981, pp 415–433.
23. Million RR, Cassisi MJ: Radical irradiation for carcinoma of the pyriform sinus. Laryngoscope 91:439, 1981.
24. Liebner EJ: Radiological studies of the lymphatic system of the head and neck. Otolaryngol Clin North Am 6:563, 1973.
25. Fisch V.: Lymphangiography of the cervical lymphatic system. Philadelphia, WB Saunders, 1968.
26. Alexander MV, Zajtchuk JJ, Henderson RL: Hypothyroidism and wound healing: occurrence after head and neck surgery. Arch Otolaryngol 108:289, 1982.
27. Kennedy JA: Personal communication (unpublished data), 1973.
28. Bakamjian FY: Total reconstruction of pharynx with medially based deltopectoral skin flap. NY State J Med 68:2771, 1968.
29. Daniel RK, Cunningham DM, Taylor GI: The deltopectoral flap: an anatomical and hemodynamic approach. Plast Reconstr Surg 55:275, 1975.
30. Wookey H: The surgical treatment of carcinoma of the pharynx and upper esophagus. Surg Gynecol Obstet 75:499, 1949.
31. Resano JH: Treatment of cancer of the esophagus. Bull Soc Int Chir 6:311, 1975.
32. Parker EF: Editorial: Carcinoma of the esophagus. Ann Thoracic Surg 23:391, 1977.
33. Sisson GA: Extended radical surgery for cancer of the head and neck—mediastinal resection for stomal recurrences. Otolaryngol Clin North Am 2:617, 1969.

4

LARYNX

Bruce W. Pearson, M.D.
Paul J. Donald, M.D.

The greater part of this book is devoted to a discussion of the management of large tumors that are difficult to treat. Function and form are often severely distorted, and the prognosis in many of the sites is poor. Lesions of the larynx are different. Function is usually preserved, albeit with some compromise, and the prognosis for survival is excellent. The five year survival rate of 84 per cent described by Kennedy and Krause[1] is typical of the results of conservation laryngeal surgery.

Probably the greatest area of persistent controversy between radiotherapists and head and neck surgeons is the management of limited laryngeal cancers. Limited or small cancers are those that don't cause fixation. All reporters claim startling survival figures, with radiation[2] or with surgery,[3] and so they should; these are early localized cancers.

One might conclude that since the results seem so comparable, what does it matter which treatment is chosen? The fallacy lies in building our treatment strategies on survival figures for a disease from which no one dies. Because physicians are not faced with the tragedy of a patient's dying from a small laryngeal cancer, they may be tempted to choose for initial therapy a less radical approach than they would if such lesions were potentially fatal. This can prove to be a tragic mistake for the patient with a T_1 cordal cancer who may later have to lose his larynx to save his life.[4] This is clearly an unnecessary event, since the tumor burden was miniscule at diagnosis and the instruments available for treatment were powerful.

Several different treatment philosophies characterize current reports on laryngeal cancer. Some hold that all cases should be irradiated, with surgery reserved for failure. Others recommend irradiating the small cancers, operating the larger ones, and using some combination of modalities in far advanced cases. In a third approach surgery can be performed for every laryngeal cancer, using conservation principles for small tumors and reconstructive procedures followed by speech therapy for the larger lesions. Finally we have the selective approach, in which the use of radiation or surgery is individualized and decided case by case. The same "stage" tumor may be irradiated in one patient and operated in another.

The selective philosophy has the distinct advantage of requiring the deepest assessment of the selection factors at the most important time for decision making, which is the physician's initial encounter with the disease. It resists the temptation to institutionalize popular prejudices in therapy, such as the submission of cases to tumor board deliberation after a biopsy has muddied the waters. Laryngeal cancer is several different diseases (e.g., glottic vs. supraglottic, T_1 vs. T_3) occurring in an equally complex variety of hosts (e.g., young vs. old, employed vs. retired, extroverted vs. reclusive). Our experience is that no single treatment is universally applicable or exclusively effective. Simplistic concepts applied to such diverse problems (there are at least five variations of T_1 glottic disease) are bound to result in overtreatment of some patients and undertreatment of others. The physician's obligation is to help the patient select the optimal treatment in each instance. To do this a careful study of the patient and his expectations and needs is as important as evaluation of the disease. A very honest appraisal of the experience and capabilities of the radiotherapists, surgeons, and pathologists involved is also necessary. And finally, a very critical assessment of the literature is required. Do actuarial statistics obscure the raw figures? Are dissimilar cases combined to inflate the numbers? Is the follow-up a mean or a minimum? And are the numerators or the denominators responsible for the fine figures quoted?

The preclusion of a temporary tracheostomy and the avoidance of surgical intervention are distinct advantages to radiation therapy. When radiation works, the voice is usually good. Some degree of hoarseness and a dry throat are not uncommon, and the time for completion of therapy is long, but these would be minor drawbacks if the prospect of failure and retreatment were as small as an uncritical survey of the literature would seem to suggest. Unfortunately the failures one sees in practice cannot be explained away as a statistical exception. In determining each patient's initial treatment selection, a balanced perspective on the drawbacks of the choice must always temper unrealistic enthusiasm for its attractions.

The greatest deterrent to radiation therapy is the complicated problem of tumor persistence and insidious progression. The greater the tumor volume, the more likely the cancer will recur. Men fare worse than women. Field size and dose are important. Usually, however, the reasons for unexpected failure are obscure.

Even when tumor has disappeared from the surface of the larynx, occult submucosal disease may infiltrate far beyond the confines of the original lesion before detection. Clinical reports[5] and whole organ serial section studies[6] have clearly shown this to be an intrinsic peril of radio-recurrent cancer, not just a problem of improper follow-up or cursory examination. In glottic tumors, the only indication of recurrent disease may be subtle fixation of a previously mobile cord. At the time of retreatment, a conservation operation that could have encompassed the original disease will no longer suffice, and a total laryngectomy, complete with its debilitating effects, must be employed. Supraglottic cancers are no exception; recurrence in this location is especially characterized by infiltration through the paraglottic space, which precludes a supraglottic laryngectomy.

Once the recurrence is recognized, the patient faces a more disabling operation and a lower chance of success. The surgeon is now treating a cancer whose borders are indistinct and unpredictable in a field of tissues whose resistance to infection and tolerance of wounding are compromised. Factors such as prolonged decannulation secondary to postoperative edema and delays in stomal healing or vocal shunt recovery definitely limit the success of conservation operations. A wound breakdown or a fistula complicating what is now the second major treatment for the patient's cancer imposes a need for prolonged enteral nutrition, and further hospitalization and expense. The sometimes unquestioned concept that many patients with laryngeal cancer can be irradiated and followed is not supported by the net loss of larynges or lives, the frequent necessity for a second treatment in the survivors, and the waste of the radiotherapeutic option for their second primary cancer.

When radiation seems to succeed, persistent laryngeal edema with or without pain sometimes occurs. This presents a serious diagnostic dilemma. Despite appearances, persisting cancer is frequent in those in whom edema persists 6 months or longer after therapy. The frequency of this correlation in a series by Ward et al[7] was 53 per cent. The most tragic statistic was the low surgical salvage rate of 26 per cent. After all, these patients' lesions were T_1 or $T_2N_0M_0$ in extent prior to radiation.

In patients with 5-year cures, the possible long-term carcinogenic effects of radiation assume importance. Mucosal epithelium is damaged by radiotherapy in a permanent and sometimes progressive manner, and in the younger individual, whose life expectancy might be another 25 years, the long-term possibility that a new malignancy will be promoted is probably very real. Continuous evidence from the atomic bombing of Hiroshima and Nagasaki, the effect on children exposed to radiation during the above-ground nuclear tests in the western U.S. desert, and finally the elevated incidence of thyroid cancer in individuals exposed to thymic irradiation in infancy and cerebral malignancy in those treated in early life for retinoblastoma provide startling corroborative evidence to support this concern. Some reports, such as that of Harwood et al.,[8] which examine the risk of malignancy from small doses during the period from five to ten years postradiation calculate this to be as small as 2 per cent. Lawson,[9] however, felt it was closer to 10 per cent.

Surgery for laryngeal cancer always involves a compromise between excision for cure, and conservation to preserve voice and nasal respiration. Surgical technology continues to evolve in response to new tools (e.g., the laser[10]), new concepts (e.g., near-total laryngectomy[11]), and new rehabilitative options (e.g., the duckbill prosthesis[12]). It is important to remember that unirradiated tissue in man responds better to mechanical trauma than does tissue that has been exposed to radiotherapy. Almost always, complete excision is feasible and would be curative at the first medical contact. But the dilemma in practice is to choose the proper balance between an adequate excision and conservation of function.

A purely surgical view would hold that all laryngeal cancer can be managed with three simple operations: endoscopic excision, laryngofissure with cordectomy, and total laryngectomy. The elaboration and refinement of these procedures constitute the history of laryngeal surgery.[13] In modern times the laser is the latest variation on endoscopic excision. The factors chiefly responsible for the success of transoral surgery are probably the suspension laryngoscope, the operating microscope, and the availability of immediate frozen section diagnosis. The frontolateral partial laryngectomy and the misnamed vertical hemilaryngectomy (which removes only the midportion or glottic half of the larynx and leaves the hyoid and cricoid levels intact) are contemporary expansions of the concept of laryngofissure with cordectomy. These are considered the vertical members of a family of conventional partial laryngectomies, while supraglottic laryngectomy is the horizontal representative. The incidence of total laryngectomy in supraglottic cancer has fallen as surgeons have learned to distinguish those cases in which the glottis is free. For these, a supraglottic laryngectomy provides local control rates identical to those achieved in the past when the glottis was sacrificed.[14]

Total laryngectomy is still considered whenever one of the conventional partial procedures is anatomically insufficient. The implications for the patient are odious. The standard partial operations conserve voice and a nasal airway, while the total laryngectomy spares neither. To bridge the gap between the partial and the total resection, the near-total laryngectomy was devised.[11] This is a resection that provides speech (like a conservation operation) but removes too much larynx to avoid a stoma (like a total).

Table 4–1 summarizes the surgical procedures considered by the authors to be meaningful options today. Perhaps these will change with further developments, but the basic framework has stood the test of time.

Table 4–1. SURGICAL OPTIONS FOR LARYNGEAL CANCER

NOTE: Surgery of the larynx for cancer breaks down logically into the following categories, which address increasing tumor volumes and present increasing degrees of disability. The addition of modified radical or bilateral neck dissections is an independent consideration that depends on the presence of disease in the neck.

I. Requires no external operation: completed simultaneously with the biopsy. Voice remains normal.
   A. Vocal cord stripping for premalignant lesions
   B. Transoral cordectomy for small cordal cancers
      1. By sharp dissection
      2. By dissection and cautery
      3. By laser excision
II. Preserves airway and voice, but voice is modified. For glottic lesions on mobile cords.
   A. Laryngofissure and cordectomy
   B. Vertical hemilaryngectomy
   C. Frontolateral partial laryngectomy
III. Preserves airway and voice, but swallow is modified. For supraglottic lesions without glottic involvement.
   A. Supraglottic laryngectomy
   B. Extended supraglottic laryngectomy
IV. Requires permanent tracheotomy but preserves voice. For cancers large enough to fix the vocal cord.
   A. Near-total laryngectomy (for intrinsic laryngeal cancer)
   B. Near-total laryngopharyngectomy (for extrinsic or pyriform cancer)
V. Requires a permanent tracheotomy and sacrifices voice.
   A. Total laryngectomy
   B. Total laryngectomy with partial pharyngectomy
   C. Total laryngopharyngectomy with pharyngeal reconstruction
      1. By skin flap
      2. By visceral transposition
      3. By free transplant and microvascular anastomosis

REHABILITATION

With successful radiation, one hopes to avoid the problem of rehabilitation altogether. Surgery may or may not require rehabilitative services, depending on the extent of the resection. There is a common misperception that equates laryngectomy with loss of the voice. In practice, the only operations in which voice is lost are those under category V in Table 4–1. Except in centers where radiation and, therefore, salvage surgery are widely performed, this represents a very small percentage of all laryngeal cancer. At the Mayo Clinic, for example, it comprises only 15 per cent of cases. Post–total laryngectomy rehabilitative techniques, both surgical and nonsurgical, have been developed to meet the needs of this group (Table 4–2).

Patients in Group I in Table 4–1 have less morbidity with surgery than with radiation, because both treatments require a biopsy under anesthetic. A transoral cordectomy is essentially an excisional biopsy. Radiation simply escalates the morbidity by causing additional time loss, dryness, edema, and late radiation sequelae to be added to the case. In Group II (small glottic lesions), the patient cured by surgery will have a hoarse voice, whereas the voice is virtually normal after a radiation cure for a comparable lesion. Properly done, the surgery takes less time and is easier to follow afterward. New findings are never attributed to radiation changes. There is no reliable phonosurgical management of the hoarseness after surgery. Rather, steps must be taken to reduce its severity at the time of the operation.[15]

Patients in Group III (small supraglottic lesions) retain a normal voice whether irradiated or operated. With both treatments there is some difficulty in swallowing; radiation damages the lubrication, while surgery alters the mechanics. The unirradiated patients are probably in a better position to deal with second primary cancers in this region. This is a more frequent problem in supraglottic than in glottic cancer.[16] Group IV patients—those with large cancers with fixation who received either near-total laryngectomy or radiotherapy as their treatment—pose greater rehabilitation problems. Those treated surgically need to learn the care of a tracheostomy tube. This is a skill, comparable to learning to manage dentures or a cane. It requires specific attention from a professional instructor. Once learned, it is readily incorporated into the patient's life activities. Rehabilitation after radiation for lesions of this size is minimal, because the patient avoids a stoma, and the voice is more natural. However, the rate of local recurrence in fixed glottic cancer after radiotherapy is greater than 50 per cent, and with the recurrence, the surgical treatment requirements usually escalate. Thus, over half the irradiated patients must expect graduation to Group V. Here the consequences of surgical treatment, now the only option, are a permanent tracheotomy and sacrifice of the voice. A near-total laryngectomy is usually no longer safe. In addition, one is dealing with irradiated tissues. Even with a total laryngectomy, the problems with mucosal desiccation or late carcinogenesis remain.

Table 4–2. VOCAL REHABILITATION TECHNIQUES FOR THE LARYNGECTOMEE

- I. Nonsurgical
  - A. Esophageal speech
  - B. Mechanical speaking aids
    - 1. Stoma-driven transoral reed
    - 2. Battery-driven transcervical vibrator
    - 3. Miscellaneous electromechanical devices
- II. Surgical
  - A. Multistaged reconstruction (e.g., Asai laryngoplasty[17])
  - B. Single-stage reconstruction
    - 1. External fistula (e.g., Taub air bypass method[18])
    - 2. Internal fistula
      - a. Without prosthesis
        - (1) Tracheoesophagal (e.g., Amatsu TE shunt[19])
        - (2) Tracheopharyngeal (e.g., Staffieri neoglottis[20])
      - b. With prosthesis (e.g., Blom-Singer duckbill[21])

Following a total laryngectomy, esophageal speech remains the primary rehabilitative maneuver. It is a hands-free, no-further-surgery approach that introduces no risk of aspiration and burns no bridges should a surgical solution be later requested. The quality of voice in a good esophageal speaker is astonishing. It easily rivals fistula speech in its tone. The success rate varies from institution to institution and from patient to patient, depending on the experience of the teacher, the tissue qualities of the pharyngoesophageal segment, and the motivation of the patient.

Mechanical speaking aids, of which there are many varieties, have special applications in special situations. Some are battery-powered vibrators, while others incorporate a reed in a tubular connection held between the stoma and the mouth. Sometimes they are offered as a permanent solution for the patient unwilling to have further surgery and unable to manage esophageal speech. Usually their use is temporary, however, in a patient who is awaiting further wound healing before the institution of fistula speech.

It has long been known that making a simple connection between the airway and the foodway will enable laryngectomized patients to speak. However, the problem of how to control the aspiration through the connection has limited the application of this principle. Asai, Amatsu, Staffieri, and others reported ingenious methods of doing it, and quite a few procedures were based on their methods.[17–20] But enthusiasm was rarely sustained. Fistulas open enough to allow speech were also open enough to permit aspiration, and fistulas tight enough to avoid aspiration were prone to stenose.

To enable a greater percentage of laryngectomized patients to utilize the fistula speech principle, Singer and Blom,[21] Panje,[22] and others have incorporated a prosthesis in the connection between the airway and the foodway. Their techniques begin with the creation of a simple puncture-connection between the trachea and the esophagus. The problem of stenosis is solved by maintaining the opening with a special plastic prosthesis, known as the duckbill in Singer's procedure and the voice button in Panje's. The aspiration problem is managed by incorporating a one-way valve into the prosthesis. With proper postoperative instruction, most patients can learn how to handle and replace their prostheses successfully. In North America, the simplicity and reliability of these techniques have led to their general acceptance. As of 1982, they have replaced, to a major extent, all the nonprosthetic post–total laryngectomy vocal rehabilitation techniques mentioned above.

THE CLINICAL BASIS FOR SELECTING AN APPROPRIATE SURGICAL OPTION FOR PARTICULAR CANCERS OF THE LARYNX

Transoral Cordectomy

This section is the first of several explaining selection and management. Endoscopic resections are used for glottic cancer when the following three criteria can be fulfilled:

1. The vocal cord is completely mobile.
2. The lesion is sharply localized on the membranous cord.
3. The borders of the lesion can be completely exposed at laryngoscopy.

Expert use of a suspension laryngoscope and the operating microscope is essential. The operative specimen must be removed in one piece, oriented, labeled, and submitted for a complete intraoperative frozen section evaluation of its margins. Vocal cord stripping is sometimes adequate for limited carcinomas in situ, but transoral cordectomy is not intended for diffuse multicentric disease. When cordal cancer is widespread and superficial but low in volume, a biopsy and radiotherapy are more appropriate.

There are too many small cordal lesions included under the T_1 designation of the TNM system to relate these procedures exactly to the AJCC classification.[23] In our own practice, approximately one third of early glottic lesions receive irradiation, a third are treated by transoral cordectomy or stripping, and a third receive conventional conservation operations as described later in this chapter.

Endolaryngeal Laser Surgery

Coherent light from a CO_2 laser source can be directed through the laryngoscope to vaporize cancer with a minimum of bleeding. There is no decisive advantage to this method over the cold-steel technique. Moreover, use of the laser adds weight to the microscope, expense to the patient, regulations to the operating room, smoke to the field, and time to the procedure. The laser cannot cut around corners, and there is no tactile feedback to the operator. There are two instances in which its use might be expedient: in the partial resection of an obstructing glottic cancer to secure an airway without a tracheotomy, and in the partial resection of a bulky supraglottic cancer to visualize the lower margins.

Conventional Open Conservation Surgery of the Larynx

This section discusses several operations for limited glottic and supraglottic cancers that do not sacrifice voice and do not necessitate a permanent tracheostomy. The cricoid ring must be preserved to prevent airway stenosis, and a valve must remain that can function adequately to permit swallowing. Cordectomy, hemilaryngectomy, and supraglottic laryngectomy are the procedures that meet these criteria. These operations are "conventional" in the sense that they have been thoroughly studied and debated, the indications and results are fairly clear, and the techniques have been refined by use.

The indications for conservation laryngectomy are often described in anatomic terms. Hemilaryngectomy is offered for T_1 and T_2 glottic cancers, and supraglottic laryngectomy for T_1 and T_2 supraglottic lesions. Bear in mind that the TNM system is simply a method of classifying tumors for reporting purposes. *It is not a prescription for therapy.* The principal contraindications to a conservation laryngectomy may involve not just the extent of the tumor but also the patient's general health.

In determining the geometry of laryngeal cancer, function and fixation are the chief criteria for tumor depth. If a glottic cancer is fixed, a hemilaryngectomy is not usually safe. In supraglottic cancer, if the voice sounds normal, a supraglottic laryngectomy will usually be possible.

Not more than a decade ago, conservation operations were reserved for patients under the age of 60. However, the important factor is not age, but the status of the patient's respiratory system. This is particularly true for the supraglottic operation. Leonard and Litton[24] showed that at least 66 per cent of their postoperative supraglottic patients demonstrated cineradiographic evidence of aspiration. They had to convert 12 per cent of their patients to a total laryngectomy for this reason. Furthermore, they found evidence of aspiration in 20 of 37 patients who had a hemilaryngectomy, although this complication was far less severe than is usually seen in the supraglottic procedure and was usually subclinical.

Unfortunately, chronic obstructive pulmonary disease (COPD) is commonly present in patients with laryngeal cancer. The addiction to cigarette smoking that is at least partly responsible for the genesis of the neoplasm is also integral to the development of this respiratory ailment. Predicting how well an individual with mild to moderate COPD will do with a supraglottic laryngectomy is most difficult. The patient with dyspnea at rest or on slight exertion is definitely not a candidate for this operation. Pulmonary function indices such as the FEV_1 are helpful to assess obstructive and restrictive pulmonary disease, and the blood gases indicate the seriousness of a ventilation-perfusion mismatch. The old-fashioned "two-flight test" is still a good predictor of success also. If a patient can climb two flights of stairs without being unduly short of breath, he will most likely tolerate a supraglottic laryngectomy without significant respiratory trouble.

In most instances, the patient's physiologic age is much more relevant than the chronologic. Howver, even though a septuagenarian may appear robust and healthy, he may not have the flexibility of mind or habit to adjust to the alterations of voice, swallowing, and airway that may follow partial laryngectomy. This is true even with the cordectomy or hemilaryngectomy. A 72-year-old vigorous, healthy patient in my experience (PJD) had a small cordal lesion that failed to be cured with radiotherapy. A hemilaryngectomy with an otherwise uneventful postoperative course was marred by the patient's insistence that he could not swallow or breathe, despite the fact that when observed he could swallow without apparent obstruction, pain, or aspiration, and had a clear airway, albeit a hoarse voice. This finding was supported by fluorographic studies. The patient was so insistent on his disability that he required periodic admissions to the hospital because of inanition. A more thorough preoperative investigation into his psychologic status might have revealed some clue to his rigidity and lack of adaptability. However, this exemplifies the problems with partial laryngectomy in the elderly.

Laryngofissure and Cordectomy

In broad generalities, glottic cancers are early or late; the critical and distinguishing feature is the presence or absence of vocal cord mobility. Laryngofissure with cordectomy is curative for selected patients in whom the vocal cords remain mobile. Except at the anterior commissure, which is a fixed point anyway, mobility is an important guide to the absence of deep infiltration. The implication of a mobile cord is that the cancer remains well localized, and thus it is unlikely that curative surgery eliminating speech or requiring a permanent tracheal stoma will be necessary.

Hemilaryngectomies, nothing more than variations on the theme, are not to be construed as substitutes or replacements for this operation. Laryngofissure with cordectomy is an extremely successful procedure when it is applied strictly to those patients for whom it was designed, that is, primarily those with unilateral cancers on a mobile cord. Horseshoe lesions involving both cords, multicentric cancer, and poor general health should exclude patients from this approach; in these radiation would be preferred. Neel et al[25] reviewed 182 laryngofissure and cordectomy cases from the Mayo Clinic series and reported that the probability of a patient's surviving 15 years was 95 per cent, or approximately the same as that expected for an age- and sex-matched population without laryngeal cancer. There were only 4 cases of local recurrences in this series, 2 of which were salvaged by laryngectomy. There were 3 deaths, 2 from distant metastases and 1 from disease in the neck. Thirty-three of these patients were followed for less than 3 years, but the median follow-up for the whole group was 6 years. Including patients with a short follow-up might bias the results in a favorable direction, but during the same period an approximately equal number of patients were treated with transoral cordectomy. Therefore these results were obtained after the most favorable T_1 lesions had already been selected out of the series.

Certain basic principles applying to the performance of cordectomy bear emphasis here:

1. Whenever the tumor approaches or involves the anterior commissure (about one third of cases) an overlying strip of thyroid cartilage, Broyles' anterior commissure tendon, and a tiny piece of the opposite cord should be included.
2. The surgical pathologist should provide immediate frozen section histopathologic confirmation of the surgical margins.
3. Very occasionally, second carcinomas or carcinomas in situ on the opposite cord may be treated by associated procedures, such as stripping or transoral removal.

The complications of laryngofissure and cordectomy include subcutaneous emphysema, problems with the temporary tracheotomy, and pulmonary aspiration. The hospitalization averages 6 days. Granulomas develop in 10 to 15 per cent of cases but usually resolve within several months of the procedure. Unquestionably the voice is disturbed. The incidence of significant dysphonia depends on the criteria of the observer and the size of the resection, particularly anteriorly.

Since the expense of laryngofissure and cordectomy is comparable to that of biopsy and radiotherapy, but the time lost from work is shorter and the likelihood of preserving life and voice is higher, the main justification for offering radiotherapy—a better voice—without deference to this classic procedure should be greeted with skepticism.

Hemilaryngectomy

There are several concepts that require discussion under the heading of hemilaryngectomy. The name itself is a misnomer, since neither the cricoid nor the hyoid levels are removed on the "hemilaryngectomized" side. The conceptual difference between a laryngofissure and cordectomy and a hemilaryngectomy is one of degree. Some would include all cordectomy procedures that include a cartilage strip under the heading of hemilaryngectomy. However, the term should probably be reserved for those cases in which all the glottic and ventricular soft tissues are removed in continuity with the thyroid ala on the involved side. The shift in some centers away from laryngofissure and cordectomy to the more extensive hemilaryngectomy operation may represent a logical alternative to radiotherapy. If more surgical cases fall into the radio-recurrent category, the need for an operation that avoids leaving denuded cartilage in the field may seem more apparent.

The performance of a vertical, partial laryngectomy should be limited to those patients whose lesions are confined to the membranous cord and in whom cordal mobility is retained. The true vocal cord may be involved as far as the apex of the ventricle. The cartilage excision accommodates the fact that the saccule prolapses out over the thyroarytenoid muscle to contact the inner surface of the thyroid ala. Tumors do vary in their degree of invasion, even among those with a mobile cord. Some are unirradiated, exophytic, and discrete. Others are postirradiated, ulcerated, and pervasive. An exophytic cancer that rises to the ventricular band may remain suitable for a hemilaryngectomy, whereas an irradiated invasive lesion of identical apparent surface dimensions may not.

Subglottic extension is a much more ominous threat than supraglottic spread. Attempts at hemilaryngectomy are ill-advised if the neoplasm extends any more inferiorly than 5 mm from the free edge of the true cord.

Discussion over how much posterior involvement militates against conservation surgery continues. The problem is what constitutes adequate surgical excision of the intrinsic laryngeal muscles attached to the arytenoid. As in consideration of the ventricle, superficial invasion is not much of a problem, but deep extension is probably best handled by a more radical procedure. Involvement of the vocal process requires excision of the entire arytenoid and all the immediate muscular attachments as well as the entire mucosa over this cartilage. One should always expect that intramucosal cancer will extend 2 or 3 mm beyond visible tumor.

A number of innovations have been proposed to expand the scope of hemilaryngectomy. The frontolateral vertical partial laryngectomy was developed to encompass those cordal lesions that extend across the anterior commissure onto the cord of the opposite side. The Kambič-Sedlaček reconstruction[26, 27] permits voice-saving principles to be applied to a lesion with extension up to (but not onto) the arytenoid cartilage of the other side. Applications are uncommon, because no epiglottic or extensive ventricular involvement should be present on either side, and both cords should be mobile. The subsequent reconstruction uses the epiglottis to provide support and adequate mucosa for glottic competence.

Reduced cordal mobility is regarded by some as only a relative contraindication to hemilaryngectomy. Lesinski et al,[28] Leroux,[29] and Kirchner and Som[30] collectively reported a 78 per cent determinate 5-year survival rate when they performed modified hemilaryngectomies for selected lesions with a "fixed" cord. The reasons give by Lesinski for their success is that in 14 of their 18 cases, the fixation was only because of invasion of the vocalis muscle, and not the deeper structures. What is most surprising is that the local recurrence rate he reported was so low, despite the fact that 8 of the 18 cases had positive margins.

Lee[31] has confirmed the impression that is basic to our understanding of the principles of cancer surgery in general, which is that positive resection margins are accompanied by a high local recurrence rate. Olofsson and Van Nostrand[6] have shown that cancers invasive enough to fix a vocal cord often extend to the thyroid and cricoid cartilages. Hemilaryngectomies (except for that described originally as an "extended hemilaryngectomy,"[11] and now known as "near-total laryngectomy") leave the cricoid behind, violate the pre-epiglottic space, and also leave the pyriform and aryepiglottic mucosa behind. Therefore, except for selected anecdotal cases, to offer hemilaryngectomy to patients with a fixed cord is to practice surgical brinkmanship.

Supraglottic Laryngectomy

Supraglottic laryngectomy was initially developed to manage limited cancers of the false cords and epiglottis. With time, tumor extensions into the vallecula and the pyriform regions were no longer considered absolute contraindications to this operation. In 1970, Sisson[32] recommended that the tongue base excision should extend no farther than within 5 mm of the circumvallate papillae. Since that time, the resected tongue base has been replaced with flaps, especially the musculocutaneous types, eliminating this amount of tumor extension as an inviolable restriction to the supraglottic operation. Pyriform fossa involvement, unless extremely limited, remains a serious contraindication to the procedure. The frequent occurrence of paraglottic and cartilaginous extension from pyriform sites militates against supraglottic laryngectomy, because the muscular, arytenoid, and cricoid elements necessary to the functional success of the supraglottic procedure cannot be safely preserved.

When bilateral neck metastases are present, a question arises as to whether the supraglottic operation is still advisable. If full radical neck dissections are done, the subsequent edema, bilateral denervation of the mylohyoid and digastric muscles that elevate the remnant for swallow, and possible loss of the twelfth nerve on the side of the largest metastatic involvement make both airway compromise and aspiration almost inevitable. These complications will be aggravated by the radiation therapy that is often instituted postoperatively in patients with bilateral neck disease. When the pattern of metastasis is such that both hypoglossal nerves, the suprahyoid elevators, and one jugular vein can be preserved (by modifying one neck dissection, for example) the supraglottic operation is more reasonable.

Painstaking preoperative counseling is absolutely essential before a supraglottic laryngectomy. All patients need to be apprised of certain possible eventualities. At surgery the tumor may turn out to be more extensive than originally thought, and a near-total laryngectomy, rather than a supraglottic procedure, might be required. This will preserve communication but necessitate the acceptance of a permanent tracheostomy. The patient must be aware that even if a supraglottic laryngectomy is done, there may be a need for a tracheostomy for a prolonged period of time. This is especially true if radiation is added postoperatively. The knowledge that the voice is preserved, despite the presence of the tube, helps immeasurably in the encouragement of such patients. The patient must be told to expect difficulty in swallowing, especially common after extensive tongue base resection, and even the possibility that a temporary gastrostomy may be required before swallowing is restored.

As with hemilaryngectomies, there are several versions of the supraglottic operation, depending upon the spread of the tumor. A convenient classification of supraglottic laryngectomy recognizes the basic procedure and four extensions. The basic resection separates the specimen from the glottis with a division down across both false cords, in front of the arytenoids. Then it passes forward through the ventricles, so that the epiglottis and pre-epiglottic space are resected intact. The initial opening is through the vallecula.

The first variation extends this concept to include a portion of the arytenoid on the worse side. The second, for lesions that compromise the aryepiglottic fold, includes the medial portion of the pyriform fossa. A third addresses ventricular involvement, and includes the upper surface of the vocal cord on the side at risk. The fourth variation encompasses vallecular or tongue base involvement. It enters the larynx through the ventricles first. Then the dissection proceeds up through the false cords, the specimen is inverted, and the final resection across the tongue base can be individualized under direct vision.

The basic and arytenoid-shaving supraglottic laryngectomies are reliable and reproducible procedures in terms of cancer control and the rehabilitation of swallow. Extension into the pyriform fossa or across the top of one vocal cord will be tolerated only by patient individuals with healthy lungs, since tongue base resection cases strain the swallowing potential to the maximum. In patients considered to be candidates for the extended form of supraglottic laryngectomy, the alternative of near-total laryngectomy should be carefully considered.[33] The prospects for swallowing will be greatly enhanced. Aryepiglottic fold involvement may be found at surgery to spill further into the pyriform than expected, and a supraglottic laryngectomy with partial pharyngectomy may be incompatible with swallowing. Bivalving the true cord to achieve control of ventricular extensions will increase the risk of aspiration and result in an extremely breathy voice, because the cord becomes lateralized postoperatively. While tongue base extension can sometimes be accommodated, massive involvement is bound to require use of a flap to provide the bulk needed to deflect the bolus during swallowing. Flaps should be used in most cases when a tongue base resection is combined with a supraglottic laryngectomy, but if age or chronic respiratory disease is a factor, the acceptance of a stoma and the performance of a near-total laryngectomy (which can also be combined with a flap reconstruction of the tongue base or pyriform) is probably the better choice.

SURGICAL TECHNIQUES

Transoral Procedures for Localized Cancer of the Membranous Cord

A careful mirror examination of the larynx in the office delineates the lesion and vocal cord movement, of course, but it also forewarns the operator of the degree of difficulty to be expected at direct suspension microlaryngoscopy. The more difficult the mirror exam, the more difficult the exposure. The largest possible laryngoscope is preferred for transoral surgery, but in the most difficult cases—i.e., those involving a short, stiff-necked patient with an underslung mandible and brittle projecting upper incisor teeth—a narrow anterior commissure laryngoscope must be selected. Some patients cannot have the transoral operation on technical mechanical grounds.

The large Kleinsasser or the double-bladed Weerda laryngoscope (Storz) with double fiberoptic illumination from a xenon source, and a chest brace for suspension used in combination with an operating microscope with a 400-mm objective, will secure excellent exposure in the majority of patients. The left hand is used to depress the larynx a little and tilt the anterior commissure into view. The table is tilted 20 degrees so the patient's head is higher than the feet. If the anterior commissure cannot be exposed because of prominent upper teeth or a narrow lower dental arch, the Dedo laryngoscope is used. This provides the narrowest aperture through which binocular microscopic vision can still be obtained, so the alignment of the microscope with the laryngoscope is more critical. Instrument access is reduced through this narrower tube.

A small cuffed anesthetic endotracheal tube is placed in the larynx. Under suspension, it holds the posterior commissure back while the anterior commissure is elevated with the laryngoscope. This helps to separate the arytenoids and place the vocal cords on the stretch. A No. 5 tube is small enough to lie entirely between the arytenoids and constitutes no significant interference with transoral surgery, which, after all, is confined to lesions of the membranous cord.

The teeth are protected and the laryngoscope is lightly lubricated before introduction. With the patient's neck slightly flexed, but the head itself extended on the atlanto-occipital joint, the laryngoscope is introduced. Once positioned, the appropriate suspension handle is added and then cranked into position, at which point the microscope is brought into play.

If leukoplakia is encountered, we prefer not to do a biopsy. Instead we strip the cord. This consists of grasping the cord mucosa anteriorly, rotating it medially with the angled forceps, stripping it back to the arytenoid, and pushing it down toward the trachea to complete the detachment at the vocal process. Bleeding is minimal if the larynx is topically cocainized before the cord is stripped. Suction trauma should be avoided by using a laryngeal suction with a side hole near the distal tip. To avoid tearing the specimen, the mucosa may be preincised with a laryngeal knife at the proposed anterior and posterior extremities of the specimen.

If carcinoma in situ (only) is reported in a clean stripping with normal margins, the cancer is probably removed. Both the specimen and the pathologist must be well oriented. The underlying tissues can be burned with electocautery (or the laser) to provide additional security, but the basic ingredient for success is to confine stripping to selected, sharply localized membranous cord lesions that look like unulcerated leukoplakia and do not reach the anterior commissure. The frozen-section pathologist will report the specimens as showing, perhaps in one or two different locations, carcinoma in situ. In some cases he may even be unsure as to whether the specimen represents carcinoma or just severe atypia. In any event, there is no invasion, and under microlaryngoscopy the operator is satisfied that either process is completely removed. The proper attitude in treating localized dysplastic lesions of the vocal cord is to achieve a complete excision and never settle for a mere biopsy.

Transoral excision is applicable to approximately a third of T_1 glottic cancers. Even more than with carcinoma in situ, this method of treatment depends on the immediate presence of a skilled pathologist examining a quick section. To be suitable for this procedure, a T_1 cancer must be exposed completely on all margins. It is grasped with large cup forceps and excised with scissors (Fig. 4–1). The excision includes the vocal ligament and the underlying vocalis muscle. Bleeding is controlled with cocaine, and the depth of the wound is extended by cauterizing the base. This prolongs healing but promotes the formation of a neocord by virtue of the scarring induced. It is important, of course, not to damage the anterior commissure or the opposite vocal cord. The specimen must be removed in one piece, and its orientation—

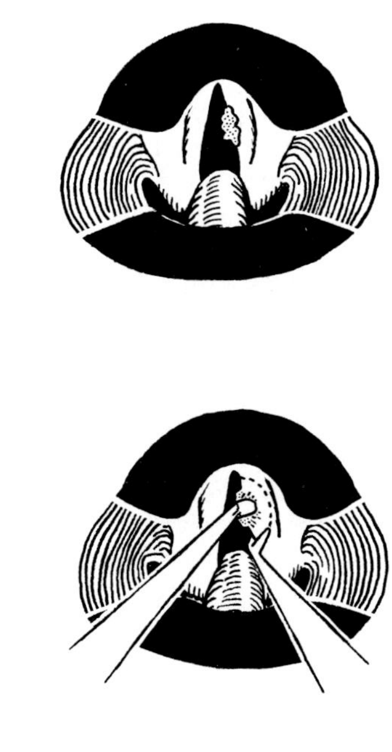

Figure 4–1. An exophytic invasive cancer of the right vocal cord meets the criteria for transoral resection. The cord is fully mobile and the lesion can be fully exposed. It does not approach or cross the anterior commissure.

anterior and posterior, subglottic and ventricular—must be maintained. The patient remains suspended until a margin-free specimen is reported.

There are probably more patients for whom this procedure would have been curative, but unfortunately many have undergone biopsy elsewhere before being referred for treatment. Critical evaluation of a cord in the biopsied state usually precludes a safe transoral cordectomy. This greatly increases the chance that radiotherapy will be recommended.

Thyrotomy and Cordectomy for Glottic Cancer

This external operation to open the thyroid cartilage and excise the cord under direct vision (which has also been called laryngofissure and cordectomy) was fully described by Morell MacKenzie[34] around 1880. Radiotherapy has not replaced it, but it has reduced the incidence and perhaps, therefore, the skill of its performance. Nevertheless, thyrotomy with cordectomy remains an important tool in every laryngeal surgeon's repertoire.

Patients come because they are hoarse, confused about the significance of their symptoms, or referred. The initial office exam is more crucial than the direct laryngoscopy that is performed later. Two questions are vital: Does the patient have vocal cord fixation, and is the anterior commissure involved? Any degree of fixation is a contraindication to cordectomy. If the cancer approaches the anterior commissure, the excision must include Broyles' tendon. Patients are forewarned of the need for a temporary tracheotomy but are assured that they are going to get a useful voice. They are offered the option of radiotherapy, as has already been noted. The successful performance of thyrotomy and cordectomy requires an outstanding surgical pathology department, readily available to analyze biopsied material on a quick-section basis.

The technique described here is the one perfected by Ken Devine over many years and is principally responsible for the results reported earlier in this chapter.[25] After a preliminary laryngoscopy and confirmatory biopsy, a tracheotomy is performed below the thyroid isthmus, and the anesthesia tubing is removed from the larynx. The larynx is exposed from the hyoid to the top of the cricoid ring through a vertical midline skin incision that is broken by one or two Z incisions, or through a collar incision. Following a midline incision, the external perichondrium is elevated laterally for a short distance. The thyroid cartilage is cut vertically with a saw, but not through the inner perichondrium, at a site decided on by the findings at the office exam (Fig. 4–2). A second cartilage cut is made up the thyroid cartilage ala on the involved side, sufficiently lateral to the midline, if one plans to include a small piece of cartilage attached to the specimen anteriorly.

The surgeon dons a headlight. The cricothyroid membrane is incised vertically in the midline and held open with skin hooks by an assistant. A small vein that is always present marks the midline and should be cauterized. The operator ascends toward the glottic level with a Frazier suction tube and a scalpel. At the level of the vocal cords the cut is off the midline so that the anterior commissure remains with the diseased cord.

On the diseased side, the internal perichondrium is cut and a slippery dissection plane between the internal perichondrium and the paraglottic soft tissues is bluntly dissected (Fig. 4–3). The thyroid alae are separated with hooks as the laryngeal interior is more carefully visualized. The specimen is retracted forward by the small piece of cartilage attached to it anteriorly, and the involved cord and ventricle are dissected free. The upper incision is usually made on the crest of the ventricular band. The subglottic incision is approximately 5 mm away from the lesion. An angled gallbladder scissors (Panzer's) is an ideal instrument for detaching the specimen posteriorly, and usually in doing so the vocal process of the arytenoid is included.

If the opposite cord is dysplastic, it is stripped with fine scissors and forceps and resurfaced with a flap from the false cord based posteriorly. This can be held in place with 6-0 mild chromic catgut. It is not necessary to suture the cartilage thyrotomy back together, as this tends to cause granulations. Rather, the soft tissues are just closed over the site. No feeding tube is necessary, and the midline wound can be closed with no more drainage than the tracheostomy provides.

Patients are told that they will have some "proud flesh" on the operated area for many weeks. The residual nodule seen at the first

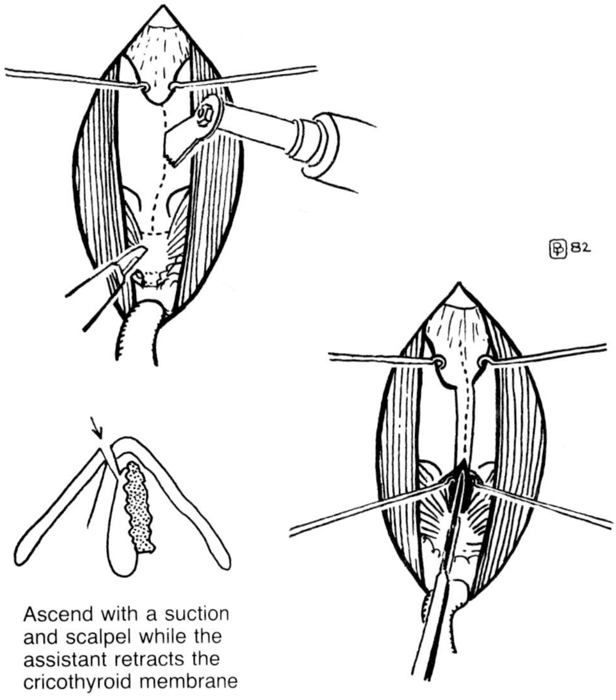

Figure 4–2. Thyrotomy and cordectomy for a right glottic cancer. The thyroid cartilage, but not the perichondrium, is split a few millimeters to the left of the midline. The cricothyroid ligament is divided with an inverted "T" in the vertical midline. Note the position of the hooks.

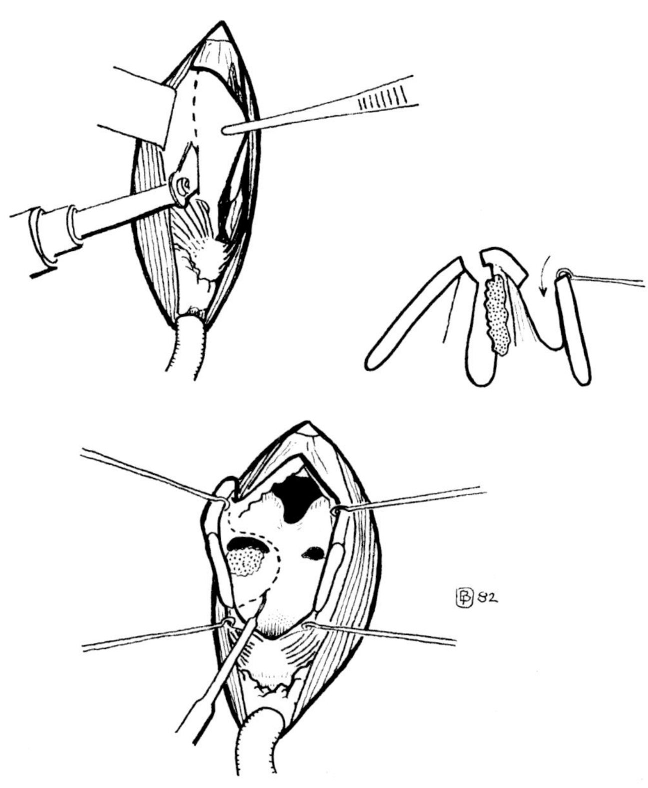

Figure 4–3. The thyroid ala is cut on the tumor side, and the posterior fragment is elevated. The specimen remains attached to a small piece of cartilage. The upper incision falls on the crest of the ventricular band when the specimen is dissected free.

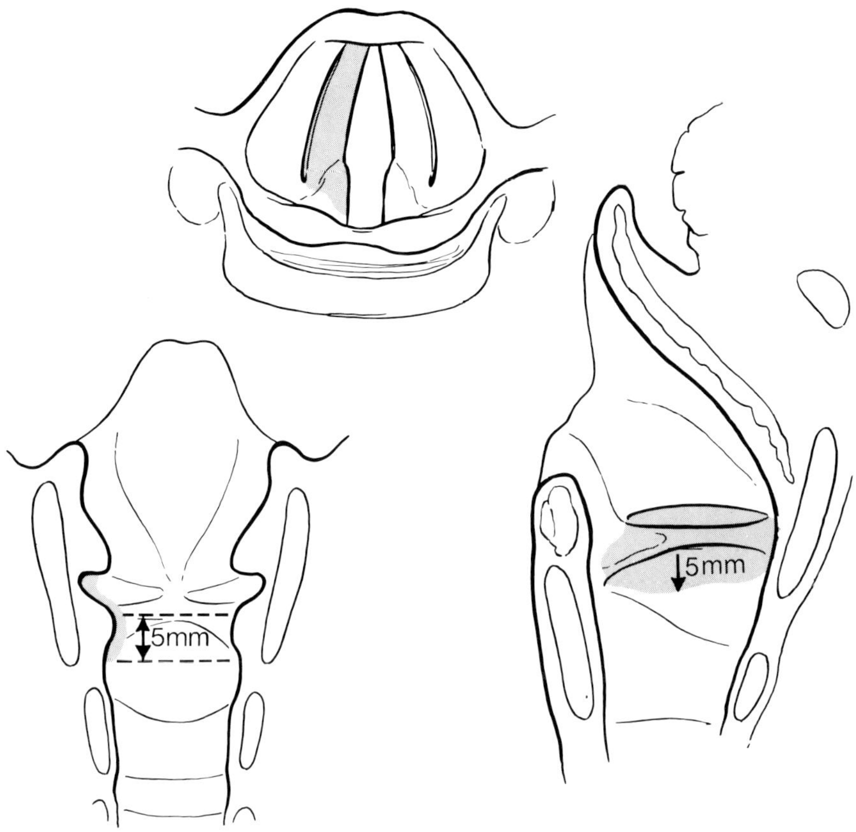

Figure 4–4. The limits of tumor extension for resection of laryngeal cancer by vertical hemilaryngectomy in superior, coronal, and sagittal views. Subglottic extension should be no greater than 5 mm.

postoperative visit usually goes away, but occasionally it requires a laryngoscopy and removal.

Hemilaryngectomy

The diagrams in Figure 4–4 outline the anatomic limitations of tumor extent within which a hemilaryngectomy can be done. The various mitigating factors previously described in this chapter must be carefully borne in mind, as the geographic extent of malignancy is only one facet of the decision-making process determining the appropriateness of hemilaryngectomy.

Hemilaryngectomy is performed following a tracheostomy done under local anesthesia. After sterile preparation, a flexible endotracheal tube is placed through the tracheostomy site and sutured in place.

A horizontal incision is made in a skin crease at the level of the cricothyroid membrane (Fig. 4–5*B*). Rarely is a neck dissection required, but if it is, a modified H incision may be used (Fig. 4–5*C*). Skin flaps are elevated superiorly and inferiorly on the plane of the strap muscles (not the subplatysmal plane). The hyoid bone is the upper limit, and the first tracheal ring is the lower. A self-retaining retractor is installed.

On the side of the tumor, the sternohyoid and thyrohyoid muscles are incised from their origin on the hyoid bone (Fig. 4–6). A clean incision down to bare bone permits the dissection of some periosteum along with the attached muscle, which facilitates suturing in the reconstruction of the neocord later on.

The thyroid perichondrium is incised along the superior border of the thyroid cartilage the entire length of the affected side, and on the opposite side a sufficient distance to give adequate exposure for the cartilage cuts. The prelaryngeal fascia and its lymph node are peeled off the larynx to the first tracheal ring and sent to the histopathologist. A vertical incision is made through the external perichondrium in the midline, from top to bot-

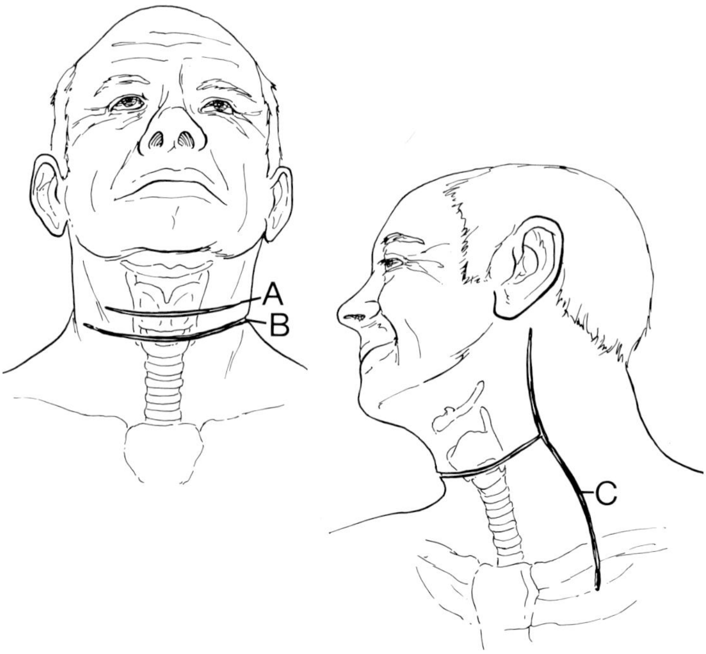

Figure 4–5. Incisions for partial laryngectomy. *A*, For supraglottic laryngectomy. *B*, For hemilaryngectomy. *C*, For radical neck dissection, when required.

tom. The perichondrium is carefully dissected away from the entire thyroid lamina of the affected side, from the midline to the posterior limit.

The cartilage cuts may be marked with dye, using a nonsiliconized needle. The markings go vertically through the midline of the thyroid cartilage and near the posterior border, with a connecting rim of cartilage left between the superior and inferior cornua, 3 to 4 mm in width (Fig. 4–7). Since this cartilage strip is primarily pharyngeal (it is part of the lateral wall of the pyriform fossa), it can safely be left behind. When the anterior commissure is involved, and marking extends about 4 mm lateral to the midline.

A sagittal saw is used to make the cartilage cuts, stopping just short of the internal perichondrium. The perichondrium is approached with great care to avoid damage by the saw. A horizontal incision is made with a scalpel in the cricothyroid membrane on the superior surface of the cricoid arch (Fig. 4–8). Bleeding from the cricothyroid artery, which crosses the cricothyroid membrane, is controlled by cautery.

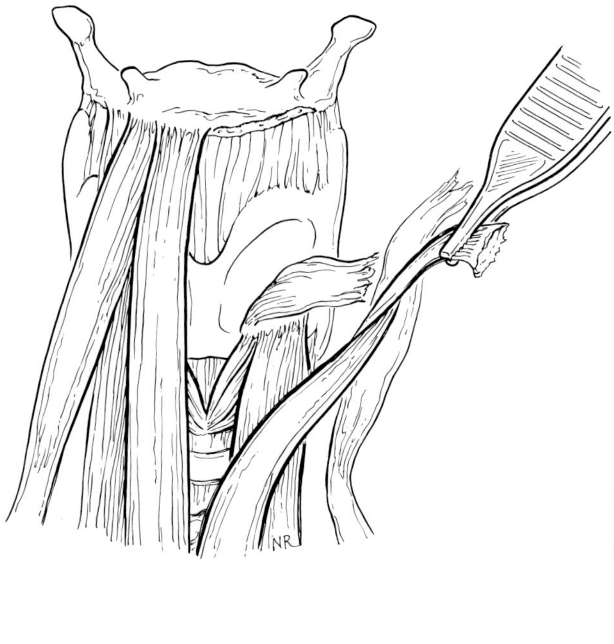

Figure 4–6. Hemilaryngectomy. Strap muscles are excised from hyoid bone, taking a little hyoid periosteum.

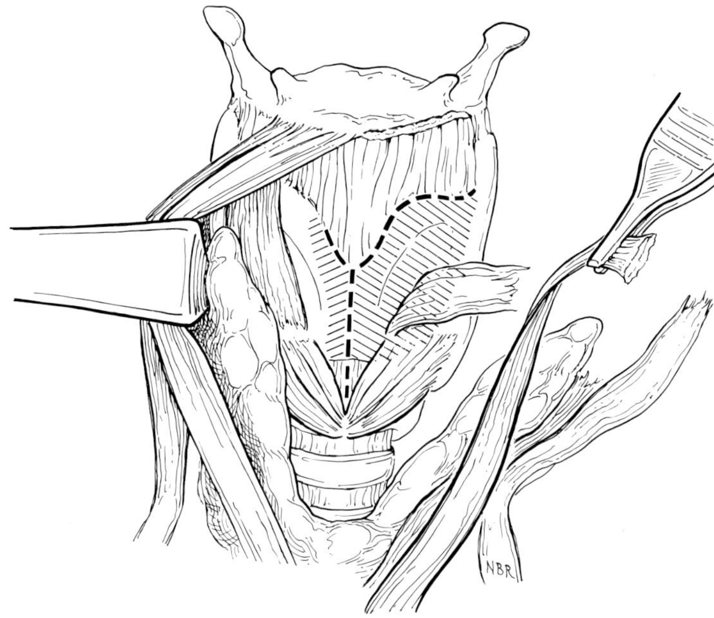

Figure 4–7. Hemilaryngectomy. Perichondrial incision over the superior aspect of the ipsilateral thyroid ala, splitting the perichondrium in the midline to the cricothyroid membrane. The incision extends superiorly 3 to 5 mm onto the other side. Crosshatched area represents the amount of perichondrial elevation.

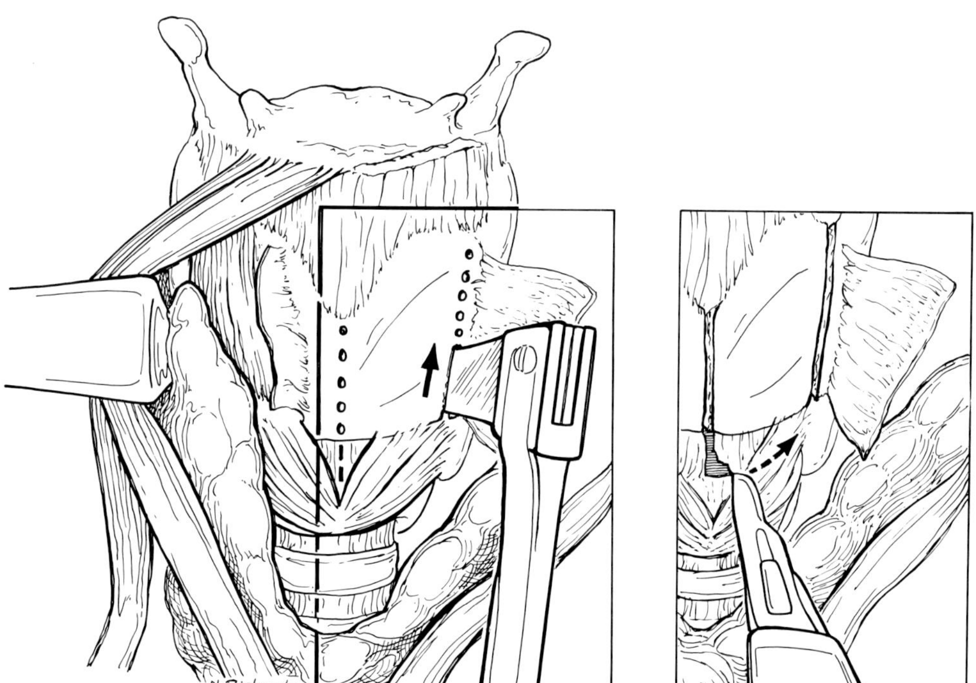

A B

Figure 4–8. Hemilaryngectomy. *A*, With the strap muscles of the opposing side retracted, the cartilage cuts are made with the oscillating saw: one in the midline and the second laterally, sparing a 3- to 4-mm strip of thyroid ala. *B*, Cartilage cuts completed. An incision is made through the cricothyroid membrane with the blade hugging the superior surface of the cricoid cartilage.

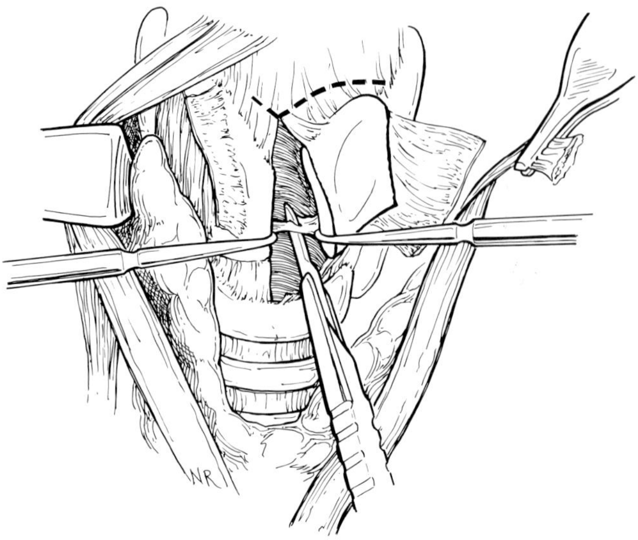

Figure 4–9. Hemilaryngectomy. The thyroid alae are held apart with hooks, and care is taken to split the anterior commissure precisely in the midline with a #15 scalpel blade. The incision need not clear the tumor by more than 1 mm.

The patient's head is further extended and a headlight is donned by the surgeon. With the cricothyroid membrane incision retracted with small skin hooks, the subglottic surface of the glottis is visualized. If the tumor extends to the sloping upper margin of the cricoid, the superior half of the cricoid cartilage should be included in the specimen. Any further subglottic extension should be managed by near-total laryngectomy.

An incision in the midline is carried from the cricothyroid membrane to just under the anterior commissure, through the internal perichondrium and endolaryngeal mucosa. If the lesion is limited to one side, the scalpel with a No. 15 blade is gently inserted between the cords and firmly cut anteriorly so that a perfect bifurcation of the glottis is achieved through the center of the anterior commissure (Fig. 4–9). This incision is extended superiorly into the petiolus of the epiglottis.

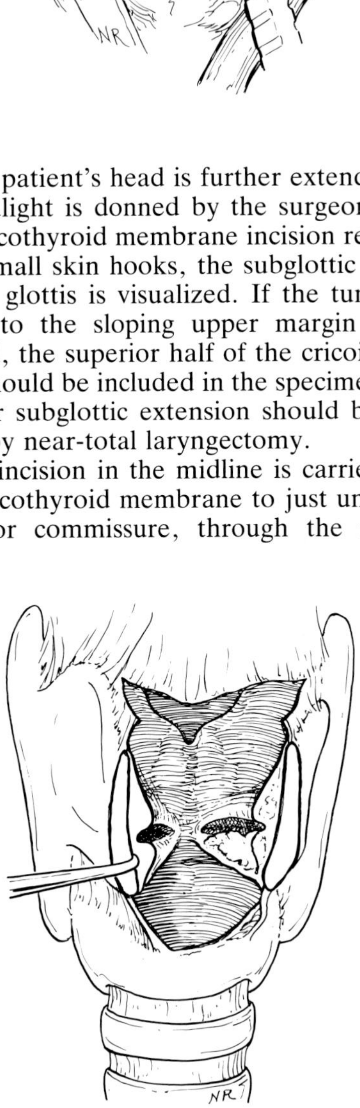

Figure 4–10. Hemilaryngectomy. The thyroid alae are held apart and the tumor extent is visualized. An incision through the thyrohyoid membrane extends into the laryngeal lumen, separating the epiglottis from the rest of the larynx.

When the lesion extends across the anterior commissure, the cords are pulled apart by hooks, and the anterior commissure as well as a 2-mm margin of involved contralateral vocal cord is included in the specimen.

The petiolus of the epiglottis is detached from its insertion into the thyroid ala. The thyroid alae can now be pulled widely apart and the tumor viewed (Fig. 4–10). Excision of the cancer is accomplished inferiorly with scissors, placing one blade inside the laryngeal lumen, and the other along the upper margin of the cricoid (or lower to include an upper margin of cricoid ring if necessary). As the arch of the cricoid sweeps toward the posterior laminae (Fig. 4–11), the cricoarytenoid joint is entered. The posterior margin of the resection is delineated with the angled (Panzer's) gallbladder scissors, with care taken to achieve an optimum margin without excising too much mucosa. Some of the arytenoid and aryepiglottic fold epithelium will be important in the reconstruction.

The final mucosal incision follows the apex of the aryepiglottic fold and connects the release of the arytenoid body to the cut through the epiglottic petiolus. This resection develops a specimen that is comparable in many ways to a cordectomy, but its volume

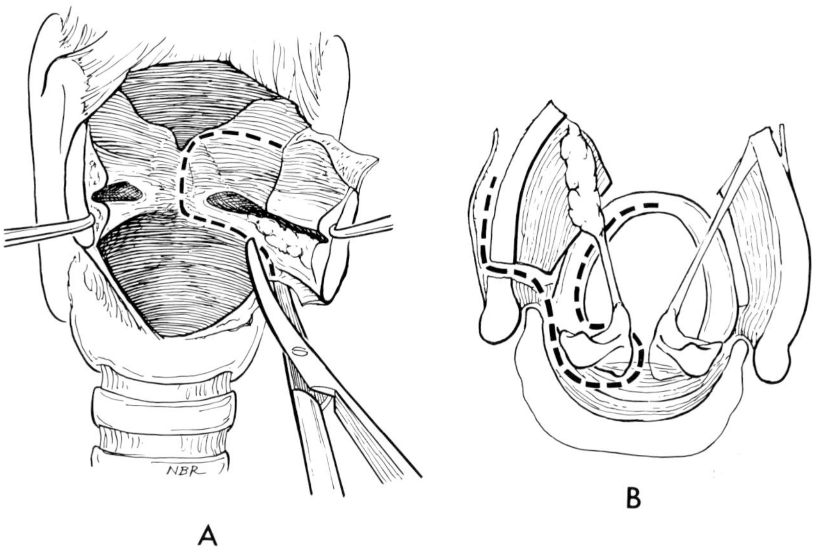

Figure 4–11. Hemilaryngectomy. *A*, The scissors hug the superior surface of the cricoid cartilage, excising the hemilarynx up to the posterior commissure. Dashed line represents the line of incision. *B*, The dashed line represents the intraluminal and extraluminal extent of resection.

is large inferiorly and superiorly and the arytenoid body and thyroid ala are included. A reasonable neocord regenerates without reconstruction following a cordectomy, provided the arytenoid remains. In the more extensive resection that we have chosen to call hemilaryngectomy, an attempt at glottic reconstruction is worthwhile. Glottic reconstruction is indicated to avoid a very breathy voice. On the other hand it carries with it the danger of postoperative airway obstruction. The surgeon ought to be a little less eager to discontinue the hemilaryngectomized patient's tracheotomy than he might be in the case of a laryngofissure and cordectomy.

To fashion a new vocal cord, the sternohyoid muscle with its attached hyoid periosteum is swung through the gap left by the excised specimen. The muscle is sutured to the laminae of the cricoid with No. 4-0 chromic catgut on a stout needle (Fig. 4–12*A*). The muscle is bulky and looks excessive, but with time it tends to shrink; thus overcorrection is justified. The remaining aryepiglottic mucosa is drawn over the posterior half of the muscle flap (Fig. 4–12*B*), but the anterior portion remains raw and must epithelialize on its own. If the anterior portion of the opposite vocal cord has been stripped, a Silastic keel is inserted between the cords to encourage epithelialization without the formation of a glottic web. The keel is left in place for about 3 weeks and removed under local anesthesia.

On the intact side, the anterior aspect of the cut true cord is sutured with 4-0 chromic catgut through two small drill holes placed in the remaining thyroid ala (Fig. 4–12*C*). The epiglottic petiole is sewn forward to the hyoid. The external thyroid perichondral flap is sutured in the midline as much as the muscle will allow (Fig. 4–13). An airtight closure is impossible, but actual fistulization is uncommon, even in irradiated cases. The wound is drained with a Penrose, and the skin is closed in layers. A light pressure dressing is applied.

Whereas cordectomy patients do not require a nasogastric tube, hemilaryngectomees usually do. Oral alimentation is usually delayed until the tenth postoperative day, and the tracheostomy is not corked before this date.

The balance between an adequate voice and a sufficient airway is difficult to achieve. A voice that is too good in the early phases often warns of an inadequate airway. Over a period of several months, the operated side tends to foreshorten. Some patients phonate against the neocord with their opposite false cord instead of their true cord. If the glottic chink is too short, especially after contralateral anterior cordal resection, it can be lengthened by a laryngotomy and insertion of a keel as a secondary maneuver. The elasticity of the tissues does not return, however, and the vocal results for "phonosurgery" following hemilaryngectomy are poor.

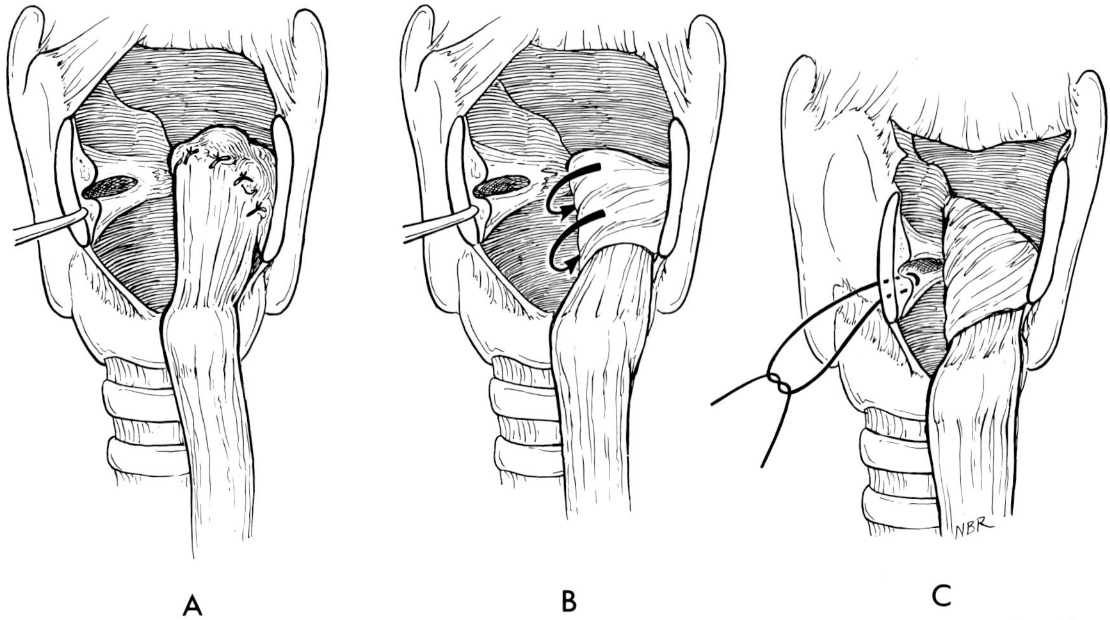

Figure 4–12. Hemilaryngectomy. *A*, The larynx is reconstructed by bringing in a muscular flap of sternothyroid and sternohyoid muscle, then suturing it to any residual arytenoid cartilage or to the raw bed over the lamina of the cricoid cartilage. *B*, A mucosal flap of aryepiglottic fold is folded over the muscle to reconstruct the "neocord." Size 4-0 absorbable sutures secure this mucosa to the subglottic mucosa. *C*, An anchoring suture draws the uninvolved vocal fold to the anterior of the larynx. The suture is secured by passing it through the two holes in the anterior extremity of the residual thyroid ala.

The same is true of a breathy dysphonia after a cordectomy. The neocord is scar tissue that is usually too tight to retain injected Teflon. The best policy in such cases is probably to make sure the patient's expectations for voice quality are realistic before the surgery is performed.

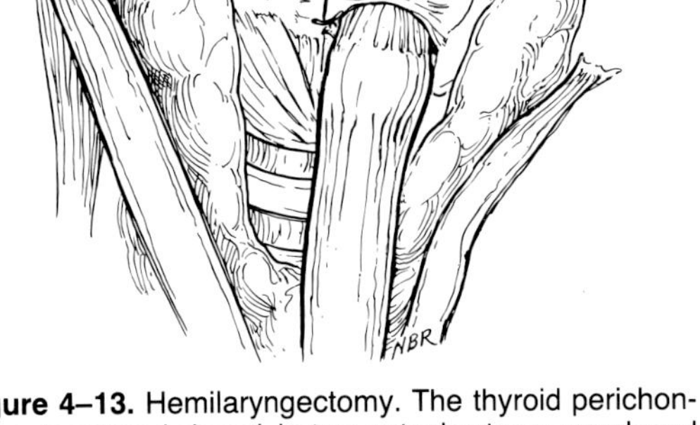

Figure 4–13. Hemilaryngectomy. The thyroid perichondrium is sutured closed, but no actual sutures are placed between it and the bulk of the muscle flap.

Frontolateral Laryngectomy

This extended form of hemilaryngectomy is used for lesions that extend from one true cord across the anterior commissure to involve the opposite cord a distance of between one half to one third of its anterior length (Fig. 4–14).

The initial stages of thyroid cartilage exposure are identical to the standard hemilaryngectomy. The sternohyoid muscle may have to be partially released from its medial attachment on the side of least involvement or it may be able to be retracted. The cartilage cut may need to extend to this side about one-third the distance from the midline to its posterior limit (Fig. 4–15).

As the soft tissue excision proceeds, the tumor is cleared by a 1- to 2-mm margin, leaving a markedly shortened cord that retracts toward the arytenoid (Fig. 4–16). A cordal anchoring that fixes it as far anteriorly as possible is done with a mattress suture through the remaining thyroid ala. The missing cord on the more involved side is reconstructed with a sternohyoid muscle flap. A keel is inserted for 6 weeks in the hope of establishing anterior re-epithelialization of both the neocord and the area in front of the

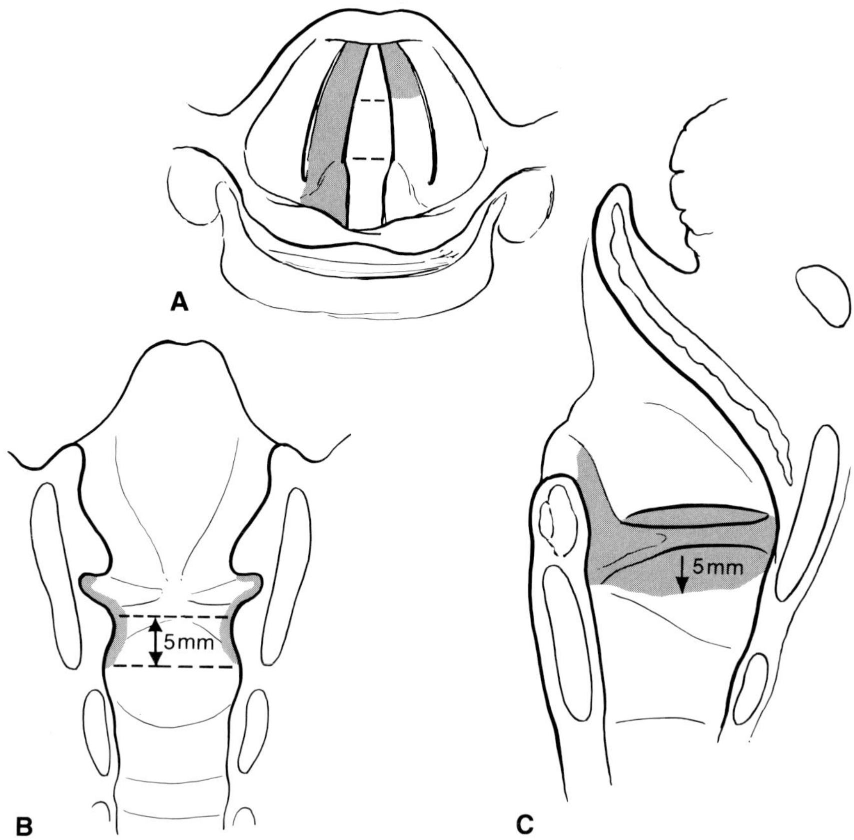

Figure 4–14. The limits of tumor extension for resection of laryngeal cancer by frontolateral vertical hemilaryngectomy in *(A)* superior, *(B)* coronal, and *(C)* sagittal views.

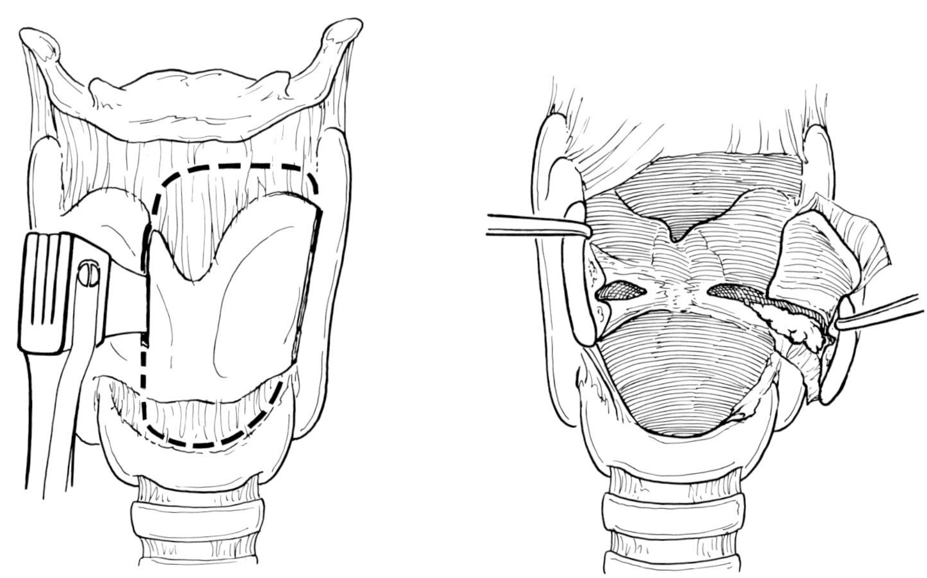

Figure 4–15. Frontolateral partial laryngectomy. *A*, The medial cartilage incision extends beyond the midline to the thyroid cartilage so that an incision through it will clear the tumor on the underlying vocal cord. *B*, The larynx is opened and tumor extent visualized. The tumor on the cord of least involvement is cleared by a 1- to 2-mm margin of healthy tissue.

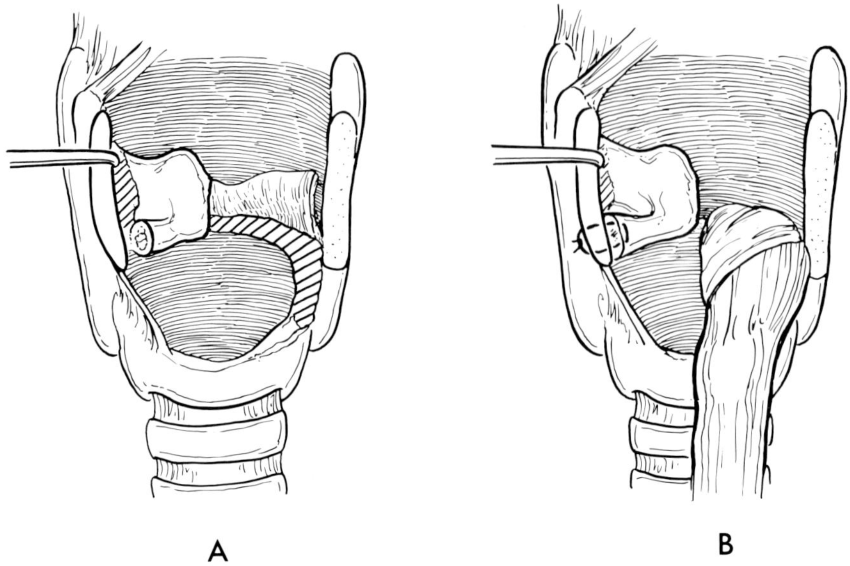

Figure 4–16. Frontolateral partial laryngectomy. *A*, Defect following resection. The tumor on the cord of least involvement is cleared by a 1- to 2-mm margin of healthy tissue. The resection of the cord of greatest involvement is similar to that for a standard hemilaryngectomy. *B*, The resected cord is reconstructed with a sternohyoid muscle flap. An anchoring suture fixes the residual cord to the remaining thyroid ala.

shortened residual cord (Fig. 4–17). Any subsequent web formation may have to be managed by the reinstitution of a keel following laryngotomy or by excision with the CO_2 laser.

Extended Frontolateral Laryngectomy with Epiglottic Laryngoplasty (Kambič-Sedlaček-Tucker Technique)

Since 1965, Sedlaček[26] and more recently Kambič[27] have been doing a form of hemilaryngectomy that has extended well beyond what have been generally considered standard limits. The lesions that can be encompassed by this procedure can involve one arytenoid and extend to the opposing cord to almost the tip of the vocal process (Fig. 4–18). The laryngeal structural support lost by the excision is supplanted by the now redundant aryepiglottic and false vocal cords as the epiglottis is brought into the supportive framework of the larynx.

The approach is identical to that for a frontolateral laryngectomy. The perichondrium is split in the midline and incised both superiorly and inferiorly throughout its length. The cartilage cut on the most affected side is unchanged and on the least involved side is carried around almost to the same extent (Figs. 4–19 to 4–27). Superiorly an incision is made in the inferior aspect of the thyrohyoid membrane, completely separating the insertion of the epiglottis from the thyroid

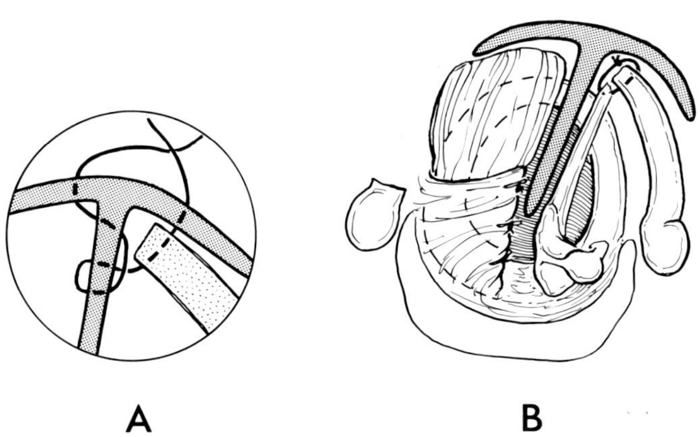

Figure 4–17. *A*, Residual cord is anchored with a suture through the thyroid cartilage remnant. *B*, The completely resected cord is reconstructed with a sternohyoid muscle flap. A Montgomery Silastic umbrella keel is inserted to prevent anterior web formation.

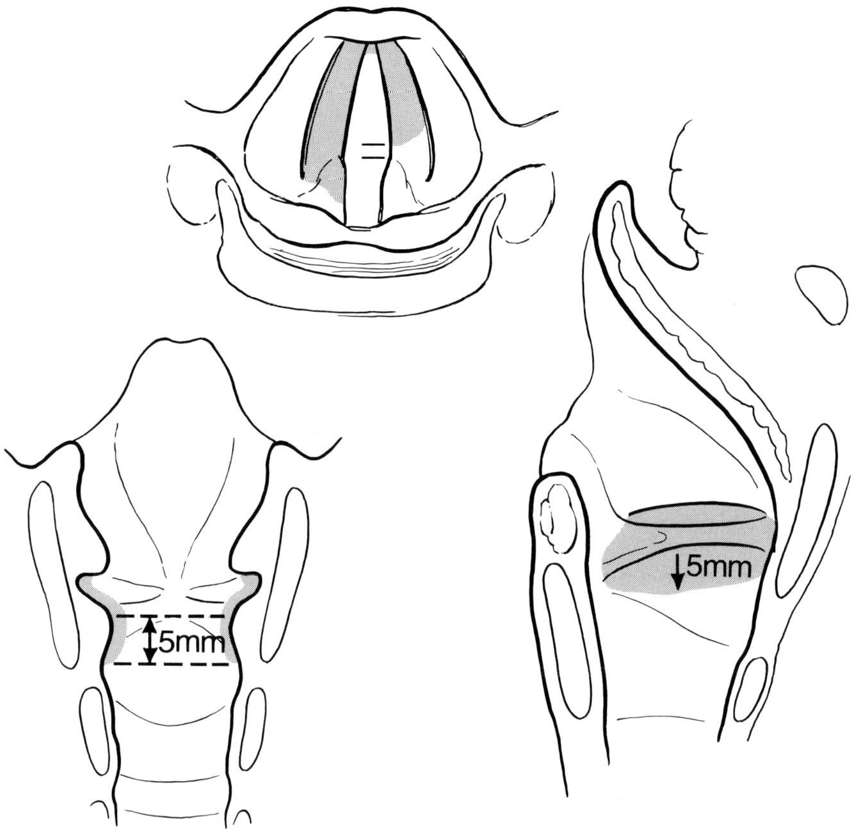

Figure 4–18. The limits of tumor extension for resection of laryngeal cancer by the extended hemilaryngectomy operation with epiglottic laryngoplasty. (Kambič-Sedlaček-Tucker procedure.)

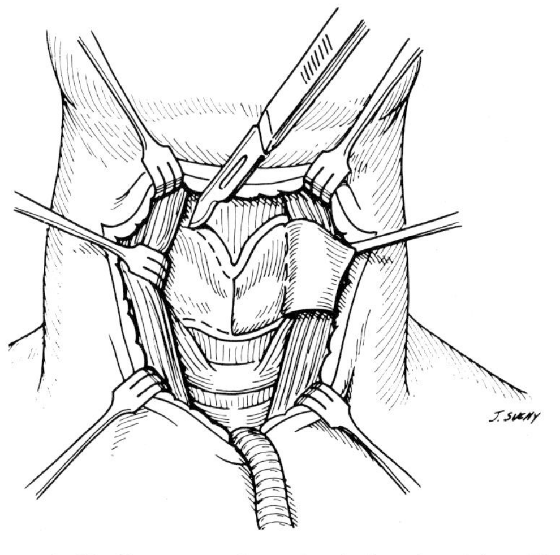

Figure 4–19. Strap muscles retracted and perichondrial cuts being made. (From Tucker HM, Wood BG, Levine H, et al: Glottic reconstruction after near total laryngectomy. Laryngoscope 89:609, 1979.)

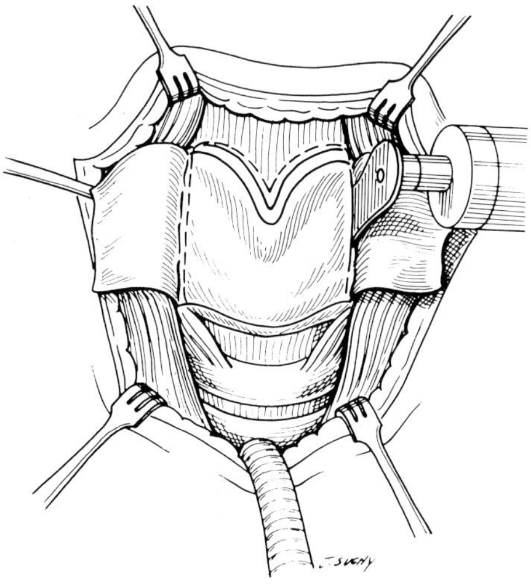

Figure 4–20. Cartilage cuts being made with saw. (From Tucker HM, Wood BG, Levine H, et al: Glottic reconstruction after near total laryngectomy. Laryngoscope 89:609, 1979.)

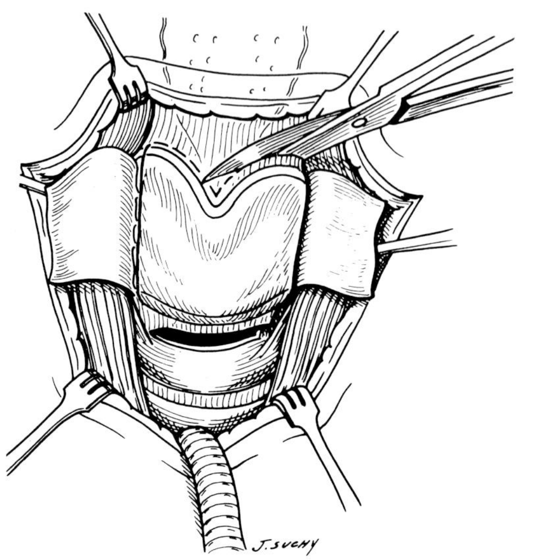

Figure 4–21. Cricothyroid membrane incised and left thyrohyoid membrane being cut with scissors. (From Tucker HM, Wood BG, Levine H, et al: Glottic reconstruction after near total laryngectomy. Laryngoscope 89:609, 1979.)

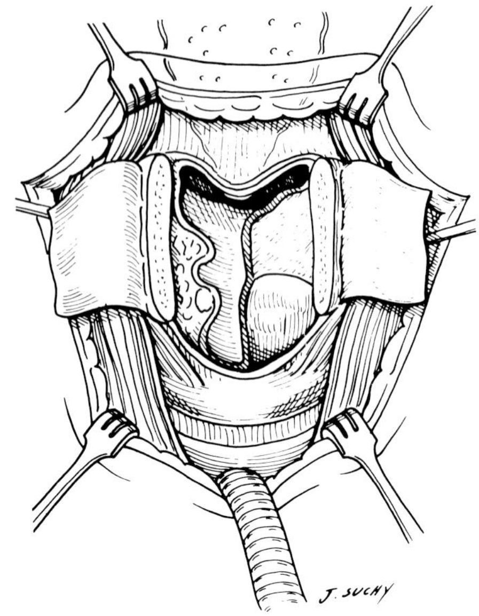

Figure 4–22. Surgical defect after completion of near-total laryngectomy. (From Tucker HM, Wood BG, Levine H, et al: Glottic reconstruction after near total laryngectomy. Laryngoscope 89:609, 1979.)

cartilage. Inferiorly the cricothyroid membrane is incised horizontally. Using this incision, the most involved site is cut with scissors along the cricoid arch, through the cricoarytenoid joint and the interarytenoid area.

On the side of least involvement the cricoid is again hugged with the scissors, and an incision across the cord is made 1 to 2 mm beyond the lesion. The specimen is removed and it is obvious that most of the thyroid

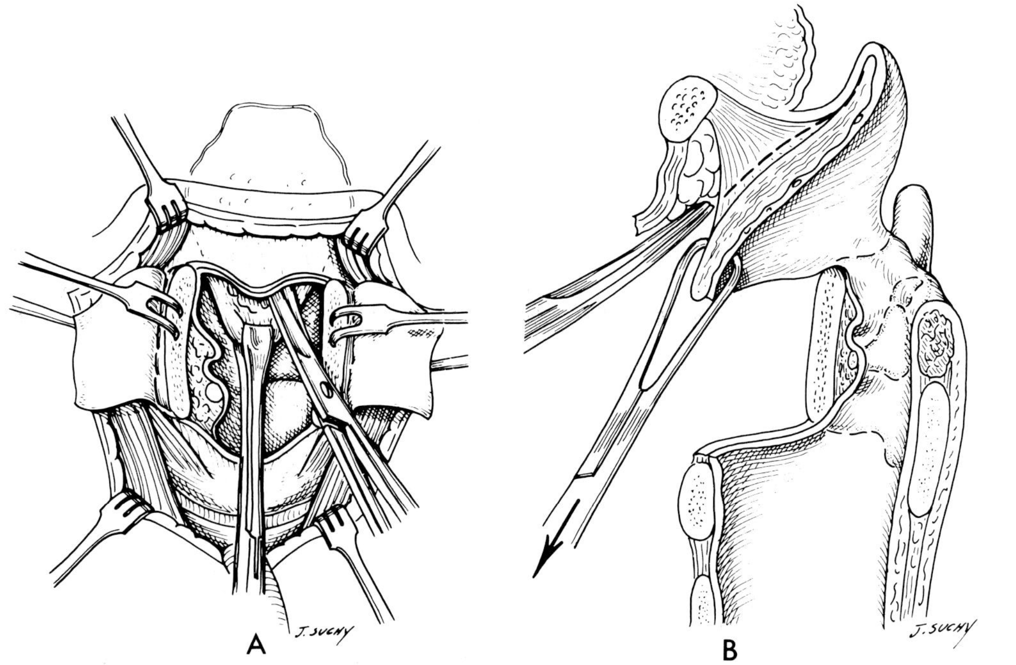

Figure 4–23. *A*, Base of epiglottis being grasped with tenaculum and pre-epiglottic space contents being dissected away with scissors. *B* Lateral view of pre-epiglottic space contents being dissected away from anterior surface of epiglottis. (From Tucker HM, Wood BG, Levine H, et al: Glottic reconstruction after near total laryngectomy. Laryngoscope 89:609, 1979.)

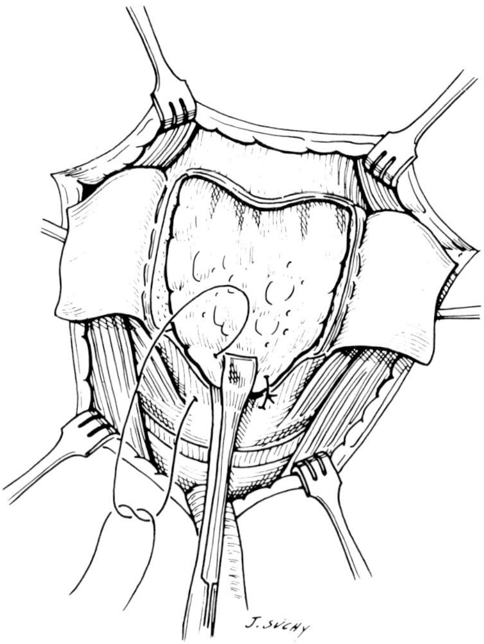

Figure 4–24. Mobilized epiglottis displaced interiorly into laryngeal defect and base being sutured to cricothyroid membrane. (From Tucker HM, Wood BG, Levine H, et al: Glottic reconstruction after near total laryngectomy. Laryngoscope 89:609, 1979.)

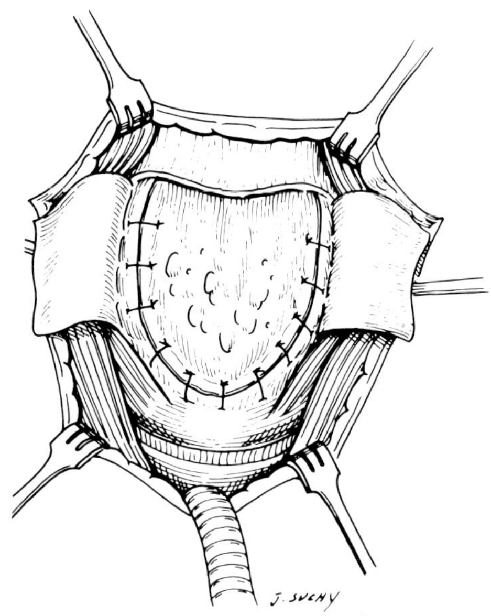

Figure 4–25. Epiglottis sutured to thyroid ala remnants and cricothyroid membrane (complete). (From Tucker HM, Wood BG, Levine H, et al: Glottic reconstruction after near total laryngectomy. Laryngoscope 89:609, 1979.)

cartilage has been excised. No attempt is made to turn muscle flaps for the reconstruction of each individual cord.

The petiolus of the epiglottis is grasped with a tenaculum and retracted inferiorly. Dissection on the anterior surface of the epiglottis into the pre-epiglottic space is done. This is a simple maneuver. Scissors dissection proceeds until the epiglottis is pulled with ease into the defect left by the thyroid cartilage excision. As the epiglottis prolapses into the gap, it pulls with it the false cords and the aryepiglottic fold mucosa, which become folded upon themselves. This redundant mucosa compensates for the lost cords, and the epiglottis for the lost structural component. The epiglottis is sewn in place with nonabsorbable suture such as Tevdek. The thyroid perichondrium is approximated, the strap muscles are returned, the wound is drained, and the skin is closed.

Speaking is discouraged for 10 to 14 days and decannulation weaning is begun at this time. Oral feeding is delayed for the same span of time. Fortunately aspiration is not much of a problem, and decannulation is usually successfully achieved.

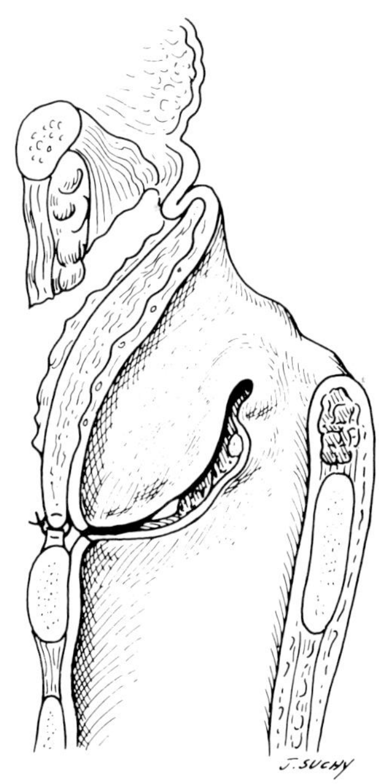

Figure 4–26. Lateral view of epiglottis sutured to cricothyroid membrane in a submucosal fashion. Also depicts close proximity of endolaryngeal mucosa, which is not sutured. (From Tucker HM, Wood BG, Levine H, et al: Glottic reconstruction after near total laryngectomy. Laryngoscope 89:609, 1979.)

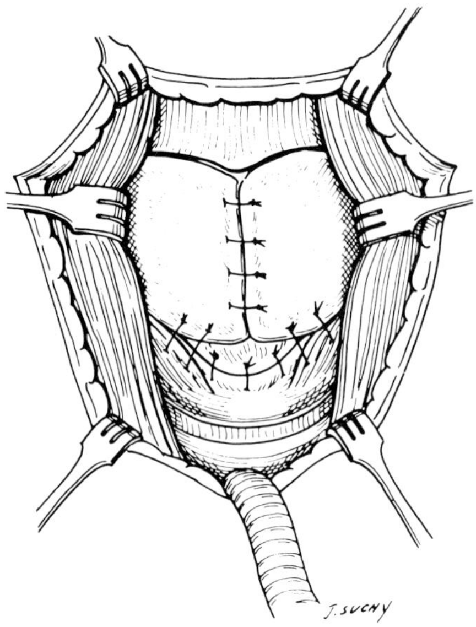

Figure 4–27. Perichondrial closure completed.

Supraglottic Laryngectomy

The diagnosis of supraglottic cancer is often delayed until the volume is great. Supraglottic laryngectomy is used to deal with more extensive cancers than those treated by hemilaryngectomy. It is usually combined with at least one radical neck dissection, and it produces a higher incidence of immediate and late postoperative complications than hemilaryngectomy. Our practice (B.P.) is always to perform a neck dissection on the side of greatest involvement, for clearance, exposure, and staging. If the primary lesion touches the midline or the primary neck dissection is reported to be positive, at least a conservation neck dissection is performed on the opposite side. An aggressive policy with regard to the neck is essential in supraglottic cancer, because this is the site most often responsible for failure. The temptation to turn to prophylactic postoperative irradiation, which has been claimed to be a serious competitor of block dissection in eliminating microscopic cancer in the neck,[35] is not justified by our own experience. After a supraglottic laryngectomy, radiation induces a persistent glottic edema that interferes with the timely acquisition of a safe airway. The dryness does nothing for the swallow, and, what is more serious, this treatment option is no longer available for use should a second primary develop. Perhaps when the cancer invades the tongue base, or is poorly differentiated, or is associated with multiple nodes with extracapsular invasion, the addition of postoperative radiation contributes hope. But it should never be relied upon to sterilize margin-positive residual disease at the primary site, or to compensate for optimistic conservatism in the neck.

In an N_0 neck, if no cancer is present, irradiation will obviously "succeed." This provides padded statistics for therapy, and no information on prognosis. If cancer was present but occult, a neck dissection, which need not be radical, removes cancer earlier and identifies its presence. This may influence the approach to the opposite neck, or to the follow-up. It educates the investigator who, after successful irradiation, will always remain in doubt about the validity of the treatment, having no information as to the true status of the neck. Sometimes either treatment fails in an N_0 neck. If it was dissected, the information gained at surgery (carotid involvement or extracapsular node invasion, for example) may provide the critical justification needed to recommend additional treatment. If it was irradiated, everything in the neck will get firm, and by the time the failure is obvious to palpation, the time for a successful salvage operation will be past.

At the editor's (P.J.D.) institution, prophylactic irradiation appears to be as effective as radical neck dissection in eliminating microscopic neck disease[36] and equal or even superior to conservation neck dissection. Unfortunately the irradiation induces a good deal of laryngeal edema that interferes with the early acquisition of swallowing and airway competence. However, when the lesion invades the tongue base or has an appreciable extension over the so-called marginal area, the addition of postoperative irradiation adds a margin of insurance.

The geographic limits safely encompassable by a supraglottic laryngectomy are outlined in Figure 4–28. Assuming, then, a policy of supraglottic laryngectomy plus unilateral or bilateral neck dissection for selected supraglottic carcinomas, the operation proceeds as follows.

A tracheostomy under local anesthesia is followed by the preparation and introduction of a wire-spiral endotracheal tube. The incision is made in a skin crease running through the thyroid tubercle (Fig. 4–5*A*) and is extended to the mastoid for the associated radical neck dissection. Unless positive nodes are present along the accessory nerve, it is

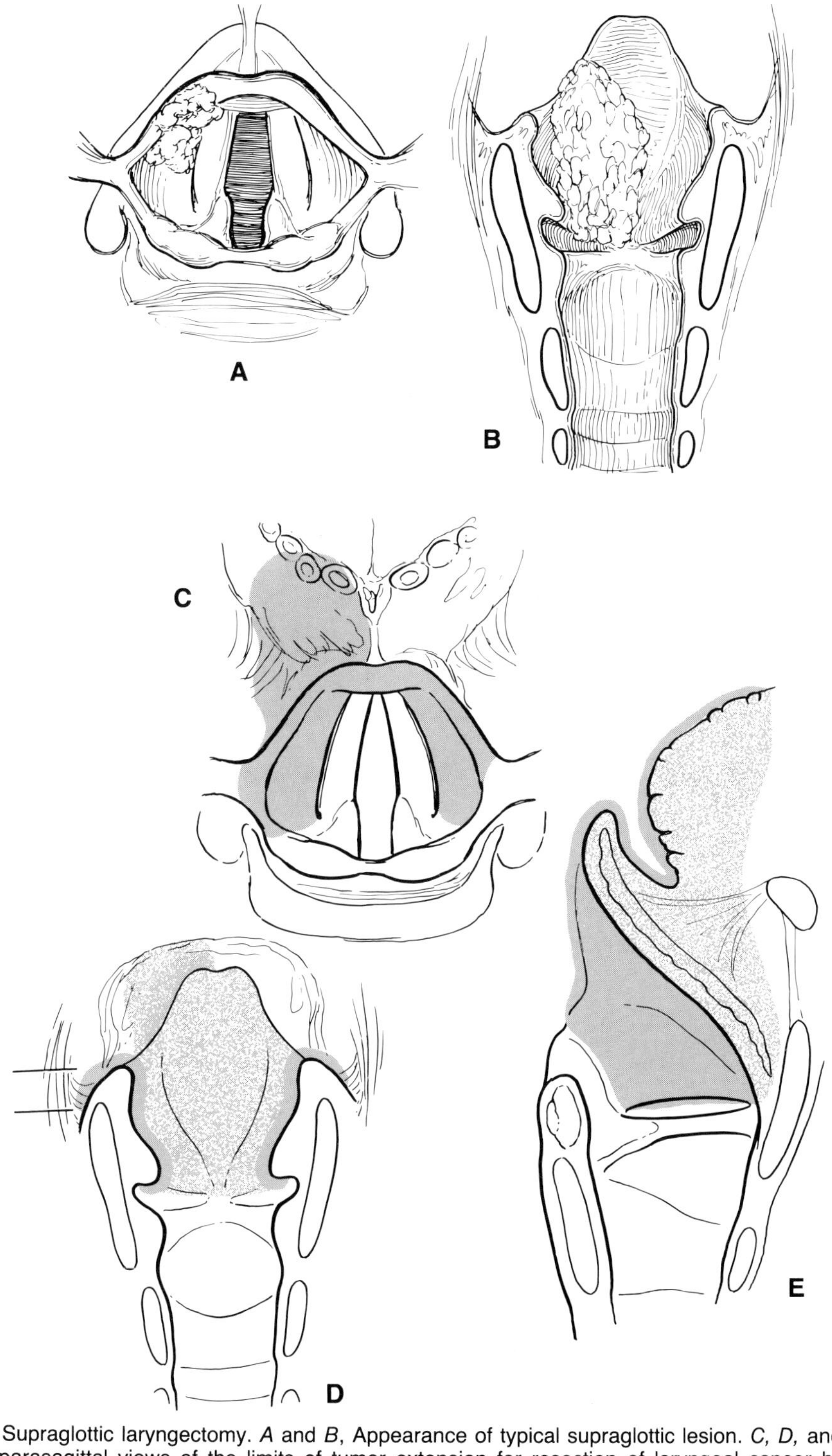

Figure 4–28. Supraglottic laryngectomy. *A* and *B*, Appearance of typical supraglottic lesion. *C, D,* and *E*, Superior, coronal, and parasagittal views of the limits of tumor extension for resection of laryngeal cancer by supraglottic laryngectomy.

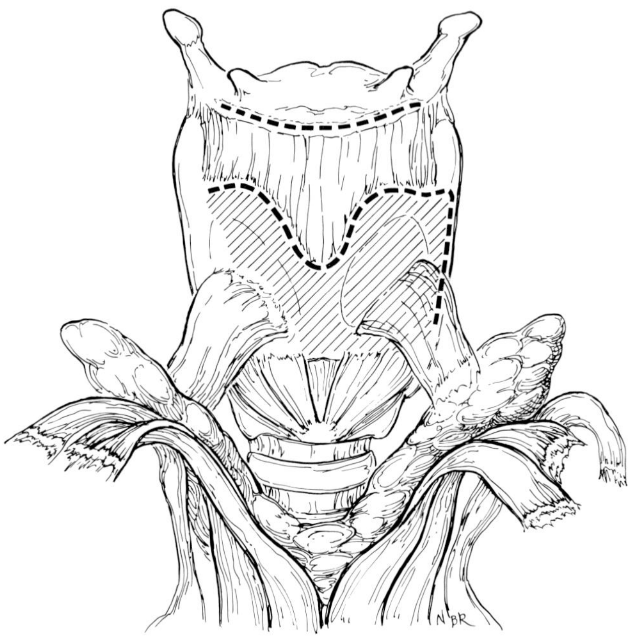

Figure 4–29. Supraglottic laryngectomy. Strap muscles are dissected from the hyoid bone along with some hyoid periosteum (upper dashed line incision). Perichondrial incisions are outlined on the thyroid alae. Shaded area represents amount of perichondrial elevation.

not necessary to include this structure in the neck.[37] A more common problem is the presence of disease near the hypoglossal or vagus nerves, since loss of these nerves during the neck dissection limits the patient's ability to resume swallowing. With appropriate individualization, an adequate dissection to remove all the lymph node–bearing tissues of the first neck is accomplished. The pedicle of the bloc is only the omohyoid muscle and its fascia, and there is little point obstructing access to the larynx by preserving it.[38] Once this pedicle is well developed, it may be incised and the neck specimen removed for frozen-section assessment. The findings, reported during the laryngeal operation, may influence the surgeon to consider simultaneous conservation neck dissection on the other side.

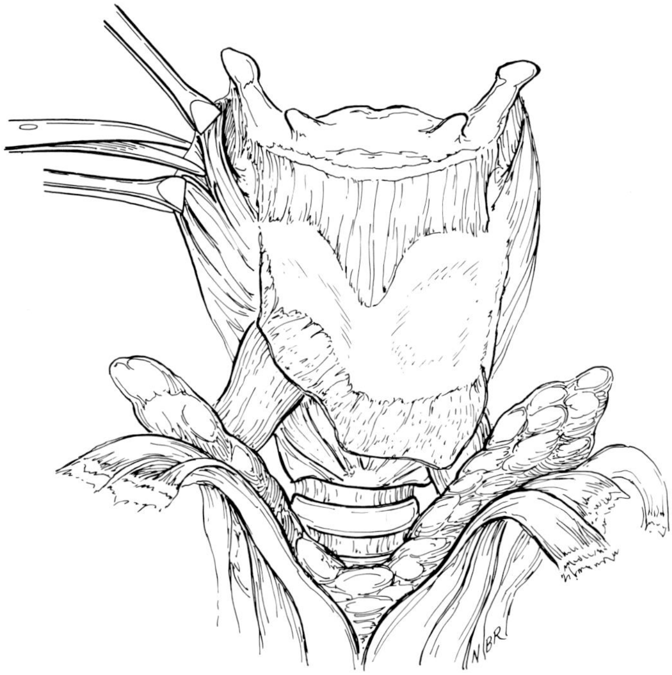

Figure 4–30. Supraglottic laryngectomy. Perichondrium reflected.

Attention is now turned to the larynx, which is exposed from the submental triangle to about the level of the cricoid cartilage. The tracheostomy site is kept out of communication with the operative field.

The strap muscles are dissected from the hyoid, with great care taken to detect and avoid any carcinoma that presses forward in the pre-epiglottic space under the thyrohyoid membrane (Fig. 4–29). The perichondrium is incised along the entire superior border of the thyroid cartilage and is reflected inferiorly to expose the upper two thirds of the thyroid laminae (Fig. 4–30). The only eventual closure with any substance will be between this layer and the tongue base.

Cartilage cuts are marked in methylene with an unsiliconized needle. They should be situated at the level of the laryngeal ventricles and above the insertion of Broyles' anterior commissural tendon. A good deal has been written about the level of the true vocal cords, the miniscule difference between males and females, and the division of the thyroid cartilage into fractions and millimeters in the hope of guiding the surgeon.[38] From a practical standpoint, there are two crucial points. First, extreme care must be taken not to injure the anterior commissure, or the patient may never swallow. Second, it must be recognized that the level of the anterior commissure is almost as high as the thyroid notch. Once the supraglottic folds are gone, the patient depends on the competence of the glottis to effect swallowing. Loss of cord tension resulting from an inadvertent anterior commissure injury, quite apart from its effects on the voice, is a critical blow to deglutition. At least the lower three quarters of the thyroid angle, the midline cartilage joining the two thyroid alae, should be preserved.

The Stryker saw is used to make the cartilage cuts down to the internal perichondrium. The incision should be carried directly horizontally to the posterior extremity of the thyroid ala on the side of greatest involvement. On the opposite side, the incision proceeds horizontally to the middle of the ala and then slants obliquely to the superior border (Fig. 4–31). In preparation for the soft tissue resection, the patient should now be given a potent muscle relaxant, in adequate dosage to assure complete relaxation of the vocal cords.

When the tumor is limited to the supraglottic endolarynx, the suprahyoid musculature is incised and an entrance to the hypopharynx is made into the vallecula on the best side. If the base of the tongue or the vallecula is involved with cancer, the entrance is usually through a pharyngotomy in the opposite pyriform fossa (Fig. 4–32). The hyoid is not skeletonized; the suprahyoid cuts are made as the lingual extent of the tumor is directly visualized.

The patient's head is maximally extended. The surgeon puts on a headlight. The epiglottis is grasped with a tenaculum, and skin hooks are used to retract the false cords and confirm the limitation of the tumor to the supraglottic larynx. Once adequate exposure of the larynx and the tumor has been achieved, the soft tissue resection begins. The

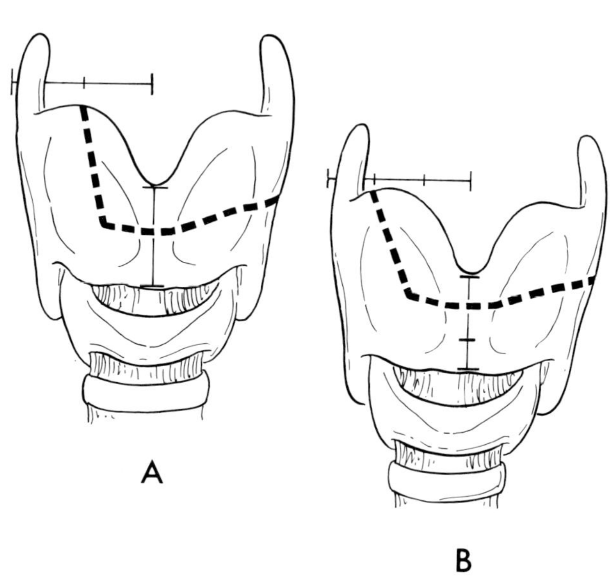

Figure 4–31. Supraglottic laryngectomy. Cartilage cuts outlined in *(A)* male and *(B)* female.

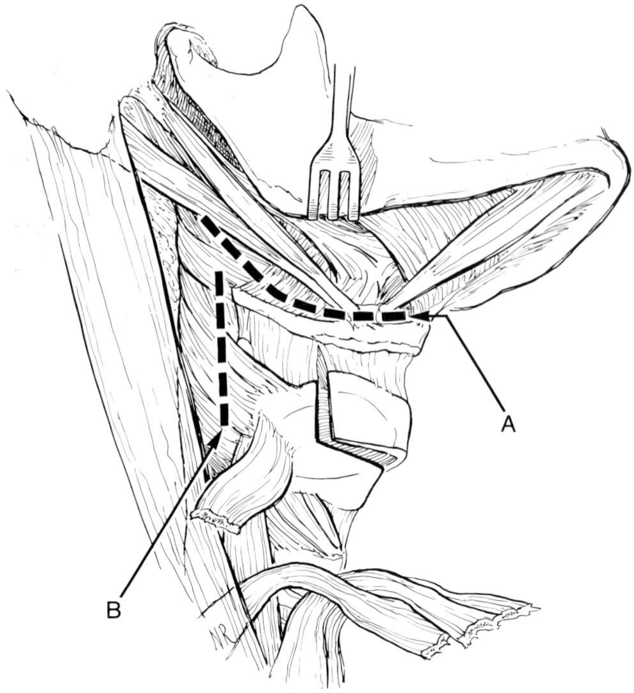

Figure 4–32. Supraglottic laryngectomy. Line *A* represents a vallecular approach, used when the lesion does not extend onto the lingual aspect of the epiglottis. The pyriform fossa entrance *(B)* is used if there is lingular epiglottic, vallecular, or tongue base invasion.

mucosal resection begins on the apex of the aryepiglottic folds and angles across the false cords obliquely into the ventricle. It is important to remember that the ventricles begin above the tip of the vocal processes (Fig. 4–33). On the most involved side, the lateral wall of the pyriform fossa is released from the superior cornu of the thyroid cartilage. The internal blade of the scissors cuts across the cuneiform down toward the vocal process tip at the level of the true cord, and then turns forward to carry into the ventricle at its apex. The external blade traverses the medial pyriform sinus mucosa until the anterior apex of the sinus is reached. At this point the external blade continues out of the pharynx and into the soft tissue until it slips under the thyroid perichondrium into the cartilage cut.

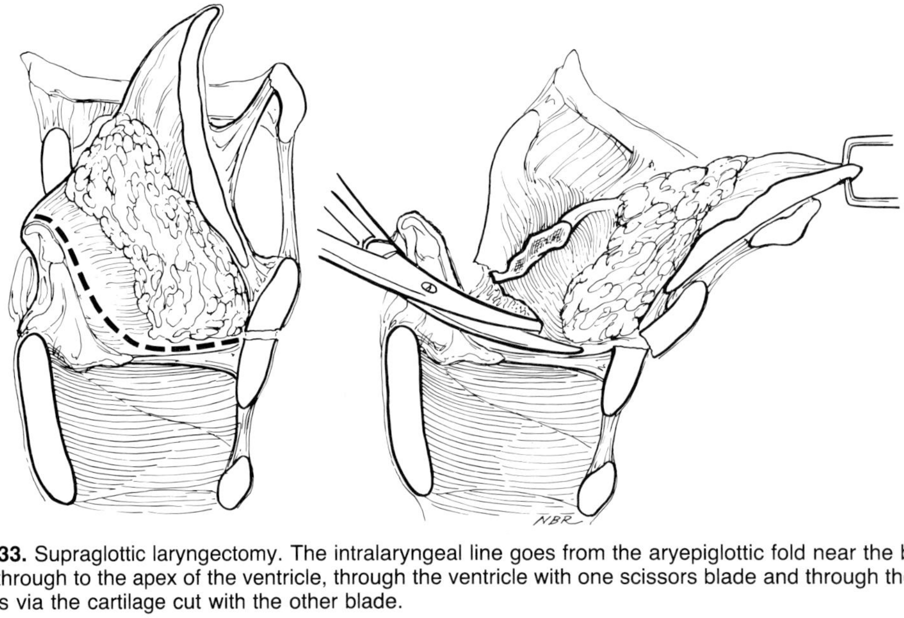

Figure 4–33. Supraglottic laryngectomy. The intralaryngeal line goes from the aryepiglottic fold near the body of the arytenoid through to the apex of the ventricle, through the ventricle with one scissors blade and through the laryngeal soft tissues via the cartilage cut with the other blade.

The scissors now continue cutting, one blade proceeding forward in the ventricle and the other in the cartilage cut.

The specimen is retracted superiorly, and visualization of the anterior commissure and the better side is aided by unfolding the specimen a bit. The scissors cross the midline above the anterior commissure, enter the opposite ventricle, and carry on up the oblique cut of the thyroid cartilage on this side. The cut through the aryepiglottic fold and the pyriform on that side is carefully distanced from the posterior margin of the tumor (Fig. 4–34). The inferior separation of supraglottis from glottis has now been made. In the case in which the pyriform fossa was the site of entry, it remains to establish the superior resection margin, which is connected inferiorly by an incision through the lateral pharyngoepiglottic fold (Fig. 4–35). This is accomplished and the specimen is delivered.

By careful dissection, it is usually possible to identify and preserve much of the superior laryngeal nerve on the less involved side. On the more involved side, an attempt to preserve this structure is usually thwarted by the need for an adequate resection, and there is little arytenoid mucosa left to justify its preservation in any case. On the side of least involvement, it is tempting to cut across the hyoid and leave the greater cornu lateral to the pyriform. However, if a portion of the hyoid is left in a slim neck, this presents the problem of a persistent mass to an unwary examiner in the follow-up months. It is probably better to grasp the horn of the bone with an Allis clamp, carefully avoid the nearby twelfth nerve, and with vigorous retraction, cut all the attachments off with a scalpel. The specimen, including the entire hyoid bone, may then be removed.

When the base of the tongue is involved, a wide margin of excision threatens the hypoglossal nerves and lingual arteries. They can usually be preserved, at least on one side, if the suprahyoid anatomy is clarified. The nerve is deep to the myohyoid; the artery is deep to the hyoglossus. Sacrifice of both arteries is not always incompatible with survival of the tongue remnant. However, the rehabilitation of swallowing after supraglottic laryngectomy is difficult when a large portion of the tongue base is removed (Fig. 4–36).

Excessive tongue base involvement does not mandate total laryngectomy for swallowing purposes. Near-total laryngectomy will allow a wide tongue resection, and will preserve the voice. It does leave the patient dependent on a permanent tracheostomy, but swallowing is superior to that achievable with the upwardly extended supraglottic procedure.

While the supraglottic laryngectomy specimen is undergoing quick-section analysis, a

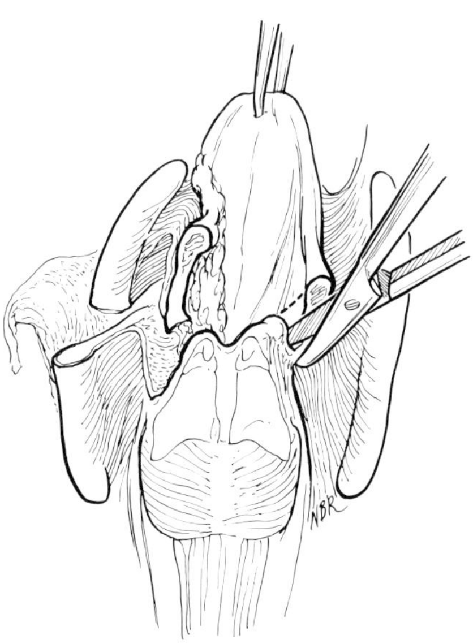

Figure 4–34. Supraglottic laryngectomy. The scissors now engage the aryepiglottic fold on the least involved side. The start of this incision is usually further anteriorly on the fold than on the side of greatest tumor involvement. This facilitates the passage of the outer scissors blade through the more anteriorly placed cartilage cut of the least involved side. This incision meets that of the opposing side, and the tumor of the supraglottis is removed from the rest of the larynx.

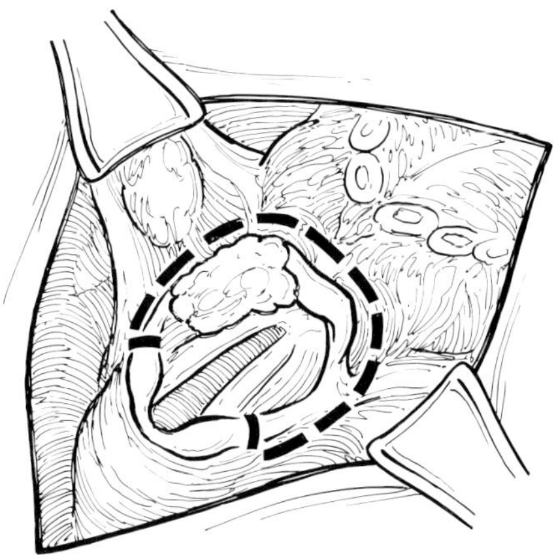

Figure 4–35. Supraglottic laryngectomy. Resection proceeds superiorly, conserving pyriform sinus mucosa wherever possible. In lesions extending no further superiorly than the laryngeal surface of the epiglottis, the resection is carried just above the vallecula, with the tongue base musculature cut off at the level of the hyoid bone.

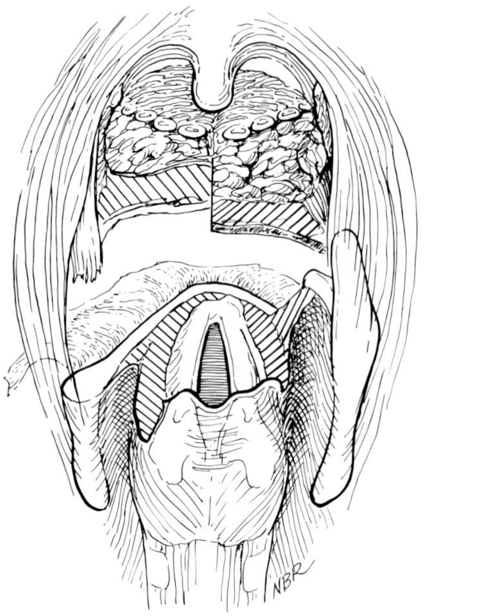

Figure 4–36. Supraglottic laryngectomy. If the vallecula or tongue base is involved, a generous margin of healthy tongue is mandatory. Illustration shows defect remaining following supraglottic laryngectomy with substantial tongue base resection.

cricopharyngeal myotomy is done. The index finger is placed in the pharynx, and a scalpel cut is made through the full thickness of the cricopharyngeal fibers of the inferior constrictor that remain attached to the cricoid. A 1-cm wide segment of this muscular ring may be excised. The remaining mucosa will appear perilously thin, but is durable and will not spontaneously perforate. Care is taken to make this excision in the posterior aspect of the pharynx, thus avoiding trauma to the recurrent laryngeal nerve.

Careful closure (Fig. 4–37) is the key to low fistulization rates and the successful rehabilitation of swallow. Mucosal approximation is not the object. The goal is to elevate the remaining larynx as high as possible and position the tongue base in an overhanging configuration. The primary closure is basically in one layer, and all sutures are placed before any are tied. With the patient's head still in the extended position, the closure is begun internally by suturing, for as far as possible, the medial pyriform mucosa to the residual arytenoid mucosa, using light catgut (Fig. 4–38). An unclosed area of considerable extent is left anteriorly to re-epithelialize spontaneously. External closure is accomplished by suturing the thyroid perichondrium to the raw tongue base, using interrupted nonabsorbable mattress sutures. The closure begins with approximation of the lateral pharyngeal walls (Fig. 4–37) using 3-0 chromic catgut or Vicryl. The perichondrium-to-tongue sutures of 3-0 silk or Tevdek are tagged with mosquito hemostats while waiting to be tied. Each one penetrates the tongue about 1 cm from the cut edge of the mucosa (Fig. 4–39*A*). This allows a part of the cut surface of the tongue to abut the raw surface of the excised false cord area.

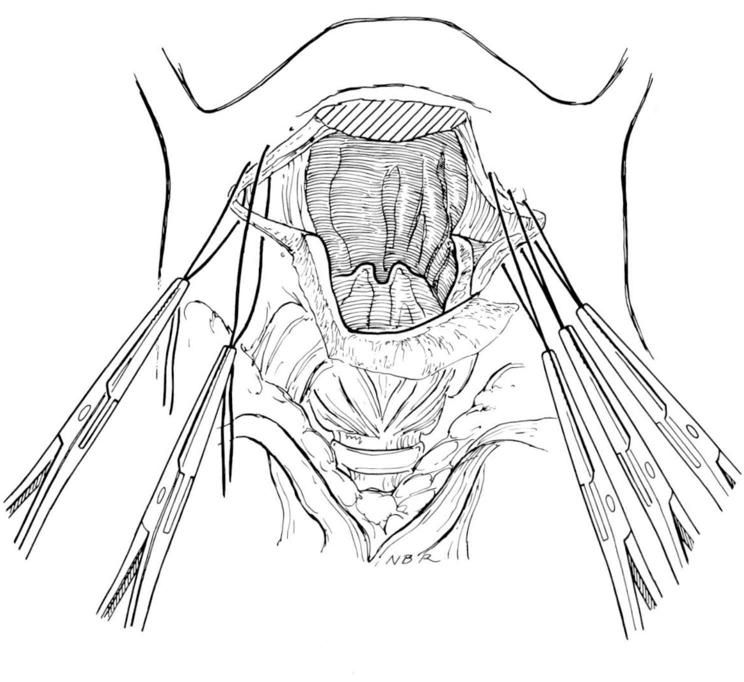

Figure 4–37. Supraglottic laryngectomy. The pharyngeal closure is begun by inserting sutures in the lateral pharyngeal wall, approximating pyriform fossa mucosa to itself up the thyroid perichondrium.

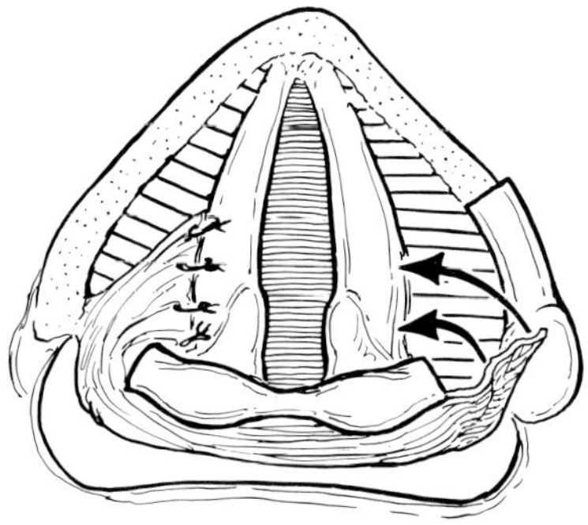

Figure 4–38. Supraglottic laryngectomy. The medial pyriform sinus mucosa is elevated and approximated to the arytenoid and ventricular mucosa as far as possible without undue tension. The remaining area anteriorly is left raw.

The head is now sharply flexed and the sutures are tied sequentially. As much of a second layer closure as possible is attempted with the strap muscles (Fig. 4–39*B*). These are approximated to the suprahyoid muscles with 2-0 chromic. However, the strength of the repair is in the approximation of the perichondrium to the base of the tongue. An internal suspension may be created by placing nonabsorbable suture through the cricothyroid ligament and sewing it under tension to the median mylohyoid raphe. The wound is drained with suction drains and the skin is closed. It may be helpful to keep the patient's head in the flexed position for approximately 10 days, and some surgeons go so far as to attach a wire to the mandible and secure it to the sternum during this period. The low-pressure tracheotomy tube cuff should be inflated to prevent aspiration as the patient regains consciousness.

The excision of significant tongue base requires some type of flap reconstruction to preclude aspiration. A pectoralis major myocutaneous flap, a deltopectoral flap (Fig. 4–40), or a trapezius flap (Fig. 4–41) may be used. The disadvantage of the deltopectoral flap is the need for a pharyngocutaneous fistula to admit the pedicle. This must be closed secondarily. A gentle bulge of the flap into the hypopharynx can be created by sewing part of the underside of the flap to itself. The musculocutaneous flaps[39] have the dual advantage of requiring no fistula and of bulging naturally into the upper airway because of their greater bulk. With time the muscle bulk diminishes because of denervation atrophy.

Fistula rates are quite low with supraglottic laryngectomy except for patients who were previously irradiated or in whom a deltopectoral flap reconstruction is required. Fortunately, when fistulas do develop they are usually small and close spontaneously. A fistula is heralded by an unexplained low-grade fever. The neck wound develops a

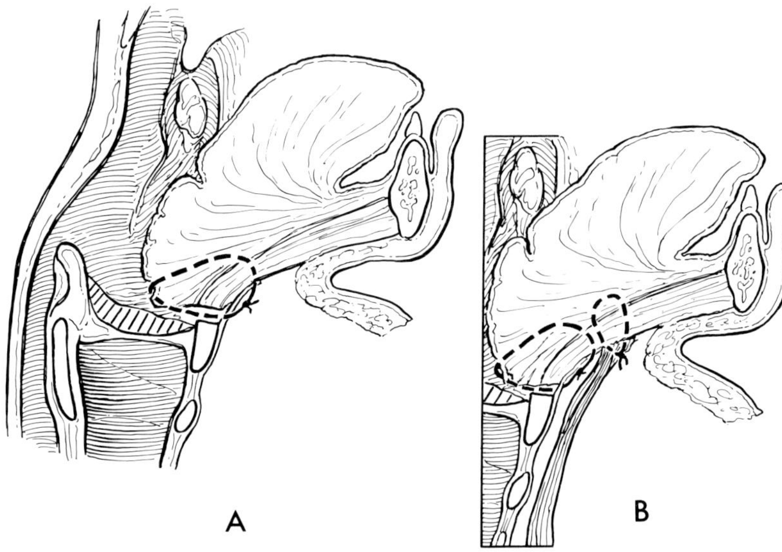

Figure 4–39. Supraglottic laryngectomy. *A,* The remaining closure is achieved by suturing the perichondrium to the tongue base. No attempt is made to achieve a mucosa-to-mucosa approximation. All sutures are placed, and then the head is flexed acutely forward and all the sutures are tied at once. Tongue base sutures must pass through mucosa and full-thickness muscle to securely anchor the laryngeal remnant. *B,* A second layer consisting of strap muscles sutured to the tongue base musculature adds a little support.

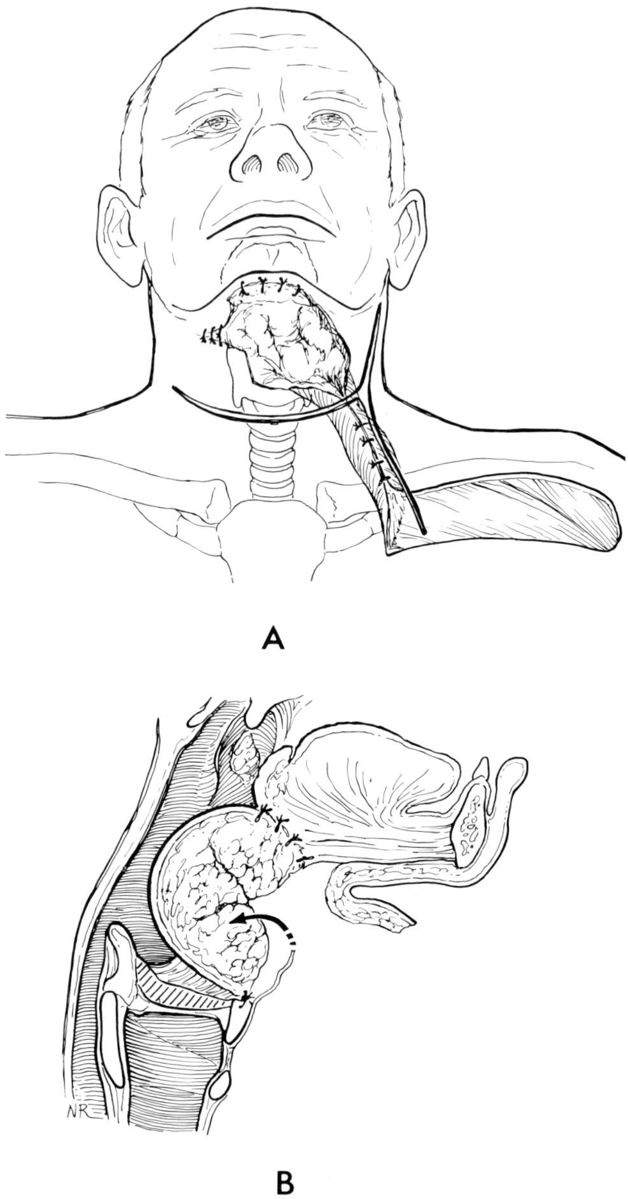

A

B

Figure 4–40. Supraglottic laryngectomy. *A,* A deltopectoral flap used to reconstruct the tongue base when an extensive lingual base resection is necessary. *B,* The flap is sutured to itself to produce a bulge to deflect the bolus during deglutition, which helps prevent aspiration. The distal flap is sutured to the cartilage remnant, with the perichondrium overlapping a portion of the new undersurface of the flap.

reddened area, and a small part of the incision either swells or dehisces. Packing with gauze soaked in dilute acetic acid or povidone-iodine usually results in rapid resolution of the problem.

The onset of planned postoperative radiation need not be delayed because of a fistula unless the carotid artery is exposed. There is some indication in the literature that to be useful, postoperative radiation should be given within 4 to 6 weeks following surgery. The best insurance against both a fistula and ineffective radiation is a complete and adequate resection at the time of the operation.

As previously mentioned, aspiration during deglutition is the most troublesome complication of supraglottic laryngectomy. Thin liquids are the most difficult test of function. Most patients can begin swallowing at about 12 to 14 days if soft, smooth-consistency

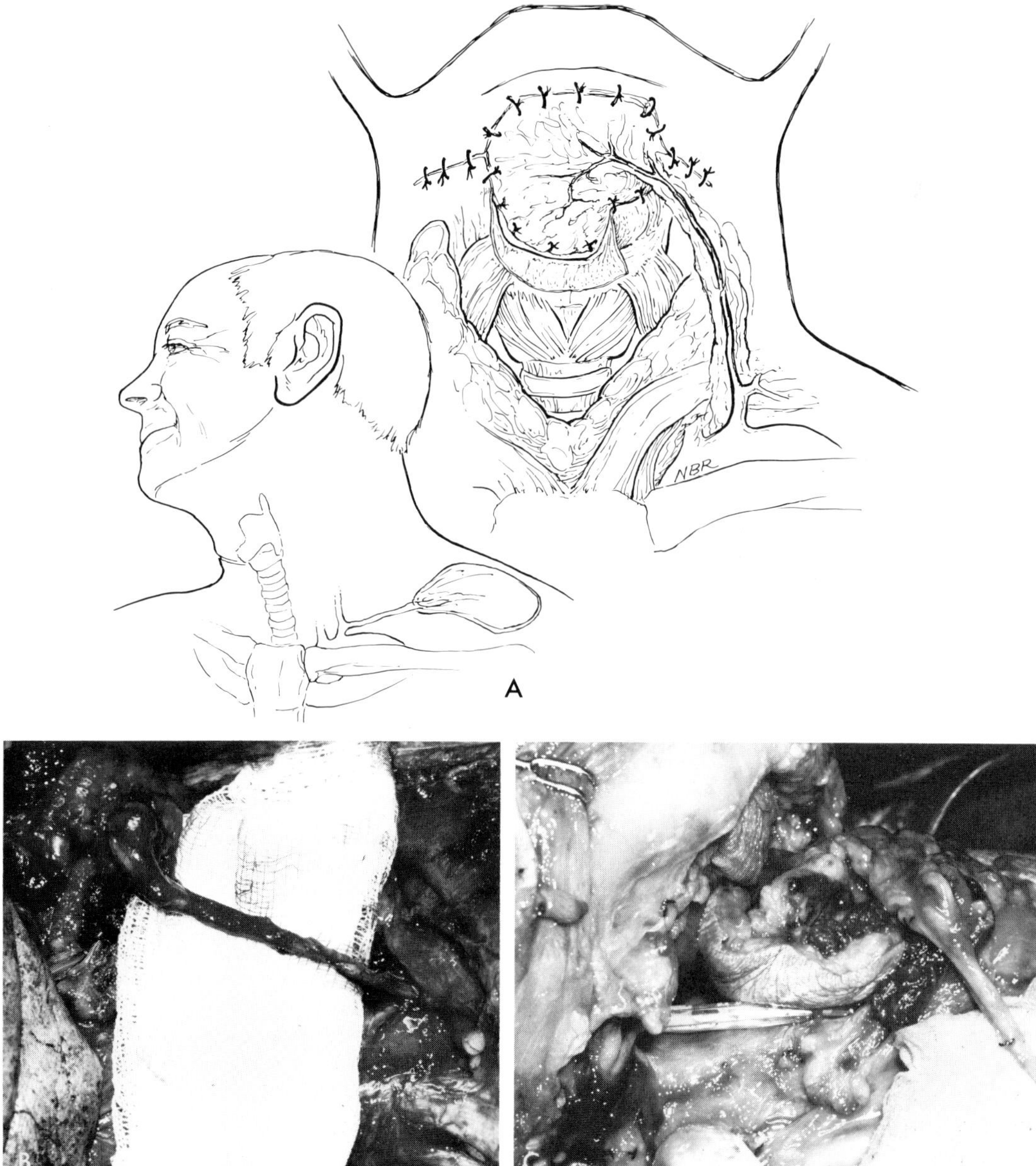

Figure 4–41. Supraglottic laryngectomy. *A,* A trapezius musculocutaneous flap is used to reconstruct the tongue base. The flap is pedicled on the transverse cervical artery and rotated into position in a one-stage procedure. *B,* Trapezius flap based on the transverse cervical vascular pedicle. *C,* Flap rotated into place. Note the flap's bulge, which simulates the base of the tongue.

foods such as applesauce or pudding are used at the start. Empathetic counseling and special instruction are vital to the success of reinstituting oral alimentation (see Chapter 16). Using half teaspoonfuls of food, the patient practices the drill of: inhale—hold your breath—swallow—swallow—cough—swallow—breathe. The tracheostomy is corked, the airway cleared, the food placed in the mouth, and the drill initiated. A speech pathologist familiar with laryngectomy patients and with swallowing problems in the neurologically impaired can often provide the time and encouragement necessary to shepherd a patient through a difficult rehabilitation. From pureed foods the patient progresses to those with a more particulate consistency. Fluids, especially those with effervescence, are the most difficult to handle. Once swallowing with minimal aspiration is accomplished, the drill may be abandoned either in part or entirely.

It is important to understand that the presence of the nasogastric and tracheostomy tubes makes swallowing much more difficult. The nasogastric feeding tube can be used to maintain adequate nutrition during the first few days of intake, when the patient's attempts at swallowing are merely to get the process started. It is helpful to get rid of the tracheostomy tube, and indeed, successful deglutition is sometimes delayed until this is done. However, the goal of decannulation must be balanced against the arytenoid and glottic edema usually present in the first few postoperative weeks. Full decannulation should not be performed until the larynx has been examined with a mirror, and the patient has demonstrated he can sleep in a recumbent position with the tube plugged.

Extended Supraglottic Laryngectomy

In selected patients it is possible to combine a supraglottic and hemilaryngectomy once a true cord lesion extends onto the ventricular fold and a hemilaryngectomy is therefore inadequate to safely encompass the cancer (Fig. 4–42). Because of the cross-flow of lymph in the supraglottic larynx, both false cord areas, the epiglottis, and the pre-epiglottic space must be removed. In the extended operation the supraglottic region is removed along with one entire true cord. This creates a significant problem regarding aspiration. In the standard supraglottic laryngectomy the only protective sphincter remaining in the upper airway is that of the intact mobile true vocal cords. In the extended procedure this last guardian of the airway is compromised by the removal of one cord. The neocord replacing it must be substantial in size and the remaining cord fully mobile in order to avoid aspiration. It is even possible to resect the anterior one third of the contralateral cord, but some of these patients cannot be safely decannulated.

The skin incision is the same as that for a supraglottic laryngectomy, and a radical neck dissection is usually required. The perichondrium is widely elevated from top to bottom and side to side. It is split in the midline to facilitate dissection and later reconstruction of the neocord. The cartilage cuts entail entire removal of the lamina on the most involved side; then a horizontal bisection of the opposing side to halfway along the thyroid lamina; then an oblique cut angling to the superior cornu (Fig. 4–43). Entrance into the hypopharynx is usually through the uninvolved vallecula. The soft tissue incision through the laryngeal mucosa on the least involved or uninvolved side is similar to that for a supraglottic laryngectomy. When the anterior commissure is reached it is bisected with the scalpel and the excision is extended inferiorly to the cricothyroid membrane, then carried along the superior rim of the cricoid cartilage. As the anterior apex of the pyriform fossa is reached, the cut is connected superiorly to the vallecular incision. Now the internal or endolaryngeal blade of the scissors is cutting through the internal mucosa along the rim of the cricoid arch as it sweeps up to become the lamina, and the extralaryngeal blade is cutting through the mucosa on the medial wall of the pyriform sinus (Fig. 4–44). This excision continues up the cricoid lamina, through the cricoarytenoid joint and through the interarytenoid muscles. Once the medial wall pyriform fossa cut on the least involved side is connected to the vallecula on that side, the specimen is removed.

On the hemilaryngectomized side, the principal difference in the defect between that remaining after an extended supraglottic procedure and that after the standard hemilaryngectomy is that there is no redundant aryepiglottic fold mucosa left to nicely pull over and cover the neocord. Elevation over the lateral and lateroposterior aspects of the cricoid will free some mucosa up for advancement, but the major portion of the covering

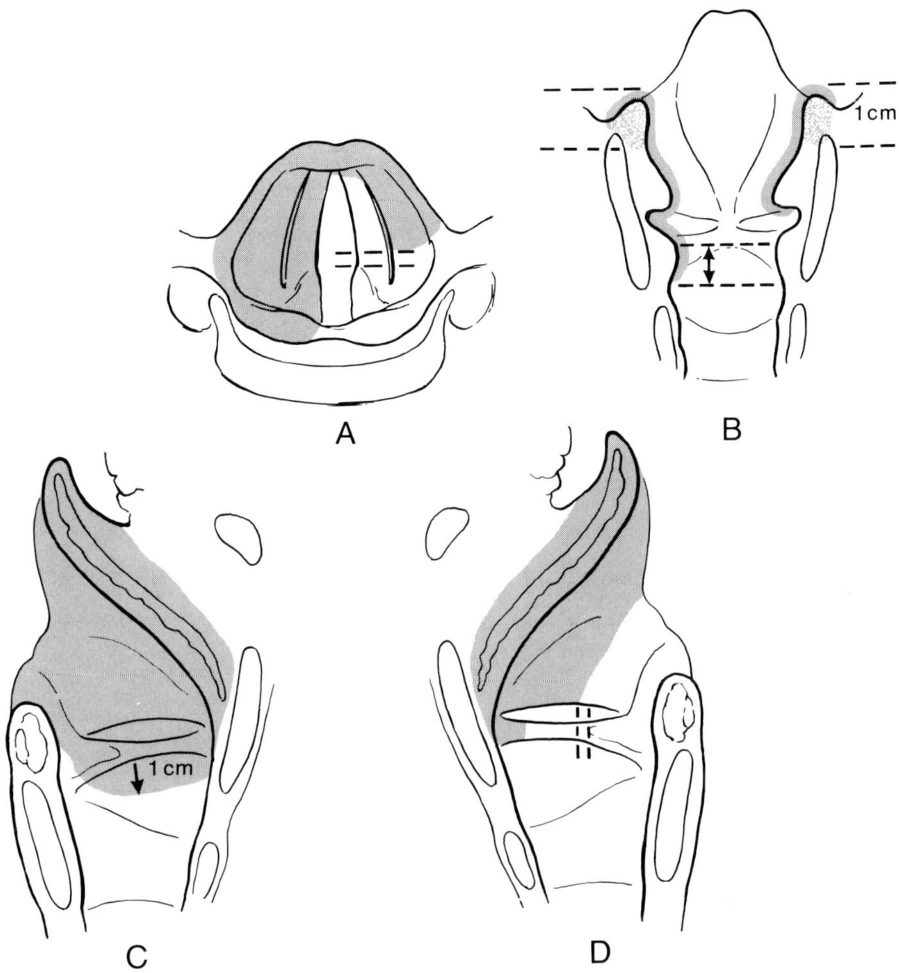

Figure 4–42. Limits of tumor extension resectable by extended supraglottic laryngectomy. *(A)* Superior, *(B)* coronal, and *(C)* and *(D)* opposing sagittal views.

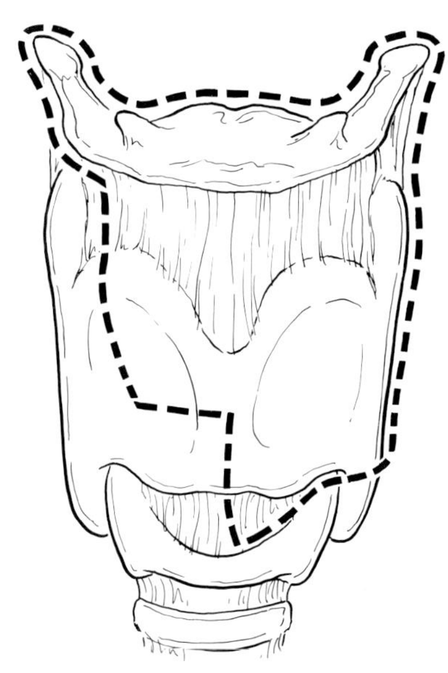

Figure 4–43. Suprahemilaryngectomy. Almost the entire thyroid external perichondrium is elevated. Cartilage incisions require the excision of most of the thyroid lamina on the side of greatest involvement, leaving only a vertical 3-mm cartilage posterior strip between the superior and inferior thyroid cornua. The contralateral ala is incised horizontally to its midportion, then inclined obliquely upward. The thyroid cartilage is also cut in the midline from top to bottom, to facilitate dissection.

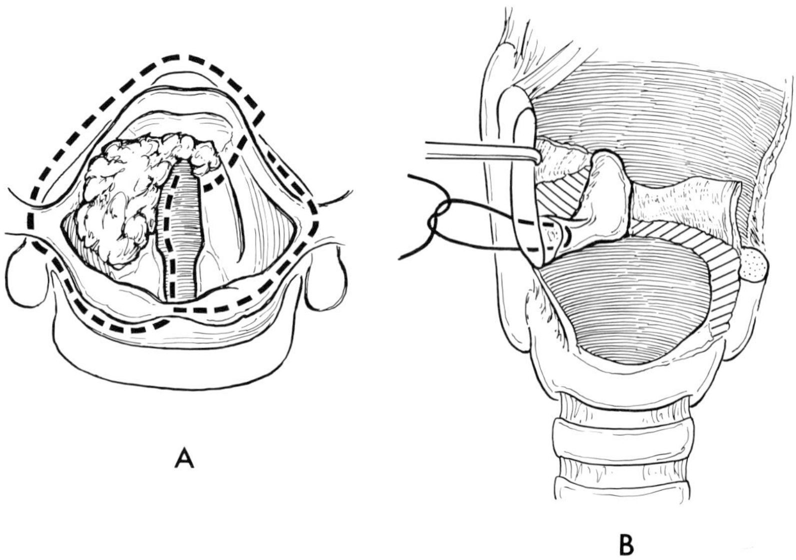

Figure 4–44. Suprahemilaryngectomy. *A,* On the side in which the vocal cord is not involved with tumor, the incision is made similarly to the supraglottic laryngectomy cut on the side of least involvement. When the anterior commissure is reached, it is bisected and the membranous incision is carried through to the cricothyroid membrane. The superior surface of the cricoid is hugged with the scissors, but now the outer blade cuts through the medial wall of the pyriform sinus at the level of the cricoid. In the hypopharynx, a vertical incision connects the one through the vallecula with the one previously mentioned in the medial pyriform wall. This connecting incision usually runs through the lateral pharyngoepiglottic fold and anterior pyriform fossa apex. *B,* Larynx with residual cord following extended supraglottic laryngectomy.

mucosa will have to come from a flap cut from the pyriform sinus mucosa.

A large flap of sternohyoid muscle is used for the neocord, and if the muscle is insufficient it is augmented with a slip of muscle from its fellow in the opposite side (Fig. 4–45). The remaining cord is anchored with a suture to the remaining thyroid cartilage near the midline.

Closure is the same as for a supraglottic laryngectomy. A cricopharyngeal myotomy is done. Vacuum drains are placed and the skin is closed. The head is maintained in a flexed position for 10 to 12 days. The time needed

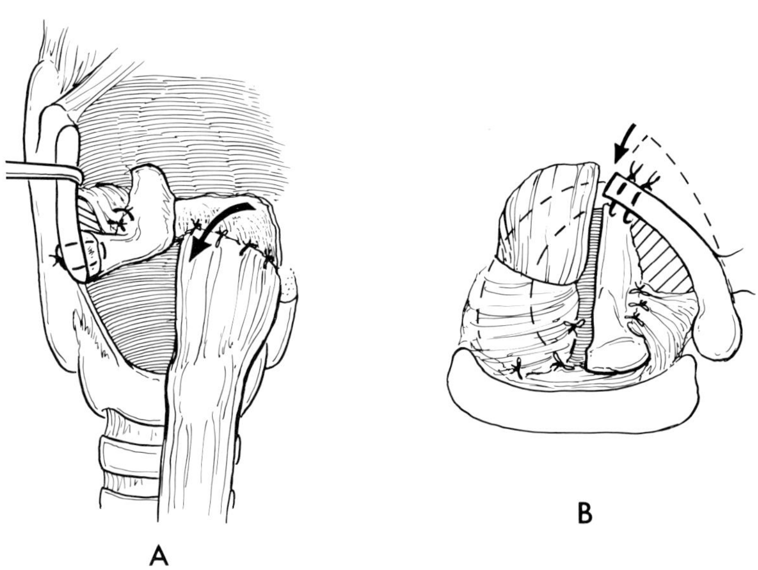

Figure 4–45. Suprahemilaryngectomy. *A,* A large neocord fashioned from as bulky a flap of strap musculature as possible is sutured into the defect created by the excision on the side of greatest involvement. It is sutured posteriorly as closely as possible to the remaining cord. *B,* A flap of pyriform fossa and postcricoid area mucosa is sutured over the neocord.

to achieve adequate swallowing may be prolonged, and decannulation may be delayed or not achievable.

Near-Total Laryngectomy

The term near-total laryngectomy is used here to mean resection of the entire larynx except for a narrow strip connecting the airway and the pharynx over the uninvolved arytenoid.

The conventional partial laryngectomies (cordectomy, hemilaryngectomy, and supraglottic laryngectomy) are contraindicated when the vocal cord is fixed. Fixation means deep invasion, and therefore requires wide local resection. While controversy exists over whether a patient with a fixed cord should have surgery first[40] or radical radiotherapy with surgical salvage,[41] little disagreement has been voiced over the extent of the surgery that is required, which is total laryngectomy. A total laryngectomy, however, excises more larynx than is necessary to control the cancer.[30] It escalates the rehabilitative problems from a situation (with conventional partial procedures) in which voice and nasal breathing are preserved to one in which voice and nasal breathing are destroyed.

Near-total laryngectomy[11, 33] focuses on resecting the cancer, not the whole larynx. Partway between conventional partial and classic total laryngectomies, it requires a stoma but preserves a voice. The voice is dependent on preserving just enough endolarynx to create a sphincteric mucosa-lined tracheopharyngeal speaking shunt over one remaining arytenoid. Inability to do this safely constitutes the principal indication for total laryngectomy.

Near-total laryngectomy is expressly designed to encompass carcinoma that fixes one vocal cord. The origins matter little. The cancer may arise from the vocal cord itself or fix it by extension through the paraglottic space from the subglottis, the supraglottic larynx, or even the pyriform fossa. The principal contraindications are involvement of the postcricoid or interarytenoid regions. Sometimes near-total laryngectomy must be rejected in favor of a total procedure in cases of radio-recurrent disease, because the margins are obscured and the safety of preserving the contralateral arytenoid is questionable. In some directions, near-total laryngectomy can actually be extended beyond the margins of a simple total laryngectomy. It can, for example, encompass tumor extensions to the trachea, the pyriform fossa, or the base of the tongue.

Without near-total laryngectomy, two practical problems arise for the surgeon. The first is that patients who could have had surgery are submitted to radical irradiation and surgical salvage; and the salvage is total laryngectomy. The second is that a whole host of overextended conventional partial operations, such as three-quarter laryngectomy or extended supraglottic laryngectomy, must be retained for possible use, despite the fact that they are performed too infrequently to be perfected. Under these circumstances reliability and predictability falter, and the control of voice, aspiration, and perhaps even the cancer, is uncertain. It must be emphasized, however, that in the experience of one of the authors (P.J.D.), three-quarter and extended supraglottic operations in patients with the appropriate indications have proved to be good cancer extirpative procedures that preserve voice, avoid significant aspiration, and obviate the need for a permanent tracheostomy. Moreover, not one of these procedures has required a tracheal stoma or conversion to total laryngectomy.

The preoperative workup for a near-total laryngectomy includes a chest x-ray, blood count, urinalysis, chemistry profile, VDRL, tuberculin test, fungal serology, and a preanesthetic medical evaluation. We have not found preoperative laryngograms or CT scans to add enough information consistently to justify their expense. A presurgical consultation with the speech pathologist is invaluable. Surgery should be delayed if necessary for alcoholic detoxification, platelet function recovery after heavy aspirin use, or a pulmonary preparation. Blood is cross-matched, with one unit retained for the neck dissection. Antibiotics are initiated preoperatively.

At the beginning of the procedure, the larynx is carefully examined to confirm the extent of the cancer. It is essential to make sure the ventricle on the good side is free, since this will be the point of entry into the lumen. The typical glottic case will deeply ulcerate the true cord and involve the arytenoid posteriorly, the anterior commissure and opposite cord anteriorly, the false cord superiorly, and the cricoid ring inferiorly. After the biopsy, a feeding tube is placed in the nose and directed into the esophagus. With the head comfortably extended, a tracheotomy is performed below the thyroid isthmus, and the anesthesia is continued through this location.

By extending the incision across the sternomastoid and up to the mastoid process, flaps are elevated in the prevenous subplatysmal plane. The associated neck dissection removes all fat and lymph nodes from the neck on the involved side, along with the sternomastoid, digastric, and omohyoid muscles, the submandibular gland, the internal jugular vein, the sensory cervical nerves, and the enveloping fascia. The carotid arterial system and the accessory, vagus, hypoglossal, phrenic, and marginal mandibular nerves are carefully preserved.

On the tumor side, the procedure for a near-total laryngectomy is identical to that for a total laryngectomy (Fig. 4–46). The pedicle, comprising the superior laryngeal nerve and the superior thyroid vascular supply, is divided. The greater horn of the hyoid is skeletonized. The suprahyoid muscles attached to the greater horn and body of the hyoid are released. The strap muscles are cut low on the tumor side, exposing the thyroid. The lobe is elevated to expose the inferior neurovascular pedicle for resection, and the recurrent laryngeal nerve is divided. The larynx is rotated aside and skeletonized along the posterior border of the tumor-side thyroid cartilage and the cricoid, from the upper trachea to the hyoid.

The distinctive steps of a near-total laryngectomy are now taken on the nontumor side (Fig. 4–47). The fascia near the medial edge of the sternohyoid muscle is incised and elevated to expose muscle. The medial edge of the muscle is retracted until the thyrohyoid membrane is visible above and the cricothyroid below. The prelaryngeal soft tissues, including the Delphian nodes, must stay with the specimen. The sternohyoid and medial half of the thyrohyoid muscles are cut free from the hyoid bone on the good side and reflected to the oblique line of the thyroid ala. The thyroid gland is divided at the junction of its isthmus, which goes, and the good side lobe, which stays. The good cricothyroid muscle is elevated from the cricoid ring with a scalpel, and the leash of blood vessels connecting the cricothyroid arcade and the laryngeal interior, which passes through the cricothyroid triangle, is cauterized.

The larynx is entered on the nontumor side by means of the following steps (Fig. 4–48).

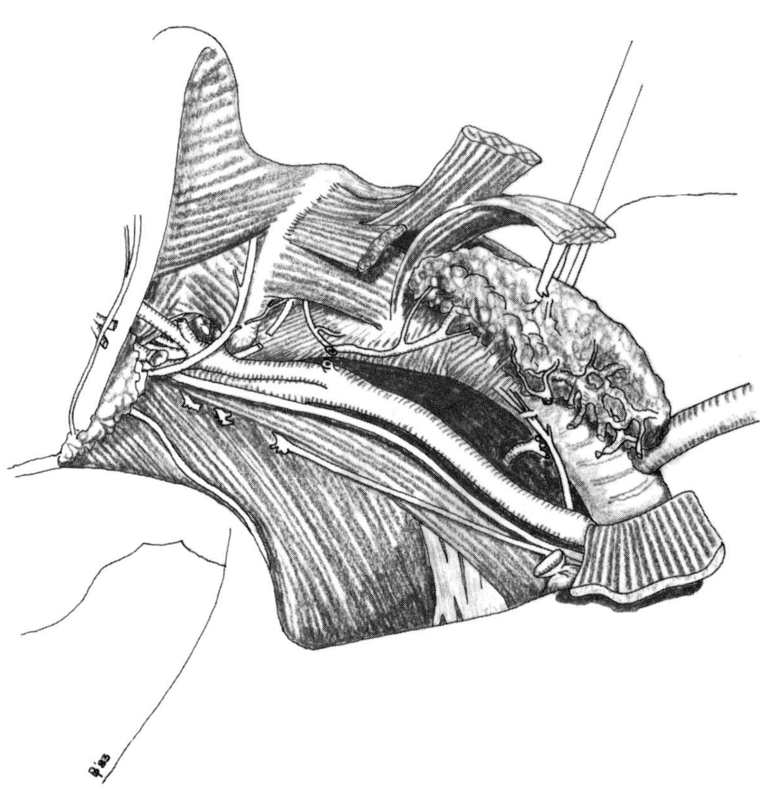

Figure 4–46

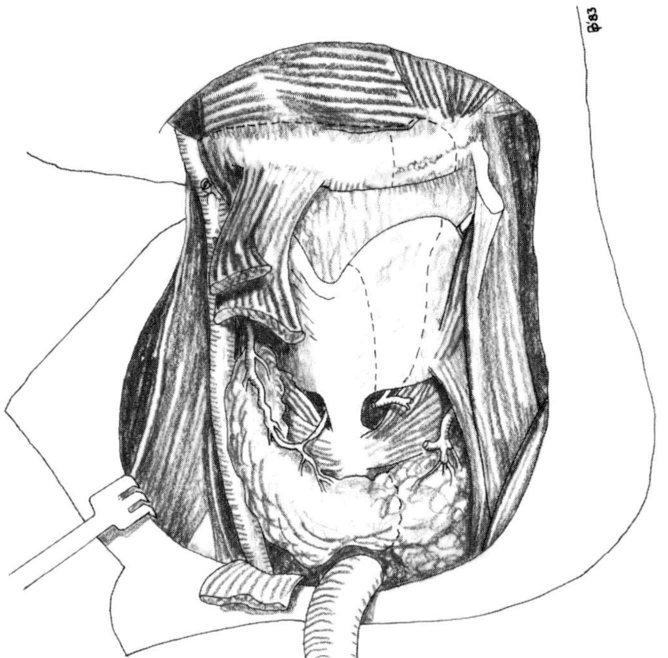

Figure 4–47

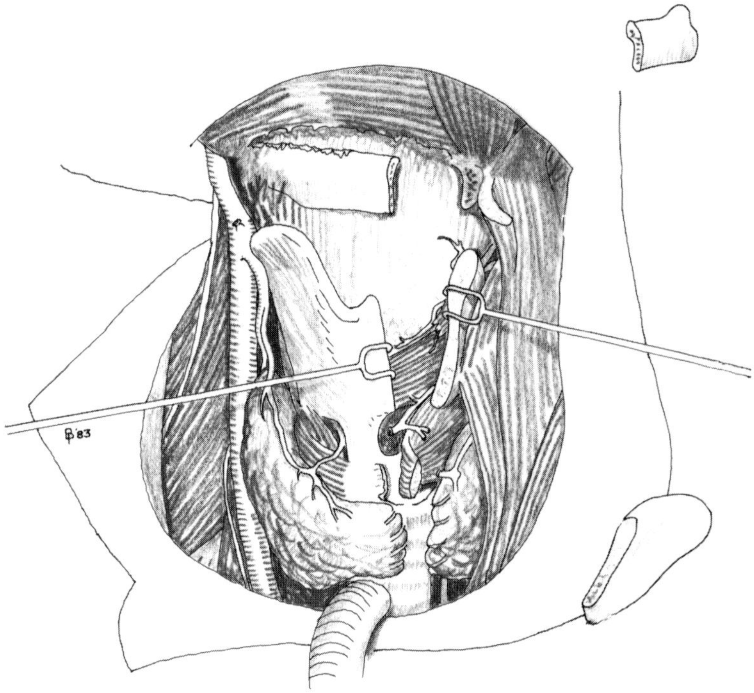

Figure 4–48

A segment of hyoid bone is removed with a rongeur at the junction of the body and the greater horn. An offside wedge of thyroid ala is removed. (Remember that this is on the nontumor side, and the ventricle is known to be clear.) The ventricle is opened at the upper border of the thyroarytenoid muscle (Fig. 4–49). The assistant spreads the ventriculotomy with hooks, and the operator visualizes the undersurface of the ventricular band. A heavy scissors is directed upward with one blade in the ventricle and the other outside the larynx (Fig. 4–50). The blades close to divide the ventricular band and false cord. This division is continued superiorly until the epiglottis can be clearly identified and retrieved. The scissors transsection is continued across the vallecula, with the body of the hyoid and the entire pre-epiglottis space kept with the specimen (Fig. 4–51).

A muscle relaxant is given. With an Allis clamp on the epiglottis and a double hook on the cut edge of the false cord, the laryngotomy is opened to allow direct visualization of the tumor, which is principally situated on the opposite side (Fig. 4–52). The scissors is then directed downward to straddle the better vocal cord at the optimal division between tumor and normal tissue. The cord is divided and subglottic visualization is gradually improved (Fig. 4–53). The exact site of the cord cut is determined by the lesion. In the extreme case it approaches the vocal process of the arytenoid; in others it is closer to the anterior commissure. As the cut descends, it angles to fit the tumor, crosses the anterior cricoid arch, and reaches the first tracheal ring. If necessary, a portion of the trachea on the tumor side is included in the specimen.

Hooks are used to separate the anterior cricotomy, and good visualization of the subglottic lumen, the tumor, and the posterior cricoid plate is obtained (Fig. 4–54). The cricoid is split posteriorly in approximately the midline with a No. 15 blade. As soon as this cut passes through the anterior lamina of the cricoid plate, the cricoid fractures in the midline through its cortical portions under the stress of the traction (Fig. 4–55). Now the entire larynx is open like a book. The tumor-bearing portion is elevated to allow the final release across the pyriform fossa to be carried out under direct vision (Fig. 4–56).

While the specimen margins (Fig. 4–57) are being studied in the surgical pathology lab, the anterior portion of the remaining cricoid arch is resected from the patient (Fig. 4–58*A*). The resection is submucosal. A finger in the pyriform sinus is useful to elevate

Text continued on page 136

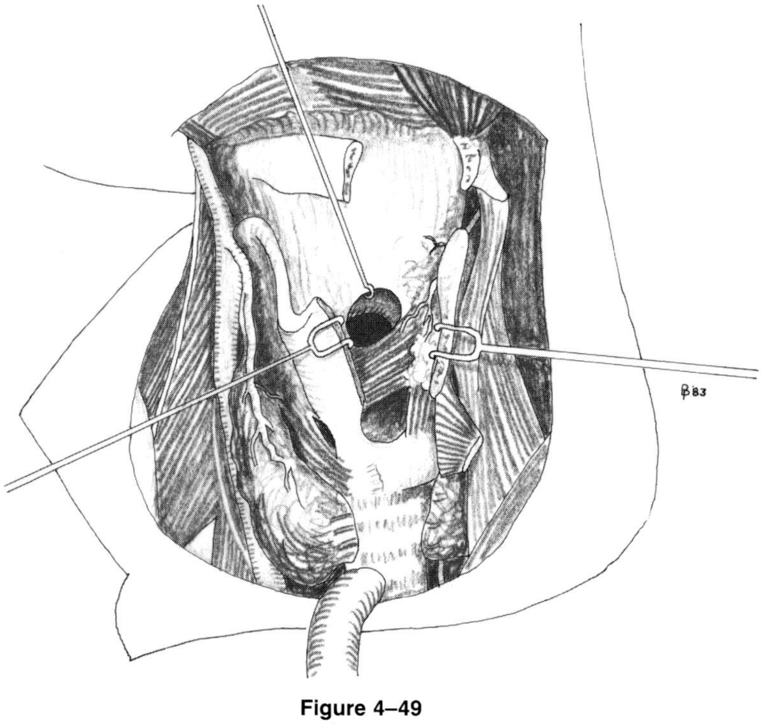

Figure 4–49

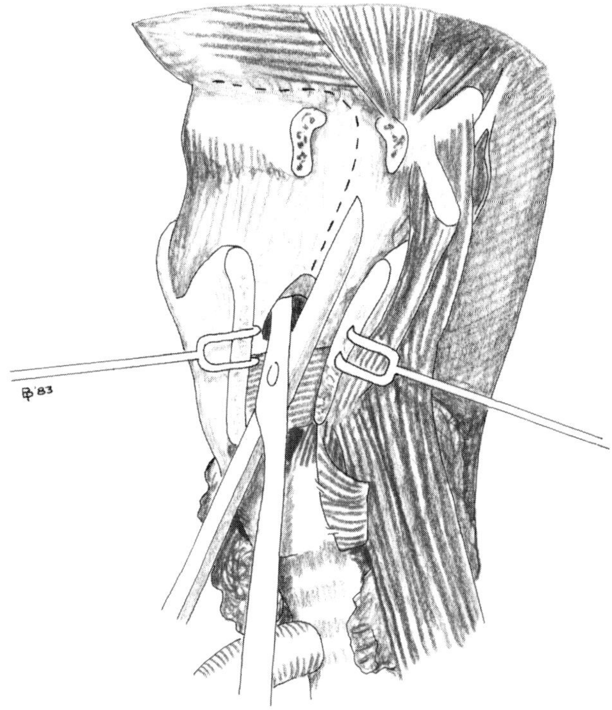

Figure 4–50

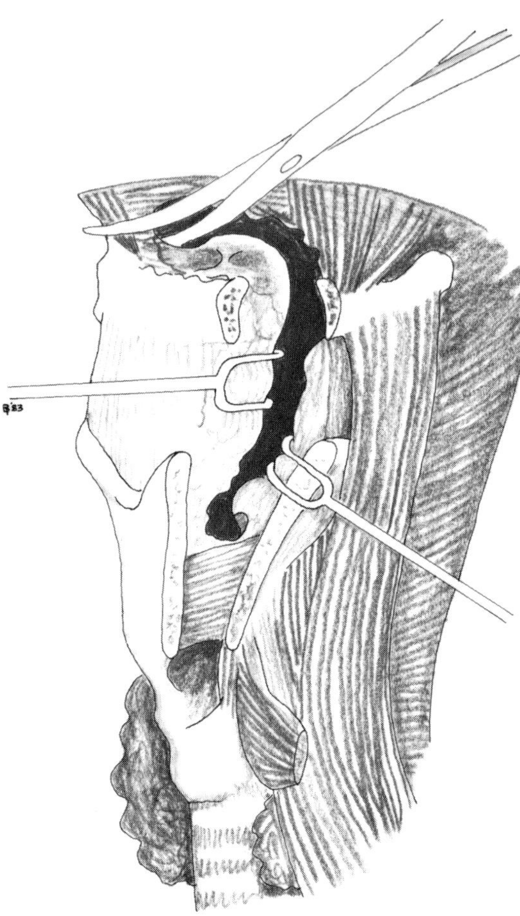

Figure 4–51

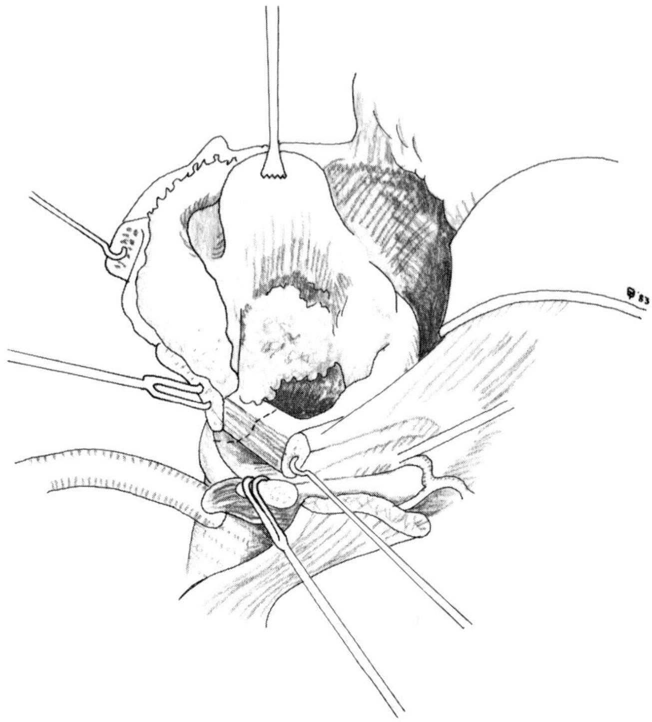

Figure 4–52

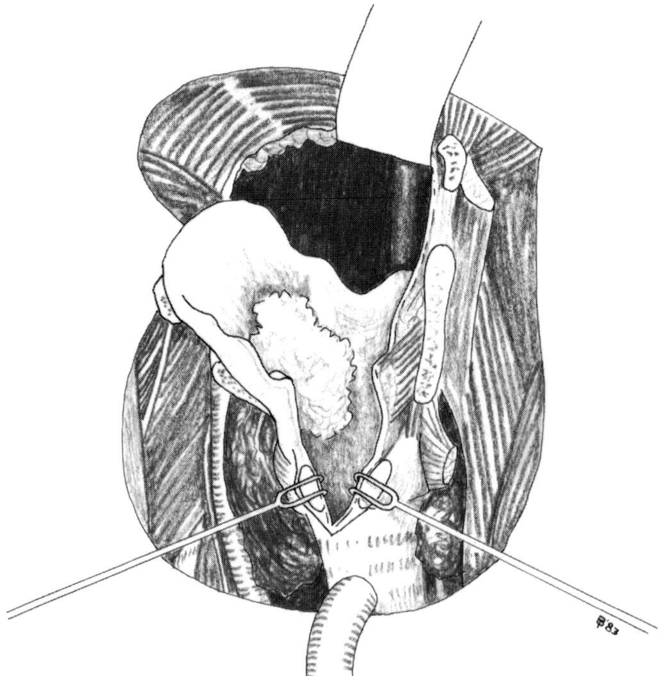

Figure 4–53

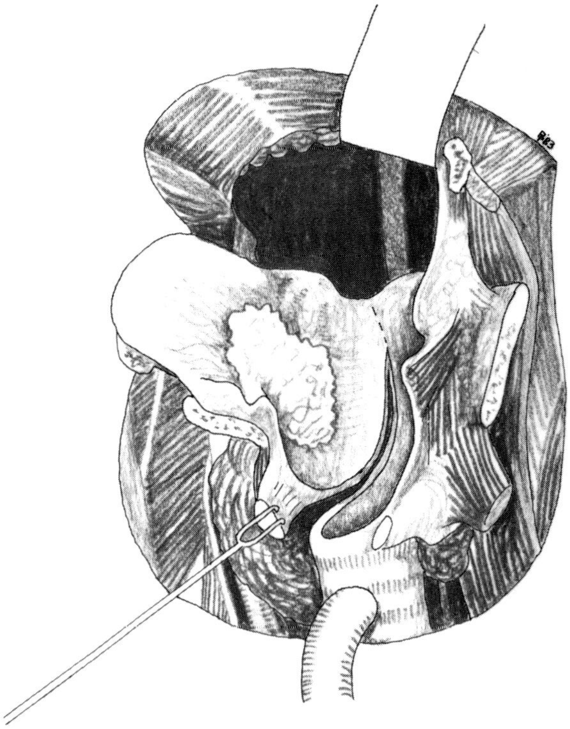

Figure 4–54

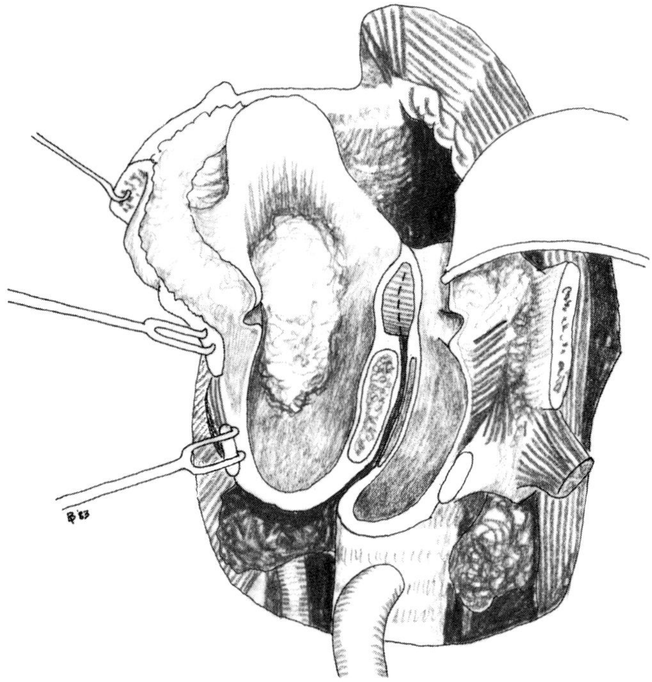

Figure 4–55

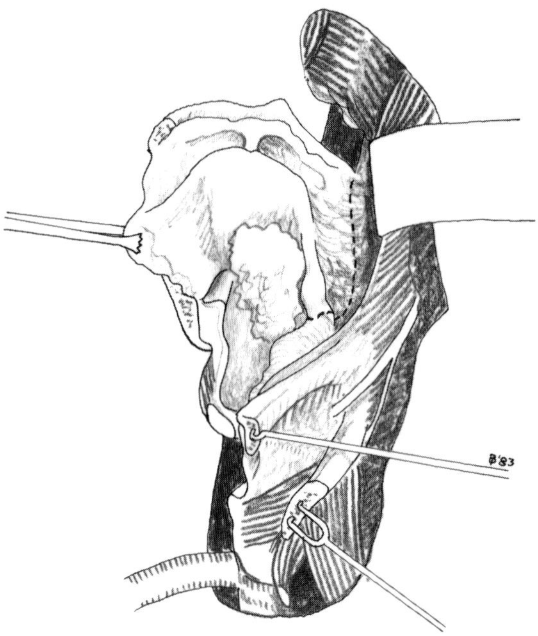

Figure 4–56

and stabilize the cartilage for this maneuver. All of the remaining glottic and subglottic soft tissues are preserved during this resection, which does not include *all* of the cricoid remnant but just enough to allow the mucosa to be tubed. Injury to the recurrent laryngeal nerve still supplying this small musculomucosal complex is avoided by preserving the

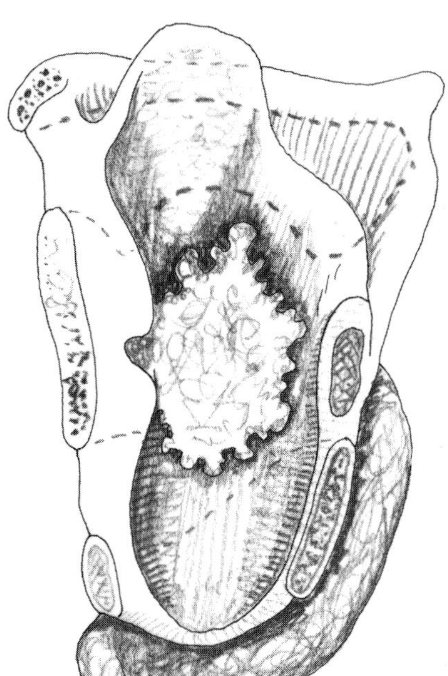

Figure 4–57

cartilage deep to the inferior thyroid cornu. Some additional cricoid plate is resected submucosally from the midline margin posteriorly, and the posterior strip of thyroid cartilage (both cornua and the oblique line and posterior border) is preserved on the good side.

The operator is now faced with a pharyngotomy, connected to the trachea by a strip of endolaryngeal mucosa. The mucosa joins the pharynx over the remaining arytenoid. By resecting the cricoid, sufficient flaccidity has been achieved that this endolaryngeal remnant can be tubed. It is often not wide enough to encircle a No. 14 French catheter (the measuring device used to assure an adequate shunt lumen). Therefore a narrow strip of "lateral" pharyngeal wall (posterior pharyngeal wall if the entire pyriform sinus is gone) is transposed down to augment the endolaryngeal remnant (Fig. 4–58*B*). Its mucosal surface automatically faces the shunt lumen. The base of this flap should be level with the remaining arytenoid, and its medial margin is sewn to the posterior midline margin of the laryngeal strip. The entire complex is then rolled into a tube to make the vocal shunt. Starting at the tracheal end, the mucosa of the shunt is approximated with 3-0 chromic catgut. The No. 14 French catheter used to gauge the lumen is removed; no stenting or supportive device is left in place that might damage the mucosa.

The pharyngeal opening is closed in a T with 2-0 chromic catgut, similar to closure in a total laryngectomy (Fig. 4–59). The cricothyroid muscle is incorporated into the shunt wall. The strap muscles from the good side are retrieved and sewn across the upper portion of the closure, where they reach the suprahyoid muscular remnants (Fig. 4–60). These two additional measures are aimed at reducing the possibility of aspiration, the first by adding to the sphincteric capacity of the shunt; the second by restoring some dynamic elevation. The wound is thoroughly irrigated, two Hemovac drains are led out through stab wounds to suction, and the apron flap is closed (Fig. 4–61). The skin at the stoma is sewn to the tracheal wall margin, and a metal tracheotomy tube is installed.

For the first postoperative week the patient is managed as if he had had a total laryngectomy. A mechanical instrument is useful for communication in the initial postoperative period. Valving the stoma too early, in a premature effort to initiate voice, only serves to delay healing at the stomal site. Attempts

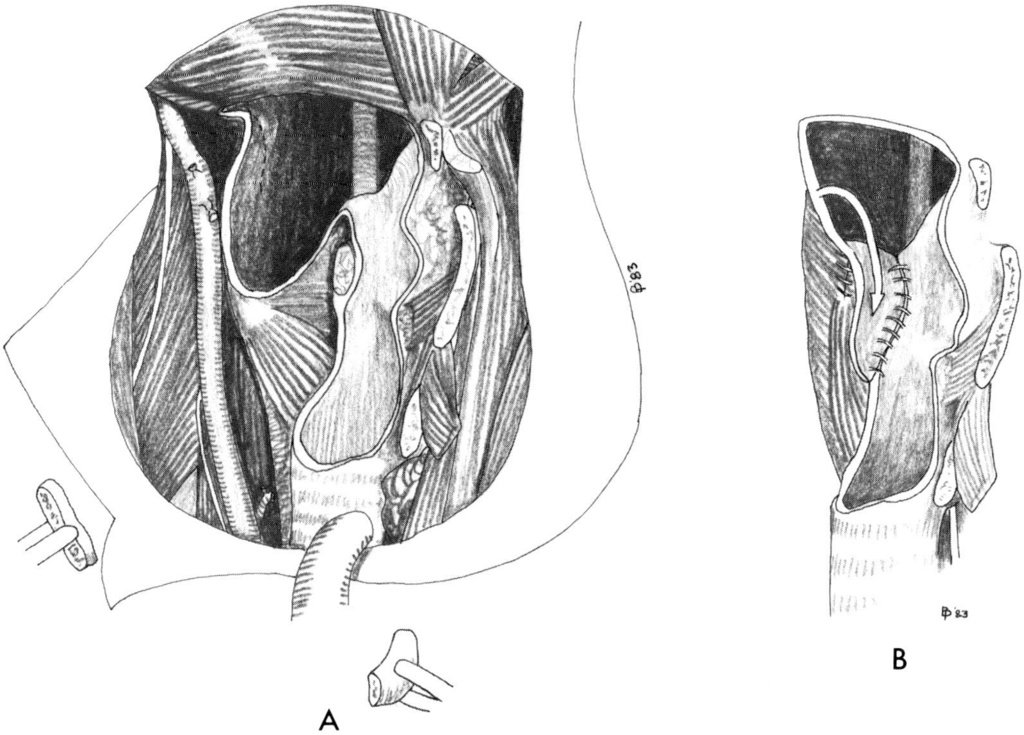

Figure 4–58

to use the shunt are usually not made before the second week. The patient starts by simply occluding his stoma and exhaling when he is engaged in changing his tracheotomy tube. At this time the pressures are usually high, and only a small squeak of air will come up. Sometime around 8 weeks postoperatively, if healing has progressed satisfactorily, use of this shunt for a voice may commence. A speech pathologist will prove invaluable in dealing with the patient's early frustrations (and subsequent successes) in acquiring shunt speech. Technical errors that have to do with valving, articulation, speaking rate, and pro-

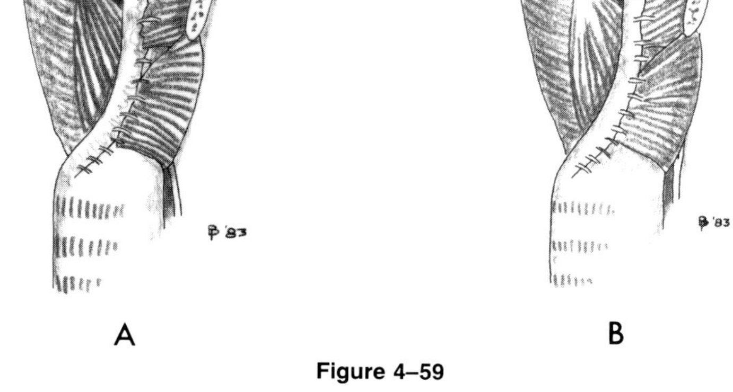

Figure 4–59

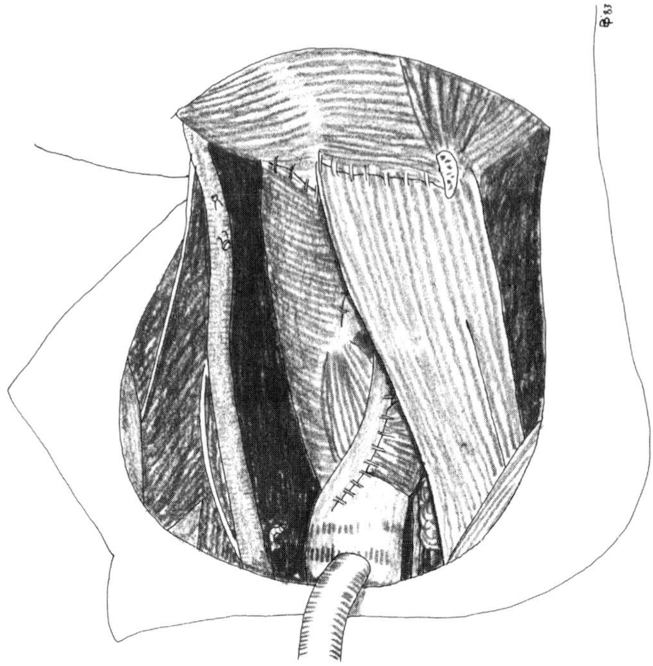

Figure 4–60

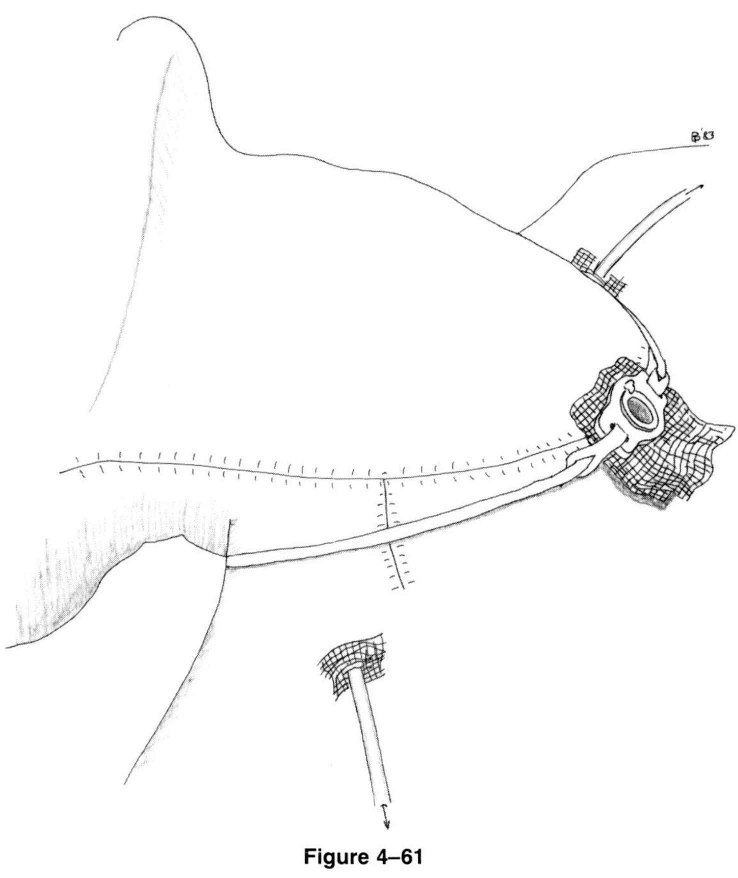

Figure 4–61

ficiency should not be overlooked after this procedure, since they are readily identified and corrected with the help of the rehabilitation team.

Problems with the tracheal stoma need to be addressed as well. More delays due to granulation are to be expected with an anterior wall stoma than with the end-on stoma of a total laryngectomy. This is compounded by the patient's need to valve. The secret of stomal healing is meticulous regional hygiene, i.e., frequent tube changes, clean dressings, and use of local peroxide and/or povidone-iodine until the skin-mucosal junction is stable.

After many months, the stoma loses its tendency to contract. The tracheotomy tube may be removed (unless the patient prefers to continue using it for the advantages it may have over his own stoma when he valves). In the absence of a tracheotomy tube, the stoma may be fitted with a Blom-Singer tracheostoma valve[42] (not to be confused with the Blom-Singer tracheoesophageal voice prosthesis). This frees the patient of the need to use his hand during speech; the valve closes at the stoma automatically on phonation.

Total Laryngectomy

A total laryngectomy is indicated when fixation of the vocal cord with cancer is complicated by invasion of the interarytenoid space, the subglottic circumference, the postcricoid region or both arytenoids. In unirradiated patients, extensive posterior bilateral or circumferential involvement, or both, is not too common. For tumor to have reached these proportions in the airway, the symptoms must have been woefully neglected. In such cases, a total laryngectomy will often be performed solely on the basis of cord fixation. The fact that near-total laryngectomies have been conducted successfully on a few radiation failures should not obscure the more frequent need for a total laryngectomy in this situation.

The principal indications for neck dissection in fixed cord cancers are spread to adjacent areas with rich lymphatics (the supraglottic larynx, for example), the presence of a neck mass, and a poorly differentiated endophytic primary. A thick neck and an unreliable patient are factors that will delay prompt recognition of cervical metastasis, so these may be relative indications. Over half the deaths following laryngectomy are attributable to failure to control disease in the neck.[43] This fact places a heavy responsibility on the surgeon (and the patient) whenever the neck is violated to perform a laryngectomy *without* using the same opportunity to remove the nodes.

Since the larynx is to be removed in its entirety, little attention need be paid to its intrinsic anatomy. A knowledge of the direct extralaryngeal routes of spread of laryngeal cancer is more germane.[44] Cancer of the ventricle and supraglottic region can penetrate the thyrohyoid membrane and spread directly itnto the neck in the vicinity of the superior laryngeal nerve. Pain and a slight fullness in this area are ominous clinical warnings. Radio-recurrent cancer can spread from the anterior commissure to the Delphian node anteriorly, and thence into the overlying fascia and even the skin of the neck. The skin over the thyroid angle ought to be included with the specimen when its mobility is questionable. Cordal cancer may spread into the paraglottic space, then out between the cricoid and thyroid cartilages into the lobe of the thyroid gland. It is prudent, therefore, in removing the thyroid lobe (and isthmus) with the specimen, to maintain its apposition to the larynx. Ventricular cancer backs up against the floor of the pyriform fossa. The implications for the hypopharyngeal resection line are obvious, especially when one considers the possibilities for submucosal spread downward into the narrower parts of the gullet. Subglottic cancer spreads circumferentially and downward to involve the trachea. This threatens the tracheal lymph nodes bilaterally. The surgeon must section the trachea at the appropriate level, and include the surrounding paratracheal nodes in his resection.

Prior to a laryngectomy it is vitally important to counsel the patient and the family on the expectations of a tracheotomy, a nasogastric feeding tube, an intravenous line, and wound suction in the early postoperative period. Good handbooks are available to familiarize everyone with the details of stomal management and the potential for vocal rehabilitation through esophageal speech.[45] The basic concepts and the proof of hope can be detailed in a preoperative consultation with the speech pathologist. The medical preparations for surgery are identical to those mentioned under the near-total procedure.

In a patient with stridor, the airway is

established by performing the tracheotomy under local anesthesia, then inducing the anesthetic. Patients without stridor can be intubated. When quick-section diagnosis is flawlessly reliable, one may conduct the laryngoscopy and confirmatory biopsy and proceed on the basis of the frozen-section report. The dividends are time saved in the hospital, the avoidance of a second anesthetic, and a minimal period of anxiety. It must be remembered, however, that misdiagnosis is always a possibility. Each report should be discussed with the pathologist in depth. Histoplasmosis,[47] radionecrosis,[48] tuberculosis,[49] leprosy,[50] Wegener's granuloma,[51] and polymorphic reticulosis[52] can all look like cancer in the office. Furthermore, pseudoepitheliomatous hyperplasia over a myoblastoma[53] or blastomycosis[54] can be misinterpreted by the pathologist as cancer. Pseudosarcoma[55] may mask an associated squamous carcinoma. Verrucous cancer[56] is notoriously benign in its microscopic appearance, and a little clinical prompting may be an important ingredient in the diagnosis. A few malignancies other than squamous cell cancer occasionally turn up in the larynx also, such as small cell carcinoma,[57] metastatic adenocarcinoma,[58] primary adenoid cystic cancer,[59] and local invasion from the thyroid.[60] The option must always be kept open that the procedure may terminate with the biopsy.

Ten steps are needed to accomplish an orderly and rapid total laryngectomy.[46] Briefly stated, these are:

1. Establish an airway.
2. Make the incision and raise the flaps.
3. Ligate the superior neurovascular pedicles.
4. Cut the strap muscles.
5. Mobilize what thyroid you need.
6. Free the hyoid margins.
7. Transect the trachea and remove the larynx (from below upward).
8. Close the pharynx.
9. Create the stoma.
10. Close the neck and dress the wounds.

A U-shaped incision may be planned to include the permanent tracheostoma site. Alternatively the transverse limb of the U may cross the larynx at the cricoid level so the tracheotomy site can be subsequently centered in an infinity-shaped skin excision in the middle of the lower flap. Radical neck dissection is performed discontinuously, and the accessory nerve is preserved only when the exigencies of the metastatic disease permit. Considerable judgment must be exercised in this regard, and an over-radical approach is recommended in cases where doubt exists. The significantly higher failure rates seen when an overly conservative neck dissection is done in order to preserve the accessory nerve make it clear that such conservatism is to be decried.

The deep cervical fascia near the hyoid and along the sternomastoid muscle is opened to visualize the carotid triangles. This is a good opportunity to palpate for nodes in cases in which a neck dissection has not been done. The superior vascular pedicles are identified by blunt dissection and divided. The superior laryngeal nerves, which can be identified by separating the hyoid and thyroid cornua with hooks, are also divided.

The sternohyoid and sternothyroid muscles are cut low over the thyroid with a knife, avoiding the gland itself. The lower segments are reflected downward to reveal the lower poles of the gland, and the paratracheal fat.

The thyroid lobe on the involved side is elevated with its paratracheal fat and nodes, together with the inferior thyroid artery, exposing the posterior border of the thyroid cartilage. This border is skeletonized by dividing the inferior constrictor all along the cartilages (cricoid as well as thyroid).

The hyoid is retracted inferiorly with a Kocher forceps and the suprahyoid muscles are released. Several large veins can be cauterized as they are exposed. The lesser horns and the greater horns are freed so the entire hyoid will exit with the specimen. The thyroid gland is divided lateral to the isthmus on the uninvolved side, and the lobe to be preserved is elevated laterally until the inferior laryngeal artery and recurrent nerve are exposed at the inferior thyroid cornu. Here they require clamping and ligation.

The trachea is severed on a bevel. The entry incision is usually between the third and fourth rings, but it bevels upward to approach the inferior edge of the cricoid posteriorly. By pulling the larynx strongly forward and completing the beveled airway transection at the lower edge of the posterior cricoid plate, the release of the larynx is initiated. It is usually possible by blunt dissection to elevate up under the cricoid, thus preserving the postcricoid mucosa of the hypopharynx. With strong traction toward the ceiling, the whole postcricoid area is skeletonized up to the arytenoids, and the apices of both pyriform fossae come into view. The larynx is pulled to the involved side, the superior thyroid cornua are freed, and the pyriform mucosa is cut into with a knife. The rest of the pyriform fossa is opened and the retroarytenoid mucosa is transected with scissors. Continuing the traction upward inverts the larynx, and the epiglottis flips into view. This is grasped with an Allis clamp and one then cuts across the vallecula. Now the larynx is free to fold outward, like a book, hinged on the ipsilateral pyriform fossa. The laryngectomy is completed by dividing this final pharyngeal attachment with scissors.

Careful attention must be paid to closing the pharyngotomy, to avoid a fistula. Chromic catgut corner tags help maintain orientation. The object is to close the pharyngotomy transversely or in a T, with a running 2–0 chromic catgut. Vertical closures cause a hypopharyngeal web. A second layer of interruptued sutures through the muscular layer helps support the mucosal closure. The wound is heavily irrigated, and immaculate hemostasis is secured. Drains are placed so their tips shun the suture line. An airtight wound is created by closing the subcutaneous tissues with catgut and reapproximating the skin with nylon sutures.

The postoperative course will be greatly simplified if the stoma is created properly. An infinity shape is cut from the skin of the lower flap to create a continuously smooth-edged opening with minimal loss of skin. The lower lip is sewn to the anterior tracheal wall with heavy chromic catgut. The sutures are "simple" with respect to the trachea and grasp at least one ring. They are "mattress" with respect to the skin, and they draw the skin toward the cut edge of the trachea so that no bare cartilage is left exposed. The endotracheal tube (which is crossing through the neck wound at this point) is removed and passed through the stomal opening in the skin, into the trachea. This allows sufficient access to complete the skin closure to the tracheal sides and posterior wall.

Patients are nursed postoperatively, with the head of the bed elevated. Adequate mist and suctioning are provided to maintain a clear tracheostomy tube. Feeding through the nasogastric tube is begun on the second postoperative day, with the patient starting very slowly to avoid the risk of vomiting against the pharyngeal closure. By gradually increasing the strength and the volume, a full tube feeding formula is reached by the fifth postoperative day. The dressing is removed the day after surgery; drains are usually left for approximately 72 hours. The staples and nasogastric tube can usually be removed on the twelfth day. The patient should be relatively free of pain, afebrile, and able to swallow his own saliva.

Prior to discharge most laryngectomy patients should have their hemoglobin, electrolytes, and calcium evaluated. They should be fully capable of looking after their tracheostomies alone or with the help of their families. A home vaporizer or suction, or both, should be supplied if necessary. Specific arrangements for speech therapy are clarified before dismissal.

With proper hygiene, stomal healing is usually complete by 4 months. Once the wound has healed, the patient is gradually weaned off the tube, omitting it for one hour one day, and escalating to two hours and so on, so long as there is no difficulty with reinsertion. Gradually and safely the patient demonstrates whether the stomal caliber is stable, but breaks the escalation for a week or so if contraction remains. Once the tube can be omitted for 24 hours, yet replaced smoothly at the end of this period, the stoma no longer requires its support. If satisfactory esophageal speech is not well under way by this time, the puncture-prosthesis method of vocal rehabilitation is advised.

VOCAL REHABILITATION SURGERY

Tracheoesophageal Fistulae for Speech

The voice loss suffered by a laryngectomee is a psychic blow that often exceeds the trauma of surgery. This has spurred surgeons to develop surgical procedures and mechanical contrivances to produce a vocal tone. After laryngectomy, of course, the articulators of speech (tongue, lips, and palate primarily) remain. If a communication is established between the airway and the foodway, the patient will speak. Air from the lungs provides 400 cc of breath support as opposed to the 90 cc by the esophagus. Air in the esophagus, as esophageal speakers show, sets the pharyngoesophageal soft tissues (the "PE segment") into vibration and establishes an acceptable vocal tone. The problems are to maintain the opening free of stenosis, to have the patient valve it on swallowing to prevent aspiration, and to arrange for exhaled air to be impeded from exiting the stoma when the patient wants it to pass into the esophagus for speech.

The history of vocal rehabilitation surgery is long and interesting. It begins with Gussenbauer's attempt to rehabilitate a laryngectomy of Billroth's with a reed-containing device around which the tracheopharyngocutaneous wound could granulate. Many ingenious contrivances were subsequently constructed, but the natural materials available at the turn of the century (metal, ivory, leather, etc.) were hard to adapt to the healing wound and the salivary conditions in which they were expected to function.

Every subsequent generation of surgeons rediscovered the concept of a vocal shunt. Guttman in 1935 reported a spontaneous case that occurred in an individual following a suicide attempt.[61] Attempts to reproduce the physiology were made in 1958 by Conley,[62] and in 1965 by Asai[17] and others.[63] But the skin tubes used to connect the two visceral tracts were not very dependable, and by 1979, Woods[64] had demonstrated that cutaneous shunts would never supersede esophageal speech in terms of their frequency of success. In more recent times mucosal techniques developed by Calcaterra[65] and by Staffieri with modifications by Komorn[66] and Griffiths[20] and others rekindled enthusiasm for fistula techniques by showing that some degree of success was possible without a second stage and without dependence on large skin flaps. The tendency toward aspiration continued to thwart these developments, however; in addition, when a fistula was open enough to permit speech, it leaked, and when modifications were employed to tighten the fistula, it stenosed.

By the late 1970's, Sisson[67] and others[68] had shown that, once it had been totally sacrificed by a laryngectomy, rebuilding a biologic connection between the airway and the foodway was an unpredictable venture. Attention shifted to a prosthetic solution again, and advantage was taken of materials and concepts that had not been available to Gussenbauer.

Blom and Singer[12] and others[22] solved the problem of stenosis by obturating the tracheoesophageal fistula with silicone rubber tubes. The problem of aspiration was overcome by fitting the tube with a one-way valve. When sufficient attention is paid to the details of postoperative management and instruction, these methods now supersede esophageal speech in terms of the frequency of communicative success. The question of whether they should be deferred until after an attempt at esophageal speech has failed remains debatable. Esophageal speech uses the same vibrator (the PE segment), is free of any operative risk, and avoids the use of the hands, a prosthesis, or the stoma valve.

Patient requirements for successful puncture rehabilitation are sufficient coordination to plug the stoma with a finger, and the willingness and ability to clean and reapply the prosthesis on a daily basis. Prior radiotherapy, repeated surgery, or previous surgical complications do not constitute contraindications.

A Taub test[69] should be performed prior to a tracheoesophageal fistula procedure. A red rubber catheter is placed through the nose into the upper esophagus and connected to an office airjet. While the operator insufflates air, the patient attempts to phonate. This suggests the spasticity of the cricopharyngeal region under airflow and the ease with which sound might be generated. Failure of this test suggests the need for repetition under fluoroscopic control, with the addition of contrast media. If the pharyngoesophageal segment is open at rest, but spastic contraction is seen in response to the insufflation of air, an associated cricopharyngeal myotomy will be required if a tracheoesophageal puncture is to succeed.

Technique of Tracheoesophageal Puncture, and Subsequent Management

The initial puncture can be performed under local or general anesthesia. We have found Singer's technique to be reliable; under general anesthesia an esophagoscope is introduced with the beveled end facing forward and the longer lip against the posterior pharyngeal wall. The room is darkened, the light is located at the upper end of the posterior tracheal wall, and the anterior lip is palpated through the tracheal stoma. The upper posterior tracheal wall is punctured with a smoothly precurved 14G intercath needle, and the catheter in its lumen is passed up through the esophagoscope into the mouth (Fig. 4–62). The esophagoscope is removed. At the stoma, a curved, pointed hemostat grasps the catheter, and as the catheter is

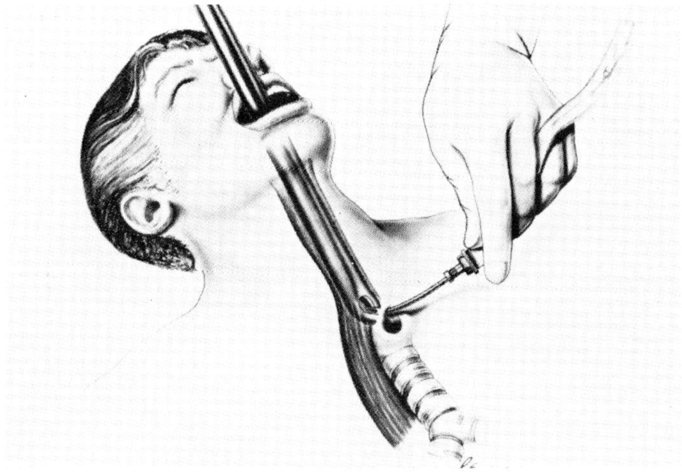

Figure 4–62. Esophagoscope placed with the distal flange facing anteriorly. The tip is situated just below the upper lip of the tracheostoma. A 14G French intracath needle is punctured through the party wall and threaded into the esophagoscope lumen. (From Johns ME, Cantrell RW: Voice restoration of the total laryngectomy patient: the Singer-Blom technique. Otolaryngol Head Neck Surg 89:82, 1981.)

pulled up at the mouth, the hemostat follows the puncture into the esophagus. A large enough opening is made, with a few spreading movements, to enable a No. 14 red rubber catheter to be introduced. The No. 14 catheter is tied to the intercath and pulled up until it is visible in the mouth. The intercath is removed. This leaves the No. 14 red rubber catheter passing like a keeper through a puncture wound in the tracheoesophageal wall. The catheter may be brought out through the nose and secured to itself with a silk tie (Fig. 4–63).

Alternatively, the catheter is repositioned so that it is directed down the gullet; its tip is lubricated and placed in an endotracheal tube and the endotracheal tube is advanced down the esophagus, well past the puncture. The endotracheal tube is then simply withdrawn. Gentle movements up and down on the catheter can confirm that it is properly positioned down the esophagus. The skin is carefully dried around the stoma and painted with tincture of benzoin. The catheter is taped very securely to the lower neck, and one must make sure that the length of free catheter is as short as possible. This is vital to ensure that the catheter is not dislodged from the puncture by regurgitation. If this happens inadvertently, the opening will rapidly close. The catheter stents the puncture for 2 weeks, during which time the patient may return home. When the patient returns to the hospital for a fitting of the Singer-Blom prosthesis, 3 days are allowed for troubleshooting and for instruction in the care and cleaning of the device. These activities are managed in the department of Speech Pathology.

The prosthesis itself varies in length from 2.2 to 3.6 cm and is made of medical grade silicone rubber. The open tracheal end has

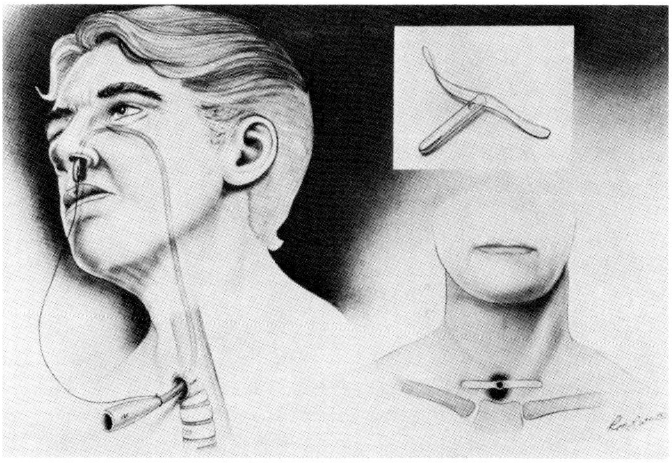

Figure 4–63. Red rubber catheter left in situ secured by a heavy silk ligature. *Left inset:* Singer-Blom prosthesis. *Right inset:* Prosthesis in place. (From Johns ME, Cantrell RW: Voice restoration of the total laryngectomy patient: the Singer-Blom technique. Otolaryngol Head Neck Surg 89:82, 1981.)

two flexible tabs that are taped to the skin (Fig. 4–63). A double-sided tape bonds the deep side of the tab, while paper surgical tape overlaps the outside to produce extra security. The blunt-tipped esophageal end features a very thin retention flange and a razor-thin slit that permits the passage of air but not the admission of saliva. There are two openings at the tracheal end, an end-lumen for cleaning, and a small side port that is positioned to face downward into the tracheal lumen. When the tracheostomy (and the end-lumen) are occluded, air will enter the prosthesis through this port to pass up into the esophagus.

Before fitting the prosthesis, the therapist removes the rubber catheter and establishes that voice is present through the unsupported fistula. If sound is obtained, this provides the initial elation the patient seeks and also excludes the diagnosis of pharyngoesophageal spasm if there are subsequent difficulties. The puncture is gauged for depth with a marked catheter, and the prosthesis is fitted. Several factors may interfere with its immediate success. These include inserting the prosthesis upside down, so the port faces upward; overfitting, or pushing too hard on the stoma so that the valve impinges against the posterior esophageal wall; underfitting, or using too short a prosthesis, so that the tube does not traverse the whole fistula; and neglecting to check the slit valve, which may not be adequately patent.

Once a successful fitting is obtained, the patient is instructed in off-site emergencies. The biggest danger is that during the first few months, at the time of a prosthesis change (which is conducted daily) the patient will lose the puncture. This may happen because he swallows when the prosthesis is out, aspirates saliva, and induces a prolonged coughing fit. Rough attempts to reinsert the prosthesis traumatize the posterior tracheal wall, and the wound closes when successful navigation is abandoned. In anticipation of this problem, the patient should carry a short length of catheter reinforced with a wooden Q-tip. This is used to probe and reopen the puncture if a temporary period elapses without the prosthesis in place.

The problem of occluding the tracheal stoma for speech has traditionally been handled manually. Recently, however, Blom and Singer[42] developed a tracheostomal vent, available commercially from the same source as the tracheoesophageal prosthesis, that relieves many patients of this restriction. The vent consists of two parts: a housing that is bonded to the skin near the stoma, and a valve that is fitted with an internal diaphragm capable of closure on exhalation. At the low pressures of normal breathing, the valve remains open. With slightly stronger exhalation, as in speech, it closes. During a cough, it can be blown out completely without unseating the housing. The patient simply needs to pull the valve from the housing and readjust the diaphragm to resume normal use.

Pharyngeal Myotomy

Occasionally the tracheoesophageal fistula procedure is unsuccessful in producing significant voicing, or the prognosis for speech development is considered poor on the preoperative insufflation test. Recently Singer and Blom[70] reported on their 3-year experience with 16 speech failures in 119 patients in whom the voice shunt had been attempted. Of these, 14 patients consented to further investigation concerning the cause of their failure. Cine contrast fluoroscopy with air insufflation through a No. 14 French catheter placed in the pharyngoesophageal segment showed pharyngoesophageal spasm as the main reason for poor voice production. A parapharyngeal nerve block with lidocaine from C2 to C5 was done transcervically (Fig. 4–64) and the insufflation test was repeated. All patients achieved adequate voicing once the pharyngeal muscle spasm was relieved by the block. Subsequent pharyngeal myotomy in these patients resulted in successful speech in all 14 patients.

Surgical Technique

Under general anesthesia, a Hurst bougie is placed in the hypopharynx and cervical esophagus to act as a guide. A horizontal incision is made in a skin crease, preferably through the scar from the previously done laryngectomy. Skin flaps are developed superiorly and inferiorly to expose the pharynx from the level of the oropharynx to the cervical esophagus. The carotid sheath is identified and retracted laterally. The bougie can be palpated through the pharyngeal wall. The pharynx usually is encased in a layer of fibrous tissue, the residuum of the previous dissection. The pharynx is dissected free from the paraspinal muscles via the prevertebral

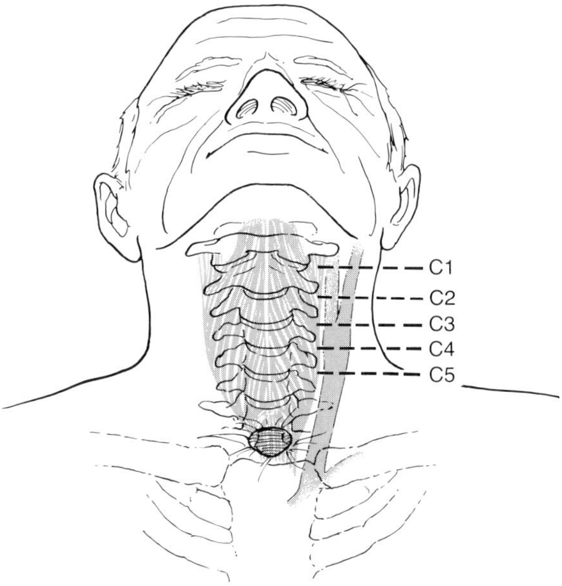

Figure 4–64. Transcutaneous cervical block of the parapharyngeal plexus through the retropharyngeal space. A spinal needle is used. Block is induced by infiltration from C2 to C5.

fascia. The fibrous layer is split posteriorly throughout the length of the pharynx. The pharynx is turned and the sphincters are cut in the posterior midline from as high as possible down into the cervical esophagus (Fig. 4–65). The muscles are cut completely through so that the submucosa bulges through the incision. If accidental penetration of the mucosa occurs, the perforation is closed with 3-0 or 4-0 absorbable suture. The wound is closed in layers and drained.

The tracheoesophageal shunt is now done and stented with a No. 14 French catheter. The shunt tube is placed about 48 to 72 hours postoperatively, at which time oral feeding is reinstated as well.

IRRADIATION

It would not be appropriate to end this chapter on laryngeal carcinoma and surgical technique without reminding readers that laryngeal cancer is not entirely a surgical disease. Radiation should be strongly considered when a lesion is too small for a

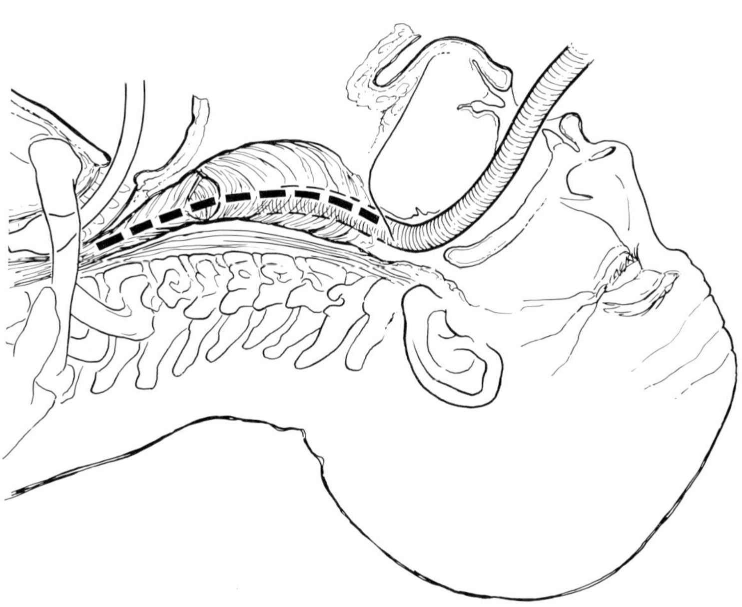

Figure 4–65. The pharynx is rolled to the side and a generous posterior myotomy is made from near the tongue base to the esophageal inlet.

laryngectomy or a near-total laryngectomy, yet unsuited for a conventional partial operation. Examples might be bilateral cord anterior commissure lesions with normal mobility, or bilateral lesions in heavily inflamed larynges, as seen in patients referred after previous stripping and biopsies have plowed under the carcinoma and rendered its extent indeterminate. Selected low-grade microinvasive cancers and verrucous cancers that cover the laryngeal interior extensively may involve much of its surface but almost none of its deep tissues. These may constitute an indication for radiotherapy, since the tumor volume is low and the surgery would be extensive, and the appearance of the surface epithelium of the larynx is more meaningful at the follow-up examinations.

For the reasons outlined under supraglottic cancer (p. 116) we do not depend on radiotherapy to manage the neck. For clinically negative necks, the therapist receives no information from the treatment, and for positive necks, the volume is usually a problem. When partial fixation suggests carotid involvement, no plan has a high rate of success, but reliance on radiotherapy after a dissection in which tumor was stripped from the carotid is especially disappointing. Local ^{125}I or ^{192}Ir implantation has been put forward to boost the radiation flux on the arterial wall,[71] but no convincing pattern of efficiency has emerged. Fortunately, partial fixation of metastases is not often present at the initial encounter with laryngeal cancer, and thus the neck dissections required for such fixation are done at a time removed from that of the laryngeal treatment. This means that the metastases are usually not contaminated into the pharynx, and the opportunity for internal carotid resection exists. With proper preparations, this is the course of action we would prefer. An angiogram and oculoplethysmograph are obtained preoperatively. Intraoperative EEG and xenon cerebral bloodflow monitoring is prearranged. After the specimen is resected, the neurovascular surgeon enters the case and resects the carotid (usually the bulb area and a segment of vagus nerve, and sometimes the hypoglossal) and repairs the defect with a short saphenous vein graft from the ankle.

COMBINED THERAPY

Toxic new chemotherapeutic drugs, which have made important differences in the treatment of lymphomas and rhabdomyosarcomas, have had little impact to date on the management of laryngeal carcinoma. The promise of combined therapy for advanced disease is predicated on the belief that the therapeutic benefit to be derived from two potentially curative treatments might summate. If we look more closely at the application of this principle in advanced laryngeal cancer, however, we must ask ourselves how it would help. The incidence of local recurrence after selective (usually surgical) treatment is too low to allow much room for improvement from a treatment program which itself risks major morbidity. Perhaps the addition of chemotherapy offers promise in the prevention of regional lymph node recurrence. Most deaths from laryngeal cancer are caused by the metastatic tumor in the neck, but at the moment no convincing data exist to show that combined treatment improves the likelihood of cure over adequate surgery alone. This is often ascribed to the difficulty of doing a meaningful study when we don't know who is at risk, i.e., who would have developed recurrence had they not received chemotherapy. This problem, the argument suggests, could perhaps be resolved by double blind studies on large numbers of patients. At the moment most physicians have a hard time randomizing their cases in a prospective study on these modalities. To do so, they have to overrule the wishes of the family and the referring physicians, and the social and economic factors presented by a specific patient. The principal difficulty, however, is not the statistical study, but the lack of knowledge regarding the potency and specificity of the drugs that makes such a study necessary.[72]

If we had evidence that combined therapy prevented pulmonary metastases, and could readily identify the patients at risk for this development, there might be some basis for advising a combined therapeutic program. However, only 2 per cent of patients die because of distant metastases alone, if cured of their local-regional disease. Therefore, in our present state of knowledge, there is too little improvement to justify such treatment; even if 1 of the 2 out of 100 patients who would potentially benefit from it could be saved, that would have to be balanced against the cost in morbidity and dollars to the remaining 98 patients who received combined therapy with no advantage over a single treatment modality alone.

CONCLUSION

This chapter should make it abundantly clear that the validity of surgery in laryngeal cancer has grown apace with cancer treatment in general. The following statement made by Trotter in 1931, and requoted by Devine in 1963,[73] 40 years after the introduction of radiation therapy for laryngeal cancer, remains pertinent today: "Radium has given us a new and very powerful addition to our means of attack, but so far from simplifying the attack it has made it more than ever dependent on experienced judgment and expert handling." The natural voice is important, but life and communication are even more important. No treatment exists to the exclusion of all others, and the initial treatment choice may well be the pivotal decision in a patient's life. The responsibility to keep the options as broad as the problem falls heavily upon the teachers and surgeons who peruse these pages.

References

1. Kennedy JT, Krause CJ: Survival rates in conservation surgery of the larynx. Arch Otolaryngol 99:274, 1974.
2. Constable WC, White RL, El-Mahdi AM, et al: Radiotherapeutic management of cancer of the glottis, University of Virginia, 1956–1971. Laryngoscope 85:1494, 1975.
3. Lillie JC, DeSanto LW: Transoral surgery of early cordal carcinoma. Trans Am Acad Ophthalmol Otolaryngol 77:92, 1973.
4. Hawkins NV: The treatment of glottic carcinoma: an analysis of 800 cases. Laryngoscope 85:1485, 1975.
5. DeSanto LW, Lillie JC, Devine KD: Surgical salvage after radiation for laryngeal cancer. Laryngoscope 86:649, 1976.
6. Olofsson J, Van Nostrand AWP: Growth and spread of laryngeal and hypopharyngeal carcinoma with reflections on the effect of preoperative irradiation. Acta Otolaryngol (Stockh), Suppl 308, 1973.
7. Ward PH, Calcaterra TC, Ragan AR: The enigma of post irradiation oedema and recurrent residual carcinoma of the larynx. Laryngoscope 85:522, 1975.
8. Harwood AR, Hawkins NV, Keane TJ, et al: Radiotherapy of early glottic cancer. Laryngoscope 90:465, 1980.
9. Lawson W, Som M: Second primary cancer after irradiation of laryngeal cancer. Ann Otol 84:771, 1975.
10. Vaughan CW, Strong MS, Jako GJ: Laryngeal carcinoma transoral treatment utilizing the CO_2 laser. Am J Surg 136:490, 1978.
11. Pearson BW, Woods RD II, Hartman DE: Extended hemilaryngectomy for T_3 glottic carcinoma with preservation of speech and swallowing. Laryngoscope 90:1950, 1980.
12. Wetmore SJ, Johns ME, Baker, SR: The Singer-Blom voice restoration procedure. Arch Otolaryngol 107:674, 1981.
13. Silver CE: Surgery for Cancer of the Larynx and Related Structures. New York, Churchill Livingstone, 1981, pp. 1 –11.
14. Bocca E, Pignataro O, Oldini C: Supraglottic laryngectomy: 30 years of experience. Ann Otol Rhinol Laryngol 92:14, 1983.
15. Thawley SE: Epiglottic reconstruction of the vocal cord following hemilaryngectomy. Laryngoscope 93:237, 1983.
16. Wagenfeld DJH, Harwood AR, Bryce DP, et al: Second respiratory tract neoplasms in supraglottic carcinoma. Arch Otolaryngol 107:135, 1981.
17. Asai R: Laryngoplasty after total laryngectomy. Arch Otol 95:114, 1972.
18. Taub S, Bergner LH: Air bypass voice prosthesis for vocal rehabilitation of laryngectomees. Am J Surg 125:748, 1973.
19. Amatsu M: A new one stage surgical technique for postlaryngectomy speech. Arch Otol Rhinol Laryngol 220:149, 1978.
20. Griffiths CM: Neoglottic reconstruction after total laryngectomy. Arch Otolaryngol 106:77, 1980.
21. Singer MI, Blom ED: An endoscopic technique for restoration of voice after laryngectomy. Ann Otol Rhinol Laryngol 89:529, 1980.
22. Panje WR: Prosthetic vocal rehabilitation following laryngectomy. Ann Otol 90:116, 1981.
23. Staging of Cancer of Head and Neck Sites and of Melanomas. American Joint Committee on Cancer, 55 East Erie Street, Chicago, 1980.
24. Leonard JR, Litton WB: Selection of the patient for conservation surgery of the larynx. Laryngoscope 81:232, 1971.
25. Neel HB, Devine KD, DeSanto LW: Laryngofissure and cordectomy for early cordal carcinoma: outcome in 182 patients. Otolaryngol. Head Neck Surg. 88:79, 1980.
26. Kambič V: Epiglottoplasty—new technique for laryngeal reconstruction. Radiologia Ivgoslavika, Suppl II: 33, 1977.
27. Sedlaček, K: Předná laterální rekonstrukĕní laryngektomie se stažením epiglottis. Cesk Otolaryngol 14:328, 1965.
28. Lesinski SG, Bauer WC, Ogura JH: Hemilaryngectomy for T_3 (fixed cord) epidermoid carcinoma of the larynx. Laryngoscope 86:1563, 1976.
29. Leroux RJ: La chirurgie conservatrice dans le cancer du larynx. Ann Otolaryngol 74:40, 1957.
30. Kirchner JA, Som ML: Clinical significance of fixed vocal cord. Laryngoscope 81:1029, 1971.
31. Lee, J.G.: Resection margins of carcinoma of the oral cavity, oropharynx, hypopharynx and larynx: a clinical study. MS Thesis, University of Iowa, 1973.
32. Sisson GA, Goldstein JC, Becker GD: Surgery of limited lesions of the larynx (past and present). Otolaryngol Clin North Am 3:529, 1970.
33. Pearson BW: Subtotal laryngectomy. Laryngoscope 91:1904, 1981.
34. MacKenzie M: Diseases of the pharynx, larynx and trachea. New York, William Wood, 1880.
35. Fletcher GH: Elective irradiation of subclinical disease in cancer of the head and neck. Cancer 29:1450, 1973.
36. Carenfelt C, Eliasson K: Cervical metastases following radical neck dissection that preserved the spinal accessory nerve. Head Neck Surg 2:181, 1980.

37. Montgomery WW: Surgery of the Upper Respiratory System, Vol II: Philadelphia, Lea & Febiger, 1973, pp. 514–541.
38. Ogura JH, Biller HF: Conservation surgery in cancer of the head and neck. Otolaryngol Clin North Am 2:641, 1969.
39. Ariyan S, Cuono CB: Myocutaneous flaps for head and neck reconstruction. Head Neck Surg 2:321, 1980.
40. Miller D: Management of glottic carcinoma. Laryngoscope 85:1435, 1975.
41. Harwood AR, Bryce DP, Rider W: Management of T_3 glottic cancer. Arch Otolaryngol 106:697, 1980.
42. Blom ED, Singer MI, Hamaker RC: Tracheostoma valve for postlaryngectomy voice rehabilitation. Ann Otol Rhinol Laryngol 91:576, 1982.
43. Jesse RH: Evaluation of treatment of patients with extensive squamous cancer of the vocal cords. Laryngoscope 85:1424, 1975.
44. Van Nostrand AWP, Brodarec I: Laryngeal carcinoma—modifications in surgical technique based on our understanding of tumor growth characteristics. J Otolaryngol 11:186, 1982.
45. Keith RL, Shane HC, Coates HLC, et al: Looking Forward . . .. A Guidebook for the Laryngectomee. Rochester, MN, Mayo Foundation, 1977.
46. Schwartz AW, Hollinshead WH, Devine KD: Laryngectomy: anatomy and technique. Surg Clin North Am 43:1063, 1963.
47. Reibel JF, Jahrsdoerfer RA, Johns MME, et al: Histoplasmosis of the larynx. Otolaryngol Head Neck Surg 90:740, 1982.
48. Chandler JR: Radiation fibrosis and necrosis of the larynx. Ann Otol Rhinol Laryngol 88:509, 1979.
49. Bailey CM, Windle-Taylor PC: Tuberculous laryngitis: series of 37 patients. Laryngoscope 91:93, 1981.
50. Kaur S: Respiratory system involvement in leprosy. Int J Lep 47:18, 1979.
51. McDonald TJ, Neel HB III, DeRemee RA: Wegner's granulomatosis of the subglottis and the upper portion of the trachea. Ann Otol Rhinol Laryngol 91:588–592, 1982.
52. McDonald TJ, DeRemee RA, Harrison EG Jr, et al: The protean clinical features of polymorphic reticulosis (lethal midline granuloma). Laryngoscope 86:936, 1976.
53. Compagno J, Hyams VJ, Ste-Marie P: Benign granular cell tumors of the larynx: review of 36 cases with clinicopathologic data. Ann Otol Rhinol Laryngol 84:308, 1975.
54. McCune MA,Rogers RS, Roberts GD: Laryngeal presentation of blastomycosis. Int J Dermatol 19:263, 1980.
55. Lambert PR, Ward PH, Berci G: Pseudosarcoma of the larynx: a comprehensive analysis. Arch Otolaryngol 106:700, 1980.
56. Ferliot A, Recher G: Ackerman's tumor (verrucous carcinoma) of the larynx: A clinicopathologic study of 77 cases. Cancer 46:1617, 1980.
57. Vrabec BT, Bartels LJ: Small cell anaplastic carcinoma of the larynx: review of the literature and report of a case. Laryngoscope 90:1720, 1980.
58. Freeland AP, Van Nostrand AWP, John, AF: Metastases to the larynx. J Otolaryngol 8:448, 1979.
59. Olofsson J, Van Nostrand AWP: Adenoid cystic carcinoma of the larynx. A report of four cases and a review of the literature. Cancer 40:1307, 1977.
60. Lawson, VG: The management of airway involvement in tumors. Arch Otolaryngol 109:86, 1983.
61. Guttman MR: Tracheo-hypopharyngeal fistulization. Trans Am Laryngol Rhinol Otol Soc 41:219, 1935.
62. Conley JJ, DeAmerti F, Pierce JK: A new surgical technique for the vocal rehabilitation of the laryngectomized patient. Ann Otol 67:655, 1958.
63. Fredrickson JM, Bryce DP, Williams GT: Laryngeal reconstruction to prevent aspiration. Arch Otolaryngol 97:457, 1973.
64. Woods RD II, Pearson BW: Alaryngeal speech and development of an internal tracheopharyngeal fistula. Otolaryngol Head Neck Surg 88:64, 1980.
65. Calcaterra TC, Jafek B: Tracheo-esophageal shunt for speech rehabilitation after total laryngectomy. Arch Otolaryngol 94:124, 1971.
66. Komorn RJ: Tracheoesophageal shunt vocal rehabilitation. Can J Otolaryngol 4:563, 1975.
67. Sisson GA, Goldman ME: Pseudoglottic procedure: update and secondary reconstruction techniques. Laryngoscope 90:1120, 1980.
68. Leipzig B: Neoglottic reconstruction following total laryngectomy. A reappraisal. Ann Otol Rhinol Laryngol 89:534, 1980.
69. Taub S: Air bypass voice prosthesis for vocal rehabilitation of laryngectomees. Can J Otolaryngol 4:579, 1975.
70. Singer MI, Blom ED: Selective myotomy for voice restoration after total laryngectomy. Arch Otolaryngol 107:670, 1981.
71. Goffinet DR, Martinez A, Pooler D, et al: Brachytherapy renaissance. Front Radiat Ther Oncol 15:45, 1980.
72. Cregan ET: Cyclophosphamide, Adriamycin and cisplatinum II in the treatment of patients with advanced head and neck cancer. Cancer 47:240, 1981.
73. Devine KD: Laryngectomy: Vicissitudes in the development of a good operation. Arch Otolaryngol 78:816, 1963.

5

NOSE AND PARANASAL SINUSES

Paul J. Donald, M.D.

Paranasal sinus carcinoma generally carries a poor prognosis. The principal reasons for this are the dearth of clinical signs and symptoms until the lesion has obtained considerable size, and the proximity of the sinuses to the brain. In addition, palpable cervical lymph node metastases, although uncommon, are frequently accompanied by nonpalpable retropharyngeal lymph node metastases.

ANATOMY

The intricate interrelated anatomy of the nasal fossae and paranasal sinuses must be thoroughly understood in order to appreciate the pathophysiology of the tumors contained therein. Further, the relationship of these sinuses to the floor of the cranial cavity is integral to the conceptualization of en bloc resection of these malignancies. Increased knowledge of these anatomic principles resulted in the evolution of craniofacial surgery, a procedure that has markedly improved the prognosis in paranasal sinus cancer.

Whereas the relationship of the maxillary sinus to the lateral wall of the nose, the orbital floor, the alveolar ridge, and the hard palate is commonly understood, appreciation of the proximity of the lateral and lateroposterior wall to the inferior aspect of the infratemporal fossa is less often considered (Fig. 5–1). The buccal fat pad as well as the anterior and posterior superior alveolar neurovascular bundles approximate the periosteum at this point. Slightly more lateral are the temporalis and pterygoid muscles. As the narrow posterior sinus wall is approached, the internal maxillary artery is encountered as it enters the pterygomaxillary space through the teardrop aperture of the pterygomaxillary fissure. The artery ascends to this point from its course deep to the mandibular neck, often insinuating itself between the two heads of the lateral pterygoid muscle. The troublesome bleeding so commonly encountered in maxillectomy is often due to a severance of this vessel as well as disruption of the pterygoid venous plexus that invests and drains the pterygoid musculature.

The posterior wall of the maxillary sinus forms the anterior wall of the pterygomaxillary space in its superior half, and the site of articulation of the ascending process of the palatine bone and the pterygoid plates in its inferior half. The maxillary tuberosity extends below the plates for 5 to 7 mm, allowing a point of surgical entry into the sinus in less radical operations in which the pterygoid plates are spared. The maxillary sinus roof medially forms the floor of the ethmoid labyrinth. Tumors of either region commonly extend into the other.

The thin osseous laminae that compose the medial walls of the orbits permit early penetration of ethmoidal carcinoma into the orbit. The roof of the ethmoid sinus, the fovea ethmoidalis, is only slightly thicker than the lamina papyracea and may make up a significant portion of the medial aspect of the anterior cranial floor (Fig. 5–2). The cribri-

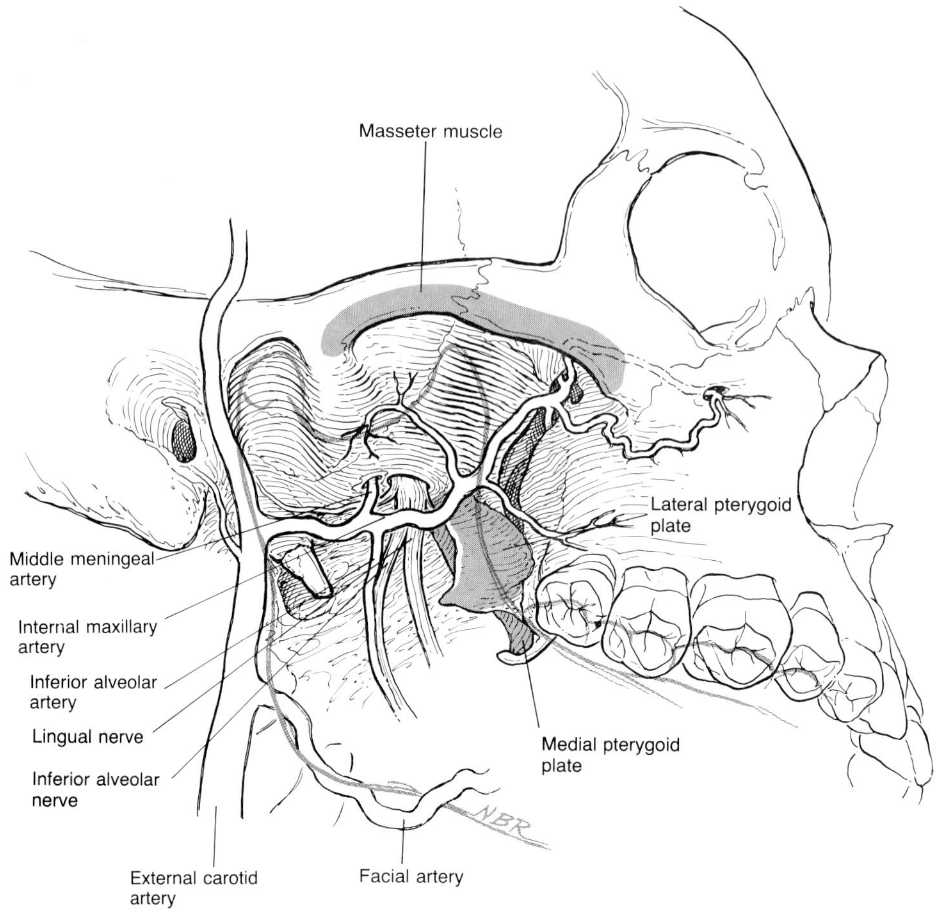

Figure 5–1. Oblique view showing the anatomic relations of the lateral and posterior walls of the maxillary sinus to the infratemporal fossa and skull base structures.

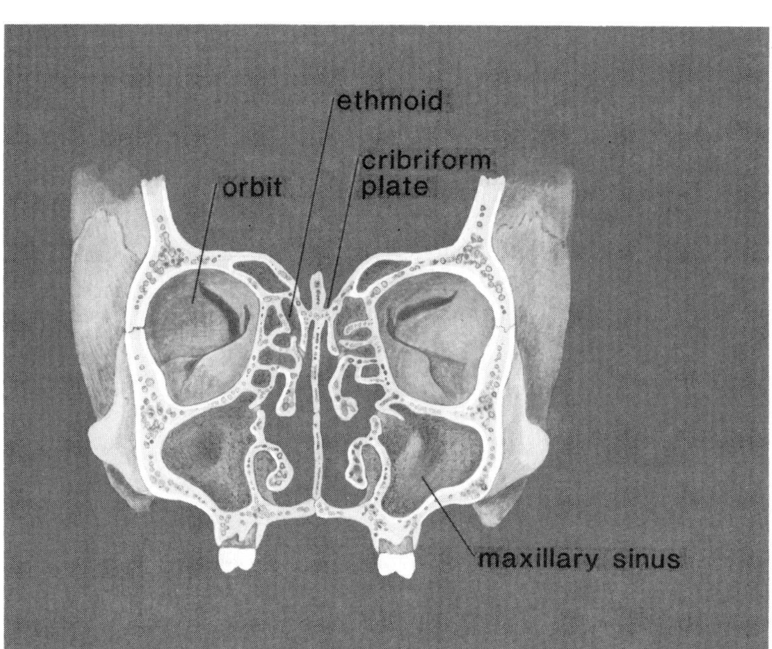

Figure 5–2. Coronal section of ethmoid sinuses. The cribriform plates and fovea make a considerable contribution to the anterior cranial fossa floor.

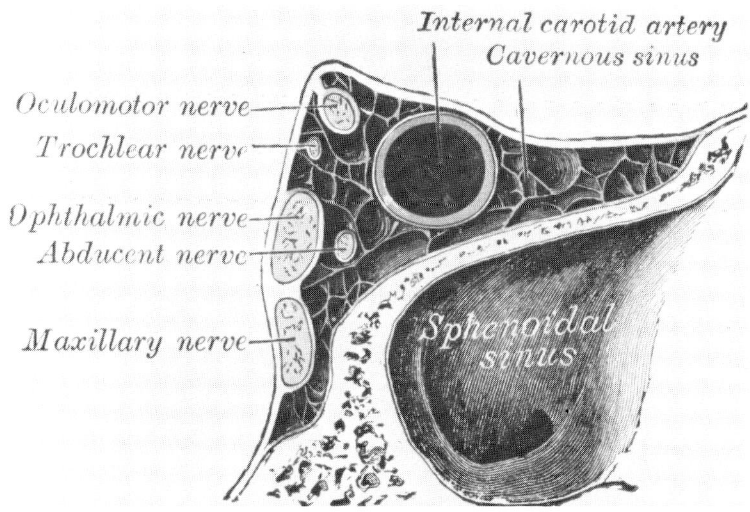

Figure 5–3. Oblique section of the sphenoid sinus with its relationship to the cavernous sinus and the internal carotid artery. (From Goss CM: Gray's Anatomy of the Human Body, 29th ed. Philadelphia, Lea & Febiger, 1975.)

form plates, which form the bony connection between the ethmoid blocks of the right and left sides, also connect both foveae. Olfactory filaments that are extensions of the subarachnoid space penetrate the cribriform plates, creating an easy access route for tumor spreading from the ethmoid sinus directly into the subdural compartment. The number of ethmoid cells is highly variable, ranging from 4 to 17, with an average of 9.[1] As an anteroposterior progression is made, the cells become larger. The posterior cells may even encircle the optic foramena, thus increasing the vulnerability of the eye to the spread of carcinoma. The most posterior ethmoid cells abut the lateral aspect of the sphenoid sinus. The posterior aspect of the ethmoid labyrinth is much wider than the anterior.

The sphenoid sinus is the most surgically inaccessible of the paranasal sinuses. It ranges in size from a mere dimple in the basisphenoid (conchal pneumatization) to extensive pneumatization of the sphenoidal lesser wing. Tumors originating in or invading the sphenoid sinus present a serious therapeutic dilemma because of the plethora of vital anatomic structures approximating its walls. The internal carotid artery lies directly on the bone of the lateral wall posteriorly, often producing an appreciable bulge into the sinus cavity (Fig. 5–3). This portion of the artery lies within the cavernous sinus. The posterior roof of the sphenoid sinus is the sella turcica, which produces another, more pronounced bulge that protrudes inferiorly into the sinus lumen. Just anterior to the pituitary gland is the optic chiasm, on the cranial side of the sphenoid sinus anteriorly. From the chiasm the optic nerves pass anteriorly and slightly inferiorly to gain the optic canals. In this course the optic nerves are intimately related to the posterosuperior aspect of the lateral wall of the sphenoid sinus (Fig. 5–4).

The bone that extends anteriorly from the optic chiasm to the cribriform area is called the planum sphenoidale (Fig. 5–5). It is made up of the sphenoid sinus roof as well as the fovea ethmoidalis. This is often a critical area of excision in craniofacial resection and a crucial area of identification from below by the head and neck surgeon. The intimate relationship of this region to the optic chiasm and optic foramina make the close cooperation of neurosurgeon and head and neck surgeon absolutely essential for the safe conduct of surgery in this area. Crucial decisions regarding the patient's sight and the safety of the internal carotid arteries arise when tumors encroach upon this vital area.

The frontal sinus is related inferiorly to the anterior ethmoidal cells so closely that one of the theories of origin of the frontal sinus is that it is simply a superior extension of the ethmoid labyrinth into the frontal bone.[2] Tumors originating in the anterior ethmoid cells have a tendency to invade superiorly to the frontal sinus via the frontonasal duct; since the latter is actually merely a foramen in 85% of individuals,[3] it provides even a shorter journey for the tumor. The thin bone of the posterior wall provides a weak barrier to the penetration of malignancy to the frontal dura and underlying brain.

The superior sagittal sinus takes origin in the frontal vein as it exits the foramen caecum

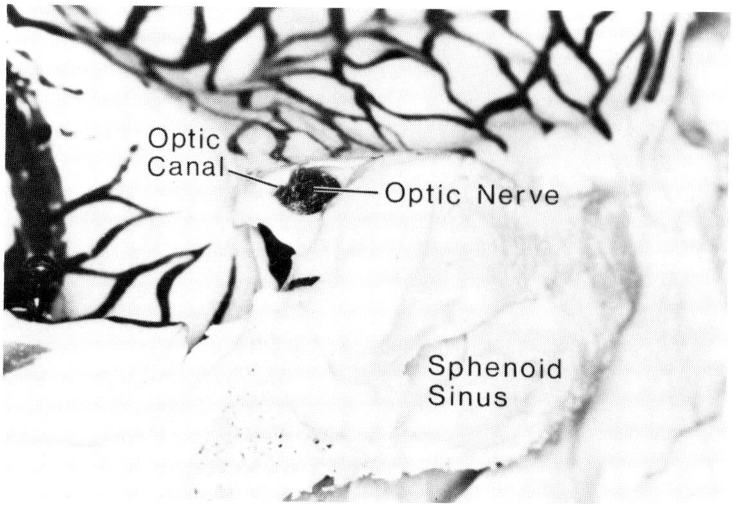

Figure 5–4. Dried skull showing the relationship of the optic nerve to the sphenoid sinus. (From Donald PJ: Recent advances in paranasal sinus surgery. J Head Neck Surg 4:152, 1981.)

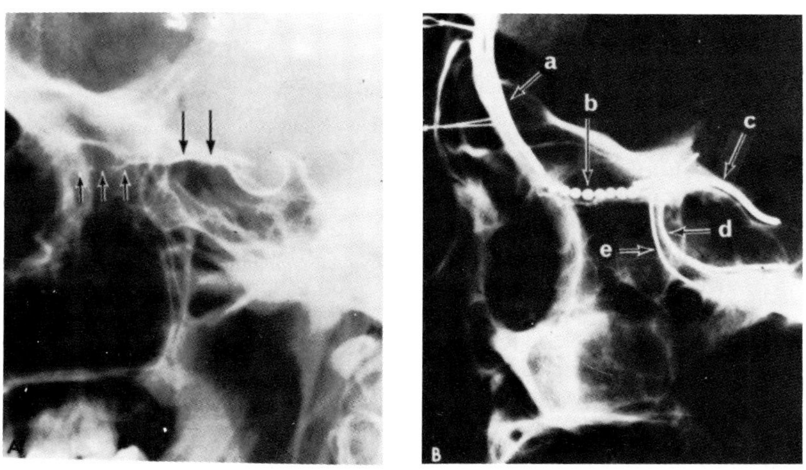

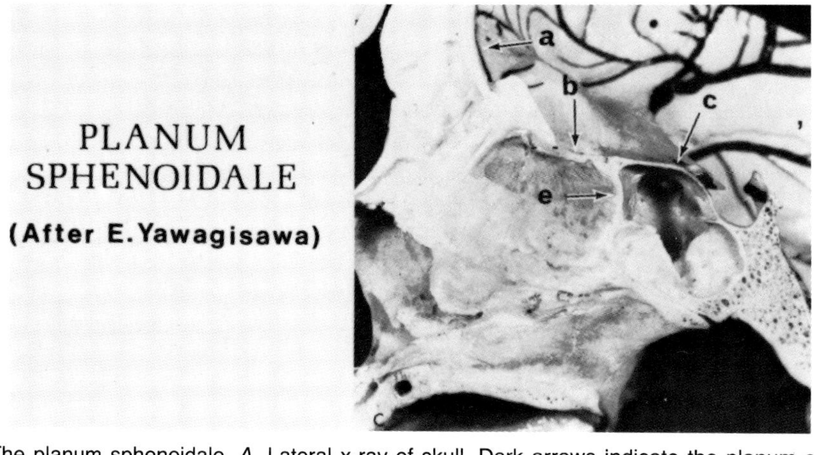

Figure 5–5. The planum sphenoidale. *A,* Lateral x-ray of skull. Dark arrows indicate the planum sphenoidale. The white outlined arrows point to the cribriform plate. *B,* X-ray of dried skull with BB shot on cribriform plate: *a,* posterior wall frontal sinus; *b,* cribriform plate; *c,* planum sphenoidale; *d* and *e,* anterior walls of sphenoid sinuses. *C,* Dried skull; *a,* posterior wall frontal sinus; *b,* cribriform plate; *c,* planum sphenoidale; *d* and *e,* anterior walls of sphenoid sinuses. (Modified from Yawagisawa E, Smith HW: Radiographic anatomy of the paranasal sinuses and related structure. *In* English GM (ed): Otolaryngology. Vol 2. Hagerstown, MD, Harper & Row, 1967.)

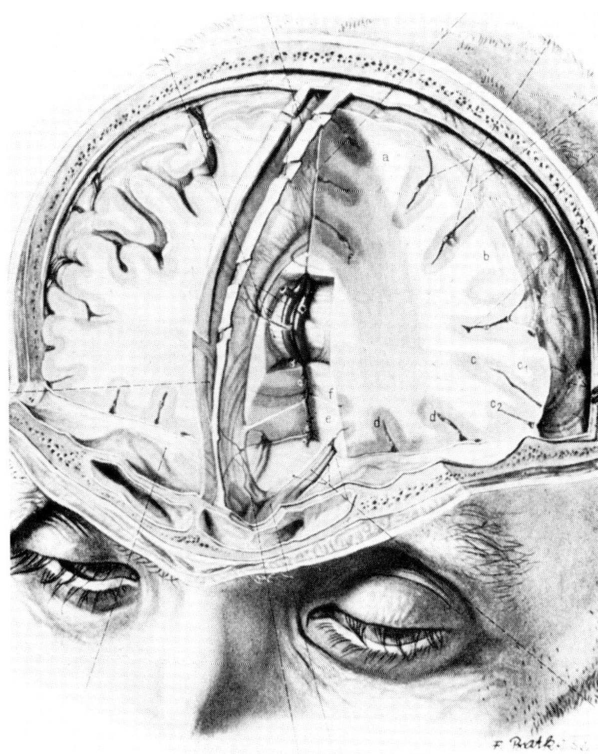

Figure 5–6. Relationship of superior sagittal sinus to posterior frontal sinus wall.

and ascends on the anterior wall of the anterior fossa (Fig. 5–6), on the spine of the posterior frontal sinus wall. Fortunately this large venous sinus can safely be tied below the coronal suture without any untoward effects.[4] In older patients the dura of this region tends to be thin, brittle, and adherent to the frontal bone. Because the superior sagittal sinus runs within the dura of the frontal lobe, it may be necessary to resect both sinus and dura at this level in order to achieve a satisfactory resection margin.

Lymphatic Drainage

The lymphatics of the nasal skin and anterior third of the nasal cavities drain into the submandibular nodes,[5] while those of the maxillary and ethmoidal sinuses drain in a manner similar to the posterior two thirds of the nasal cavities. Approximately 50 per cent of these vessels coalesce in the peritubal lymphatic plexus adjacent to the eustachian tube and then pass to the lateral pharyngeal and high retropharyngeal lymph nodes or alternatively directly to nodes of the superior deep cervical chain. The remaining 50 per cent bypass the peritubal network and go directly to these latter cervical nodes.[5, 6] The wisdom of combining irradiation and surgery either pre- or postoperatively to eradicate microscopic tumor foci in this region is readily apparent.

Although one would assume that the mucosal lymphatic drainage of the sphenoidal and frontal sinuses would follow that of the nasal mucosa adjacent to it—namely to the peritubal lymphatics or directly to the nodes of the jugulodigastric area—the precise anatomy of the lymphatic system in this area remains obscure.

PATHOLOGY

Because paranasal sinus tumors are so rare, making up only between 0.2 and 0.5 per cent of all body tumors,[6, 7, 8] any significant degree of experience in their management is unfortunately limited to a few surgeons in large regional centers. Maxillary sinus cancers are the most common, representing about two thirds to three fourths of paranasal sinus tumors in most series, with malignancies of the ethmoid bloc making up most of the rest. Frontal and sphenoidal sinus malignancies are very rare.[6, 9] Table 5–1 lists a large series of cases compiled by Batsakis,[10] showing the distribution of paranasal sinus and nasal fossa carcinomas.

Table 5–1. CANCER OF THE NASAL CAVITY AND THE PARANASAL SINUSES*

	Anatomic Site of Origin				
Author(s)	*Maxillary Antrum*	*Nasal Cavity*	*Ethmoid Sinus*	*Sphenoid Sinus*	*Frontal Sinus*
Ireland and Bryce	124	22	33		4
Osborn and Winston	63		31		
Frazell and Lewis	261	113	40	1	1
Tabah	36		14	1	1
Conley	60	15	15	2	3
Lederman	356	154	172		4
Lewis and Castro	451	237	75	3	6

*From Batsakis JG: Cancer of the nasal cavity and the paranasal sinuses. *In* Tumors of the Head and Neck—Clinical and Pathological Considerations. Baltimore, Williams and Wilkins, 1974.

Squamous cell carcinoma and its variants, *transitional cell carcinoma* and *lymphoepithelioma,* make up 50 to 80 per cent of all sinus tumors.[6, 10, 11] As a general rule the more anteriorly located tumors (e.g., those in the anterior aspect of the maxillary antra and the nasal cavities) tend to be more well differentiated histologically, whereas those in the posterior regions are more anaplastic.[6] *Inverting papilloma,* a locally aggressive but generally nonmetastasizing tumor, carries a 10 to 15 per cent incidence of frank malignant degeneration.[6] This degeneration is characterized mainly by the appearance of atypical cells and/or a marked increase in the number of mitotic figures. Often these changes occur as one or multiple foci in a tumor that otherwise is characteristic for inverting papilloma. The orderly cellular maturation pattern of squamous epithelium with considerable acanthosis and endophytic growth typifies this lesion. The erosion of bone is said to be caused by pressure rather than infiltration.[12] Squamous cell cancer, on the other hand, is characterized by direct invasion of bone by chords and islands of tumor cells. Late diagnosis is so common that bone destruction is present in 70 to 80 per cent of cases.[9]

Adenocarcinoma is seen in 10 to 14 per cent of cases. According to Batsakis[13] even histologically benign lesions behave in an aggressive manner. Cohen and Batsakis[14] found that even oncocytomas of the maxillary sinus act clinically in an uncharacteristically malignant way. Adenocarcinomas arise in the minor salivary glands of the sinonasal tract. Most of them are adenoid cystic in type and develop in the maxillary sinus.[6, 13] They express their usual behavior of local infiltration and extension along nerve sheaths, with the proximity of the cranial nerves of the sinuses to the skull base allowing early extension of these neoplasms toward the brain. Of the remaining adenocarcinomas, Batsakis et al[15, 16] have identified and described three distinct growth patterns: papillary, sessile, and alveolar-mucoid. These lesions favor the ethmoid sinuses and superior nasal vault as their site of origin. Those of the nasal cavity have a more favorable prognosis than ones involving the sinuses. Of the three types, the papillary variety, whose cells resemble those of the respiratory epithelium, has the best prognosis. The sessile variety features a more anaplastic cell and is widely based. The alveolar-mucoid tumors arise presumably from the seromucinous gland below the lamina propria of the epithelium.

Adenocarcinomas are extremely aggressive locally and tend to metastasize by blood rather than lymphatics. Unlike the more commonly occurring adenoid cystic carcinoma, metastases from the other varieties are less frequent, and prolific direct spread is their principal malignant feature. However, Rafla[17] reported distant metastases in 8 of 15 patients. Local recurrence following resection is common, and the tumors are relatively radioinsensitive. The prognosis is poor, with 5-year survival rates on the order of 20 per cent.[15]

Melanoma makes up only 1 per cent of the total number of nasal and paranasal sinus malignancies, but this site is second in frequency to only the oral cavity for mucosal melanoma of the head and neck. The multicentric nature and satellitosis of these tumors render them difficult to resect. Melanomas of the nasal cavity have a better prognosis (44 per cent 5-year survival) than those arising in the sinuses (0 per cent 5-year survival).[18] Radiation response is poor and should be reserved for those cases that are unresectable or for attempted control of local recurrences.

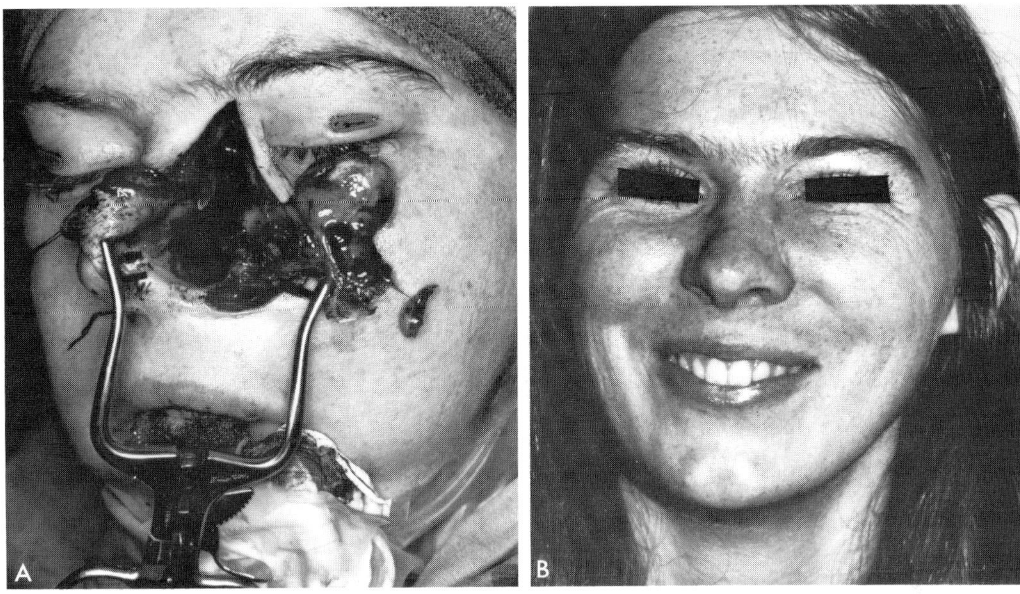

Figure 5–7. *A,* Young woman with an esthesioneuroblastoma of the superior meatus of the nose. Craniofacial resection was not necessary. *B,* Photograph following full course of planned postoperative irradiation.

Esthesioneuroblastoma is a rare malignancy that may arise anywhere in nasal olfactory epithelium. It originates in cells of the neural crest rather than in the esthesioneuroblast as once thought.[19, 20] This lesion may appear in the valut of the nose, in the superior meatus, or on the superior turbinate. According to Obert et al,[21] in all the cases they reviewed, the esthesioneuroblastomas occurred high in the nose. In our experience, one lesion originated on the middle turbinate and extended into the maxillary sinus. The histologic picture is characteristic of that of a neuroblastoma, featuring neurocytes and neuroblasts with rosette and pseudorosette formation. Electron-microscopic features of neurites and secretory granules containing biogenic amines help to differentiate this tumor from other sarcomas and anaplastic carcinomas.[22] The biologic behavior of this tumor belies its seemingly benign histology. Local recurrences and regional and distant metastatic disease are not uncommon, with cervical lymph nodes and the lungs being the most frequent sites of metastases.[23] The tumor typically extends into the ethmoid sinuses, orbit, maxillary sinus, and superiorly through the cribriform plate and fovea ethmoidalis.

Resection using the craniofacial technique is the most commonly employed treatment for esthesioneuroblastoma. Occasionally the lesion clears the nasal vault and ethmoidal fovea sufficiently to permit successful transfacial excision through a lateral rhinotomy, sparing the patient a craniotomy (Fig. 5–7). A combination of surgery and posteroperative irradiation is recommended.

The 5-year survival rate is reported to be 50 per cent, but the 10-year rate only 30 per cent.[23] We have, however, seen a patient who lived with persistent tumor for 20 years (Fig. 5–8).

DIAGNOSIS

One of the primary reasons for the poor prognosis in paranasal sinus cancer is its lack of early symptoms. The few symptoms that do occur—i.e., purulent drainage, nasal obstruction, and epistaxis (Fig. 5–9)—are so commonly encountered in benign diseases that carcinoma of the sinonasal tract may not be suspected. Late signs of proptosis, chemosis (Fig. 5–10), lateral displacement of the eye (Fig. 5–9), facial swelling (Fig. 5–11), or frank erosion through the skin (Fig. 5–12) signify a poor prognosis. Maxillary sinus lesions may erode inferiorly into the palate (Fig. 5–13) or alveolar ridge, producing loose teeth, a swelling, or an ulcer.

Vigilance on the part of the physician in detecting and pursuing the cause of nasal bleeding of undetermined origin, the reasons for unilateral nasal obstruction of recent onset, or the source of purulent drainage that

Text continued on page 159

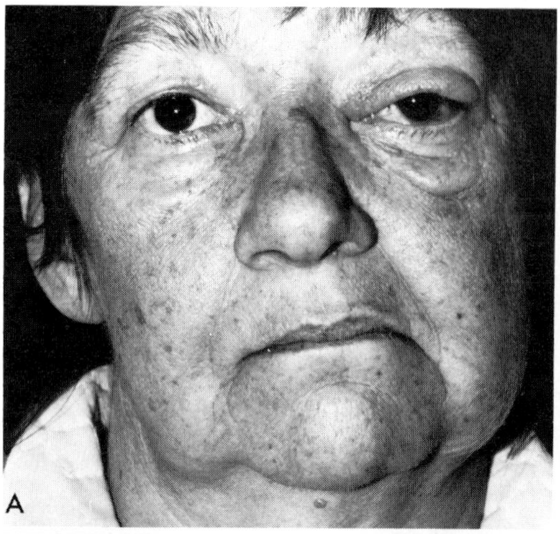

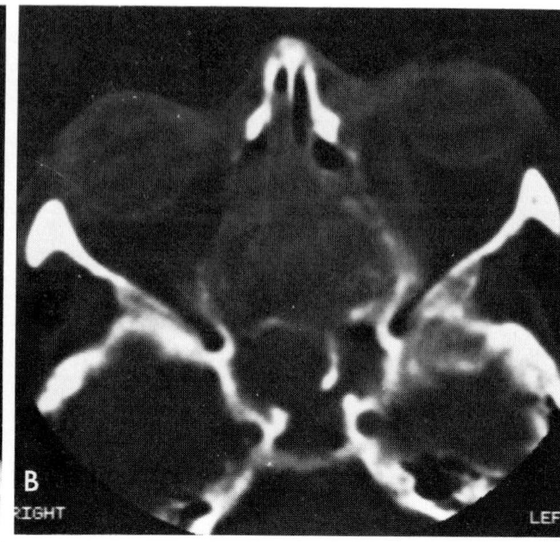

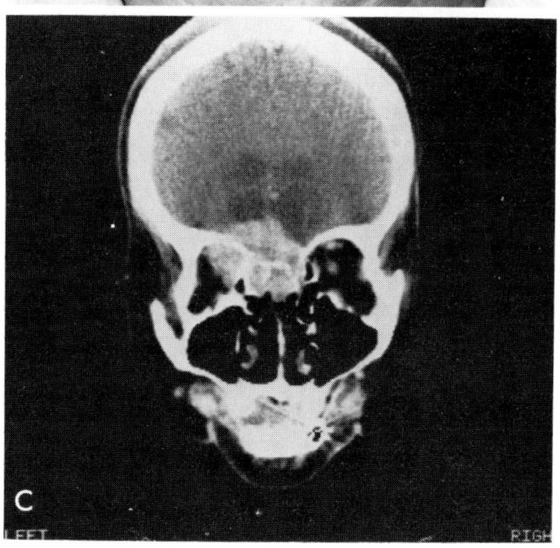

Figure 5–8. *A,* Sixty-five-year-old woman with an esthesioneuroblastoma of the ethmoid sinuses for 20 years. Note displacement of left globe. *B,* CAT scan showing horizontal section through both orbits. Large tumor fills the superior nasal cavities and ethmoid sinuses. The left orbit is full of tumor and the right orbital apex is involved but to a lesser degree. *C,* CAT scan in coronal section showing intracranial extension.

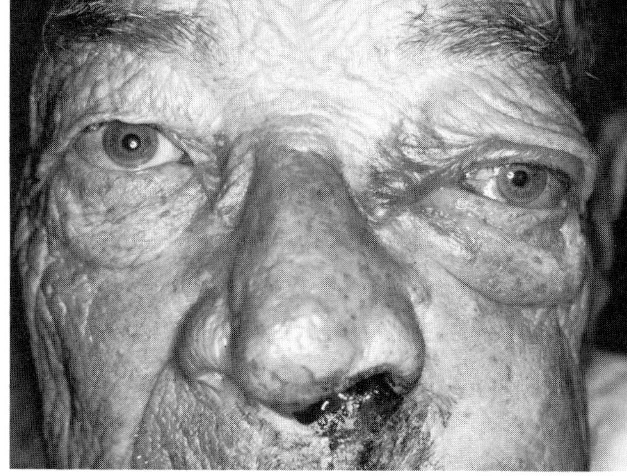

Figure 5–9. Advanced carcinoma of the ethmoid sinus in an elderly man presenting with epistaxis, nasal swelling, and orbital displacement.

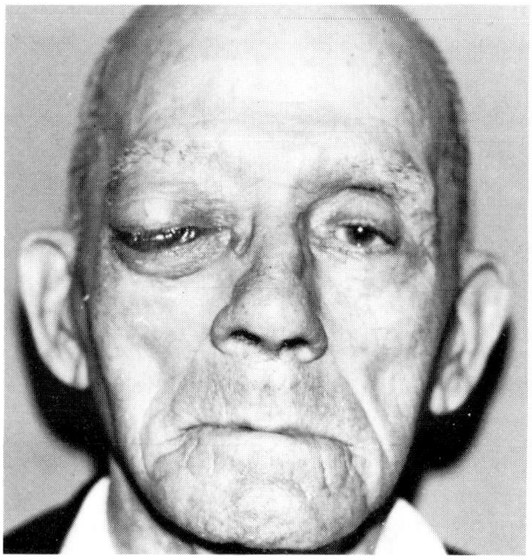

Figure 5–10. Carcinoma of the ethmoid sinus in an 82-year-old man who presented with chemosis and proptosis. The cause of these ocular symptoms remained undiagnosed for months until finally routine sinus x-rays were obtained.

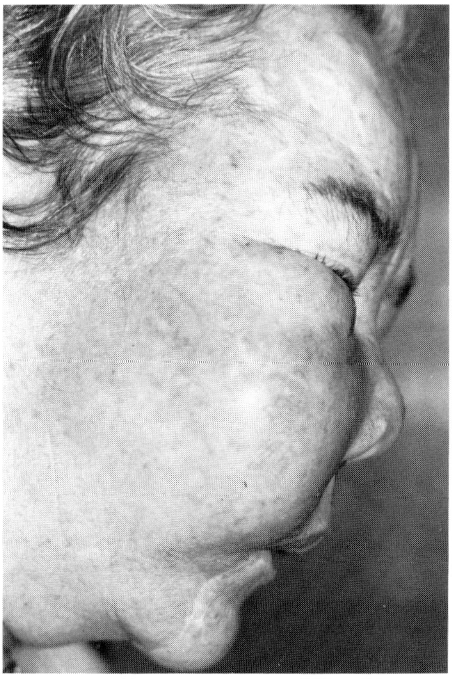

Figure 5–11. Profound facial swelling in a woman of late middle age. A carcinoma of the maxillary sinus had breached the anterior sinus wall and infiltrated the overlying soft tissue.

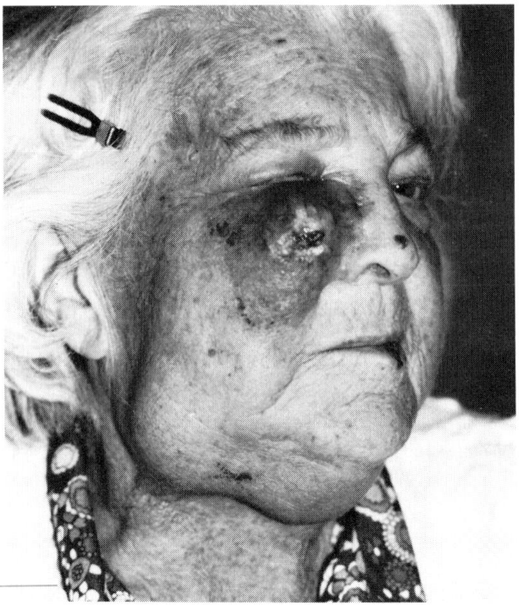

Figure 5–12. An elderly woman with a large maxillary carcinoma that remained undiagnosed until it ulcerated through the skin.

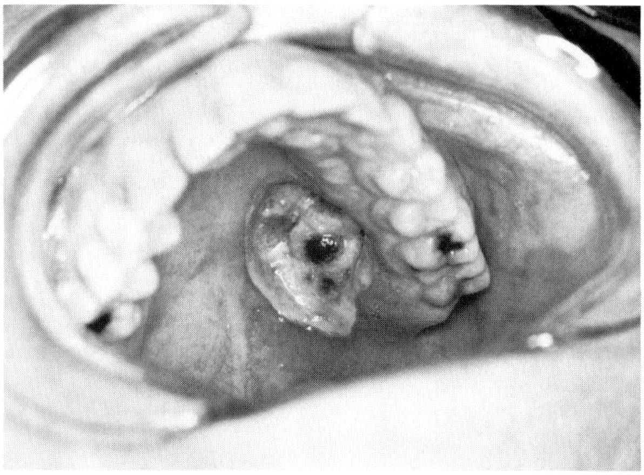

Figure 5–13. A maxillary sinus carcinoma ulcerating through the palate.

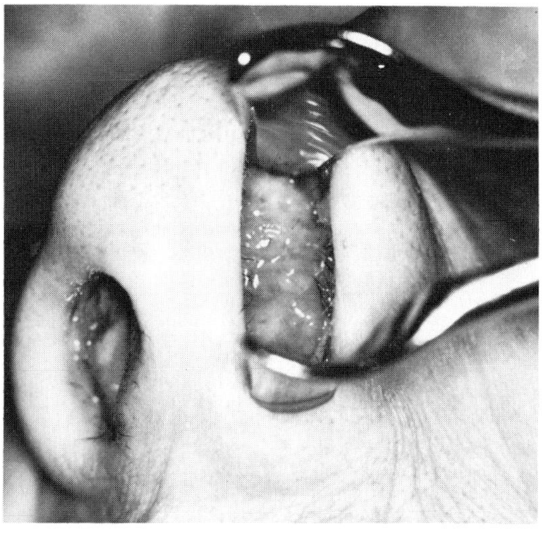

Figure 5–14. Extensive maxillary sinus carcinoma presenting in the nose, producing nasal obstruction.

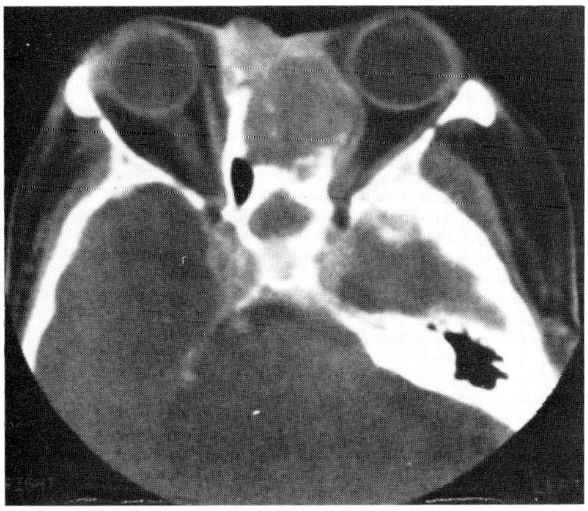

Figure 5–15. CAT scan of a middle-aged man with a large recurrent ethmoid sinus carcinoma. The sphenoid sinus is opacified and filled with thick mucus but not tumor.

is refractory to antibiotic therapy is necessary in order to make an early diagnosis. Although intranasal examination may reveal the tumor in some cases (Fig. 5–14), in others the lesion may remain obscure within the sinus cavities and be detectable only by radiographic exam. The average delay from onset of symptoms to final diagnosis is 6 months.[24]

As a screening device, standard paranasal sinus x-ray examination is helpful, since 80 per cent of patients with maxillary sinus tumors have evidence of bone erosion.[9] However, as a means of judging tumor extent the standard examination is extremely limited. One of the biggest problems in managing paranasal sinus cancers is the determination of tumor extent. Even with computerized tomography, diagnostic errors are frequent, because although the primary site of involvement may be obvious, the degree of tumor extension is often obscure. Robin and Powell[25] analyzed 282 cases of paranasal sinus malignancy and found an error in estimate of tumor extension in one third of the cases. A serious source of diagnostic error in our own experience is the difficulty in interpretation of a density in a sinus cavity on the CAT scan (Fig. 5–15). Plugging of a sinus ostium by tumor can result in the accumulation of secretions that are indistinguishable on the scan from tumor even by densitometry.

The radiographic findings suggesting a diagnosis of malignancy are (1) sinus opacification, (2) a soft tissue mass, (3) sclerosis of bony walls, and (4) erosion or destruction of bony walls.[26] None of these findings alone is diagnostic, a soft tissue mass with bone destruction being the most suggestive combination of signs. Tomography in both the sagittal and coronal planes is extremely helpful, especially in detecting the superior extent of tumor. The presence and extent of cranial floor erosion is critical to the planning of a craniofacial procedure. It is not uncommon for polytomography to produce a more accurate appraisal of encroachment on the cranial floor than the CAT scan (Fig. 5–16). On the other hand, soft tissue invasion by tumor can be detected by tomography but is much more accurately assessed by CAT scanning.

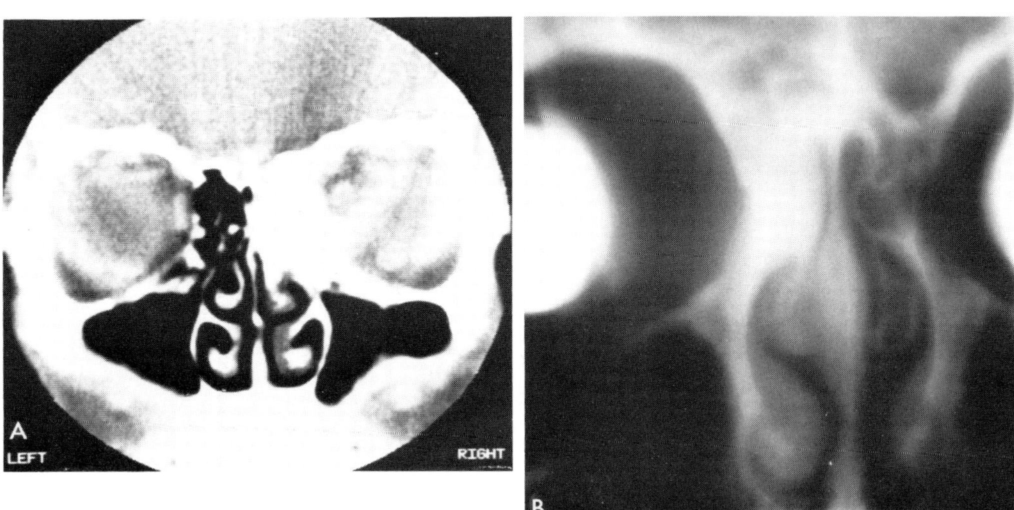

Figure 5–16. *A,* Coronal CAT scan of an osteoblastoma of the ethmoid sinus, showing tumor invasion of the fovea. *B,* Coronal polytomograph of same patient delineating an air interface between tumor and fovea, which more accurately depicts the actual situation at surgery.

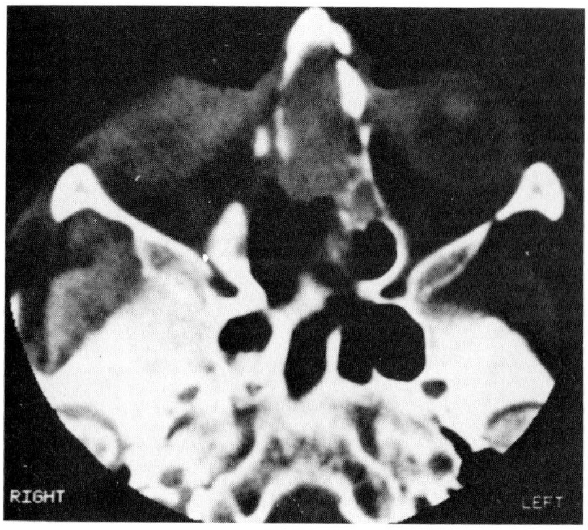

Figure 5–17. Horizontal CAT scan of an elderly woman with malignant melanoma of the nasal cavity extending into both ethmoid sinuses. Sharp depiction of precise tumor extent is seen.

Tumor invasion of the cheek from the maxillary or ethmoid sinus will obliterate the usual low density shadow produced by fat. Invasion of cheek skin lymphatics will produce thickening of the skin. Excellent contrast between tumor and air in the nasal cavity produces an accurate picture of intranasal extent and septal involvement (Fig. 5–17). Soft tissue thickening along the mucosa adjacent to the medial pterygoid plate is strong suggestive evidence of pterygoid involvement and possible nasopharyngeal extension. Early involvement of the eustachian tube torus is hard to determine, but rigidity of the tube may be assessed by utilizing the modified Valsalva maneuver and observing for changes in the torus.[27]

Tumor extension through the posterior antral wall will show up on CAT scan as bone erosion and will also obliterate the thin fat plane surrounding the lateral pterygoid muscle. Since even chronic infection rarely blurs this fine cleavage plane, its obliteration strongly suggests pterygoid muscle involvement. Invasion of this structure signifies infratemporal fossa extension requiring a massive surgical undertaking. Destruction of the base of the plates is a firm indication of invasion of the pterygomaxillary space. Orbital extension of tumor superiorly from the maxillary antrum is best seen with the scan taken in the coronal plane. The axial plane produces an excellent display of orbital involvement and erosion of the lamina papyracea. Loss of the fat plane around the optic nerve indicates involvement of Tenon's capsule and extraocular muscle invasion. Because of proximity to the ophthalmic vein this may mean direct extension to the cavernous sinus.[27]

Perineural spread of cancer can be assessed by both CAT scanning and conventional tomography; it is seen as an expansion of the bony foramen through which the nerves travel.

Despite use of the most modern diagnostic techniques, often the establishment of the extent of tumor can be determined only at the time of resection. If resectability can be established only at the time of surgery, the patient must be so apprised. As the surgery proceeds, great care is taken to perform mainly a debulking procedure without compromising any major function or producing any major cosmetic defect. If the lesion is deemed unresectable, as much gross tumor is removed as possible and postoperative irradiation is done once healing has taken place.

TREATMENT

Nasal Vestibule Lesions

Lesions of the vestibular region of the nose (Fig. 5–18) are sneaky. Whereas even squamous cell cancers of the nasal dorsum are not regarded with much apprehension, because local resection and the application of a skin graft are usually sufficient to eradicate the disease and reconstruct the defect, the vestibular area of the nose is distinctly different. Extension of a seemingly innocuous tumor on the nasal sill or columella into the premaxilla and for a considerable distance along the nasal floor is a common finding. Resection of a generous margin of tissue in the region of the nasal tip, nasal floor, premaxilla, and upper lip is important. If the alveolar bone is to be spared (Fig. 5–19) the patient must be warned that he will likely lose the vitality of his upper central teeth.

A skin incision outlining the tumor by at least 2 cm is done (Fig. 5–20). This invariably results in the loss of the nasal columella, one or both alae, and the superior central part of the upper lip. Intranasally a much wider resection of up to 4 cm from the visible edge of the tumor is done along the septum, nasal floor, and even the anterior maxilla. A lateral rhinotomy (Fig. 5–21) may be required for improved exposure. The premaxilla is excised

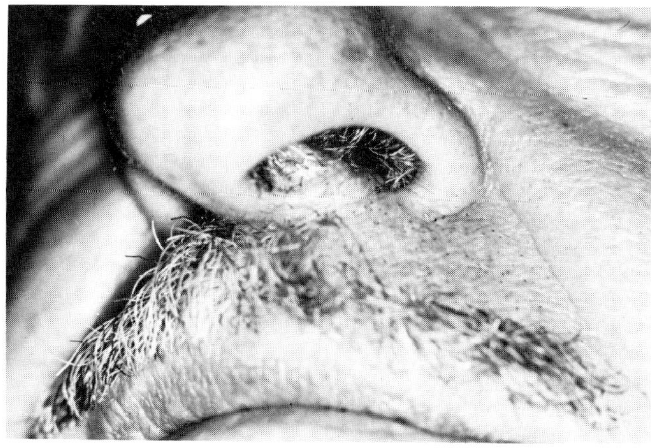

Figure 5–18. Squamous cell carcinoma of the nasal vestibule.

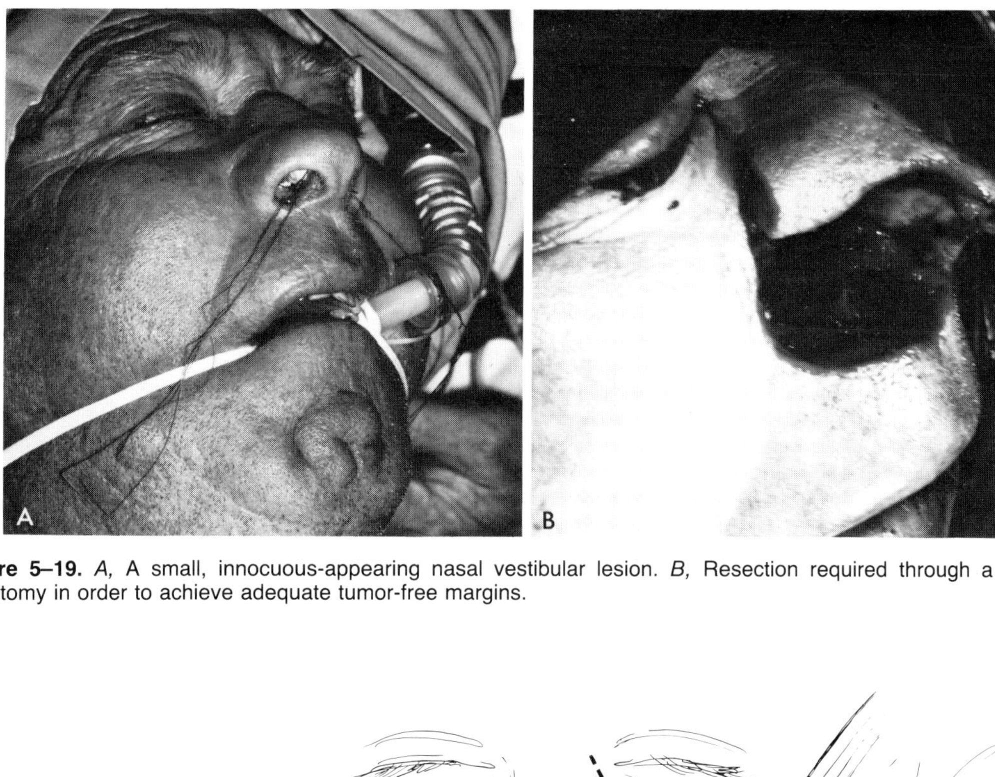

Figure 5–19. *A,* A small, innocuous-appearing nasal vestibular lesion. *B,* Resection required through a lateral rhinotomy in order to achieve adequate tumor-free margins.

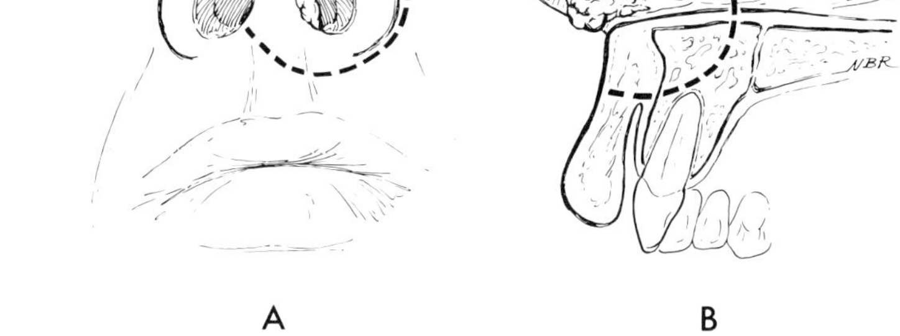

Figure 5–20. Resection of nasal vestibular cancer. *A,* Outline of area of resection, frontal view. *B,* Parasagittal view outlining resection of premaxilla, columella, and septum.

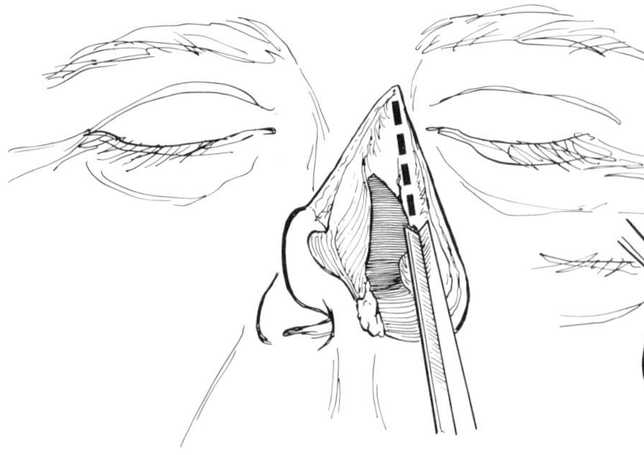

Fig. 5–21.

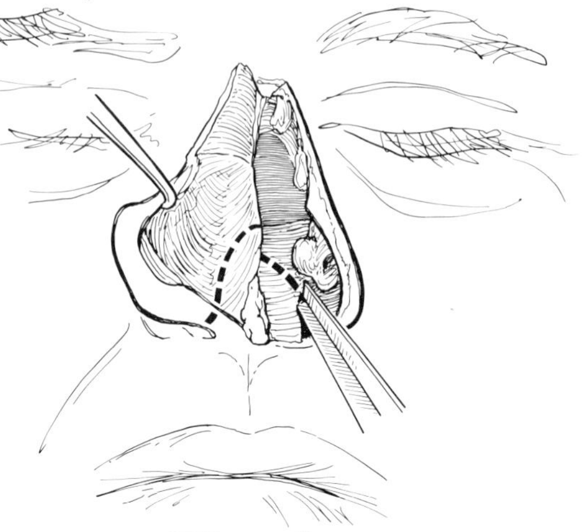

Fig. 5–22.

Figure 5–21. Lateral rhinotomy.

Figure 5–22. Osteotome used to resect the nasal floor portion of the premaxilla.

(Fig. 5–22) using a power saw. Bleeding from the incisive artery is controlled with bone wax or cautery. The upper lip is approximated and the raw area covered with a split-thickness skin graft. The postoperative cosmetic appearance is usually quite acceptable (Fig. 5–23), and further reconstruction should be delayed for at least a year because of the danger of local recurrence. At that time, a nasolabial flap with a previously implanted cartilage graft for structural support of the nasal ala is used for reconstruction (Fig. 5–24). The conchal cartilage of the ear provides an excellent source for a composite graft (Fig. 5–25). It beautifully mimics the nasal alar curve, and the cosmetic impact on the donor site is minimal.

If the defect is larger, and especially if it involves all or part of the nasal lobule, reconstruction of the tip as a unit is best done utilizing a midline forehead flap (Fig. 5–28). Tip support is essential for good esthetic restoration, and grafts of cartilage or bone are necessary to shore up the framework. When reconstructing the nose it is also vital to remember to provide an internal as well as an external lining. The internal lining can be contributed by the skin of a composite graft or it can be contributed by the nose itself. Millard has developed an ingenious method of reconstructing the support of the nasal tip. If a sufficient portion of the nasal septum remains, an L-shaped chondromucosal flap is constructed that when advanced will provide tip support. The flap is pedicled superiorly on the mucoperichondrium, the cartilage cut subperichondrially under this pedicle, and the strut swung forward on this hinge (Fig. 5–27). Septal mucosa is advanced to cover all raw cartilage, and all otherwise exposed areas are lined with split-thickness skin. At the next stage, deficient nasal lining is replaced by utilizing the skin of the dorsum, which is cut, elevated to the rim, and turned

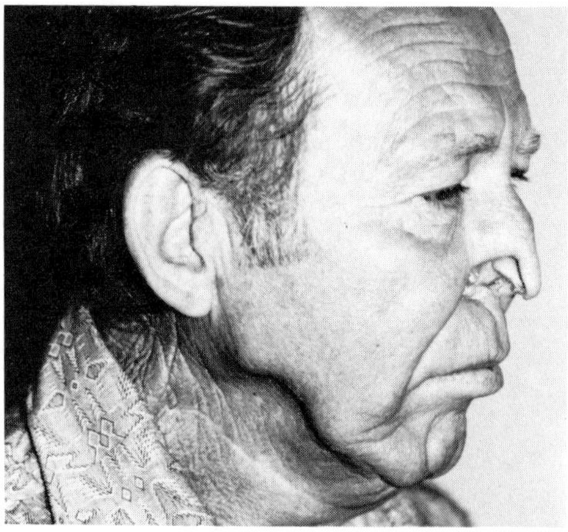

Figure 5–23. Postoperative appearance following resection of nasal vestibular carcinoma. Delay in reconstruction of 1 year is necessary in order to detect early recurrences.

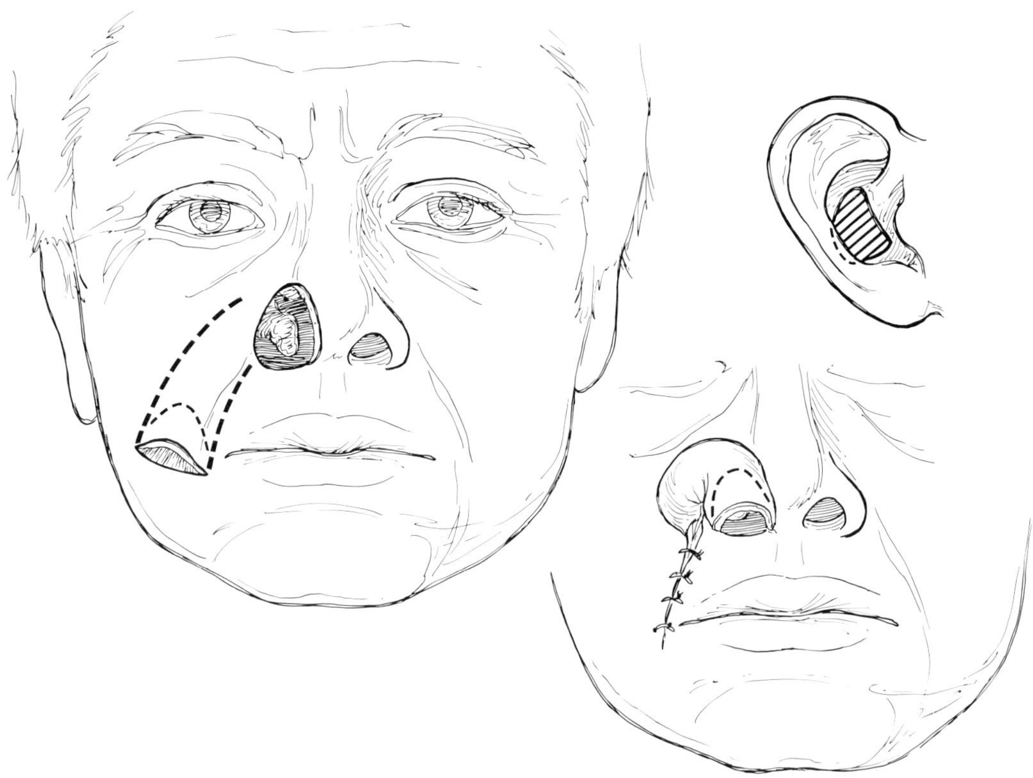

Figure 5–24. Staged nasal alar reconstruction using a nasal labial flap and conchal composite graft.

under. A midline forehead flap pedicled on either the supratrochlear or supraorbital arteries or both is turned to cover the raw area and to refashion the nasal alae, columella, and lobule.

In the delayed case, the skin of the nasal dorsum is used to provide the inner lining as just described (Fig. 5–28). The midline forehead flap is used for the external coverage and formation of the nasal tip (Figs. 5–26, 5–28). It may be created as a regular cutaneous or as an island flap. If the latter is used, a subcutaneous tunnel may be made in the residual nasal skin through which the flap may be introduced. Alternatively, the skin bridge can be split, the flap rotated into place, and continuity restored over the pedicle (Fig. 5–26). The advantage of the island flap is the elimination of a second stage. The disadvantages are bulkiness in the glabella-nasion region and the risk of pedicle compression by subsequent edema of the skin bridge. The midline flap is rotated into the defect and the columella and tip areas reconstructed. The forehead defect is approximated in the midline. If there is much tension in the closure, large stay sutures can be placed well to the outside of the suture line. These remain for 2 to 3 weeks.

Anterior Facial Lesions

A few facial lesions acquire such a size or extent that they are beyond curative resection (Fig. 5–29). However, some that may initially appear to be hopeless can be rescued with a heroic procedure (Fig. 5–30). So many cutaneous carcinomas of either basal or squamous cell type are readily curable by limited resection, and reconstruction is simply achieved with application of a skin graft or the rotation of a small flap into the defect. Occasionally such efforts are frustrated by a pernicious lesion that persistently recurs despite repeated limited local excisions. At this point "whittling away" of the tumor must cease and a definitive resection with wide margins be done. The tumor specimen in such a case will reveal deep infiltration into the skeletal elements of the nose and even into the adjacent maxillary sinuses.

The patient in Figure 5–30 exemplifies such a case. Following numerous attempts at local

Text continued on page 167

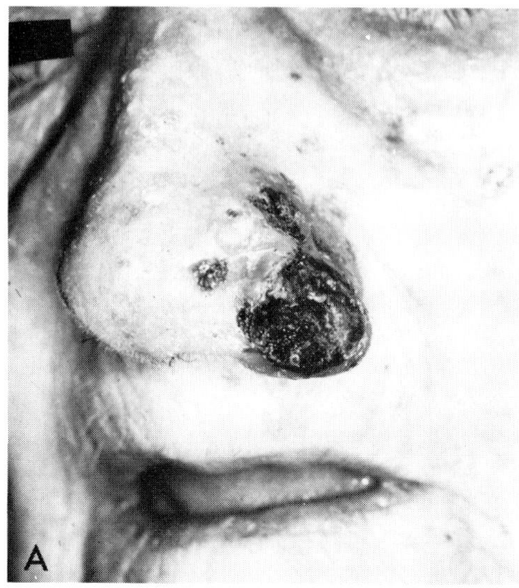

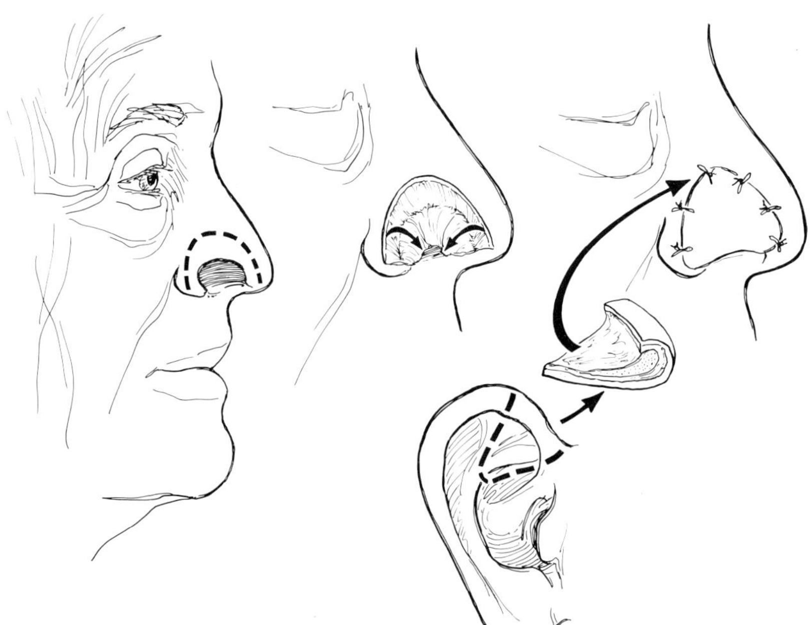

B

Figure 5–25. *A,* Lesion. *B,* Composite cartilage graft used to reconstruct the nasal ala.

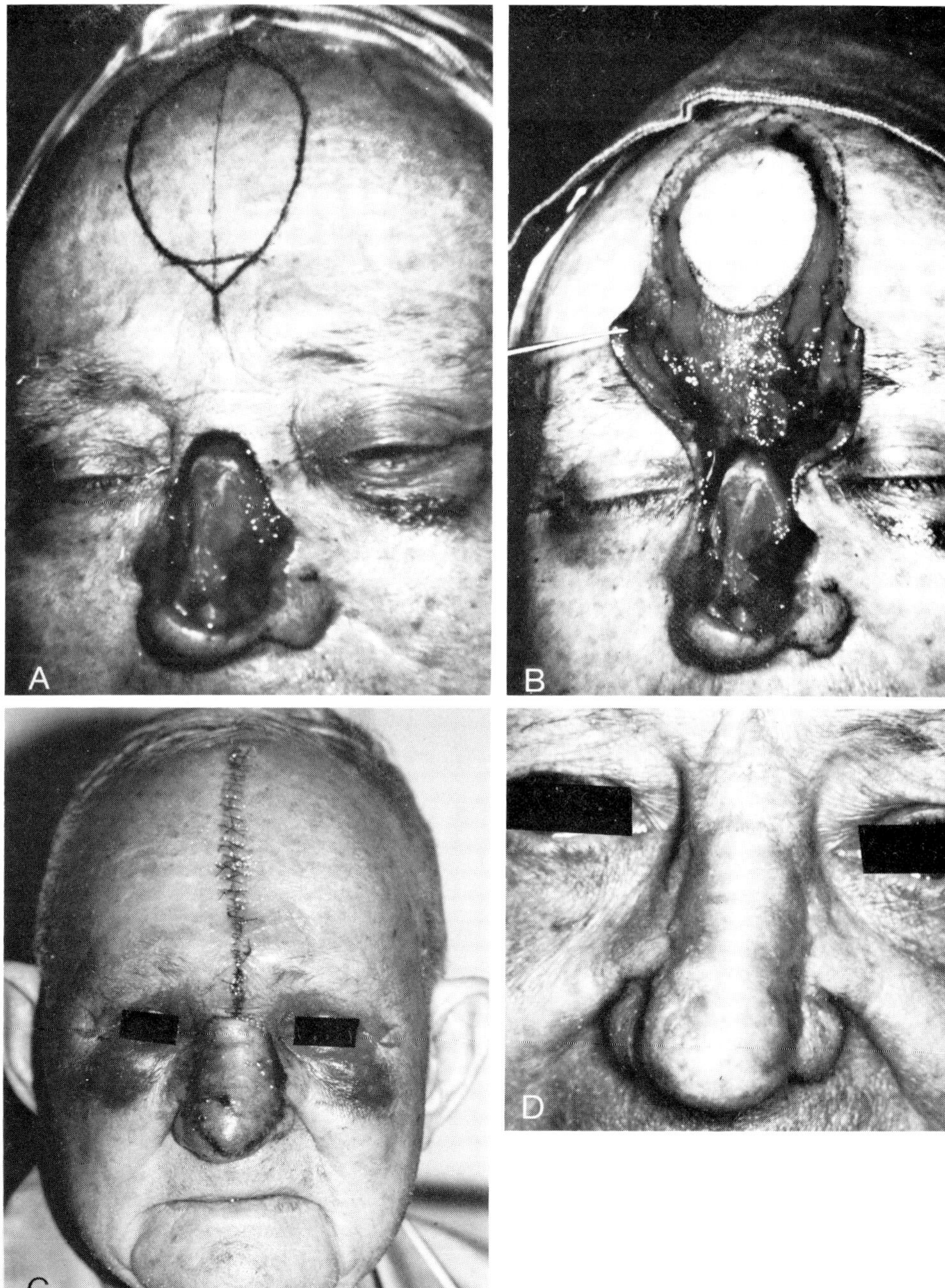

Figure 5–26. Midline forehead flap used to reconstruct the nasal dorsum. *A,* Flap outlined. *B,* Island flap pedicled on the supraorbital and supratrochlear arteries, elevated and ready to transpose into defect. *C,* Flap turned and sutured into position. *D,* Six weeks postoperatively.

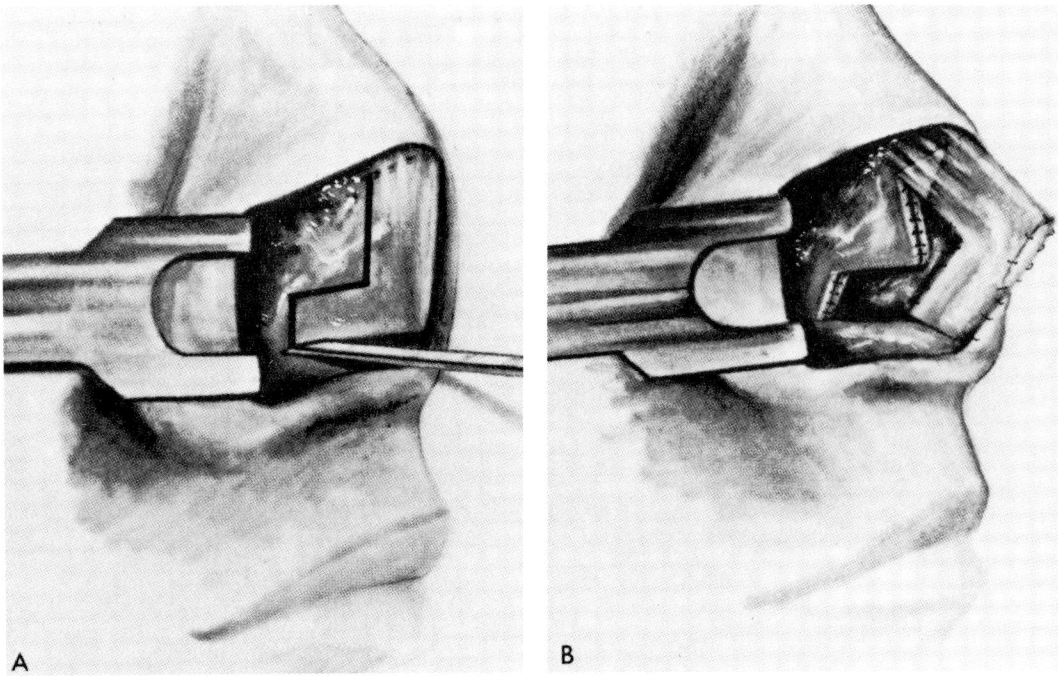

Figure 5–27. L-shaped composite strut of septal cartilage and mucoperichondrium of both sides of nasal septum. *B,* Flap is pedicled on the mucoperiosteum of the nasal dorsum and adjacent septum. Cartilage is fractured to the dorsal extent of the septum, and the flap is swung anteriorly. (From Millard R: Anesthetic reconstructive rhinoplasty. Clin Plast Surg 8:169. 1981.)

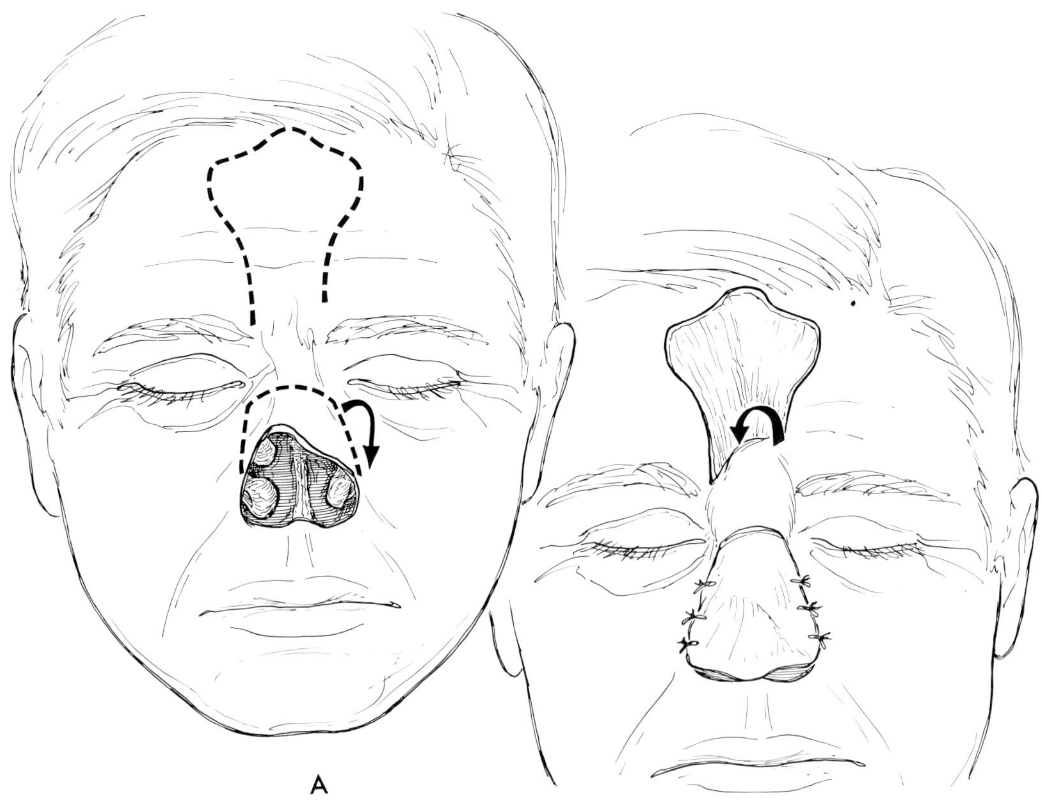

Figure 5–28. *A,* Midline forehead flap used to reconstruct the nasal dorsum. Turn-down flap on nasal tip is outlined and ready to dissect to nasal rim, where it is pedicled and used to provide the inner nasal lining. Midline forehead flap is outlined and may be delayed. Inner lining is provided by a turn-down flap of skin of the nasal dorsum. Midline forehead flap is rotated under the subcutaneous tunnel after a portion of the flap has been de-epithelialized. *B,* Flap rotated into place.

Illustration continued on opposite page

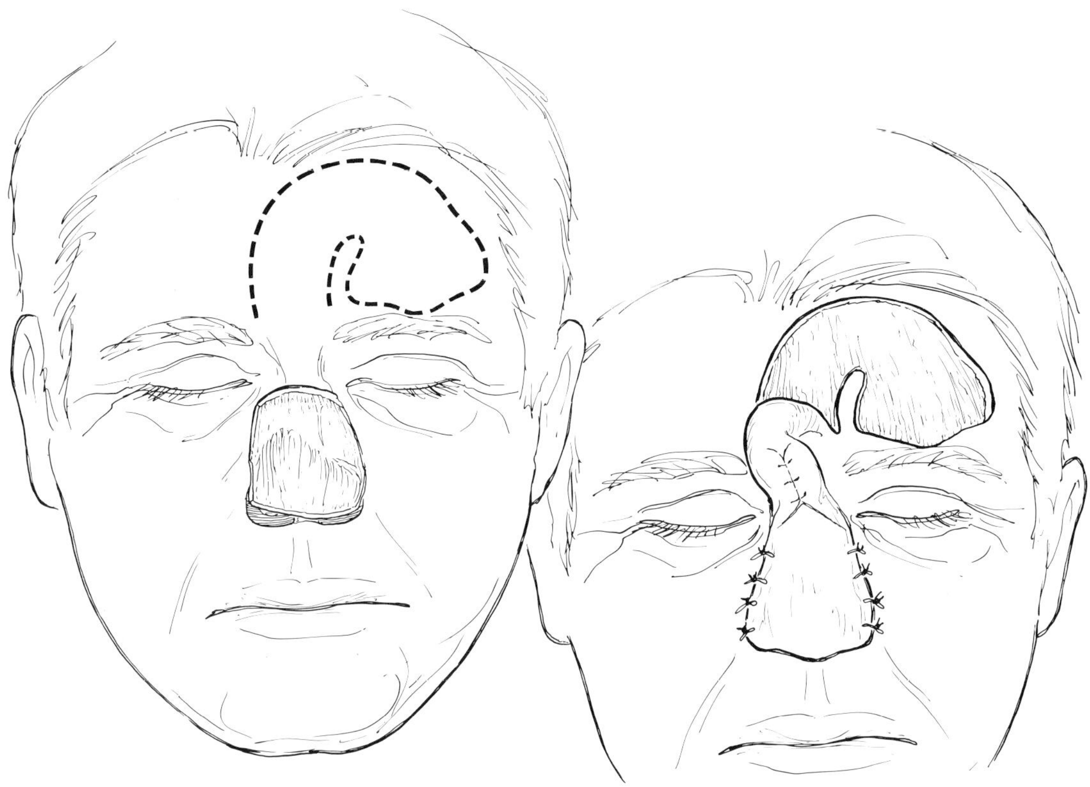

C

Figure 5–28 *Continued. C,* Alternatively the flap is rotated extracutaneously, with the pedicle then divided and returned to the forehead at a later stage. When a longer pedicle is required, an "up-down" design may be utilized.

excision the tumor had deeply infiltrated the soft tissues of the anterior part of the face and the cartilaginous portion of the nasal dorsum and had breached the anterior walls of the maxillary sinuses. The cutaneous resection margin is outlined in Figure 5–31. A wide skin margin must be taken to avoid cutting across tumor that may have infiltrated laterally into the dermis, previous scar tissue, or muscle planes, a phenomenon that is very often seen in these cases.[4] Spread along embryologic cleavage lines is another common trend in these aggressive cancers. Through-and-through excision is done into both nasal cavities and maxillary antra (Fig. 5–32). Also included is a portion of premaxilla, because of tumor infiltration into the nasal sill and vestibule.

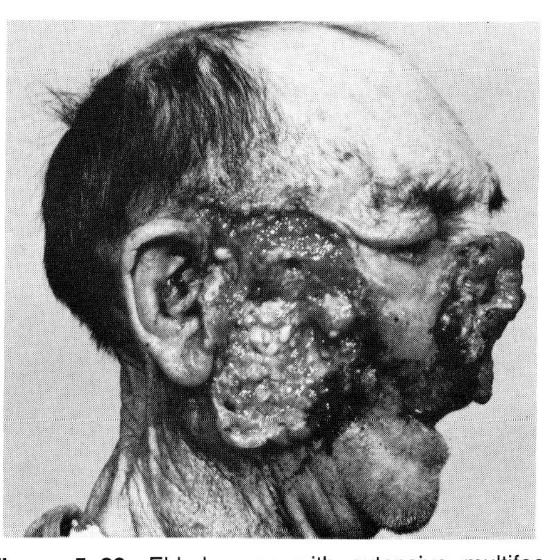

Figure 5–29. Elderly man with extensive multifocal squamous cell carcinoma of the face.

Coverage of such a defect presents a significant reconstructive challenge. An extensive rebuilding effort using flaps should be resisted, since the burying of a local recurrence under a large flap may result in the tumor's becoming unresectable by the time it is detected (Fig. 5–33). In the patient shown in Figure 5–30, coverage was achieved by local advancement of the facial soft tissue utilizing 2 large Kuhnt-Szymanowski flaps (Fig. 5–34), which permitted closure of the

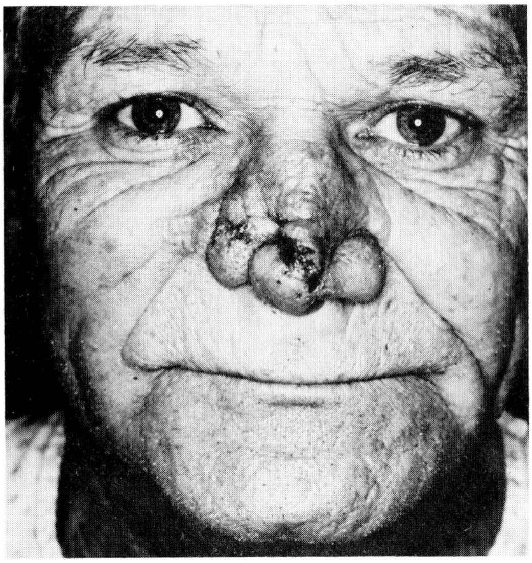

Figure 5–30. Midline nasal squamous cell cancer that had been repeatedly treated by small conservative excisions and radiation therapy. Tumor extended throughout the skin of the entire nose as well as its framework. In addition, spread to the cheek skin and underlying tissue was also palpable.

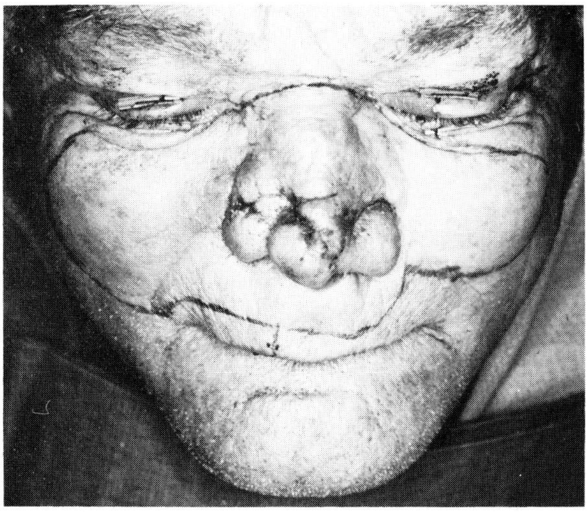

Figure 5–31. Margins of resection for patient in Figure 5–30 are outlined.

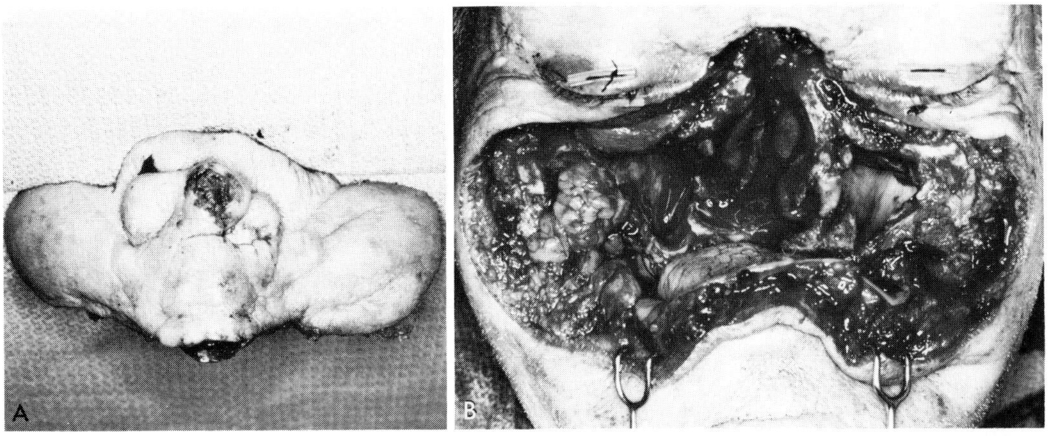

Figure 5–32. A total rhinectomy and bilateral anterior maxillectomies were necessary, as was excision of overlying facial skin. *A,* Specimen. *B,* Defect.

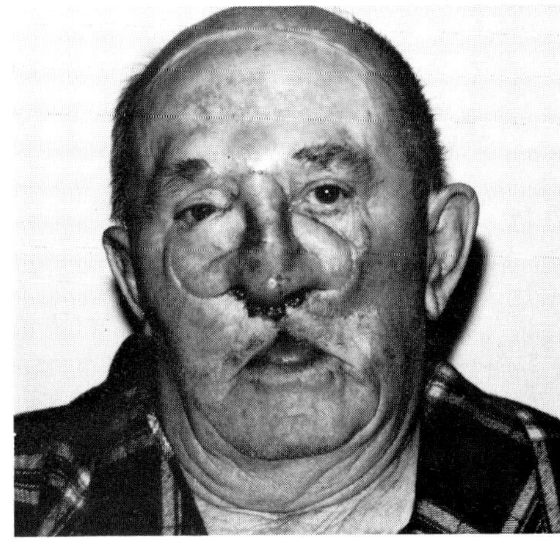

Figure 5–33. Immediate reconstruction of a similar defect in this patient, in whom a bipedicled forehead flap obscured a local recurrence that had become inoperable prior to its detection.

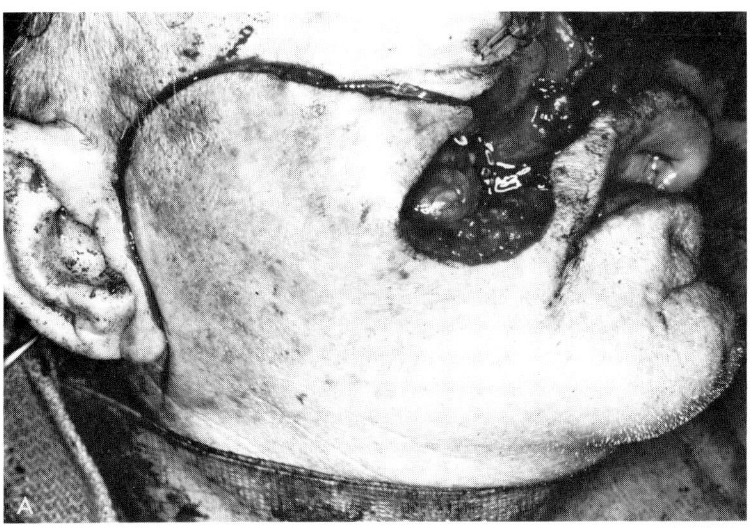

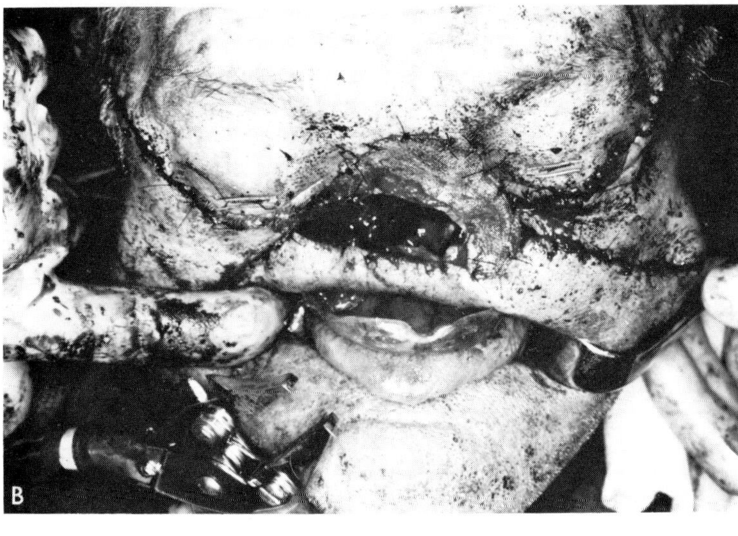

Figure 5–34. Bilateral Kuhnt-Szymanowski flaps were used to obtain closure in the patient in Figure 5–32. *A*, Flap outlined. *B*, Defect closed.

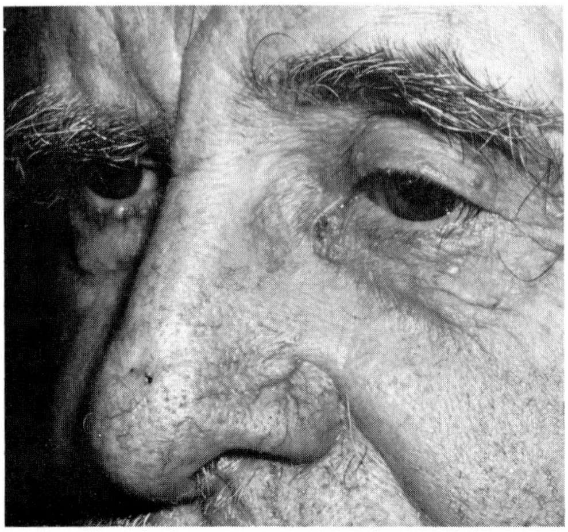

Figure 5–35. Small, innocuous-appearing basal cell carcinoma of the inner canthal skin of the eye. This is an extremely dangerous position for basal cell carcinoma.

defect and clear visualization of the resection margins on follow-up. The unsightly area of the amputated nose can be covered by a prosthesis until a 12- to 18-month follow-up ensures the absence of local recurrence. At that time the patient may even decide to retain the prosthesis rather than undergo the rigors of a nasal reconstruction.

Another site that produces substantial difficulties in management is the nasal-jugal area. This region of skin between the caruncle of the eye and the dorsum of the nose just lateral to the nasion occasionally harbors malignancies, usually of the basal cell variety (Fig. 5–35), that acquire a particularly pernicious character. They have a tendency to extend deeply and laterally from the cutaneous surface into the underlying ethmoid and even the maxillary sinuses, thereby jeopardizing the eye. The morpheaform type of basal cell tumor is common in this area, and local recurrences following conservative local resections are the rule (Fig. 5–36). Many surgeons are lulled into a sense of complacency usually engendered by their favorable experience with this lesion in other sites. However, with such tumors in this dangerous site, even rather aggressive excisions may prove unsuccessful (Fig. 5–37). Moh's fresh tissue technique (Chapter 7) has one of its most pertinent applications in these cases. It is not uncommon for the recurrent and larger lesions to require an orbital exenteration and even a craniofacial procedure.

Craniofacial Resection

The standard maxillectomy and external ethmoidectomy procedures are not covered in this chapter, as they are well described in a number of surgical atlases and texts. Although the maxillary portion of these operations can usually be accomplished en bloc, the ethmoidal part is more of a piecemeal affair. A significantly wide margin of healthy tissue is often difficult to attain, and the bony nature of the specimen makes frozen sections unobtainable. Considerable judgment is required to establish a good cancer ablative procedure at this site. Craniofacial resection facilitates the establishment of superior and often lateral tissue margins, and has significantly broadened the perspective in ethmoidal and maxilloethmoidal cancer surgery.

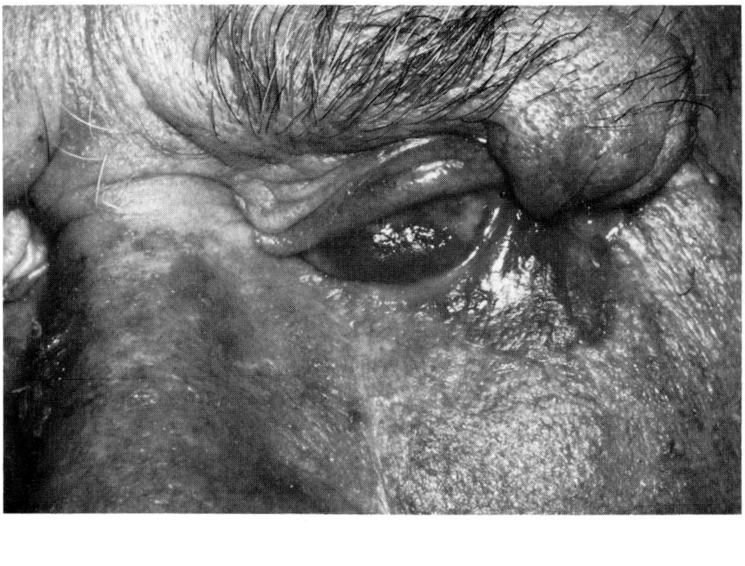

Figure 5–36. Past conservative resection of the medial canthal basal cell carcinoma shown in the preceding figure. The tumor eventually claimed this patient's eye.

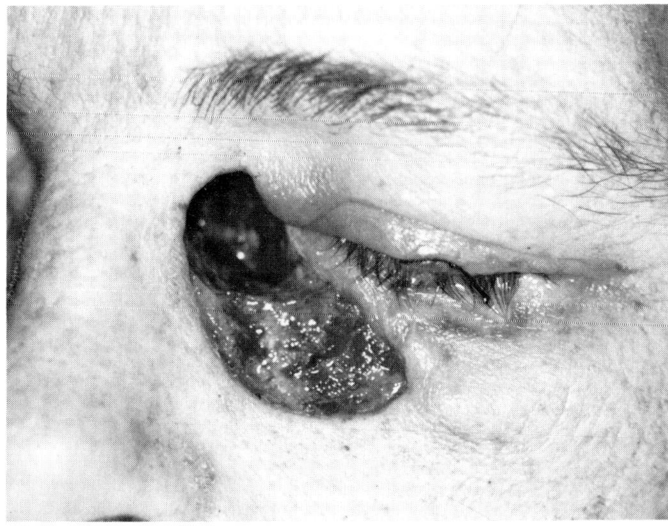

Figure 5–37. Basal cell carcinoma of the inner canthus managed by an aggressive skin excision, exenteration of the ethmoid sinus, and resection of part of the bony wall of the nose. Despite this resection, most tumor margins were positive. Curative excision required orbital exenteration and a craniofacial procedure.

Surgical resection has traditionally been the method of choice in the management of paranasal sinus cancer. Irradiation therapy is usually reserved for adjunctive therapy or palliation in patients with hopeless unresectable disease or in those who are too debilitated by intercurrent disease to operate upon. For tumors of the maxilla located below Ohngren's line, maxillectomy is the standard approach, and is often curative. Simple maxillectomy is much less successful with tumors above this line, because of their proximity to the orbit and pterygomaxillary space. A much more radical procedure is required, usually involving orbital resection. Patients with tumors in this area should be strongly considered for craniofacial resection.

Although small ethmoidal tumors can be adequately excised transfacially, usually these tumors, because of their occult nature, are not detected until quite large. Adequate excision in these instances must include the floor of the anterior cranial fossa, the medial and superior orbital walls, and often the orbital contents.

To enhance the survival rate, follow-up radiotherapy is employed. The histopathologic establishment of integrity of the surgical margins in these cases is exceptionally difficult because of the piecemeal nature of portions of the resection. The addition of radiotherapy greatly enhances the opportunity for complete tumor ablation.

Craniofacial resection is used for cancers whose geographic center may be either maxillary or ethmoidal in origin. If the lesion originated in the ethmoid sinus, occasionally a portion of the maxilla can be spared. A primarily maxillary tumor may not have as much cranial spread, thus reducing the amount of anterior fossa floor needing resection. In most instances, the eye must be sacrificed. In only one case in our own series was the eye spared; this involved a man with a small adenocarcinoma that demonstrated no bone erosion of the lamina papyracea but did encroach on the cribriform plate (see Case I, p. 181). He is alive and well 5 years following craniofacial resection. Occasionally maxillary encroachment by an ethmoid tumor is minimal, permitting salvage of the dental arch of the affected side. However, in most instances, a maxilloethmoidectomy and orbital exenteration are required. When there is cutaneous involvement, a wide margin of skin must be excised, compounding the reconstructive problem.

Preparation

Preparing the patient for surgery requires the coordinated efforts of the head and neck surgeon, neurosurgeon, and maxillofacial prosthodontist. The planning and timing of each surgeon's step in the procedure is anticipated and agreed upon ahead of time. Each participant should plan to be present for most of his partner's contribution to the procedure, as the most difficult aspect of the operation is to establish clear surgical margins. Both surgical participants contribute to and jointly decide on the determination of these margins, which are especially crucial in the region of the fovea ethmoidalis and planum sphenoidale. The patient needs to understand the gravity of the procedure and that he is going to have "brain surgery" with its possible after-effects as well as the attendant problem of the usually inevitable facial deformity. Many patients with substantial amounts of resected anterior fossa floor experience agonizing headache for a number of weeks postoperatively. This is because of traction on the dura as the brain and its protective coverings prolapse somewhat into the facial cavity. Avoidance of radical or rapid changes in head position often will minimize this distressing symptom, while mild analgesics are usually sufficient to quell the pain.

The loss of the eye, especially if little disturbance in vision has been experienced, is an exceptionally traumatic psychological prospect for most patients. Even the eye already blinded by disease is precious, and thus orbital exenteration is a highly charged emotional consideration. Nevertheless, the surgeon must not allow his judgment to be swayed into compromising a chance of cure in these circumstances. Surgical margins must be dictated by the surgeon, not the patient. On the other hand, some patients with a longstanding aggravating problem find the afflicted eye an anathema and actually request its excision (Fig. 5–36).

Compared with loss of the eye, defects in the lower part of the face are relatively less traumatic, and the functional improvement and psychological boost a patient gets from the use of an "immediate" dental obturator is remarkable. Planning the extent of palatal, alveolar ridge, and soft tissue resection in advance with the prosthodontist allows sufficient time for a functional palatal prosthesis to be made. The dentition that is to remain is carefully checked so that any restorative work necessary can be completed preoperatively. Once the resection has been done and the closure completed, the obturator is fitted into the defect. The prosthesis forms a platform on which a bolster can be placed to support the skin graft lining the cavity (Fig. 5–38).

Procedure

General anesthesia is induced and maintained through either an oral endotracheal tube or a tracheostomy tube. The tracheostomy eliminates the nuisance posed by the tube in the mouth and may contribute to a cleaner operative field. The head may be supported on a headrest such as the Mayfield. While this restricts the mobility of the head that is desirable for the head and neck surgeon during the transfacial portion of the resection, it may be required by the neurosurgeon. It is perfectly feasible to do the entire procedure using the headrest. The only drawback is that occasional adjustments to improve visualization will be needed from time to time.

A urinary catheter is placed to monitor urinary flow. Hypotensive anesthesia is used during particularly hemorrhagic parts of the operation. In addition the patient is kept relatively dehydrated in order to minimize cerebral volume. Monitoring of urine output is critical in order to continuously assess renal function and, indirectly, vascular perfusion. Finally, the catheter is needed to drain the large volumes of urine resulting from the use of osmotic diuretics to further shrink the brain.

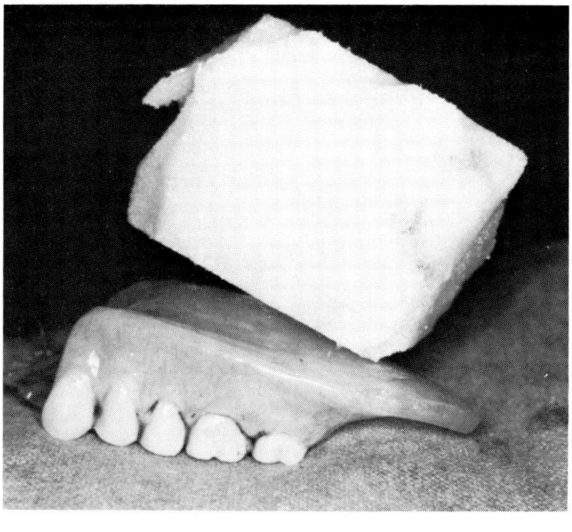

Figure 5–38. Preoperative maxillary prosthesis that restores the dental arch and can support a bolster to stent the skin grafts within the maxillectomy cavity.

Doppler monitoring of the chest is the most sensitive indicator of air embolism and is vital in these operations, since if the dural venous sinuses are violated the patient is at great risk from this complication, especially with the head tilted up. An arterial line monitors blood pressure and is essential when using hypotensive anesthesia. Cannulization of the subclavian vein monitors the central venous pressure. The tip of the central venous catheter is placed in the right atrium, to provide a ready means of extraction in case of air embolism. A lumbar drain is often used to drain cerebrospinal fluid, thus facilitating the intracranial dissection.

Before the definitive operation is done, a surgical confirmation of actual tumor resectability is undertaken. This is an essential step to avoid the tragedy of being committed to a major impairment of the patient's subsequent function by doing a massive procedure only to find at the end of the operation that the tumor is surgically unencompassable. Key areas to include in this exploration are the cavity of the sphenoid sinus, the area of the planum sphenoidale, and, if the patient finds the loss of both eyes unacceptable, the opposing orbital walls. Making this determination necessitates piecemeal removal of gross tumor, entirely violating the principle of en bloc resection. It unfortunately is the only means of determining tumor extent.

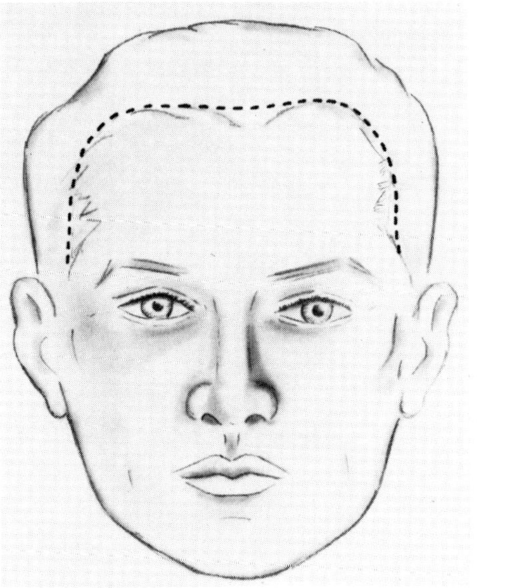

Figure 5–39. Bitemporal coronal incision commonly employed in craniofacial surgery to provide access to the anterior cranial fossa. Care is taken to avoid damage to the superficial temporal artery on the side opposite the lesion, in case the scalp flap is used in reconstruction. The pericranium is preserved as well, as it also may be employed in adding support to the cranial floor.

If there is any question about the possible inoperability of the total amount of intracranial tumor, then the craniotomy must be done first and the undersurface of the cerebrum checked to see if unresectable areas of the brain have been invaded by cancer. On the other hand, if the preoperative assessment raises a question concerning the proximity of tumor to the cranial floor, the transfacial approach is done first.

The cranial portion of the operation is usually performed first by the neurologic surgeon. A bitemporal coronal incision is made about 2 cm behind the hairline (Fig. 5–39). Care is taken to preserve the pericranium, as it will be used later in the reconstruction of the cranial floor. Rainey clips are placed for hemostasis, and the flap is turned inferiorly. Bur holes are placed with a craniotome or Gigli saw (Fig. 5–40). A skull flap is removed that is large enough to permit exposure of the anterior fossa floor back to the planum sphenoidale. Once some experience is gained with this procedure, a smaller cranial flap is sufficient for adequate resection, Ketchum et al,[29] for instance, recommend bone removal just larger than a bur hole. However, we have found such a small skull eventration too difficult to work through and impossible when there is extensive intracranial involvement. Bridger[30] uses a frontal sinusotomy approach in patients with minimal intracranial extension. He removes a portion of both the anterior and posterior frontal sinus walls, exposing a limited amount of the medial floor of the anterior fossa. The disadvantage of this approach is that, in addition to the drawback of limited exposure, the problem posed by the dead space is difficult to eliminate by flaps or grafts and was the source of a fatal brain abscess in a patient in our own series.

The dura can either be retracted after careful dissection or incised at the craniotomy site. Sisson and Becker[6] recommend an extradural approach, but the dura of the anterior pole of the frontal lobe is brittle in the elderly and prone to injury during craniotomy. In addition, the area of the cribriform plate is perforated by dural extensions surrounding the olfactory filaments and is often torn during extradural dissection. We have used both approaches, but when the CAT scan suggests intracranial invasion[6] the intradural approach makes exposure of the tumor much easier. In addition, intracerebral extension is far more easily assessed and dealt

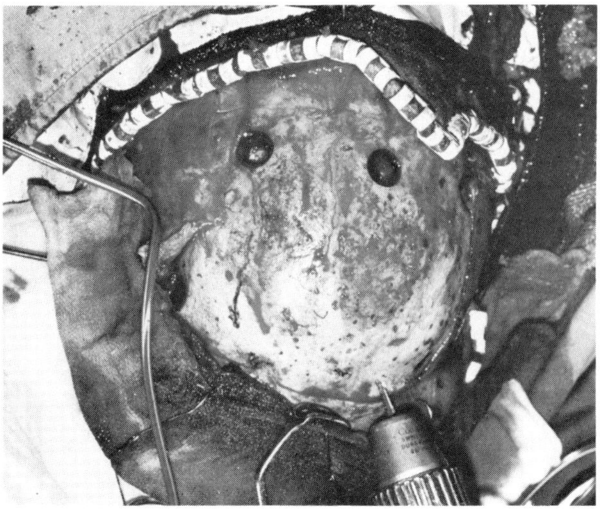

Figure 5–40. Bur holes are placed and a craniotome is used to excise a skull flap. The flap must be sufficient to allow for exposure of the anterior fossa floor all the way to the planum sphenoidale.

with when this latter exposure is used (Fig. 5–70).

The frontal lobes are gently retracted and the tumor extent determined (Fig. 5–41). Invasion of the area of the optic chiasm, the cavernous sinus, or the intracranial portion of the internal carotid artery usually indicates inoperability. However, encroachment upon the lateral aspects of the middle fossa does not carry the same restriction. If an alternative circulation can be established by creating a temporal-cerebral arterial shunt, then the middle fossa floor resection is feasible. A detailed outline of this procedure is given in Chapter 9.

A biopsy of the frontal lobe adjacent to the areas of dural penetration must be done in order to determine whether there is intracerebral invasion. A generous cuff of frontal lobe must be resected surrounding any site of such involvement. Most patients tolerate this quite well.

The area encompassing the extent of tumor into the anterior fossa is clearly exposed and outlined, and margins of uninvolved dura surrounding the neoplasm are established (Fig. 5–71). The stage is now set to proceed with the transfacial part of the operation. Hemostasis is checked, retraction released from the frontal lobe, and the Cushing's veil, if present, is reflected to cover the craniotomy wound. The headrest is adjusted and the transfacial portion may proceed.

The extent of incision on the face varies with the amount of tumor spread. An ethmoidectomy incision in continuity with a lat-

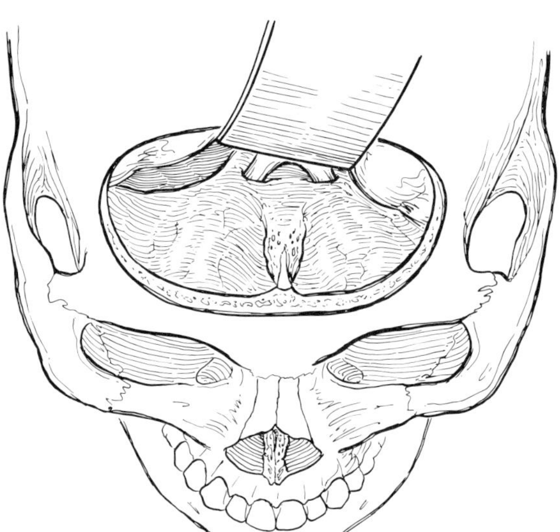

Figure 5–41. Exposure of the entire floor of the anterior cranial fossa is possible up to the lesser wing of the sphenoid by this approach.

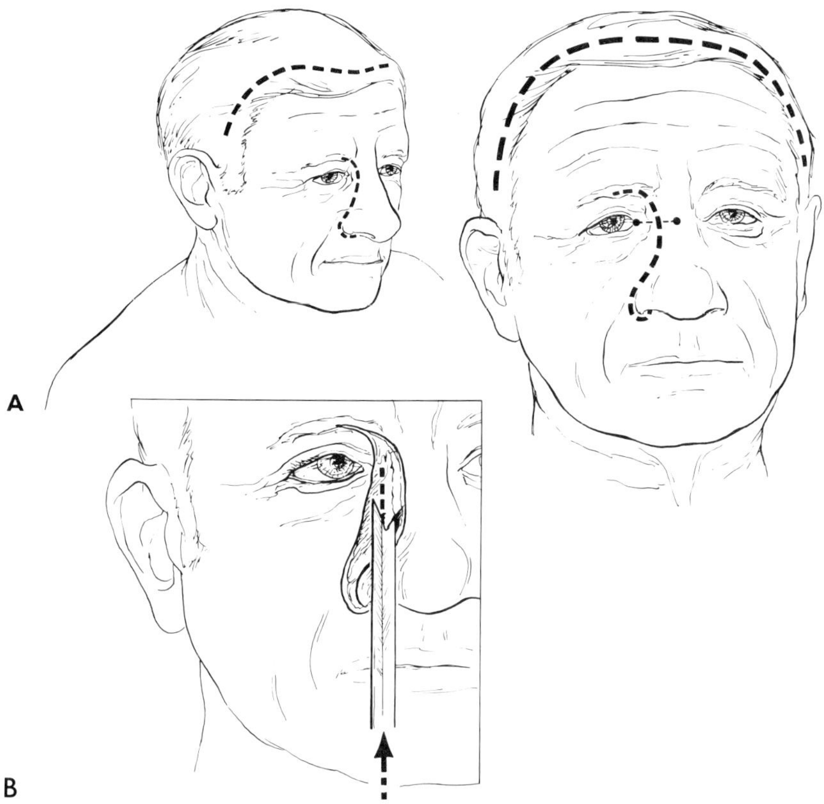

Figure 5–42. *A,* Lateral rhinotomy incision coupled with an ethmoidectomy incision provides excellent exposure for lesions limited to the ethmoid bloc, orbit, and upper maxilla. *B,* Lateral osteotomy portion of rhinotomy.

eral rhinotomy may be sufficient if the tumor is limited to the ethmoid block with no orbital and minimal maxillary invasion (Fig. 5–42*A*). The incision begins just in the inferior hairs of the medial aspect of the brow. Care is taken to angle the knife so that it parallels the hair follicles. The incision proceeds inferiorly in a gentle curve that traverses a point midway between the midline of the nose, near the nasion, and the medial canthus of the eye. The lateral rhinotomy portion of the incision extends in the natural facial cleavage line between the lateral nose and the anterior cheek skin. It courses around the nasal ala and into the vestibule of the nose. An osteotome is driven from the pyriform crest through the ascending process of the maxilla, and is then angled to the midline of the nose superiorly, as in a lateral osteotomy for rhinoplasty (Fig. 5–42*B*). With the aid of a medial osteotomy the bony nasal wall is fractured to the midline.

Excision of the lacrimal bone and lamina papyracea with biting forceps exposes the anterior ethmoidal extent of the tumor. Removal of the junction of the lateral wall of the bony nose and the face of the maxilla, similar to the Denker procedure, reveals the maxillary limits of the disease (Fig. 5–55). The exposure is enhanced by excision of as much of the maxillary face as is necessary. Piecemeal tumor removal is often required in order to visualize the superior limits of the tumor. Another factor limiting visualization is bleeding. This is usually controlled by hypotensive anesthesia and the use of an intranasal pack of 1-inch ribbon gauze soaked in 0.5 per cent lidocaine and 1/200,000 epinephrine. If possible, the nasal septum is preserved, as it will be of great value in reconstruction of the anterior fossa floor.

Once the superior margins of the tumor have been delineated, the neurosurgeon deflects the coronal flap and retracts the brain. He can then guide the head and neck surgeon who is tapping out the margins of the tumor from below. From above, the neurosurgeon protects the brain and other vital structures with a malleable Teflon-coated retractor. The two surgeons working in concert can then

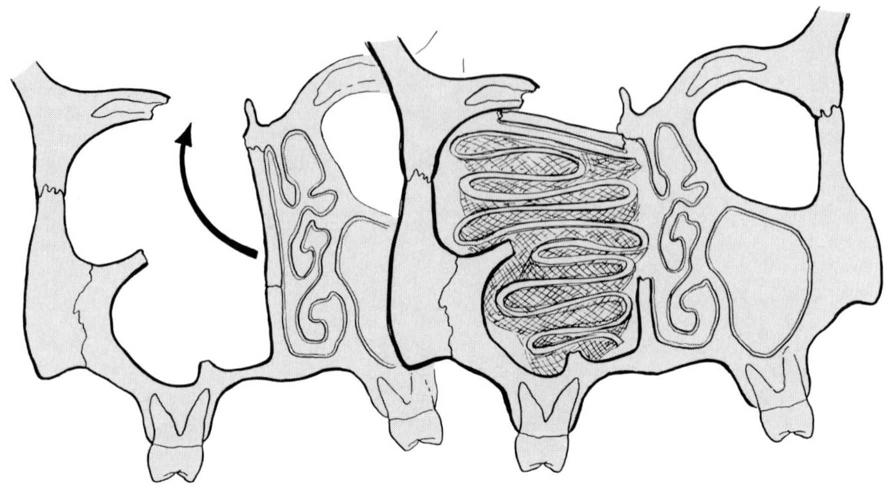

Figure 5–43. The nasal septum is denuded of mucosa on one surface and then cut from its attachments to the nasal crest and the nasal dorsum. It is greenstick-fractured at the nasal vault, and the flap is swung superiorly to reconstruct the cranial floor. The flap is held in position with packing.

clearly and safely establish the limits of resection. Once the bloc is free, it is delivered through the facial wound.

Reconstruction entails the establishment of a watertight dural seal. Careful suturing of dural rents followed by reinforcement with fascial grafts produces the best results. Temporalis fascia is preferred to fascia lata and is readily available through the coronal incision. Support for the cranial floor is best provided by a nasal septal chondralosseous-mucosal flap. The mucosa is denuded from the tumor side of the septum, and the septal flap is detached from the surrounding attachments and fractured across the nasal vault. A greenstick fracture will allow hinging of the flap on a mucoperiosteal pedicle. The flap is swung superiorly and packed into position (Fig. 5–43). A ventricular drain is placed, or the lumbar drain maintained, to control intracerebral pressure. The drain can usually be removed by the third postoperative day.

Postoperative antibiotics are a controversial subject in any area of surgery. We have elected to give a short course of a broad-spectrum antibiotic on the day prior to surgery, intraoperatively, and 3 to 5 days postoperatively. Postoperative infection has not been a problem. We have had only one case of infection, a brain abscess occurring 3 months postoperatively.

Craniofacial Resection with Maxillectomy

Most patients requiring craniofacial surgery for paranasal sinus cancer have extensive neoplasms. Orbital exenteration and maxillectomy as well as ethmoidectomy are usually necessary. The face of the sphenoid is commonly removed, and the frontal sinus may require exenteration.

The cranial portion of the operation remains the same as previously described; however, extension of tumor through the orbital roof and the frontal sinus should be anticipated. Marked restriction of ocular motility and visual impairment are danger signs indicating orbital apex involvement. Tumor extending this far requires resection of portions of the lesser wing of the sphenoid bone and a part of the middle fossa floor. The cavernous sinus and the intercavernous and intrapetrous portions of the internal carotid artery present special problems. The CAT scan is invaluable in the preoperative evaluation of this potential problem. Often the degree of tumor involvement is more extensive in these cases, with tumor extending across the nasal septum and involving both cribriform plates.

The maxillectomy is done through the standard Weber-Fergusson incision (Fig. 5–44). A triangular dart in the lip helps to prevent notching of the vermillion border later on. If there is skin involvement, a generous cutaneous margin of 3 to 4 cm is taken to ensure complete tumor encompassment (Fig. 5–45). If any doubt at all exists concerning tumor fixation to skin, the area must be resected (Fig. 5–46), since the dissemination of cutaneous tumor via skin lymphatics occurs with astounding rapidity, with subcutaneous tumor spreading wide of the primary.

The maxillectomy is performed in the usual way, but care is taken to note if the posterior

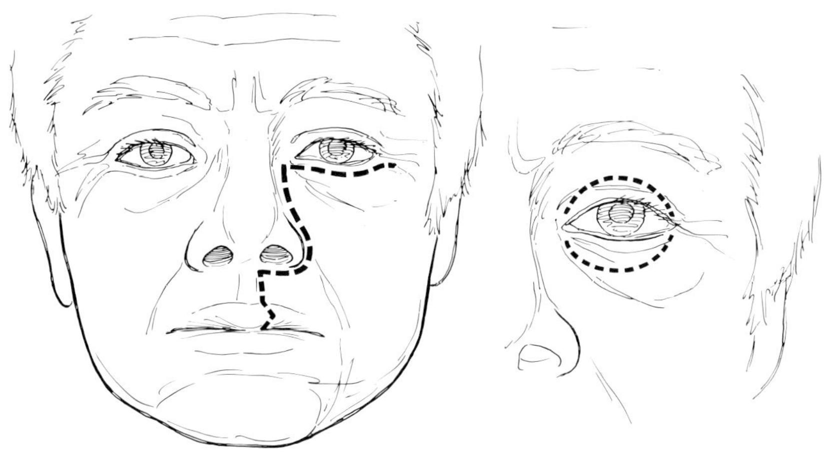

Figure 5–44. Weber-Fergusson incision with the labial incision deflected along the philtral crest and a dart placed in the lip in order to avoid a whistle deformity once healing has occurred.

wall has been transgressed by tumor. Encroachment of the pterygomaxillary space usually means a poor prognosis. Complete resection of the pterygoid muscles is then necessary, and clival resection must be seriously considered (see Chapter 9).

The amount of alveolar ridge and nasal floor to be resected is determined by the extent of tumor. Extension of disease across the septum and into the opposing sinus requires a wide maxillary excision, but unfortunately this severely compromises prosthetic rehabilitation (Fig. 5–47). (See Chapter 14.) An attempt is made to save as much alveolar ridge and as many teeth as is feasible within the limits of adequate cancer resection. Bearing in mind the same constraints, as much soft palate as possible is preserved. This helps enormously in the rehabilitation of speech and swallowing.

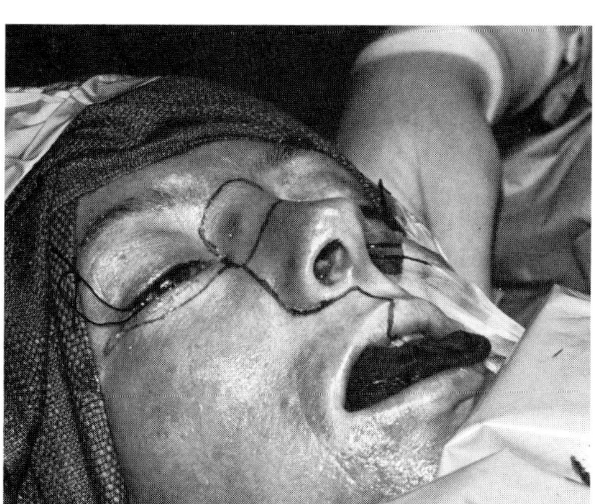

Figure 5–45. Because of skin involvement, a wide cutaneous margin was necessary in this case.

The ethmoid bloc is resected as already described. Lesions in the posterior region of the maxilla and ethmoid labyrinth present a special problem because the optic chiasm lies adjacent to the planum sphenoidale. Gentle retraction by the neurosurgeon exposes the region, and careful removal of affected bone can be done without disturbing the optic nerves. The roof and even the lateral wall of this side of the orbit may require removal.

Reconstruction of the area involves use of both flaps and free grafts. Covering the resected area with a skin flap provides excellent cutaneous surfacing, good support for the intracranial contents, and also partially obliterates the cavity. The single deterring factor to using a flap is the masking of any local recurrence, which then does not become obvious until it has reached a large and most often unresectable size. Konno et al,[31] however, argue that primary reconstruction with a deltopectoral flap produces the best cosmetic and functional result and that the covering of possible recurrences is justified by the poor prognosis of patients who develop locally recurrent cancer. Although cure is indeed difficult in this group, it is possible. Moreover, early small local recurrences of disease can be controlled for a considerable time with locally destructive methods such as cautery, cryotherapy, and laser.

Some form of cranial support is essential. The septal flap used in the more limited ethmoid resection is usually not available in this more extensive operation. A pericranial flap created at the time of craniotomy provides bulk, resilience, excellent blood supply, and close proximity for this portion of the reconstruction (Fig. 5–48). The dura is sutured and patched with temporalis fascia and

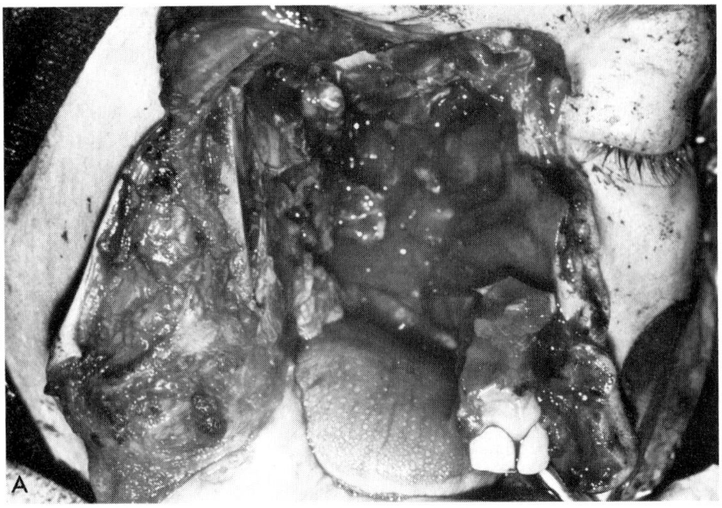

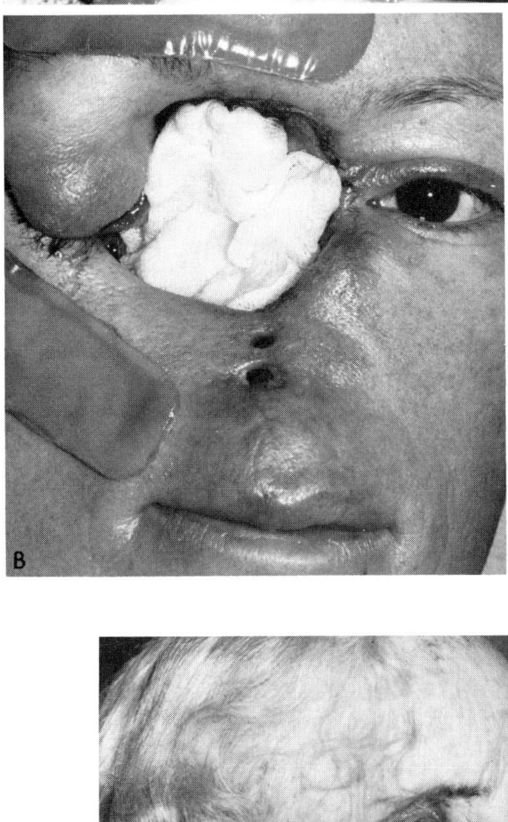

Figure 5–46. Although skin involvement was suspected, there was no fixation to tumor. Biopsy of the overlying skin showed tumor invasion, and a generous excision was required. *A,* Operative appearance of tumor from the maxilla and ethmoid bloc invading the nasal cavity and the overlying skin. *B,* Postoperative appearance. A wide resection was required to obtain a tumor-free margin.

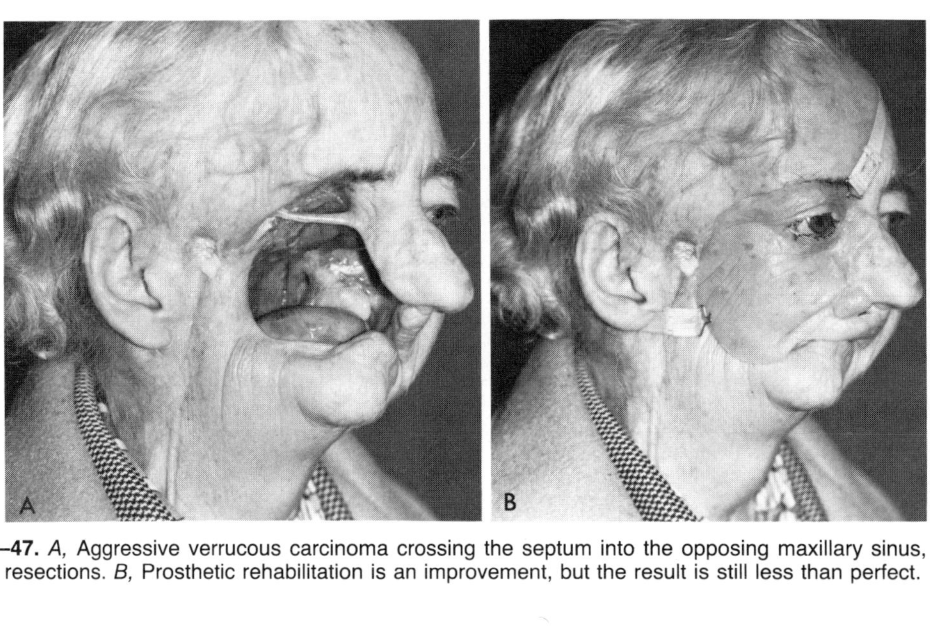

Figure 5–47. *A,* Aggressive verrucous carcinoma crossing the septum into the opposing maxillary sinus, requiring repeated resections. *B,* Prosthetic rehabilitation is an improvement, but the result is still less than perfect.

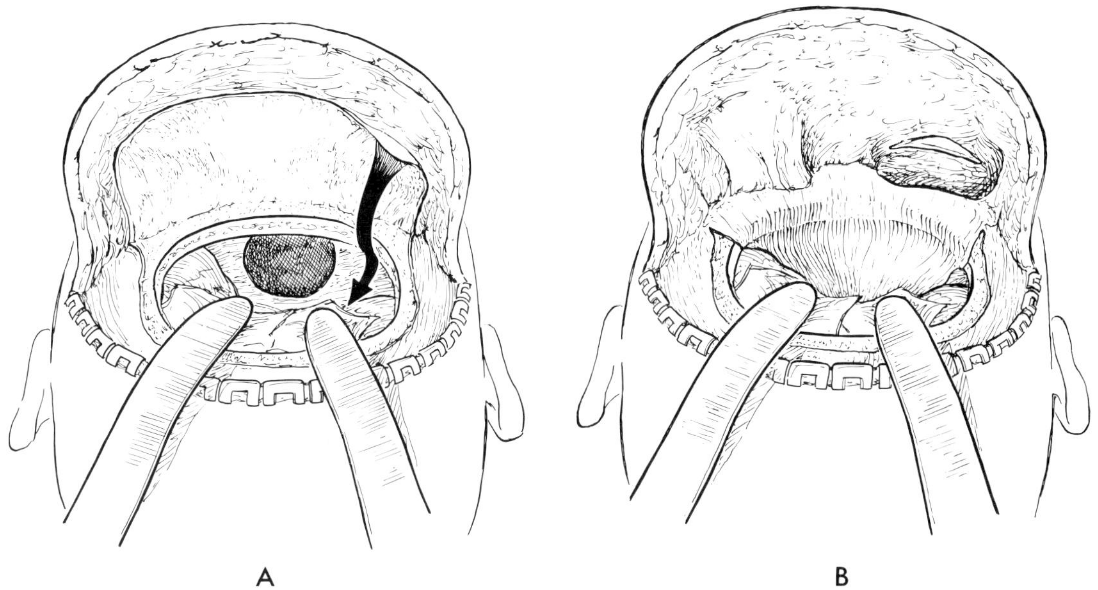

Figure 5–48. *A,* Pericranial flap is elevated at the time the scalp incision is made. *B,* Flap is brought through the craniotomy defect, folded, and tucked to lie along the defect in the floor of the anterior cranial fossa.

the pericranial flap turned into position. A split-thickness skin graft is placed against the pericranial flap; Bridger[30] suggests using a forehead flap brought through an incision just above the brow (Fig. 5–49). The remaining cavity is lined with a split-thickness skin graft. A graft of good quality is necessary against the raw cheek. Failure to resurface this area results in severe retraction of the cheek flap. The skin is held in place by a sponge bolster and packing which in turn is held in place by a prosthetic obturator.

The packing material is removed 7 to 10 days postoperatively. Careful cleansing of the cavity and frequent observations are made until the cavity is re-epithelialized.

Frontal Sinus Carcinoma

Frontal sinus carcinoma is most often mistaken for a mucocele. Because bone erosion occurs in both entities, this finding cannot serve as the important differential feature that is so relevant with lesions in the other paranasal sinuses. Robinson[32] reports that in a 4-year period, 3 of 12 patients presenting with a frontal sinus mucopyocele had an underlying carcinoma. Chronic infection commonly produces frontal sinus opacification and bony sclerosis. Unfortunately, findings of sclerosis have also been cited by a number of authors[32–34] in cases of cancer, thus eliminating another important differentiating sign.

An excellent article by Brownson and Ogura[35] reviewing 102 cases in the literature revealed pain and swelling to be the most common of the presenting symptoms of frontal sinus carcinoma. Radiographic evidence of bone erosion on plane films was seen in 48 per cent of patients. Most demonstrated anterior wall involvement, with only 17 per cent showing posterior wall erosion. However, on exploration 75 per cent of the patients in the entire group were found to have erosion of the back wall. Intracranial extension was found in 19 per cent.

Although metastases were found in only 12 per cent of cases, survival rates were miserable. This is probably due to the lack of experience of any one individual with this lesion. Because of the frequency of posterior wall penetration, a combined craniofacial excision should be employed. Both walls of the sinus, the dura, the adjacent superior saggital sinus, and the frontal lobe, if necessary, should be removed. Removal of the adjacent ethmoid sinuses and orbital contents depends on the degree of involvement. If tumor has extended into the overlying skin, wide excision followed by coverage with a scalp flap must be done.

Reconstruction of the bony defect should

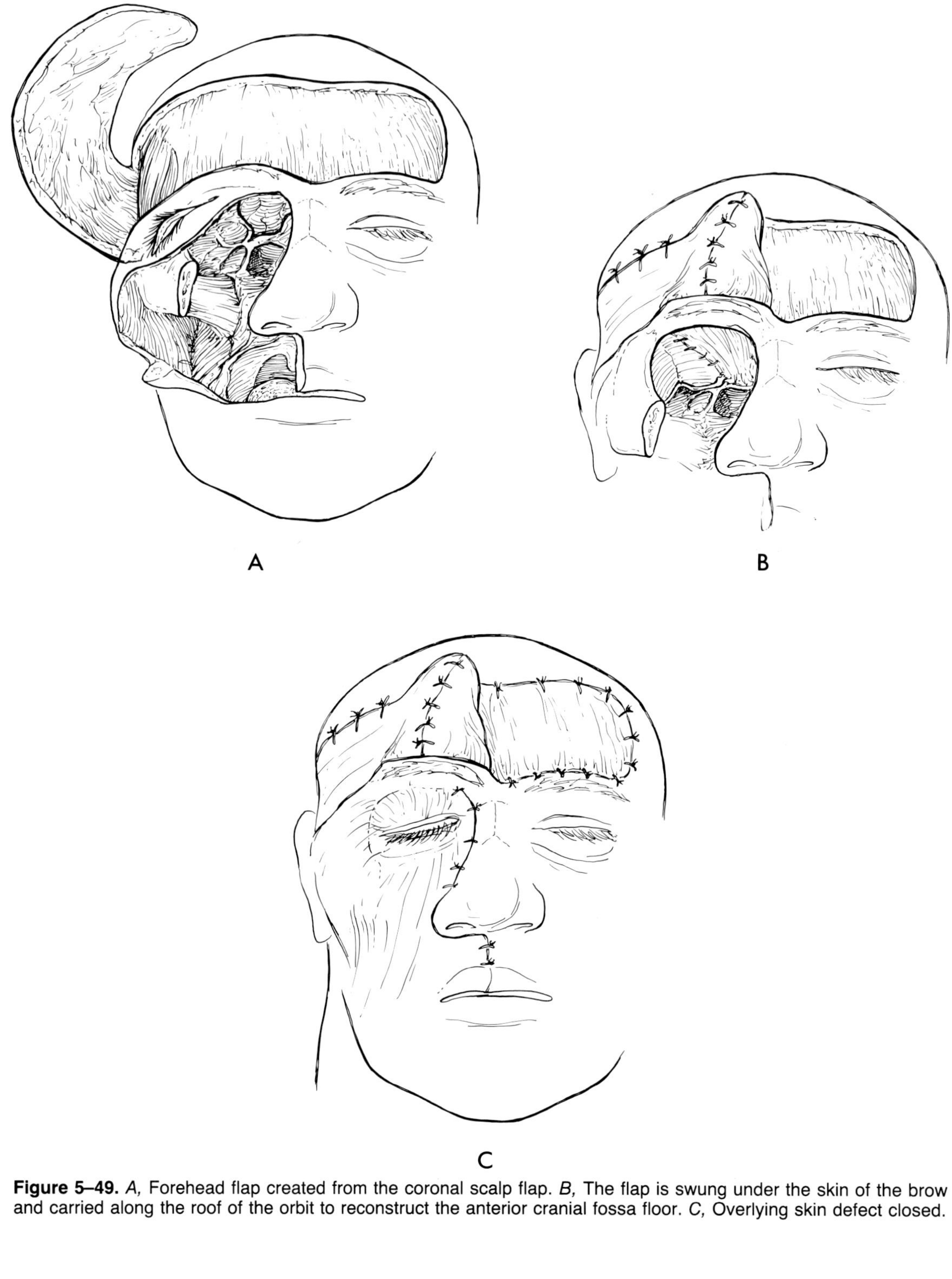

Figure 5–49. *A,* Forehead flap created from the coronal scalp flap. *B,* The flap is swung under the skin of the brow and carried along the roof of the orbit to reconstruct the anterior cranial fossa floor. *C,* Overlying skin defect closed.

be delayed 1 to 2 years to permit early discovery of local recurrences should they develop.

Sphenoid Sinus Carcinoma

Sphenoid sinus carcinoma is fortunately exceedingly rare. One of the largest published series contains only 7 patients.[36] Deep-seated head pain and ocular palsies are the most common presenting symptoms. The abducens nerve is most frequently affected, because of its proximity to the lateral sphenoid sinus wall during its traverse through the cavernous sinus. The frequency of sixth nerve palsy in these patients illustrates the problem of extension of tumor beyond the confines of the sinus prior to diagnosis, rendering the tumor in most cases inoperable and incurable.

Most tumors residing in the sphenoid are extensions from either the ethmoid labyrinth or the nasopharynx. Care must be taken in these instances not to assign an inoperable status to these patients prior to exploration. Obturation of the sphenoid sinus ostium will cause mucus accumulation and opacify the sinus on CAT scan. Without clear evidence of bone erosion and cavernous sinus extension on the scan, exploration and delineation of tumor extent must be done.

The floor of the sinus and sphenoid rostrum are the areas least frequently involved with tumor. Cancers commonly penetrate the sella turcica or extend through the lateral walls and roof of the sinus. Occasionally they protrude through the sinus ostium and present in the nose or nasopharynx.

Treatment of these malignancies has traditionally been radiation therapy. This region is remarkable in that it can withstand the rigors of more than one full course of irradiation. Only rarely is a patient cured; in sphenoid sinus carcinoma radiotherapy is usually only palliative, with the patient succumbing to the disease 6 to 24 months later. Recent advances in craniofacial surgery may make some of these patients amenable to resection. Rerouting of the cerebral circulation by a superficial temporal to middle cerebral bypass anastomosis will permit sacrifice of the internal carotid artery. This facilitates a potential clivectomy, cavernous sinus resection, and sphenoidectomy (see Chapter 9). Risk to vision in both eyes is extremely high.

CASE REPORTS

CASE I. A 61-year-old man who had worked for 20 years as a hardwood sander was initially seen with a 6-month history of right-sided nasal obstruction and blood streaking of the nasal mucus. Examination revealed no disturbance of vision or ocular motility. In the nasal cavity, a small polypoid mass was apparent in the middle meatus and on the middle turbinate (Fig. 5–50). A biopsy revealed an adenocarcinoma.

Because of the proximity of the tumor to the fovea and cribriform plate (Fig. 5–51), a craniofacial resection was designed. The facial approach was through a lateral rhinotomy. The lesion did not erode the lamina papyracea, permitting preservation of the globe (Fig. 5–52). Minimal brain retraction was necessary. To expose the fovea ethmoidalis and cribriform plate with the brain thus protected, bony incisions were made with an osteotome through the facial incision. The specimen was then delivered through the face by pushing from above. The anterior fossa floor was reconstructed with a septal flap (Fig. 5–43). The patient is alive and well without recurrence 6 years following resection (Fig. 5–53).

CASE II. A 44-year-old Chinese male was seen 9 months following a full course of irradiation for a lymphoepithelioma of the nasopharynx. His complaint of left-sided nasal obstruction and epistaxis promoted a nasal examination that revealed a large exophytic mass emanating from the nasal vault, obstructing the entire left nasal chamber. A biopsy revealed a poorly differentiated squamous cell carcinoma. No interference with ocular motil-

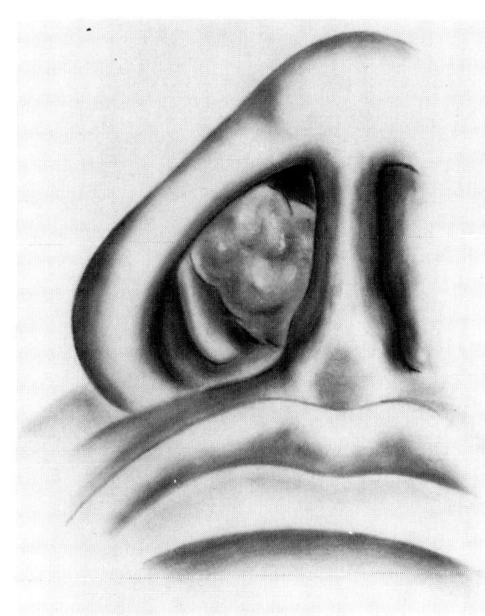

Figure 5–50. (Case I) Drawing of intranasal tumor at time of presentation.

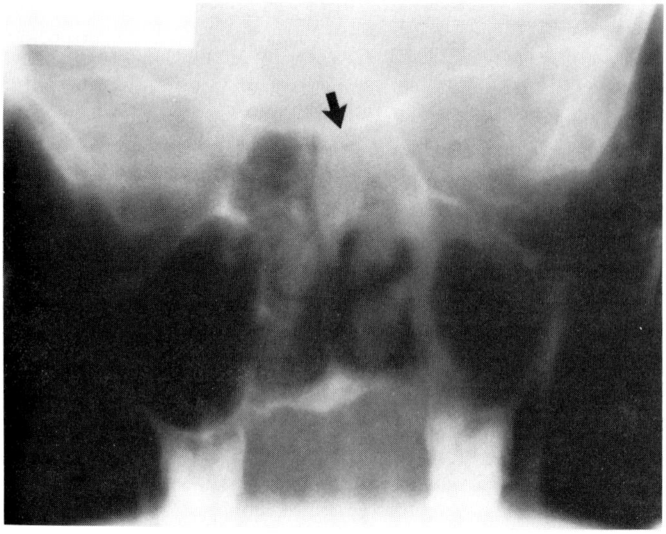

Figure 5–51. (Case I) Coronal tomograph showing proximity of tumor to the anterior cranial fossa floor.

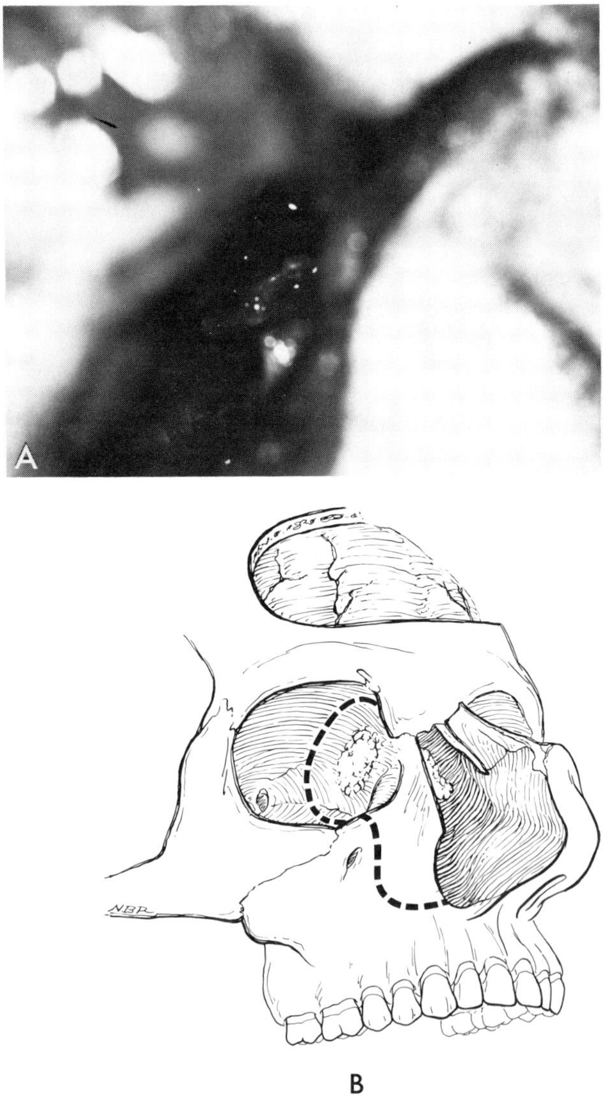

B

Figure 5–52. (Case I) *A,* Lateral rhinotomy showing a small tumor of the anterior ethmoid sinus that did not invade the lamina papyracea. The globe could be spared. *B,* Tumor in situ and resection outlined.

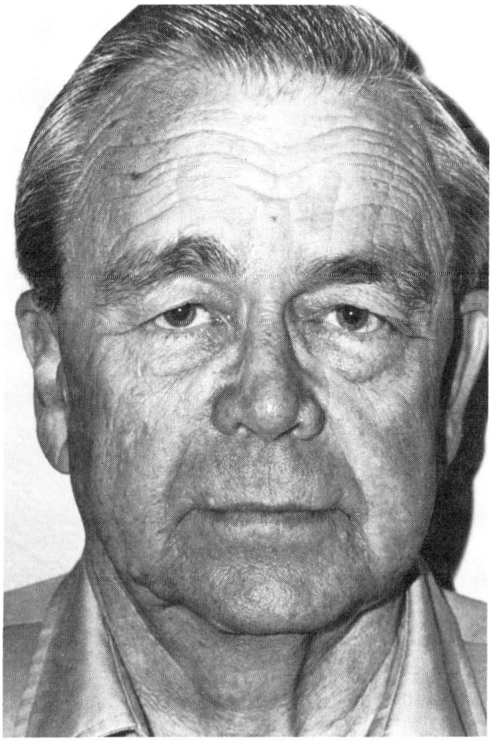

Figure 5–53. (Case I) Patient 6 years following craniofacial resection for adenocarcinoma of ethmoid sinus.

ity was seen, but a mild degree of proptosis was present. Complete stripping of the nasopharyngeal mucosa on two separate occasions revealed no evidence of recurrent cancer at this site. Tomography showed a moderate-size mass invading the left orbit and encroaching on the ethmoidal fovea (Fig. 5–54). A craniofacial procedure was then designed.

The maxilla and ethmoid bloc were exposed through a Weber-Fergusson incision. A lateral rhinotomy and Denker procedure on the maxilla revealed the extent of the tumor (Fig. 5–55). The lesion extended into the upper maxilla from the anterior ethmoids (Fig. 5–56). Once the extent of the tumor was determined and it could be established that the alveolar arch and palate could be preserved, attention was turned to the cranial part of the procedure.

A coronal flap was turned and a bifrontal craniotomy performed (Fig. 5–57). Because of the patient's youth, the dura was supple and an extradural approach was used. Retraction of the frontal lobes revealed no evidence of tumor on the dura. With ribbon retractors protecting the frontal lobes, the floor of the anterior cranial fossa in the region of the tumor was outlined through the facial wound with a 4-mm osteotome (Fig. 5–58). The left fovea and orbital roof as well as both cribriform plates were included (Fig. 5–59). The neurosurgeon by pushing inferiorly, from above, on the incised anterior fossa floor delivered the tumor through. In this way, the neoplasm could be completely excised en bloc, leaving no doubt regarding the integrity of the bony margins while at the same time protecting the dura and brain from injury.

The areas where small cerebrospinal fluid leaks occurred from cutting across the dural encasements of the fila olfactoria were oversewn. A flap of pericranium from the frontal skull was turned into the defect in the anterior cranial fossa floor to support the frontal lobes (Fig. 5–60). This was in turn reconstructed with a forehead flap developed from the original coronal skin flap (Fig. 5–61). The distal end of the flap was tunneled under the brow of the exenterated orbit. The flap must be placed as close to the orbital apex as possible while at the same time ensuring that it covers any bur holes at the superior aspect of the craniotomy (Fig. 5–62).

One esthetic drawback to this flap is the hirsutism that results from the preservation of any

Text continued on page 188

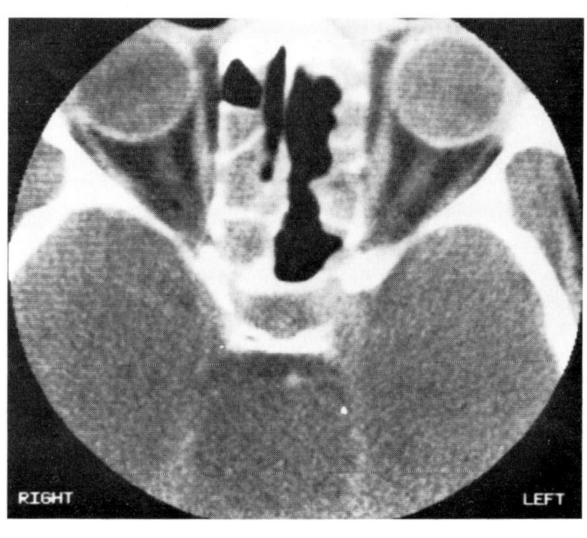

Figure 5–54. (Case II) CAT scan demonstrating a carcinoma of the left ethmoid sinus eroding into the orbit and encroaching on the fovea ethmoidalis.

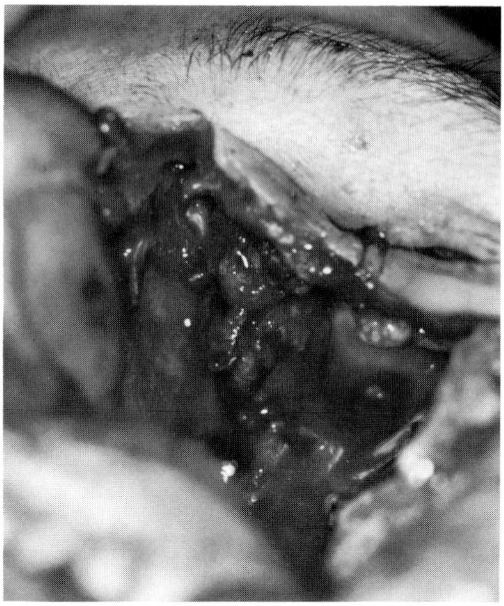

Figure 5–55. (Case II) Lateral rhinotomy and Denker procedure that excises the junction of the anterior and medial wall of the maxilla as well as much of the anterior wall. This exposure provides an excellent view of tumor extent.

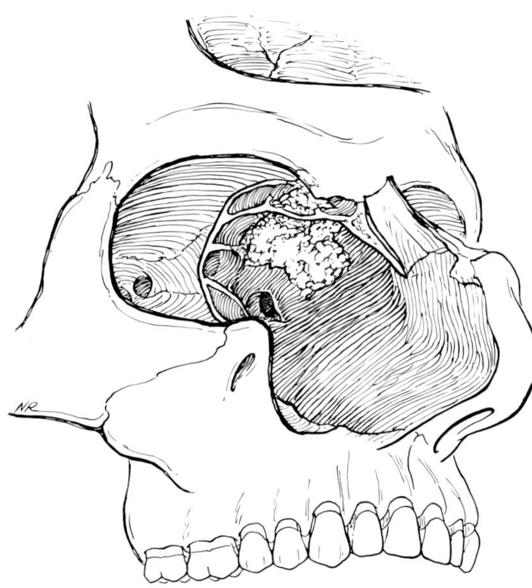

Figure 5–56. (Case II) Tumor involving the ethmoid sinuses and the upper maxilla, allowing a sparing of the alveolar ridge and hard palate. Surgical approach used is similar to that for Figure 5–52*B*.

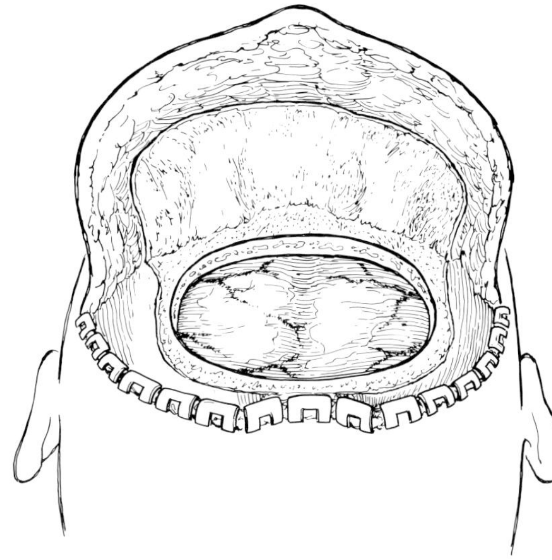

Figure 5–57. (Case II) Coronal scalp flap dissected inferiorly and bifrontal craniotomy done.

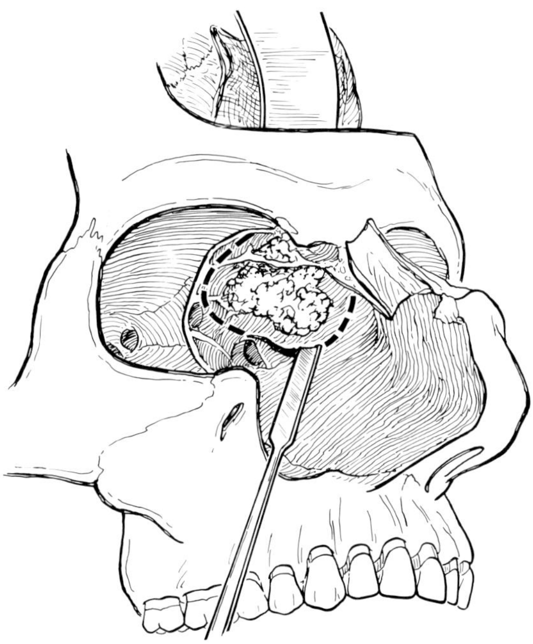

Figure 5–58. (Case II) Cranial encroachment of tumor outlined from below with a 4-mm osteotome while the frontal lobes are protected from above with malleable retractors.

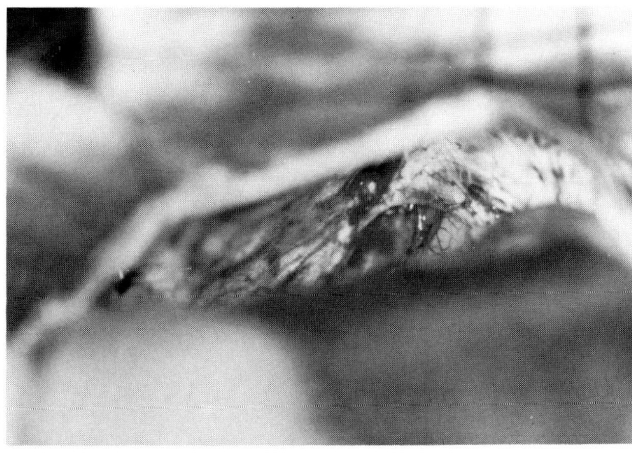

Figure 5–59. (Case II) Defect in anterior fossa floor remaining after tumor excision.

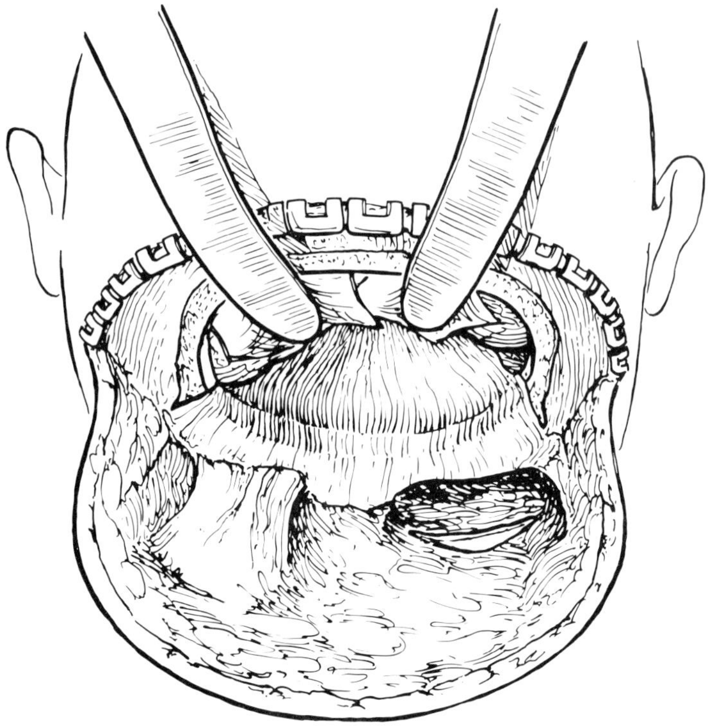

Figure 5–60. (Case II) Pericranial flap turned to reconstruct anterior fossa floor.

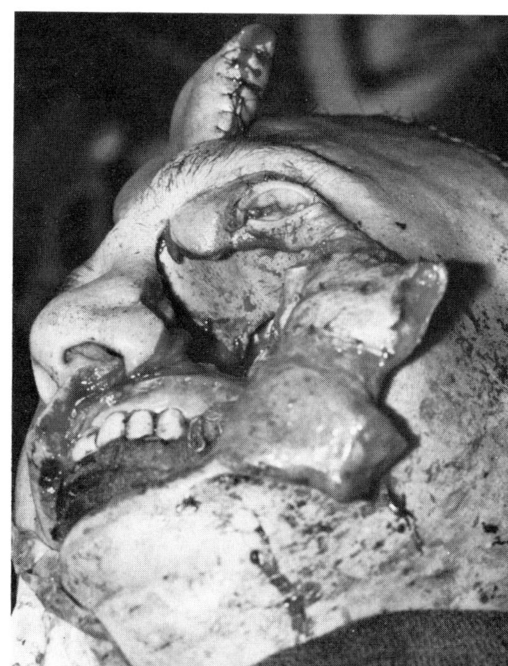

Figure 5–61. (Case II) Forehead flap developed from coronal scalp flap is used to complete reconstruction of the anterior fossa floor and line the superior aspect of the orbit and ethmoid cavity.

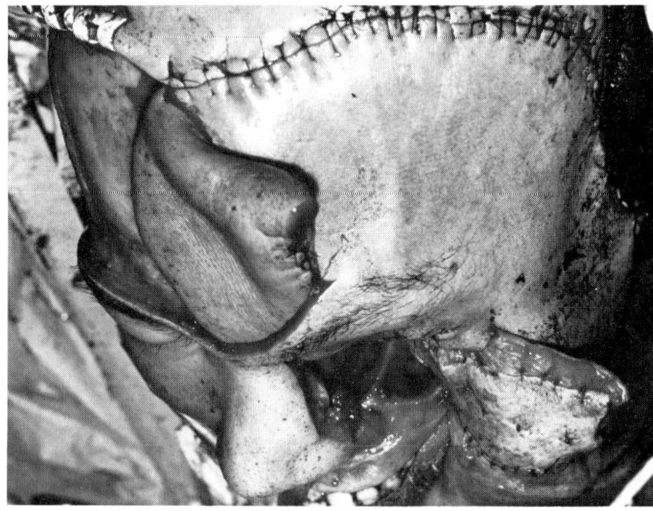

Figure 5–62. (Case II) The bur holes must be covered by the flap's pedicle. A large dog ear results that will be eliminated when the flap pedicle is incised and returned to the forehead.

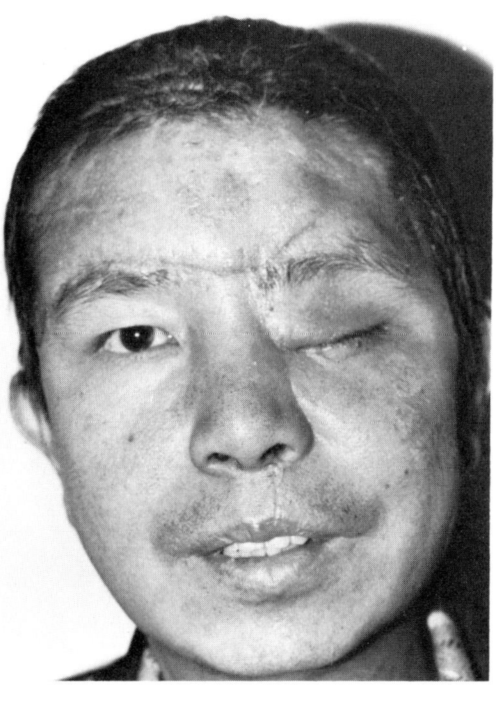

Figure 5–63. (Case II) Flap pedicle is returned to the forehead. Patient is symptom-free and has a healed cavity and acceptable cosmetic appearance.

residual hair-bearing skin at its tip. If the flap is long enough, the tip should be amputated. The large dog ear resulting from turning the flap under the brow should not be surgically attacked in any way. Once the flap is well seated and established (usually 3 to 4 weeks postoperatively) the pedicle is restored to the forehead, giving good functional support and protection to the anterior fossa floor and an acceptable cosmetic result (Fig. 5–63).

CASE III. This patient was a 48-year-old smoker, but only an occasional alcohol user, who had 7 months previously presented to his local otolaryngologist with a 3-month history of right frontal and orbital pain. Diminished vision and lateral displacement of the right globe immediately preceded this first visit. Intranasal examination revealed a mass that radiographically showed its origin in the right ethmoid sinus. A biopsy produced a diagnosis of squamous cell carcinoma. A full course of radiotherapy resulted in only a transient improvement in symptoms. Foul rhinorrhea was continuous from the time of irradiation, and 10 days prior to the patient's first visit to our Head and Neck service, his proptosis and orbital pain returned. His eye had diminished vision and motility, was proptotic, and was laterally displaced (Fig. 5–64). The right nasal chamber was filled with a necrotic mass. CAT scan and coronal tomography of the paranasal sinuses revealed an extensive tumor infiltrating the orbit and breaching the anterior fossa floor (Fig. 5–65). The tumor did not extend into the orbital apex or the sphenoid sinus. In view of the patient's age, lack of orbital apex or sphenoidal involvement, and the fact that there was no evidence of metastatic disease, a craniofacial resection was elected.

A Weber-Fergusson incision (Fig. 5–66), lateral rhinotomy, and Denker procedure revealed extensive tumor in the ethmoid and maxillary sinuses (Fig. 5–67). Once it was established that there was no tumor in the sphenoid sinus, clivus, or optic chiasm, a maxilloethmoidectomy and orbital exenteration were done (Fig. 5–68). Extensive tumor erosion of the anterior fossa floor was seen once the tumor had been debulked (Fig. 5–69). Execution of the craniotomy now proceeded. Through a bifrontal craniotomy performed via a coronal scalp incision, the dura was entered and the floor of the anterior fossa exposed. Tumor was seen protruding through dura (Fig. 5–70), and a biopsy of adjacent frontal lobe demonstrated cerebral extension. The involved brain was excised until a tumor-free margin was obtained. From below, careful excision of the anterior fossa floor proceeded using the 2- and 3-mm osteotomes, keeping the bony excision clear of visible tumor by 2 cm. Gentle retraction of brain with Teflon-coated malleable retractors provided the necessary margin of safety required to procure a clear bony resection without risking cerebral damage. Special care was exercised at the orbital apex as the optic chiasm was approached. The orbital roof on the right was almost completely removed. Both cribriform plates, most of the nasal septum, and the entire ethmoid bloc of the opposite side, including the fovea, were removed (Fig. 5–71). The specimen was delivered through the face from above (Fig. 5–72).

The dura was reconstructed with temporalis fascia and reinforced with pericranium. The cavity was lined with split-thickness skin. Despite negative margins on frozen section, within 3 months the lesion recurred locally and the patient died.

Text continued on page 194

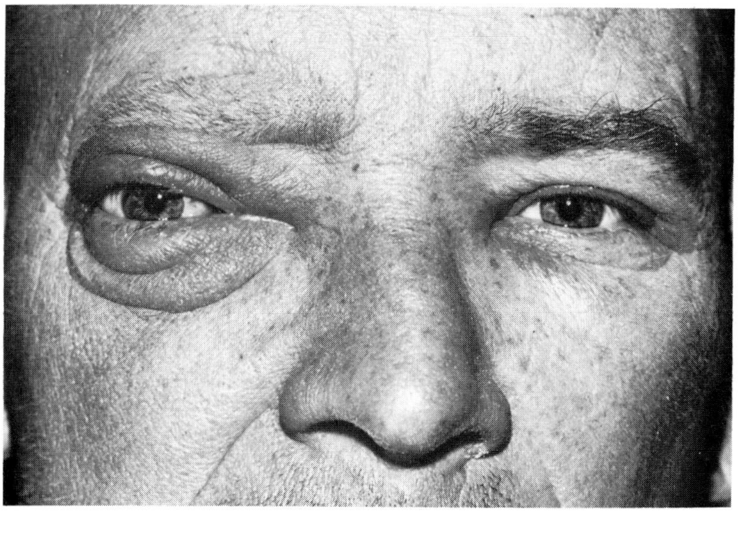

Figure 5–64. (Case III) Patient with persistent ethmoid cancer following conservative excision and irradiation therapy.

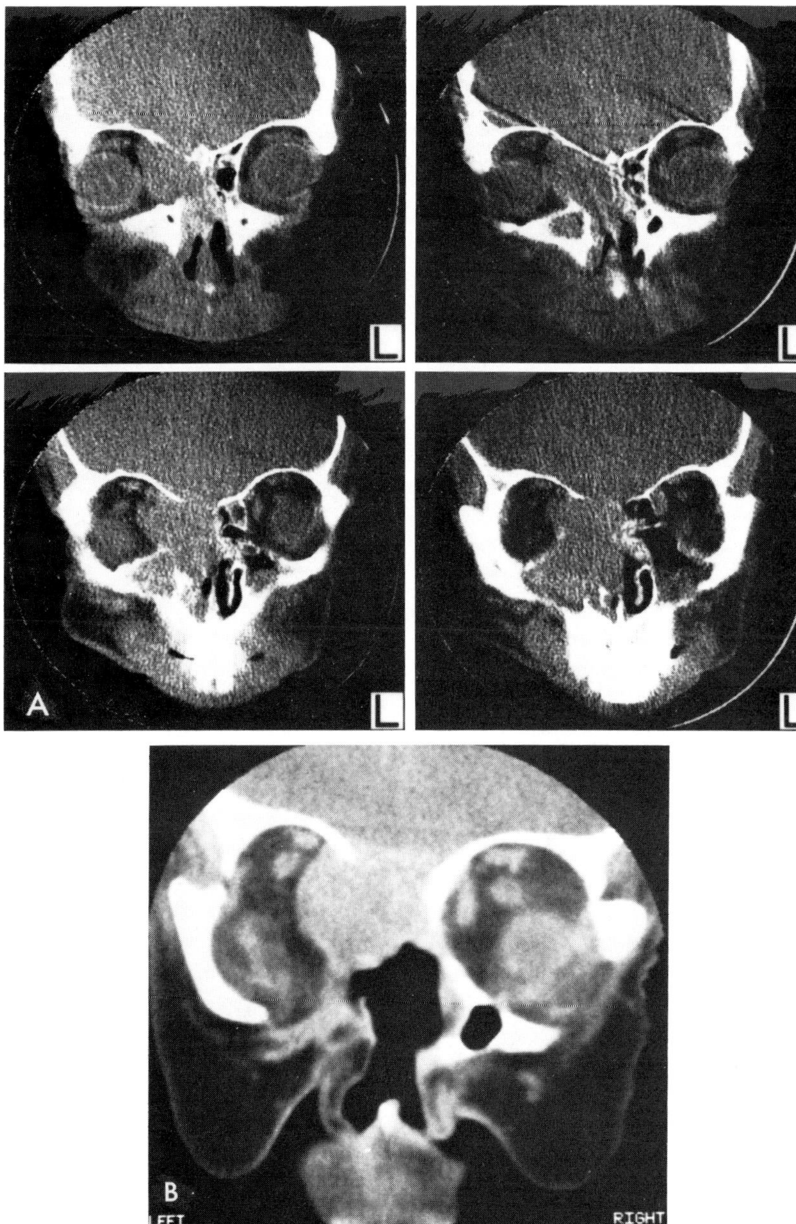

Figure 5–65. (Case III) *A,* CAT scan taken prior to radiotherapy, showing ethmoid tumor eroding the floor of the anterior fossa and invading the orbit. *B,* CAT scan taken prior to surgery, showing anterior cranial fossa invasion.

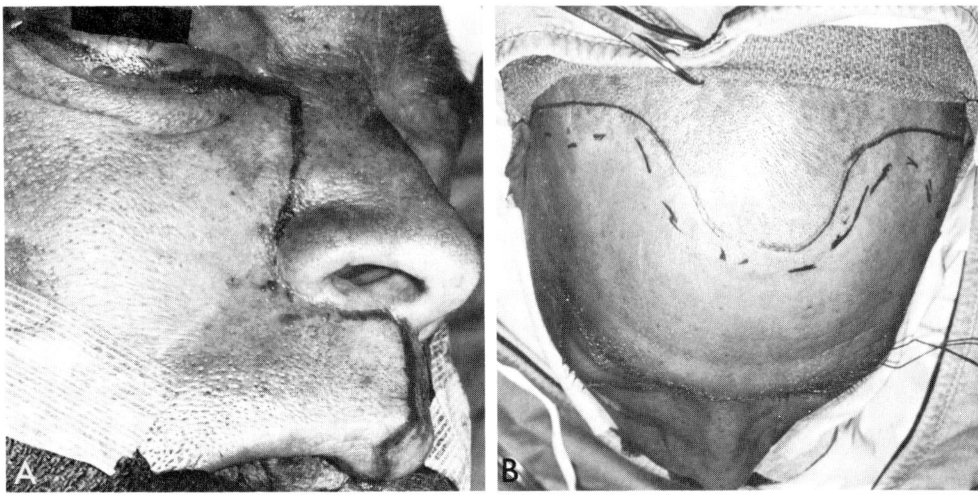

Figure 5–66. (Case III) *A,* Weber-Fergusson incision outlined. *B,* Coronal scalp incision outlined.

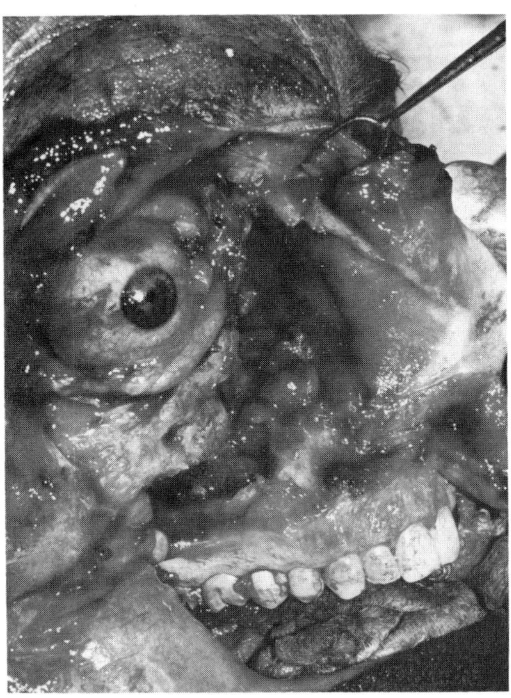

Figure 5–67. (Case III) Lateral rhinotomy and Denker procedure revealed extent of tumor.

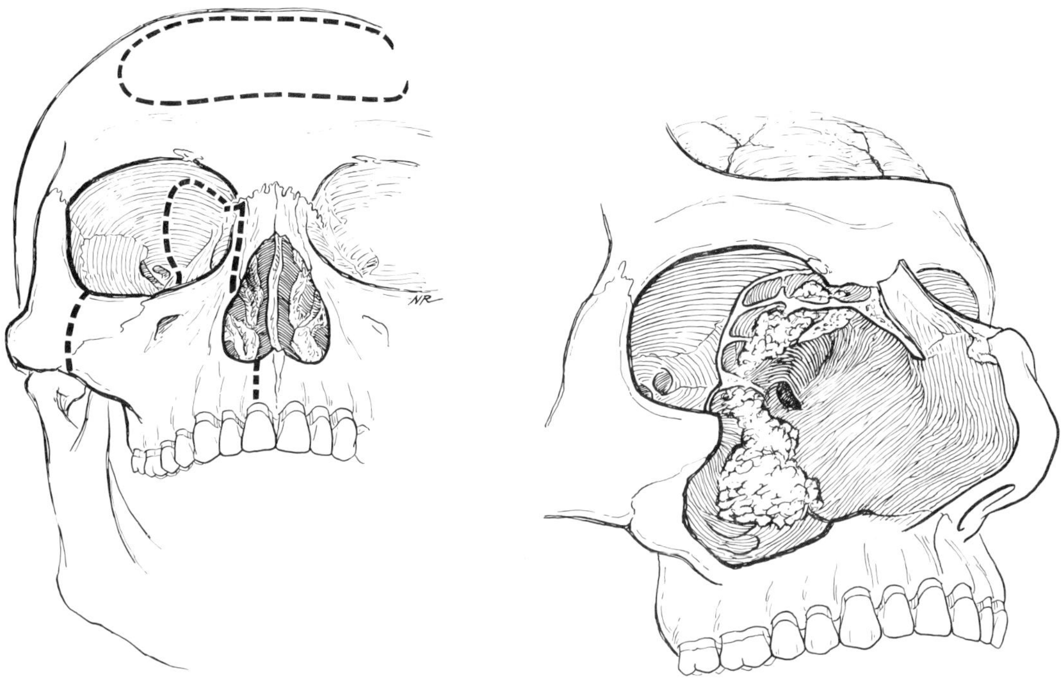

A B

Figure 5–68. (Case III) Orbital exenteration and maxillectomy done. *A*, Bony incisions. *B*, Removal complete.

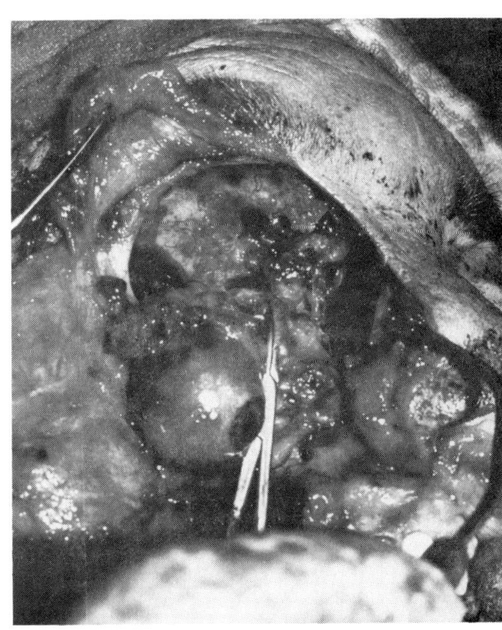

Figure 5–69. (Case III) Extensive tumor erosion through the anterior cranial fossa floor as seen from the orbital aspect.

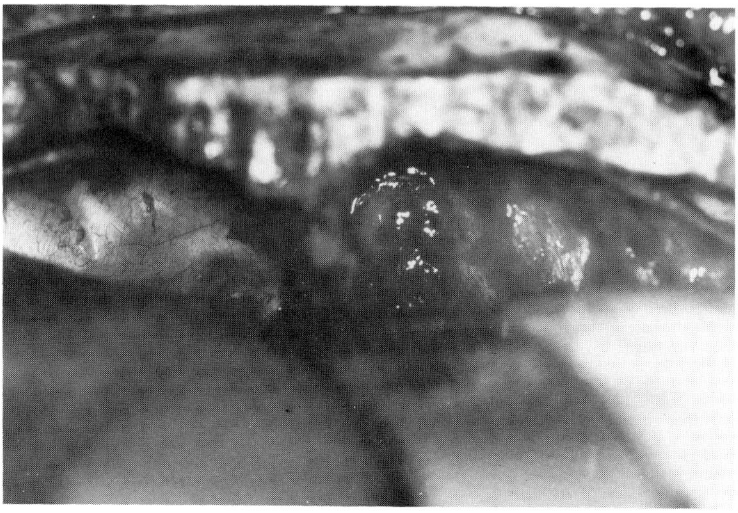

Figure 5–70. (Case III) Intracranial extent of tumor visualized through bifrontal craniotomy.

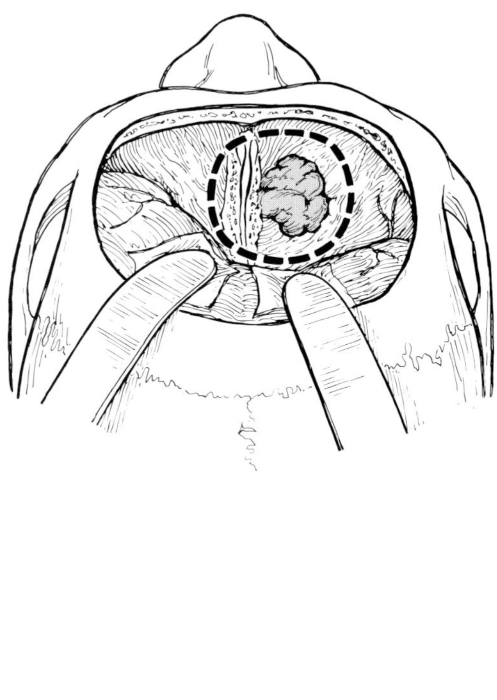

Figure 5–71. (Case III) Intracranial extent of tumor outlined from above.

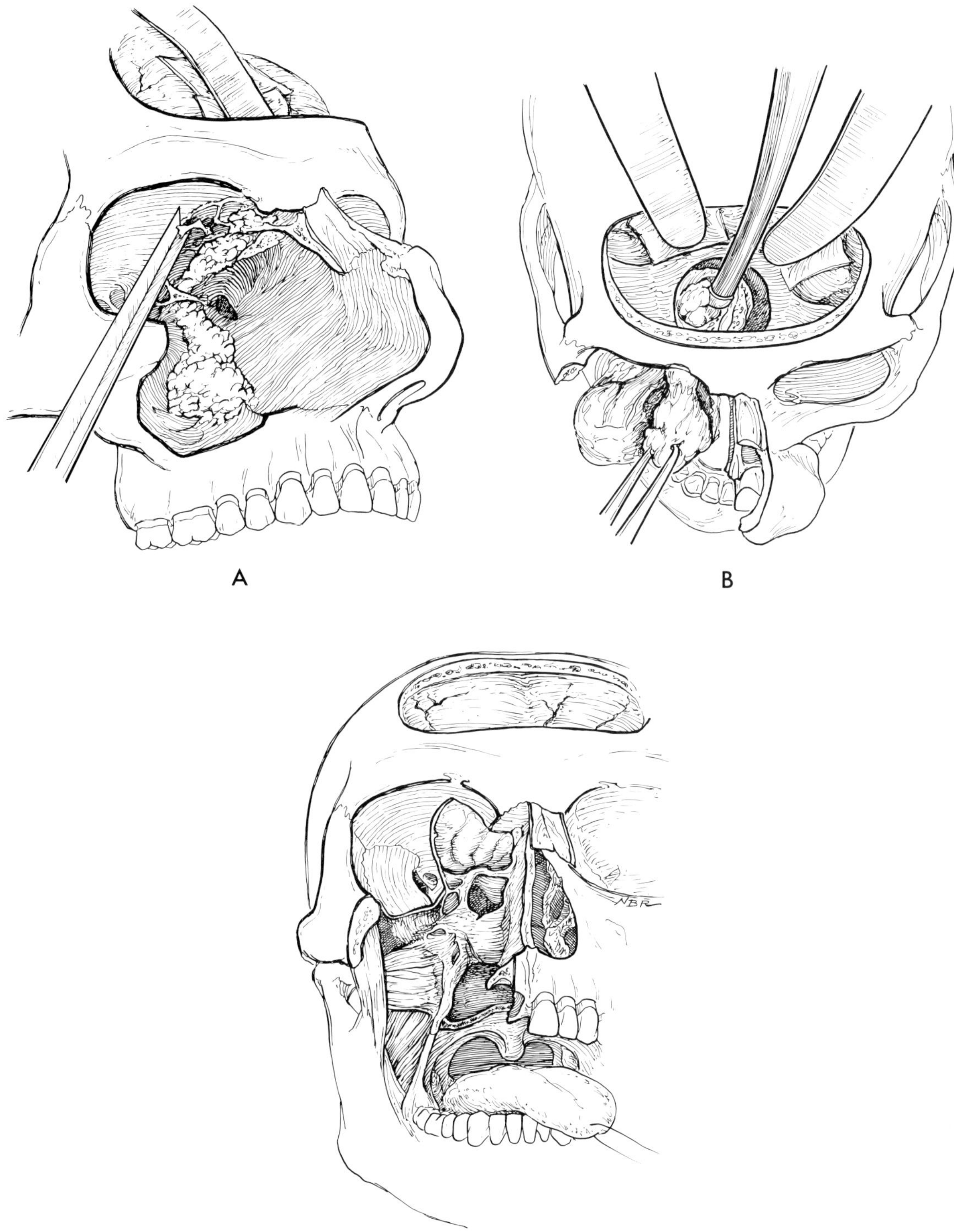

Figure 5–72. (Case III) *A,* Anterior cranial fossa floor involved with tumor, removed with osteotome from below. *B,* Once maxilloethmoidectomy is done, tumor is delivered from above, through the facial incison. *C,* Defect following maxilloethmoidectomy, orbital exenteration, frontal craniotomy, and anterior fossa floor resection.

Illustration continued on following page.

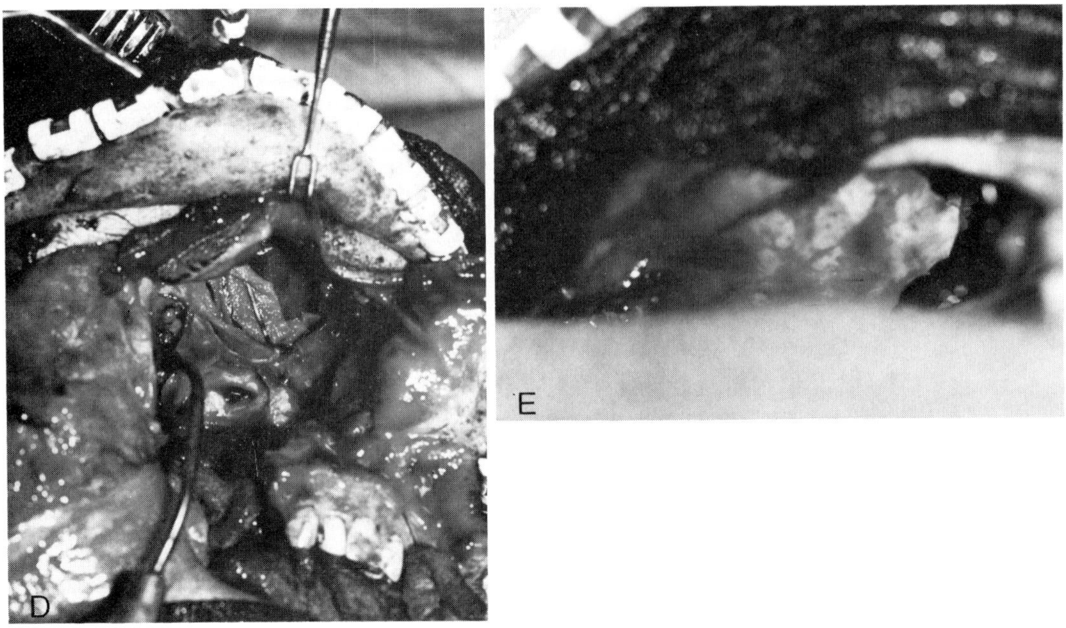

Figure 5–72 *Continued. D,* Defect as seen from facial view. *E,* Defect as seen from cranial view.

References

1. Van Alyea OE: Nasal Sinuses, 2nd ed. Baltimore, Williams & Wilkins, 1951.
2. Schaeffer JP: The Embryology, Development and Anatomy of the Nose, Paranasal Sinuses, Nasolacrimal Passageways and Olfactory Organ in Man. Philadelphia, Blakiston, 1920.
3. Montgomery WW: Surgery of the Upper Respiratory System, Vol I. Philadelphia, Lea & Febiger, 1971, pp 126–135.
4. Donald PJ: Frontal Sinus and Nasofrontal Ethmoidal Complex Fractures. Self Instructional Package #80400, American Academy of Otolaryngology, 1980, p 12.
5. Goss CM: Gray's Anatomy of the Human Body, 29th ed. Philadelphia, Lea & Febiger, 1975, p 741.
6. Sisson GA, Becker SP: Cancer of the nasal cavity and paranasal sinuses. *In* Suen JY, Myers EN (eds): Cancer of the Head and Neck. Churchill Livingstone, New York, 1981, pp 242–279.
7. Birt BD, Briant TDR: The management of malignant tumors of the maxillary sinuses. Otolaryngol Clin North Am 9:249, 1976.
8. Jesse RH, Butler JJ, Healey JE Jr., et al: Paranasal sinuses and nasal cavity. *In* MacComb WS and Fletcher GH (eds): Cancer of the Head and Neck. Baltimore, Williams & Wilkins, 1967, pp 329–356.
9. Conley J: Concepts in head and neck surgery. *In* The Paranasal Sinuses. New York, Grune & Stratton, 1970, pp 54–68.
10. Batsakis JG: Cancer of the nasal cavity and the paranasal sinuses. *In* Tumors of the Head and Neck—Clinical and Pathological Considerations. Baltimore, Williams & Wilkins, 1974, pp 112–122.
11. Chandler JR, de la Cruz A, Pickard RE: Tumors of the nose and sinuses and their surgical treatment. *In* English, GM (ed): Otolaryngology, Vol III. Hagerstown, MD, Harper & Row, 1978, pp 1–17.
12. Vrabec DP: The inverted Schneiderian papilloma: a clinical and pathological study. Laryngoscope 85:186, 1975.
13. Batsakis JG: Neoplasms of the minor and "lesser" major salivary glands. *In* Tumors of the Head and Neck—Clinical and Pathological Considerations. Baltimore, Williams & Wilkins, 1974, Chapter 2.
14. Cohen MA, Batsakis JG: Oncocytic tumors (oncocytoma) of minor salivary glands. Arch Otolaryngol 88:71, 1968.
15. Batsakis JG: Mucous gland tumors of the nose and paranasal sinuses. Ann Otol Rhinol Laryngol 79:557, 1970.
16. Batsakis JG, Holtz F, Sueper RH: Adenocarcinoma of the nasal and paranasal cavities. Arch Otolaryngol 77:625, 1963.
17. Rafla S: Mucous gland tumors of paranasal sinuses. Cancer 24:683, 1969.
18. Freedman HM, DeSanto LW, DeVine KD, et al: Malignant melanoma of the nasal cavity and paranasal sinuses. Arch Otolaryngol 97:322, 1973.
19. Cantrell RW, Ghorayeb BY, Fitz-Hugh GS: Esthesioneuroblastoma: diagnosis and treatment. Ann Otol Rhinol Laryngol 86:760, 1977.
20. Mandeloff J: The olfactory neuroepithelial tumors. Cancer 10:944, 1957.
21. Obert GH, Devine KD, McDonald JR: Olfactory neuroblastomas. Cancer 13:205, 1960.
22. Kahn LB: Esthesioneuroblastoma: a light and electron microscopic study. Human Pathol 5:364, 1974.
23. Skolnik EM, Massari FS, Tenta LT: Olfactory Neuroepithelioma. Arch Otolaryngol 84:84, 1966.
24. Harrison DRN: The management of malignant tumors of the nasal sinuses. Otolaryngol Clin North Am 4:159, 1971.

25. Robin PE, Powell DJ: Diagnostic errors in cancers of the nasal cavity and paranasal sinuses. Arch Otolaryngol 107:138, 1981.
26. Dodd GD, Jing B-S: Radiology of the Nose, Paranasal Sinuses and Nasopharynx. Baltimore, Williams & Wilkins, 1977, pp 215–276.
27. Mancuso AA: Computed tomography of the head and neck. Baltimore, Williams & Wilkins 1981, pp 203–214.
28. Millard RD: Aesthetic reconstructive rhinoplasty. Clin Plast Surg 8:169, 1981.
29. Ketcham AS, Chretien PB, Schour L, et al: Surgical Treatment of Patients with Advanced Cancer of the Paranasal Sinuses in Neoplasia of the Head and Neck. Chicago, Year Book Medical Publications, 1974, pp 187–209.
30. Bridger GP: Radical surgery for ethmoid cancer. Arch Otolaryngol 106:320, 1980.
31. Konno A, Togawa K, Izuka K: Primary reconstruction after total or extended total maxillectomy for maxillary cancer. Plast Reconstr Surg 67:440, 1981.
32. Robinson JM: Frontal sinus cancer manifested as a frontal mucocele. Arch Otolaryngol 101:718, 1975.
33. Conner, CE: Metastatic hypernephroma of right frontal, ethmoid and maxillary sinuses. Arch Otolaryngol 28:994, 1938.
34. Brunner H: Primary tumors of the frontal bone. Arch Otolaryngol 57:158, 1953.
35. Brownson RJ, Ogura JH: Primary carcinoma of the frontal sinus. Laryngoscope 81:71, 1971.
36. VanWart CA, Dedo HH, McCoy EG: Carcinoma of the sphenoid sinus. Ann Otol Rhinol Laryngol 82:318, 1973.

6

THYROID

Paul J. Donald, M.D.

Nowhere in the considerations of head and neck cancer is there more controversy than over the management of thyroid malignancy. Part of the problem is the uncommonness of the disorder, depriving any one surgeon with the wealth of data in his own experience necessary for accurate decision making. In a public health survey conducted from 1969 to 1971, only 37 new cases of thyroid carcinoma per million population were reported each year.[1] According to the Armed Forces Institute of Pathology fascicle on thyroid tumors, the attack rate for most countries averages 2 to 3 cases per 100,000 population.[2] Another factor contributing to the therapeutic enigma is the protean behavior of these tumors. Autopsy studies reveal the incidence of occult thyroid malignancy to vary from 0.08 to 5.7 per cent in individuals who were not suffering from any known history of thyroid disorder.[4, 22] On the other hand, patients have been reported who suddenly developed and quickly succumbed to widespread papillary carcinoma, a disease that usually enjoys a benign reputation.[5-11]

INCIDENCE

Despite the relatively low incidence of thyroid cancer as noted above, it does seem to have increased in frequency over the years. Carroll et al[12] showed a twofold increase in the incidence of thyroid carcinoma from 1941 to 1962 in New York State. In an extensive review of the literature, Mazzaferri[13] alludes to the increased incidence of the disease over roughly the same time period. Although part of this may be due to an improvement in diagnostic accuracy, the increased frequency has been mainly ascribed to the irradiation of the thymus so commonly done in the 1940's. This well-publicized relationship between cervical and mediastinal irradiation and thyroid malignancy is one of the best promulgated pieces of public health information in modern experience. The findings of Favus et al,[14] who discovered a palpable thyroid mass in 16.5 per cent of individuals with histories of cervical or mediastinal irradiation, are frightening. In addition, they found an abnormal ^{131}I scan in 10.5 per cent of those with a palpably normal gland. Of those who subsequently underwent thyroidectomy, 33 per cent had carcinoma.

In an analysis of 576 cases of papillary carcinoma, Mazzaferri et al[13] found a female-to-male ratio of 16 to 1. They found the peak age incidence to be in the third decade of life, with a rather constant female-to-male ratio throughout each age group. According to Sommers,[15] most children and adolescents with thyroid carcinoma have undergone prior irradiation. Becker et al[16] state that 50 per cent of children with solitary thyroid nodules have cancer. An exhaustive epidemiologic review by Clark et al[17] revealed an extremely consistent female predilection for thyroid malignancy, with females generally outnumbering the males by a ratio of 2 to 1.

It is important to note here that a much higher frequency of overall thyroid disease is seen in females as compared to males, with Clark et al[17] reporting a ratio of 5 to 1. Moreover, the incidence of thyroid nodules is significantly higher in women than in men, and carcinoma is reputed to occur in 4 to 12 per cent of patients with nodular disease.[18, 19] The implication of other thyroid diseases in the genesis of carcinoma is undecided. Meissner and Adler[20] found 5 cases of carcinoma in 226 glands that were excised primarily for Graves' disease. Olen and Klinck[21] found 53 cancers in 2000 excised hyperfunctioning glands. Of Mazzaferri's 576 patients with papillary carcinoma, 17 had Graves' disease, and two others had hyperfunctioning nodules.[13] There is some experimental evidence in animals of malignant change in thyroid glands that have been made hyperplastic.[22] There is also evidence that endemic adenomatous goiter predisposes patients to thyroid tumors. Unfortunately, in many of the areas of the world where iodine-poor diets are not treated with iodine prophylaxis, good statistics are not available. Wegelin[22] showed a higher incidence of malignancy at autopsy in Berne (1.04 per cent), where endemic goiter was common, than in Berlin (0.09 per cent), where it was not. In the modern literature, many studies conflict and fail to show conclusive evidence of this association. Although a common association between thyroiditis and thyroid cancer has been observed, the etiologic significance of this remains obscure. Hirabayashi and Lindsay[23] propose that it represents the usual inflammatory reaction observed around most tumors, or the response to a tumor-elaborated antigen.

PATHOLOGY

At present, four basic histologic forms of thyroid carcinoma are recognized: (1) papillary; (2) follicular; (3) medullary; and (4) anaplastic or undifferentiated. The distribution of tumor types is reflected in Mazzaferri's[13] review of 714 cases (Table 6–1). Fortunately the more benign varieties are by far the most common. The thyroid can be the site of rare tumors such as lymphoma, teratoma, or sarcoma, and it may also be a depository of secondary carcinoma. In Mazzaferri's series, an additional 3 cases of lymphoma were found. Of 62 metastasizing tumors described by Silverberg and Vidone,[24] 24 per cent had secondaries in the thyroid. Shimaoka et al[25] listed malignancies of the breast, lung, and kidney as common organs of origin. Malignant melanoma, because of its similar propensity to spread by blood, also frequently spreads to the thyroid.[26] The tendency of laryngeal carcinoma to directly invade the thyroid gland by direct penetration of the thyroid lamina is well known.

Table 6–1. ANALYSIS OF 714 THYROID CANCERS*

Type	*No.*	*Percentage*
Papillary	585	81.9%
Follicular	114	16.0%
Medullary	9	1.3%
Anaplastic	6	0.8%

*From Mazzaferri EL, Young RL, Oertel JE, et al: Papillary thyroid carcinoma: the impact of therapy in 576 patients. Medicine 56:171, 1977.

Papillary Carcinoma

Gross Appearance. Small tumors may appear as nothing more than a scar that is fibrotic or calcific in nature. Larger ones are generally well encapsulated, but the very large lesions usually show some evidence of invasion beyond the capsule. These larger varieties commonly have colloid-filled cysts that may be up to 4 cm in diameter (Fig. 6–1). The colloid material is usually thin, brown, and watery in consistency. Numerous papillae project into the cyst's lumina,[9] giving the epithelial surface the appearance of a shag rug. Calcification and even ossification may occur in the more heavily fibrosed areas of the tumor.

Microscopic Features. The tumors have both solid and cystic areas, the latter varying widely in size. The epithelium lining the cysts is composed of a single layer of cuboidal amphophilic cells of rather uniform size. They project into the cyst lumina on a vascularized stalk in the form of many villus-like fronds (Fig. 6–2). The cells themselves have infrequent mitotic figures and no evidence of nuclear hyperchromatism or pleomorphism, the hallmarks of malignancy in other tissues.

The more dense areas have foci of fibrosis and calcific deposits. Calcified, laminated spherules called psammoma bodies (Fig. 6–3) are usually present. Nests of cells, some of which show evidence of squamous metaplasia complete with keratin pearl formation, may be seen. In some regions the cells form actual follicles.

Lymphatic invasion is common. In the AFIP series[2] of 226 papillary carcinomas, lymphatic invasion was seen in 75 per cent of cases. Blood vessel invasion was much less common, being present in only 10 per cent.

The presence of multiple foci of tumor in

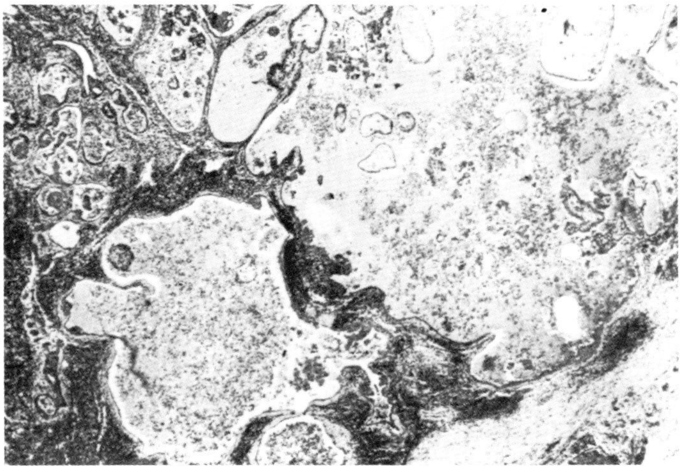

Figure 6–1. Photomicrograph of large cyst in a papillary carcinoma of the thyroid. (H & E × 48) (From Meissner WA, Warren S: Tumors of the thyroid gland. Fascicle 4, Atlas of Tumor Pathology, 2nd ed. Washington DC, Armed Forces Institute of Pathology, 1969, p 73.)

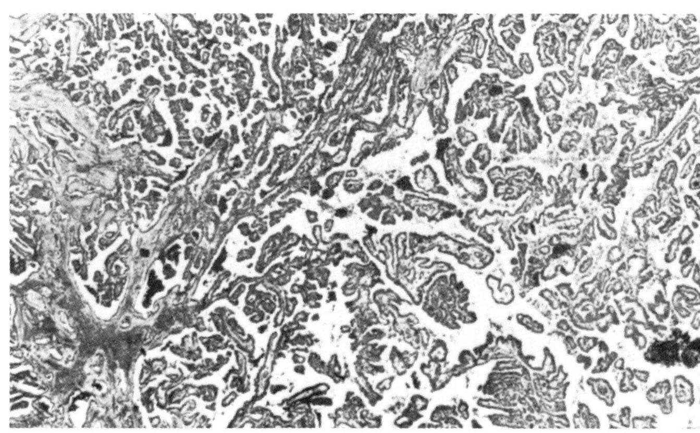

Figure 6–2. Photomicrograph of a papillary carcinoma of the thyroid showing the many villous-like fronds of tumor. (H & E × 50) (From Meissner WA, Warren S: Tumors of the thyroid gland. Fascicle 4, Atlas of Tumor Pathology, 2nd ed. Washington DC, Armed Forces Institute of Pathology, 1969, p 72.)

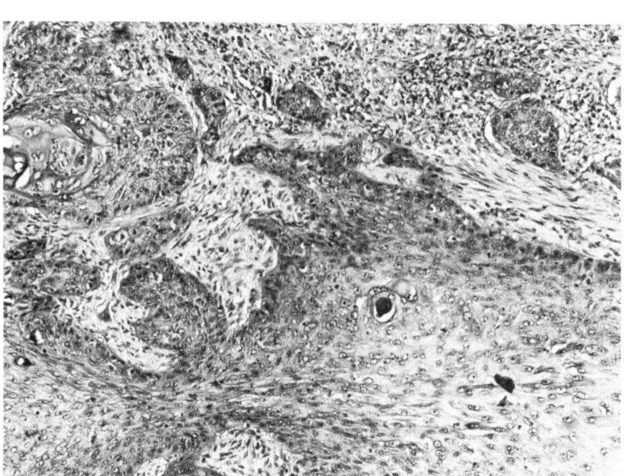

Figure 6–3. Photomicrograph of papillary carcinoma of the thyroid, showing a psammoma body. (H & E × 100)

any one gland is extremely common, having been noted in as many as 89 to 90 per cent of cases in some series.[26] This may represent multiple spontaneous foci of disease or intraglandular metastasis. This finding has strongly dissuaded many surgeons from performing only lobectomy for papillary disease.

The differentiation of benign papillary adenoma from papillary carcinoma is made on the basis of invasiveness, since the morphologic characteristics of the cells are virtually indistinguishable. The presence in carcinoma of capsular and extracapsular invasion and the permeation of adjacent lymphatics or blood vessels are the prime histologic differentiating features. Benign papillary adenomas are fortunately rare and are highly unlikely to be a precursor to malignancy. Psammoma bodies, although not a feature distinguishing a benign from a malignant tumor, are characteristic of papillary cancer and are exceedingly rare in normal thyroid tissue.[27, 28]

Pathophysiology. Papillary carcinoma is the most common and the most benign-behaving malignancy of the thyroid gland. Although early metastases to cervical lymph nodes are common, the progress of the disease is slow, with 5- to 10-year survival rates in the 90 to 95 per cent range. Even with distant metastases the progression is protracted.

One of the most common presentations of papillary adenocarcinoma is a lump in the neck. The misnomer "lateral aberrant thyroid" was applied in the past to papillary carcinoma metastatic to a lateral cervical lymph node, which was thought to arise as a mass of ectopic tissue. There are rare instances when small foci of normal-appearing thyroid follicles appear in a lymph node or even outside the nodal capsule.[29, 30, 31] However, for practical purposes, these should be considered as possible metastases and a thorough investigation as well as careful continued observation made on such patients.

Normal thyroid tissue can be found anywhere along the track of migration of the thyroid gland in its embryologic development. Because of the one-time proximity of the developing heart to the embryonic thyroid, portions of the gland may be found in the chest, in the mediastinum, aortic arch, and even the heart itself.[2] Normal thyroid tissue can be found occasionally in adjacent strap muscles and must not be misconstrued as cancer. Thyroglossal duct remnants are generally either epithelium, normal thyroid tissue, or cyst. However, more than 30 cases of carcinoma have been reported originating in a thyroglossal duct remnant.[32]

The course of papillary cancer is slow, especially in children and young adults. The tumor is often present for a long time and reaches a considerable size before invading adjacent tissues. It is not uncommon to see large papillary tumors in patients who have no hoarseness, dysphagia, or vocal cord paralysis. In Mazzaferri's series,[13] contiguous structures were involved in only 4.7 per cent of patients. However, patients over the age of 40 have a worse prognosis. In a series by Sedgwick and Bookwalter,[33] 270 cases were followed for a minimum of 10 years. The mortality rate for patients younger than 40 was 8 per cent and for those older than 40 was 30 per cent. Over 80 per cent of the patients who died were over the age of 40 when first treated.

As mentioned, lymph node involvement is very common. In a series of 393 patients by Frazell and Foote,[34] 50 per cent had cervical adenopathy and 11 per cent had bilateral disease. In Mazzaferri's group there was cervical or mediastinal involvement in 46 per cent.[13] The AFIP[2] study showed lymph node involvement in 76 per cent of patients. Lymph node disease does not necessarily mean that blood vessel invasion has also taken place, and there are also cases in which distant metastases are present and cervical involvement is limited entirely to the gland.

Follicular Carcinoma

Gross Appearance. The second most common thyroid malignancy is follicular carcinoma. It is of firmer consistency than the papillary variety, grayish-pink, gritty when cut, and tends to be solid all the way through. Often a central scar is present that may be calcified. Any cavitation is usually the result of infarction and subsequent liquefaction, but this is uncommon. Tumor tissue may invade surrounding structures and permeate lymphatics. The propensity of these tumors for blood vessel invasion is far greater than in papillary carcinoma and may even be obvious on gross examination.

Microscopic Features. The microscopic picture of follicular carcinoma may be highly variable. Follicles containing colloid may be seen, and the overall picture closely resembles that of an adenoma (Fig. 6–4). The only clue to malignancy is capsular invasion or the

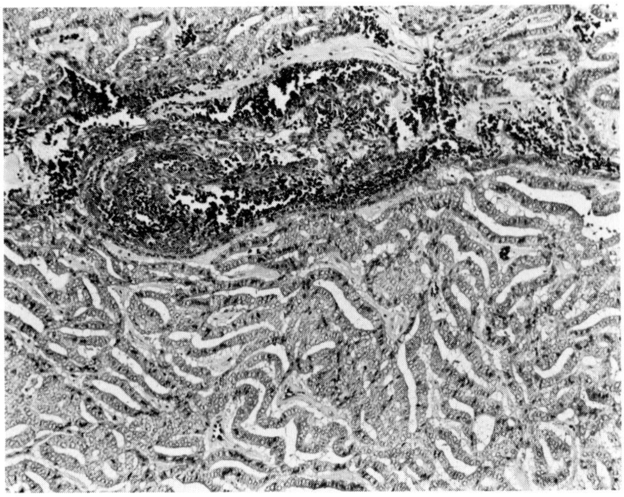

Figure 6–4. Photomicrograph of a follicular carcinoma of the thyroid, showing vascular invasion. (H & E × 100)

invasion of a blood vessel or lymphatic channel. The great variation in follicle size among these tumors has fostered a number of subclassifications based upon this parameter, and indeed there appears to be some correlation between follicle size and prognosis. Small size or no follicle formation at all is associated with aggressiveness, invasiveness, and a poor prognosis.

Generally, there is little variation in cell size in any one tumor, and few or no mitotic figures are seen. Occasionally, the histologic picture is one of packed follicular cells with no colloid formation and significant cellular pleomorphism. A cellular picture of mixed morphology is not uncommon. In an examination of 80 differentiated tumors by Russell et al,[26] a consistent follicular pattern was found in only 2.5 per cent. A mixed papillary and follicular picture and even some areas of undifferentiated tumor are frequently seen. Some authorities feel that any tumor showing a mixed picture should be described as such, whereas others state that the tumor should be named according to its most predominant component. The behavior of these tumors generally corresponds to that of the most predominant cell type.

Pathophysiology. The slowly progressive character of papillary carcinoma is somewhat characteristic of the follicular form as well. However, because of the propensity of follicular tumors for blood vessel invasion, blood-borne metastases are much more common. Follicular cancer is much more common in females and often appears to originate in an adenomatous goiter. A prolonged history of thyroid adenoma preceding the development of tumor is not uncommon. Most benign adenomas, however, remain as such. How and why a particular adenoma undergoes malignant transformation remains a total mystery.

Lymph node metastases are less common in follicular cancer than in the papillary variety. Although blood-borne secondaries are common, they may remain dormant for a considerable time before becoming symptomatic. In fact, histologic confirmation of blood vessel invasion does not necessarily mean that there are distant metastases. In 34 cases of follicular cancer followed by Warren,[35] all of whom had histologic evidence of vascular invasion, only 2 per cent died of subsequent metastasis.

Overall 10-year survival rates range from 34 to 68 per cent.[36, 37, 38] In a series of 100 cases in which the cancer was limited to the thyroid gland itself, Beahrs and Pasternak[39] reported a 10-year survival rate of 90 per cent. Meissner and Warren[2] state that with extensive invasion the 5-year survival rate is around 50 per cent. They further quote a collective series of the American Cancer Society that gives an overall 5-year survival rate of 64.7 per cent.

Medullary Carcinoma

Gross Appearance. Medullary carcinoma is a hard, dense, solid tumor of gray-white coloration occasionally marked by hemorrhages. It varies in size from 1.5 to 10 cm. Unlike the differentiated malignancies, it is not generally well encapsulated and is locally

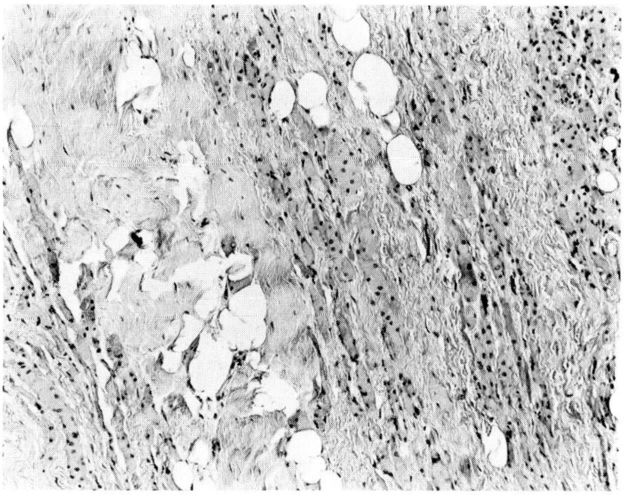

Figure 6–5. Photomicrograph showing chords of irregular cuboidal cells with hyperchromatic nuclei in a fibrous stoma characteristic of medullary carcinoma of the thyroid. Tumor is interspersed with deposits of an amorphous material that will take up a stain specific for amyloid. (H & E × 100)

infiltrative. One of its characteristic features is gross angioinvasion.

Microscopic Features. The tumor is composed of clusters or trabeculae of cells interspersed by a dense fibrotic stroma containing amyloid (Fig. 6–5). The cells are round or polyhedral, but can be spindle shaped or assume the appearance of a follicular cell. The cytoplasm is eosinophilic and granular, and the nuclei are hyperchromatic. Some parenchymal cells are binucleate, and occasionally giant cells may be seen in reaction to the amyloid deposits. Mitoses are present but infrequent. There are no colloid-containing follicles, although some of the cells may assume a follicular pattern. The cellular arrangement may be a more palisaded trabecular configuration and may even resemble a carcinoid tumor.

Electron-microscopic evidence of intracellular thyrocalcitonin granules suggests that the tumor is of C cell origin.[16] Some individuals show high levels of circulating thyrocalcitonin, and concomitant parathyroid hyperplasia is not uncommon.

The amyloid found in the hyaline stroma takes up most of the characterizing stains. Its ultrastructure reveals a composition of glycoproteins and acid mucopolysaccharides peculiar to primary and secondary amyloid deposits in other disease states. The material is commonly found in the metastases as well; however, medullary carcinoma does not result in generalized amyloidosis.

Calcium deposits are also found in the stroma, some of the them resembling the psammoma bodies found in papillary carcinoma. Some plasma cells and lymphocytes are also seen. Blood vessel and lymphatic invasion is very common.

Pathophysiology. This tumor makes up between 5 and 10 per cent of all thyroid cancers.[2, 3] It is commonly seen in patients beyond the fourth decade of life. It is usually unifocal, with the remaining thyroid gland showing little reaction to it. As with the differentiated types, the course of medullary carcinoma is slow. Metastases to lymph nodes and the bloodstream are common. Over half the cases demonstrate cervical metastases on first presentation.

The tumors are also highly locally invasive, extending into the trachea and larynx. The pharynx and cervical esophagus may be constricted by retropharyngeal encroachment of tumor (Fig. 6–6). Death occurs as a result of distant blood metastases, lymph node involvement, and local extension. Beahrs and Pasternak[39] reported an 85 per cent 10-year survival among 36 patients whose disease was confined to the thyroid gland on initial presentation. The survival rate dropped precipitously to 42 per cent among 41 additional patients who presented with lymph node involvement. In Freeman and Lindsay's series of 33 patients, 39 per cent died of their disease.[40] Hazard et al[41] reported a 30 per cent mortality rate, and Williams et al[42] a rate of 33 per cent, with most of the patients in both series being followed for at least 10 years.

Among thyroid cancers, the medullary variety is distinguished by a number of systemic peculiarities. The tumor has a strong familial tendency[43] and is associated with a number of other tumor states and endocrinopathies.

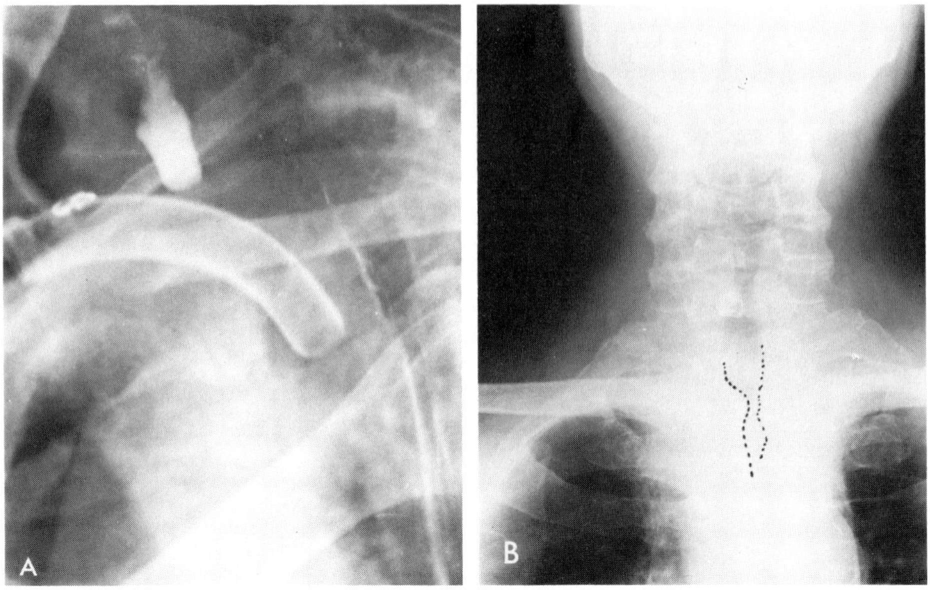

Figure 6–6. *A,* Barium swallow of an elderly patient with a longstanding medullary carcinoma of the thyroid. Note the tumor producing extensive pressure on the esophagus. *B,* Soft tissue x-ray shows marked narrowing of trachea.

A distinct clinical entity identified as multiple endocrine adenomatosis syndrome (Type II) has been identified. It is associated with pheochromocytoma that is often bilateral (70 per cent of cases).[2] Neurofibromas, of both cutaneous and mucosal origin, are frequently found. A symptom complex similar to that of carcinoid syndrome, with facial flushing and diarrhea, has also been linked to a humoral substance secreted by some medullary tumors. Ljungberg et al[43a] researched a family of 150 members and identified 7 members with medullary carcinoma and 8 with pheochromocytoma and multiple neurofibromatosis. The overall incidence of medullary cancer is thought to be around 20 per cent.[45] The inheritance mode is autosomal dominant.

Thyroid adenomas and hyperplasia are more commonly seen with medullary carcinoma than with any other cell type. The production of thyrocalcitonin linking the cell of origin in medullary cancer to the parafollicular or C cell has already been alluded to. These patients may even present with the clinical picture of hyperparathyroidism. However, many patients with medullary thyroid cancer, even with the genetic syndrome, do not have hyperparathyroidism.

Medullary tumors have been known to elaborate an adrenocortical hormone in sufficiently high amounts to produce Cushing's disease. Prostaglandins, serotonin, and histaminase have all been identified as secretory products of these neoplasms. The most consistent laboratory test for following patients with these tumors is the monitoring of thyrocalcitonin levels. Tumor production of this hormone can be stimulated by artificially inducing hypercalcemia by calcium infusions. Pentagastrin can stimulate calcitonin secretion as well, although not in all cases. Wells et al[45] used the pentagastrin stimulation test in a number of families with a genetic trait for medullary carcinoma. They operated upon four children who had elevated calcitonin levels on pentagastrin stimulation, but palpably normal thyroid glands. They found the gland in each case to be riddled by multiple foci of medullary carcinoma.

Undifferentiated Carcinoma

The incidence of undifferentiated carcinoma varies from 1 to 15 per cent.[2, 12] It is a highly aggressive neoplasm with a poor prognosis.

Gross Appearance. The tumor is a typical cancer: firm, generally solid throughout, whitish in color, and without the usual cystic or hemorrhagic areas seen in the less malignant types. Local invasion into the opposite lobe and into adjacent structures is the rule.

Microscopic Features. The predominant histologic type is either small cell or large

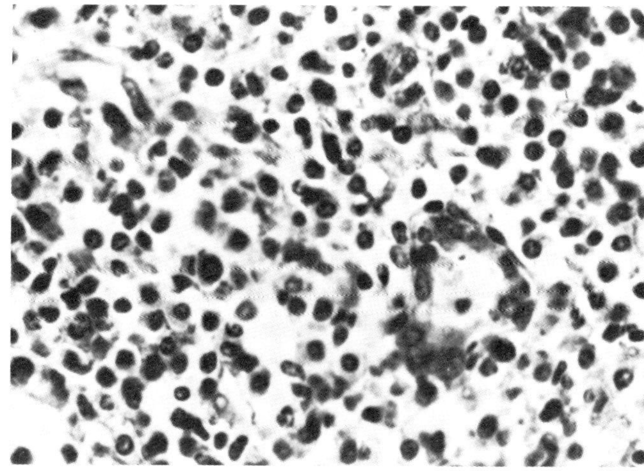

Figure 6–7. Photomicrograph of a small cell variety of undifferentiated carcinoma of the thyroid. The monotonous cellular pattern is reminiscent of a lymphoma. (H & E × 1500) (From Meissner WA, Warren S: Tumors of the thyroid gland. Fascicle 4, Atlas of Tumor Pathology, 2nd ed. Washington DC, Armed Forces Institute of Pathology, 1969, p 105.)

cell. Differentiation between the two types is important in that the small cell type has a somewhat better prognosis. The small cell variety has two forms: compact and diffuse. The compact (Fig. 6–7) shows a plethora of small cells packed together in tight clusters with an intervening stroma similar to that found in medullary carcinoma. Mitotic figures are frequent, but pleomorphism is minimal. In both this and the large cell variety, occasional follicles may be seen. The diffuse type has the small cells loosely arranged without any clear organization. The appearance is very similar to a lymphoma. Blood vessel invasion in both types is exceedingly common.

The large cell type is composed of a wide variety of large bizarre cells (Fig. 6–8). Marked pleomorphism, frequent mitoses (some of which are abnormal), and hyperchromatism of the nuclei are prominent features. The cells may resemble those of the strap cells of a rhabdomyosarcoma. Giant cell formation is also seen. The predominant large cell may be more spindle shaped and have a morphology strikingly similar to that of a fibrosarcoma (Fig. 6–9).

A mixed picture of small and large cells is not too uncommon, and foci of undifferentiated tumor in a papillary-follicular setting are also seen. It is possible that the undifferentiated variety may be a further degenerative step in the gradual progression of malignancy in a neoplasm that may even have originated as an adenoma.

Pathophysiology. Rapid lymph- and bloodborne metastasis and early progressive local invasion are the hallmarks of this extremely aggressive cancer. In a large series of 160 patients reported by Woolner et al,[46] 50 per

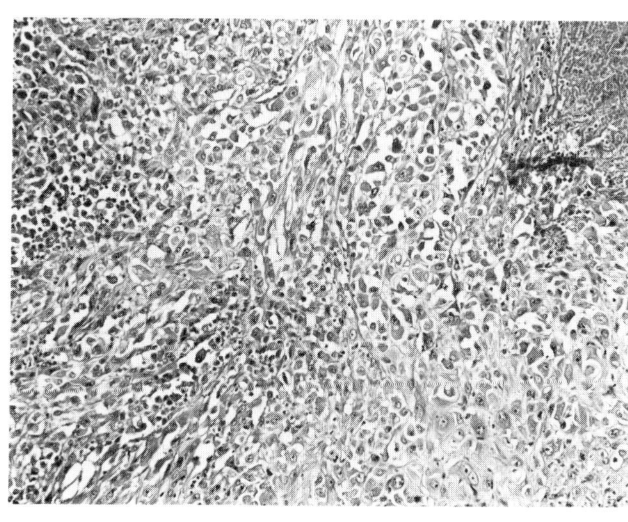

Figure 6–8. Photomicrograph of a large cell type of undifferentiated carcinoma of the thyroid. (H & E × 100)

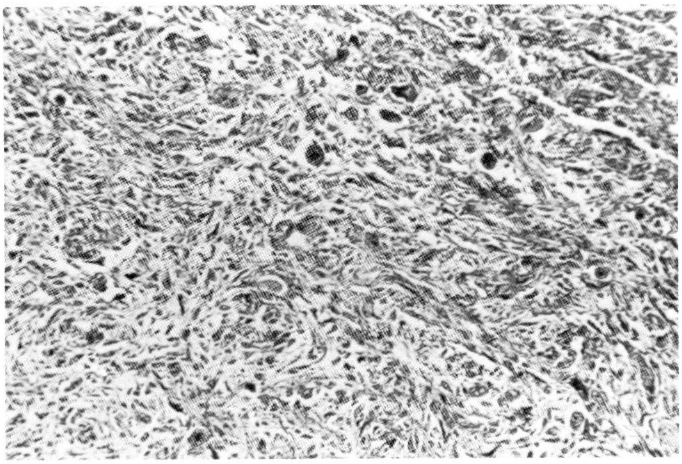

Figure 6–9. Photomicrograph of a large cell type of undifferentiated carcinoma of the thyroid wherein the predominant morphology is a spindle-shaped cell. (H & E × 100) (From Meissner WA, Warren S: Tumors of the thyroid gland. Fascicle 4, Atlas of Tumor Pathology, 2nd ed. Washington DC, Armed Forces Institute of Pathology, 1969, p 107.)

cent died within 5 months, and most by 3 years. Only 4 of the original 160 patients were alive after 5 years. In a review of 84 cases by Aldinger et al,[47] the mean survival time following diagnosis was 6.2 months and the 5-year survival rate was 7.1 per cent.

At a symposium on the management of thyroid cancer at the annual meeting of the American Academy of Otolaryngology in 1980,[48] there was universal pessimism expressed by the panelists regarding the fate of victims of this disease. Early, aggressive surgery coupled with external irradiation may be the only possible means of salvaging any afflicted patients. Unfortunately, even the most radical local attack on these tumors is usually doomed to failure because of distant metastases.

THE SOLITARY NODULE

Management of the solitary thyroid nodule is a conundrum whose precise solution has evaded medical practitioners for decades. An overwhelming number of erudite dissertations, flow-sheets, and schemata have been put forth in attempts to clarify this dilemma. Opinions have varied over the years from the philosophy of test, wait, and watch to recommendations for sugical excision of most or all of these nodules. From a general statistical standpoint, there are certain clinical and investigative factors that tend to sway the opinion toward either watchful waiting or surgical excision. However, each individual patient independent of the balancing of these factors can habor a malignancy in the thyroid gland.

Table 6–2 shows the various clinical and investigative factors that favor either malignancy or benignity. Although such information can serve as an aid in decision making, it will become clear from the following discussion that what, for example, appears to be a perfectly benign lump in a male patient in a favorable age group, with an encouraging looking scan, can indeed be malignant.

Diagnostic Factors

Age. A mass in the thyroid gland of a child must be assumed to be malignant. Although these patients most often present with cervical adenopathy and even distant metastases, the course of the disease is usually markedly protracted. Patients often survive as long as 20 years after the diagnosis is made before succumbing to the disease.

Table 6–2. FACTORS FAVORING MALIGNANCY OR BENIGNITY OF SOLITARY THYROID NODULE

Factors	*Benign*	*Malignant*
History		
Age	20–40	<20; >40
Sex	Female	Male
Previous irradiation	No	Yes
Dysphagia	No	Yes
Hoarseness	No	Yes
Airway obstruction	No	Yes
Physical Examination		
Mass consistency	Firm; cystic	Stony-hard
Extra thyroid mass	No	Yes
Vocal cord paralysis	No	Yes
Fixation	No	Yes
Pain and tenderness	Yes	No
Hyperthyroidism	Yes	No
Investigation		
^{131}I scan	Hot or warm	Cold
Ultrasound	Cyst	No cyst

A relatively equal distribution of case incidence is present from the second to the fourth decade. In patients over the age of 60, the incidence of carcinoma in a nodule is much higher and tends to be of the more malignant variety.[49] Mustacchi and Cutler[50] observed that although the incidence of papillary carcinoma changes little with increasing age, the other histologic varieties occur more frequently in the older age groups. This is especially relevant in that thyroid masses are relatively common in the elderly.

Sex. Thyroid nodules are much more common in females. Although they outnumber males in the incidence of malignant masses, the frequency of benign lumps is much higher in women than in men. The inference, therefore, is that a thyroid nodule in a male is much more likely to be cancerous than one in a woman.

Prior Irradiation. The widespread irradiation of infants for the prophylaxis of crib death due to "status thymus lymphaticus" is well-known history. The use of ionizing irradiation for the treatment of acne was also popular years ago. A thyroid nodule in an individual with such a history carries with it some ominous statistics, with as many as one third of these patients harboring thyroid carcinoma.

Numerous studies have indicated that as many as 80 per cent of all patients with thyroid carcinoma may have had prior irradiation.[51] A large study by Raventos and Winship[52] of 528 patients revealed an average latent period of 10.9 years between exposure to irradiation and subsequent diagnosis of disease.

Such statistics make it clear that a history of prior cervical irradiation in a patient with a thyroid mass is one of the strongest indications for excisional biopsy.

Symptoms. Symptoms related to a thyroid mass may develop either from compression caused by the mass or from its invasion of other structures. Adenomatous goiters and individual adenomas may reach substantial size (Fig. 6–10) and by pressure alone cause dysphagia, dyspnea, and stridor. Retrosternal adenomas are especially infamous for this because of their confinement in the upper thoracic cavity. However, most benign processes do not cause such symptoms, and complaints of dysphagia, hoarseness, or airway obstruction strongly suggest malignancy.

Hoarseness is usually secondary to invasion of one or both recurrent laryngeal nerves. It is, however, remarkable how much involvement can be tolerated without actual paralysis.

Signs. Although Graves' disease is seen occasionally with carcinoma, a thyroid nodule in a hyperthyroid patient is usually a toxic nodular goiter. In a study of 150 cases of thyroid cancer, Fitzgerald[53] could not find one tumor that would concentrate radioiodine more than a normal gland. As already mentioned, however, Meissner and Adler[20] found five carcinomas in glands from 226 patients who had Graves' disease.

Pain and tenderness are most often seen in viral thyroiditis and the early stages of Hashimoto's thyroiditis. The presence of circulating antithyroid antibodies is not helpful in ruling out carcinoma. Malignancy may coexist with both of these states.

The actual consistency of the mass is often difficult to discern because of the overlying soft tissue. A stony-hard mass definitely suggests carcinoma, as does fixation to, or infiltration of, surrounding structures (Fig. 6–11). On the other hand, a fluctuant cyst or softish mass is much more suggestive of a benign process (Fig. 6–12).

Vocal cord paralysis or a palpable mass elsewhere in the neck strongly indicates malignant disease, and the presence of a thyroid mass together with vocal cord paralysis is almost always an indication for surgery. A benign process almost never causes paralysis.

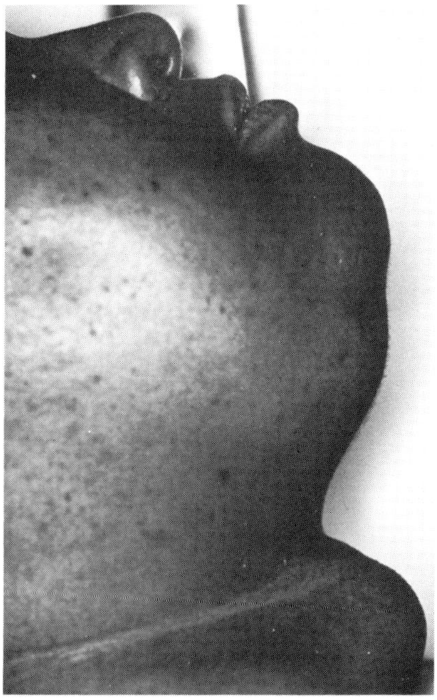

Figure 6–10. A young black male with a large firm midline neck mass that produced dysphagia and stridor but was histologically an adenomatous goiter.

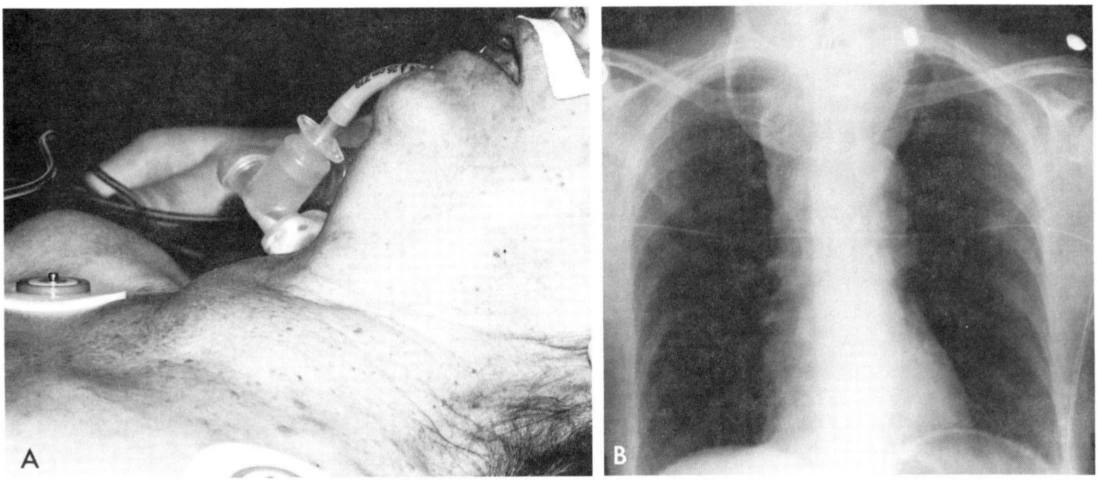

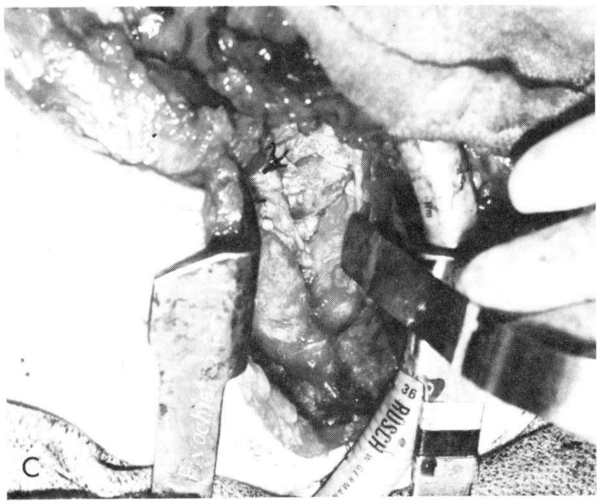

Figure 6–11. *A,* Elderly woman who presented with a 6-month history of a fairly rapidly enlarging neck mass that was stony hard. She had severe dysphagia, severe dyspnea, and stridor requiring emergency tracheostomy. *B,* Chest x-ray following emergency tracheostomy, showing mediastinal widening secondary to tumor. *C,* Intraoperative photograph of mediastinotomy illustrating a relatively avascular, hard, stony tumor. Signs and symptoms were strongly suggestive of undifferentiated carcinoma of the thyroid. Diagnosis was desmoid tumor of the neck and mediastinum.

One must bear in mind, however, the possibility of idiopathic paralysis coexisting with a benign adenoma. Conversely, the absence of paralysis in the presence of even a large tumor does not rule out carcinoma.

A palpable mass elsewhere in the neck raises alarm because of the high probability of metastasis. However, an incident in the author's experience might serve as a warning against overzealous treatment in some of these cases. A middle-aged woman with a hard thyroid mass and a 2-cm firm neck node was explored with a plan of node biopsy and lobectomy, to be followed by definitive surgical therapy based upon the pathologic findings at frozen section. The neck node revealed microscopic foci of amorphous material resembling amyloid and dense fibrous tissue but no definitely identifiable cells of thyroid origin. The pathologist suggested a diagnosis of medullary carcinoma. Thyroid lobectomy produced a frozen section diagnosis that was equivocal. The neck was closed with plans for re-exploration when a definitive diagnosis of cancer was established. Paraffin sections with Congo red stains subsequently established the amorphous deposits as hyaline in a lymph node, representing end-stage chronic inflammation, and the thyroid tumor was a follicular adenoma with densely packed cells.

Laboratory Investigations

^{131}I Scan. One of the most useful differentiating tests for diagnosing a thyroid mass is the ^{131}I scan. By analyzing the pattern of the gamma emissions emanating from the radioactive iodide trapped by the gland, nodules can be portrayed. They are classified according to ^{131}I uptake as "hot" or "cold." The hot, hyperfunctioning nodule is generally considered to be benign, although a few isolated instances of malignancy have been found in hot nodules.[54, 55, 56] A hot nodule, moreover, may screen and obscure a cold

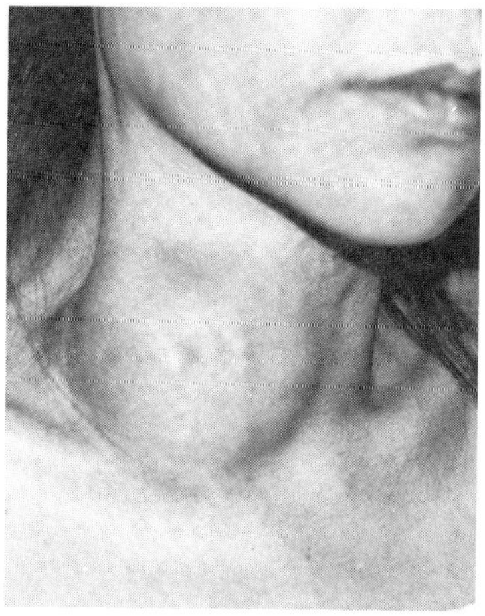

Figure 6–12. A middle-aged Laotian woman with a large cystic mass in the neck. The scar marks the site of previous incisions and drainage; one was done in her native village with a hot umbrella spoke. In the wall of the cyst was a thyroid carcinoma.

area adjacent to it. Carcinomas generally tend to be autonomous, and their radioactive iodine uptake is not influenced by the administration of exogenous thyroid. The lack of depression of ^{131}I following administration of triiodothyronine and the failure of the thyrotropin-releasing hormone test both demonstrate this autonomy.

Normal or irregular functioning is not an uncommon finding in differentiated carcinomas. In Fitzgerald's autoradiography experiment on 150 cancers, 40 of the tumors were shown to contain organified iodine. The use of ^{131}I as a means of therapy for papillary and follicular carcinoma, as well as its combination with TSH stimulation in order to elevate its uptake by the tumor, illustrates the frequency of function and coexistent malignancy in a nodule.

The cold nodule may be a cyst, a tumor of other than thyroid origin, or a carcinoma. Approximately 10 to 20 per cent of cold nodules are determined to be carcinomatous. Table 6–3 compares the various radioisotope uptake findings in benign and malignant nodules. It is somewhat disheartening to see the similarity of isotope findings between the two groups. However, a solitary solid cold nodule should be generally considered to be carcinoma until proved otherwise.

Ultrasonography. The differentiation of a solid from a cystic cold nodule can be made with 90 per cent accuracy with the B mode ultrasound scanner. Although cyst formation is a feature of both papillary and follicular lesions, these cysts are small. Furthermore, the probability of the residual solid tissue in a predominantly cystic lesion being carcinomatous is slight. For example, if the entire lesion measures less than 3 cm in size, the chance of it being malignant is only 2 per cent.[58]

Needle Biopsy. Thyroid carcinoma is often difficult to diagnose histologically. The principal problem is the differentiation of benign papillary and follicular adenomas from their malignant counterparts. As is obvious from the discussion earlier in the chapter, the major differentiating histologic features are not based on cellular morphology; rather, a diagnosis of malignancy is made on the basis of capsular, blood vessel, or lymphatic invasion. This information is difficult to extract from material procured by needle biopsy. Furthermore, the stromal component of medullary carcinoma strongly resembles the fibrosis of some of the inflammatory disorders. Small-cell anaplastic carcinoma closely resembles lymphoma, and large-cell anaplastic tumors may resemble sarcoma.

Some pathologists have acquired considerable skill in the interpretation of needle biopsy and fine needle aspiration cytology. Because of the relative rarity of thyroid cancer, it is difficult for most pathologists to acquire the degree of experience required unless they undergo special training. This is especially true concerning fine needle aspiration cytology.

Open biopsy remains the surest method of establishing the diagnosis of the suspicious thyroid nodule.

SURGICAL MANAGEMENT

The cornerstone of treatment of thyroid carcinoma is surgery. Papillary carcinoma is

Table 6–3. FINDINGS IN RADIOACTIVE ^{131}I SCANS IN TWO MAJOR GROUPS*

	Normal	*Hot Nodule*	*Cool Nodule*	*Cold Nodule*	*Multiple Nodules*
Colloid nodule	23.07%	3.6%	12.07%	58%	3.6%
Carcinoma	22.0%	3.7%	11.0%	63.0%	0.0%

*After Hoffman GL, et al: The solitary thyroid nodule. Arch Surg 105:379, 1972.

not only the most common malignancy but also the most controversial in terms of surgical management. Opinions vary from lobectomy through lobectomy-isthmusectomy to total thyroidectomy. Because of the frequency of bilateral involvement with these tumors, total thyroidectomy with parathyroid preservation is probably the safest procedure. If total thyroidectomy devascularizes the parathyroid glands, then one gland is removed, carefully diced, and implanted in the antecubital fossa of the arm. However, any tumor involvement of these glands militates against their preservation. Similarly, direct infiltration of the recurrent laryngeal nerves demands that they be sacrificed.

Cervical involvement with metastatic disease requires neck dissection. Although the limited "lumpectomizing" of cervical nodes is still advocated by some, either radical or conservation dissection is the most effective treatment.[59] For most patients with limited neck disease, conservation neck dissection with preservation of the eleventh cranial nerve, the sternocleidomastoid muscle, and even the internal jugular vein is sufficient. The internal jugular vein, if directly invaded by tumor, should be removed.

Residual disease and distant metastases can be effectively managed for a considerable time by the administration of ^{131}I. In Mazzaferri's series, in which 116 patients were treated, ^{131}I in total doses ranging from 50 to 800 mCi was given.[13] The dose was less than 200 mCi in 87 per cent of the patients and less than 300 mCi in 90 per cent. Following surgical and medical therapy, 44.8 per cent of these patients had no demonstrable ^{131}I uptake. However, in 70 individuals, representing 12.2 per cent of the entire group of 504 patients who were judged to be free of disease at the cessation of their initial therapy, the disease recurred. The recurrences were treated by revision therapy, and half of the patients in this group were given ^{131}I in addition. Four of the 8 patients with distant disease eventually died. During their prolonged period of observation, 19 patients died. Of these, 7 who had persistent tumor died of other causes and 5 died as a direct result of the carcinoma. Given these statistics, a more conservative approach to surgical management with adjunctive ^{131}I administration would appear to be an effective therapeutic combination.

Follicular carcinoma requires slightly more aggressive management, because of its increased invasive potential. Lymph node dissection is frequently required because of the common finding of cervical metastasis. Tollefsen[60] reported an overall 49 per cent incidence of neck secondaries, 28 per cent of which were manifest and 21 per cent were occult. The efficacy of conservation neck dissection in the management of follicular carcinoma is yet to be proved.[61] An important deterrent factor to the conservation procedure is the incidence of recurrent neck disease following this operation, with Black et al[62] noting a 22 per cent recurrence rate in necks thus treated. Adjunctive ^{131}I therapy is still effective because of the propensity of most follicular tumors to trap and organify the isotope. Most tumors can be safely excised without having to remove adjacent laryngeal or tracheal skeletal elements. Only when there is direct invasion of these structures need there be any resection, and then it should be of a limited nature.

Medullary carcinoma is highly invasive locally and often accompanied by cervical lymphadenopathy. In a study of 40 such cancers by Gordon et al,[63] 67 per cent of those who had a radical neck dissection survived 5 years. However, a 43 per cent survival rate was seen in those whose necks were not dissected. Occult adenopathy was present in 70 per cent of the latter group. ^{131}I is almost never taken up by the tumor and is of little value in the management of this disease. Despite the optimism of some,[63] external beam irradiation has marginal efficacy in medullary cancer.

Undifferentiated carcinoma has a dismal prognosis. The only possibility for cure may be with an aggressive combination of surgery and external beam irradiation. Millburn and Ameen[64] report cure rates of between 25 and 35 per cent in totally unresectable disease with external irradiation alone, but few therapists share their enthusiasm. The experience of Crile and Hawk,[65] who had only 1 survivor among 24 patients treated by surgery or surgery and radiotherapy, is more the rule.

Thyroidectomy

Since the standard procedure is well described in other texts,[66–68] only points of importance in the resection will be stressed. Once the diagnosis of cancer is made, total extracapsular thyroidectomy is always performed, because of the frequency of bilateral

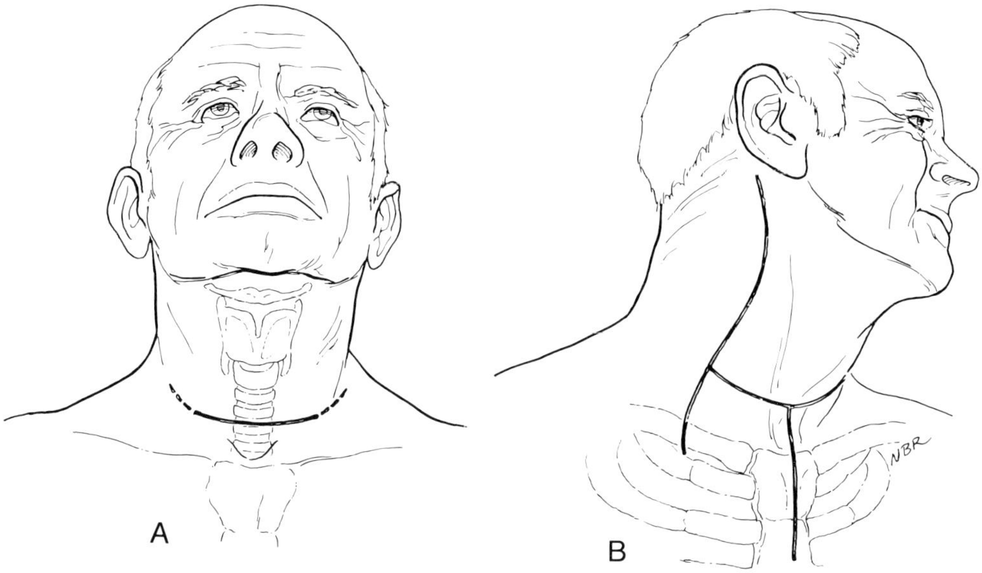

Figure 6–13. *A,* Standard thyroidectomy "collar-type" incision. *B,* Skin incision extending from the collar incision to accommodate the sternal split necessary to dissect thyroid tumor from the mediastinum.

disease. Neck dissection (either radical or conservation) if done with the thyroidectomy makes the dissection of the gland much easier. In papillary disease without internal jugular or sternocleidomastoid muscle involvement, a conservation neck dissection is done.

Incision. A "collar-type" incision is made in a crease line in the neck at the level of the inferior border of the cricoid cartilage (Fig. 6–13), approximately 2½ to 3 cm above the sternal notch. The skin incision extends about midway across the width of the sternocleidomastoid muscle on each side. The incision is carried through the platysma, exposing the superficial layer of deep cervical fascia investing the strap muscles. If a neck dissection

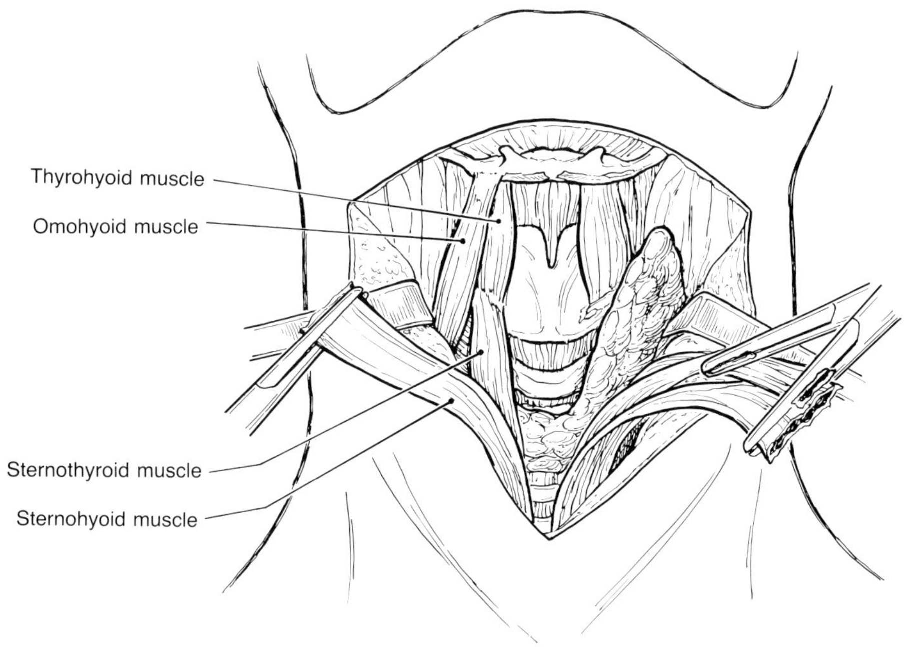

Figure 6–14. The strap muscles on the side of the tumor are cut from the hyoid bone, with care taken to preserve the nerve and blood supply that is located inferiorly. Interference with either may cause disfiguring atrophy and fibrosis.

is to be done, the "collar" incision is continued to a point 2 cm anterior to the trapezius muscle, where it is joined by a vertical incision made from the mastoid tip to the clavicle, forming a type of "half-H" incision.

Flaps are developed through this avascular plane superiorly to the level of the hyoid bone and inferiorly to the level of the sternum, and the incision is propped open with self-retaining retractors.

Strap Muscles. If the tumor is stuck to the strap muscles, they are excised en bloc with the tumor. However, if the neoplasm is restricted to the gland, the straps are either detached from the hyoid superiorly or separated in the midline and retracted laterally. Incision of the straps at their insertion into the hyoid, followed by dissection inferiorly, will preserve the blood and nerve supplies that enter the muscles inferiorly (Fig. 6–14). This facilitates dissection of the tumor and, unless the thyroid nodule is small, is probably the safest and most expedient method of exposure. The thyroid lobe on the tumor side is thus exposed.

Recurrent Nerve. In the catalog of head and neck procedures, thyroidectomy is one of the easier to perform. The principal factor that makes it difficult is the proximity of the recurrent laryngeal nerve. There is little doubt that careful dissection of the nerve and direct visualization is the surest means of its preservation.

Although it is classically described as occupying the triangle formed by the trachea and esophagus medially, the carotid laterally, and the lobe of the thyroid superiorly, the course of the nerve may be highly variable. Figure 6–15 shows the location of both recurrent nerves in their extraglandular and retroglandular courses. On the left side, the nerve usually emerges from its origin on the vagus to pass under the arch of the aorta and ascend in the tracheal esophageal groove. Behind the thyroid gland, it penetrates the inferior constrictor muscle and then dips posteriorly behind the cricothyroid articulation. The nerve commonly divides into anterior and posterior branches. In some cases, only the posterior branch assumes a course posterior to the joint. In rare instances, the nerve may divide prior to penetrating the inferior constrictor, creating the possibility of a pure abductor paralysis if only one branch is injured.

On the right side, the nerve passes under the subclavian artery and, like its left-sided counterpart, seeks the tracheoesophageal groove, ascends, and pierces the inferior constrictor to reach the larynx. It tends to be more lateral to the tracheoesophageal groove than the left. In an anatomic study by Hunt,[69] the right nerve was found in a lateral relationship to the groove 33 per cent of the time and the left 22 per cent. This lateral position renders the nerve more prone to injury during dissection.

The nerve is closely related to the inferior thyroid artery, and some authors have described this common anatomic association as a guide to its safe dissection.[70, 71] However, the profusion of anatomic variations (Fig. 6–16) should dissuade the surgeon from using this relationship as a reliable guideline. Loré[72] actually warns against using this landmark and advocates beginning the dissection at the thoracic inlet, identifying the nerve either in the groove or lateral to it, and then following it up to the gland. He advises ligating the inferior thyroid artery adjacent to the gland rather than out laterally. Not only does this avoid the danger of traumatizing the nerve if it is entangled in branches of the artery, but it may preserve the blood supply to parathyroids in the area as well.

Once dissection of the thyroid from the adjacent trachea and larynx begins, the recurrent nerve becomes obscured by a substantial sheet of fibrous tissue binding the posterior surface of the gland to the esophagus and hypopharynx. This ligament (Fig. 6–17), first described by Berry,[73] lies directly over the nerve.[74] The safest way to protect the nerve is to dissect it as one would the facial nerve in parotidectomy. A Mixter clamp is slipped over the epineurium of the nerve, gently elevated, parted, and the intervening connective tissue free of the nerve cut with scissors (Fig. 6–17).

The superior laryngeal nerve, especially the external laryngeal branch to the cricothyroid muscle, is in jeopardy during the dissection of the superior pole of the thyroid. Although the consequences of injury are not as severe as with damage to the recurrent nerve, interference with pitch modulation if the external laryngeal nerve is cut, hemilaryngeal anesthesia if the superior nerve is cut, or both, represent significant complications. The superior laryngeal nerve is high in relation to the thyroid gland proper (Fig. 6–18) and should be out of danger in most cases. However, the anterior suspensory ligament of the gland may be mistaken for a glandular

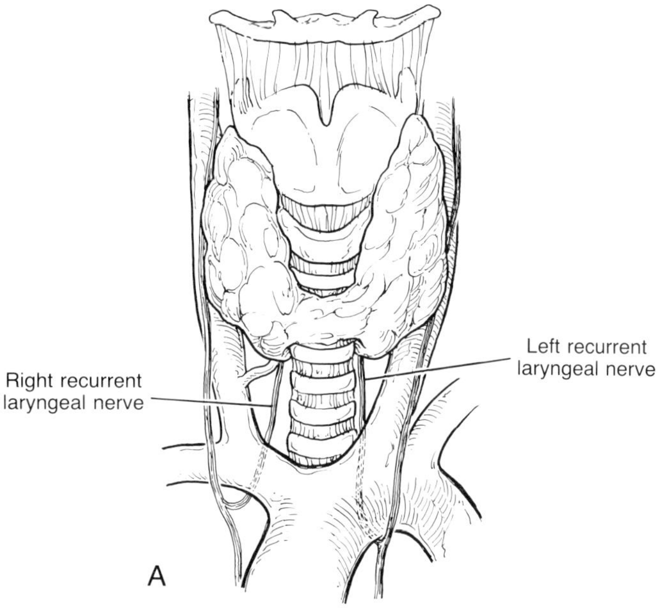

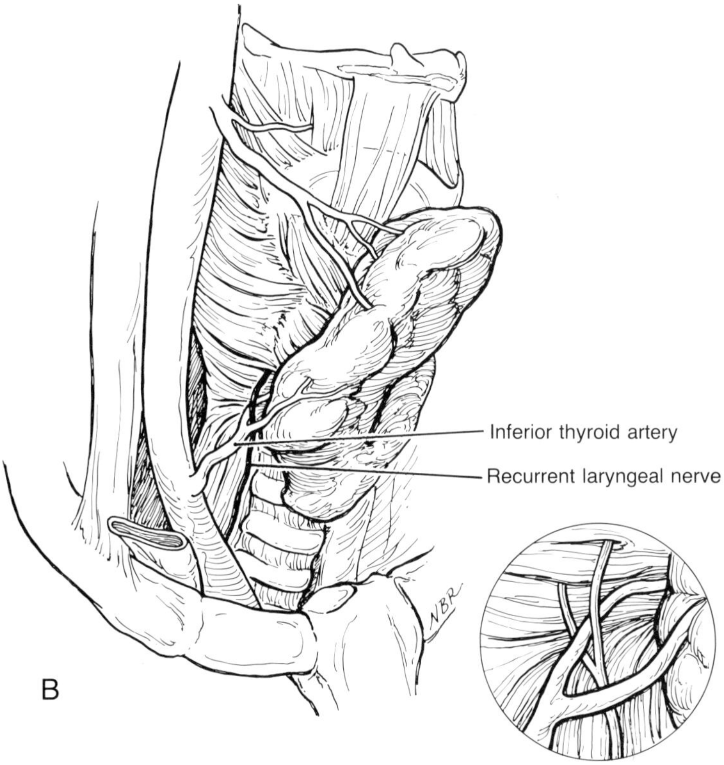

Figure 6–15. Relationship of the recurrent laryngeal nerves in *(A)* the extraglandular course and *(B)* the intraglandular course.

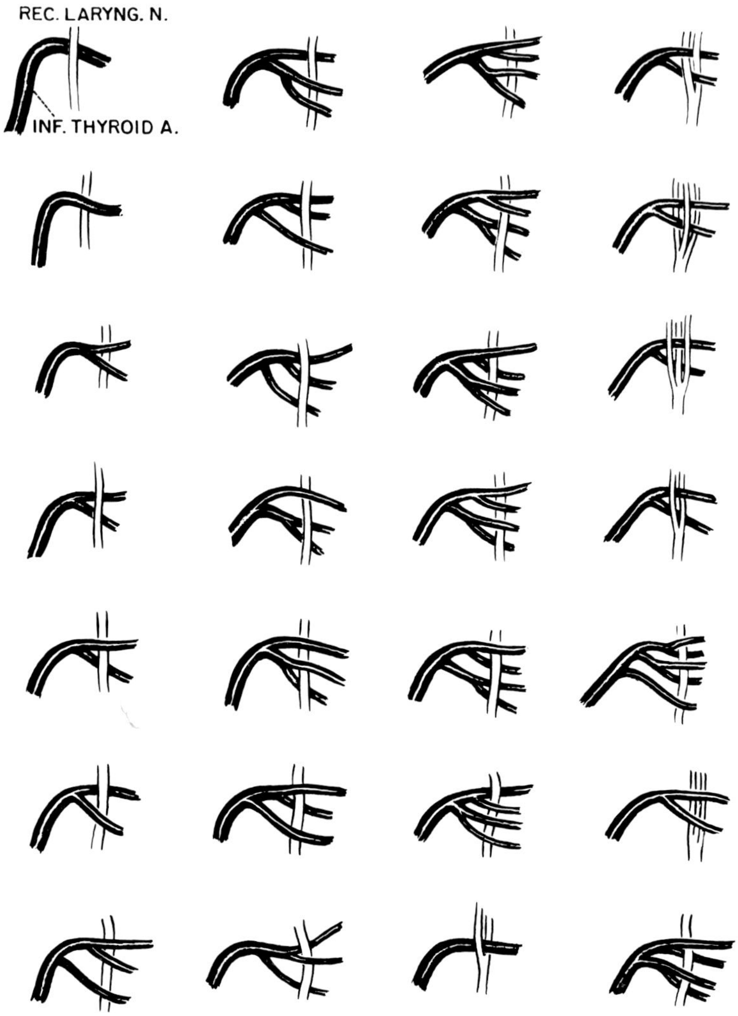

Figure 6–16. Anatomic variations of the course of the recurrent laryngeal nerve in relationship to the inferior thyroid artery. (From Sedgwick CE, Bookwalter JR: Thyroid tumors. *In* Sedgwick CE (ed): Surgery of the Thyroid Gland. Philadelphia, WB Saunders, 1974.)

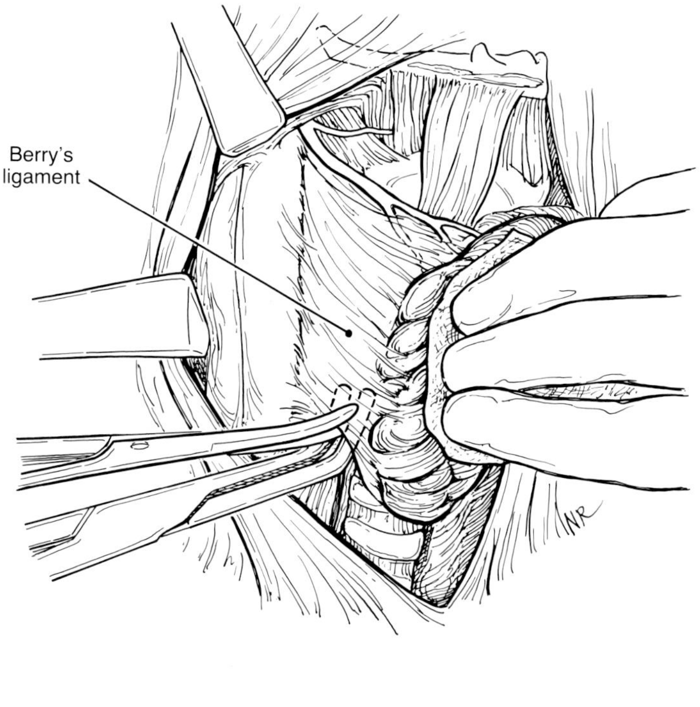

Figure 6–17. Dissection of Berry's ligament, with preservation of the recurrent laryngeal nerve.

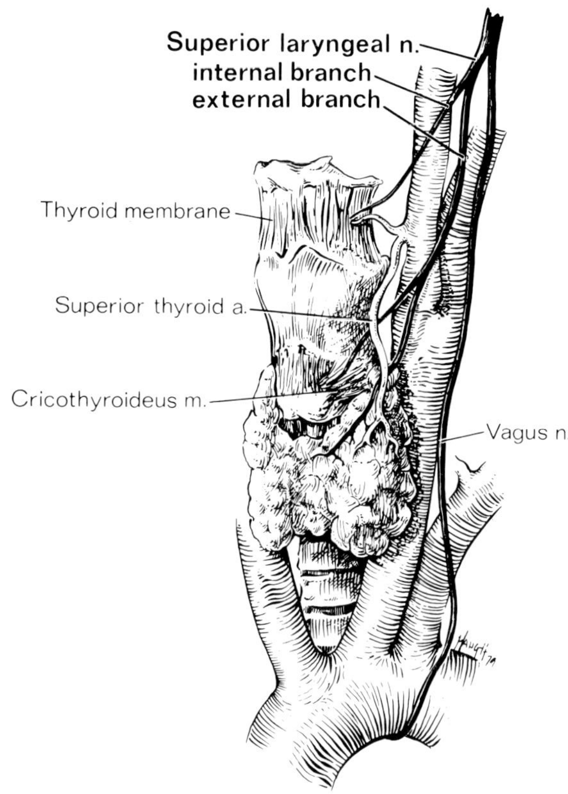

Figure 6–18. Relationship of the superior laryngeal nerve to the superior pole of the thyroid gland. (From Caldarelli DD, Holinger LD: Complications and sequelae of thyroid surgery. Otolaryngol Clin North Am 13:93, 1980.)

attenuation, and indeed such an attenuation or thyroid lingula may reach and even wrap around this nerve. The superior thyroid artery and vein should be ligated close to the glandular tissue of the upper pole. If a lingula is present, the superior laryngeal nerve is isolated and the external laryngeal nerve dissected free from the vessel and gland. Usually, careful isolation of the vessels in the ligament close to the gland with identification of the external nerve until the area of the cricothyroid muscle is past will keep these neural structures safe.

In the body of the gland, careful attention should be paid to the position of the carotid sheath. If the tumor is large, the internal jugular vein may be adherent to it. Inadvertent incision of the vein can be prevented if, following dissection of the inferior and superior poles, the middle thyroid vein is identified and ligated.

Parathyroid Glands. A careful search for the parathyroid glands is an important step in total thyroidectomy. Hypoparathyroidism is one of the most difficult of medical management problems. However, in malignant disease, especially medullary or undifferentiated cancer, preservation of these vital glands may be impossible because of tumor invasion by direct extension. Fortunately, in a high percentage of individuals the parathyroids are in an extrathyroid location. It has been estimated that in most people two thirds of the glands are in the neck, with most of the remainder located in the upper mediastinum. Although the usual number of glands is four, 33 per cent of individuals have more (usually 5 or 6).[75] The location of the two superior glands is fairly constant, usually on the posteromedial surface of the superior pole. Although they are often positioned close to the superior thyroid artery, they are usually supplied by the inferior. Dissection in the region of the inferior border of the cricoid to the cricothyroid articulation and up the inferior cornua of the thyroid cartilage will usually reveal the superior parathyroids. The inferior glands are usually found near the inferior pole of the thyroid, but are commonly extraglandular in location. A frequent location is the crossing of the inferior thyroid artery by the recurrent laryngeal nerve, but the gland is usually a little more superficial in location than the nerve. The inferior parathyroids may even be intraglandular, entrapped in a fold of thyroid parenchyma. These glands are also found in the tracheoesophageal area anywhere from the inferior thyroid pole to the pericardium.

If parathyroid preservation can be achieved

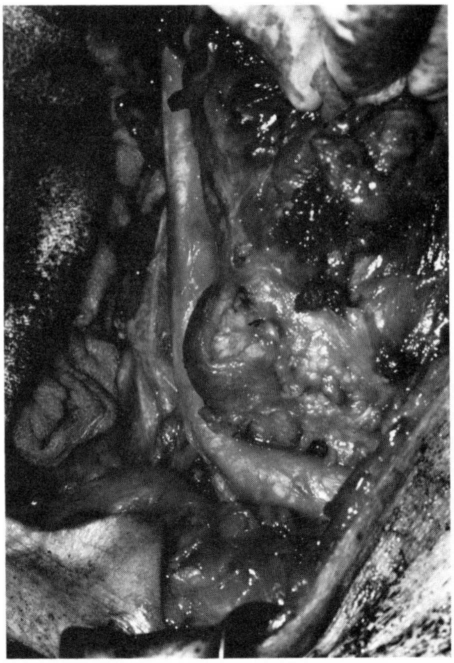

Figure 6–19. Large carcinoma of the thyroid in a 50-year-old man. Tumor displaced the right common carotid artery in the root of the neck.

but the blood supply is in jeopardy, the gland can be prepared and implanted in the sternocleidomastoid muscle or the antecubital fossa as described by Tenta and Keyes.[76] The gland is diced into 2 × 2 × 2 mm pieces, with control under the dissecting microscope if desired. A transverse crease incision is made in the antecubital fossa. Parallel furrows are cut in the flexor and pronator muscles in the forearm, and the diced parathyroid tissue is implanted. Parathyroid function can be monitored by taking serial calcium levels.

Mediastinal Resection. Resection of the thyroid gland for cancer requires removal of all adjacent lymph node and loose connective tissue. The lymphatic tissue is directly adjacent to the thyroid and drains laterally to the internal jugular chain as well as to the nodes of the pharyngoesophagus and mediastinum. Most of this tissue, even that of the upper mediastinum, can be readily dissected from a cervical approach. Figure 6–19 shows a 56-year-old man with a large papillary carcinoma of the thyroid with bilateral cervical metastases. The tumor pushed the right common carotid artery aside and hugged the brachiocephalic trunk. Complete resection was possible through a transcervical approach. No palpable adenopathy was apparent in the mediastinum, which was also negative on CT scanning.

Tumor occasionally descends into the mediastinum, and adequate resection is possible only with a trans-sternal approach (Fig. 6–20). Unlike resections for squamous cell carcinomas of the upper aerodigestive tract, the trans-sternal approach for thyroid cancer does not require removal of bone. Although mediastinotomy might appear to be radical treatment for a disease with an often somewhat benign course, it must be remembered that thyroid cancer kills.[77] Moreover, those

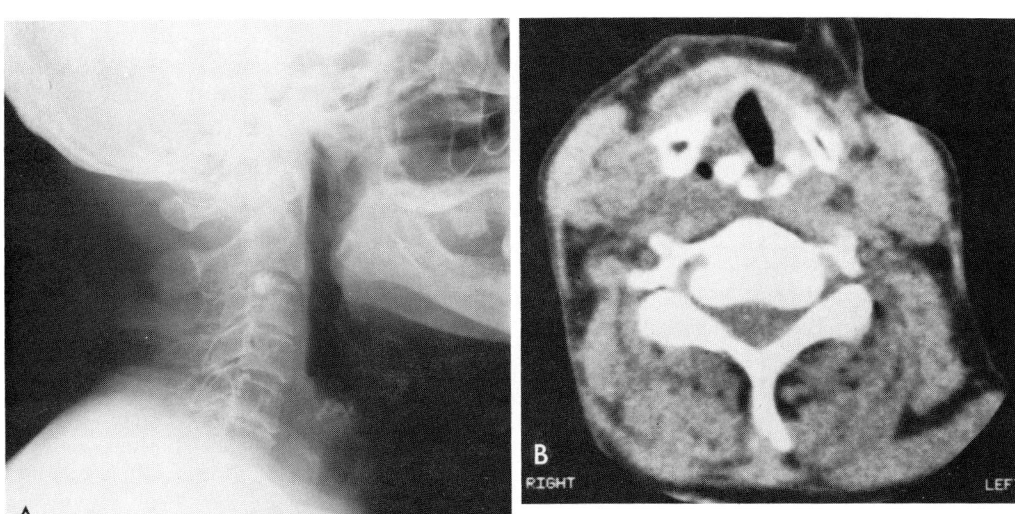

Figure 6–20. Large undifferentiated carcinoma of the thyroid gland in an elderly woman, causing erosion of the larynx and severe airway obstruction. *A,* Lateral soft tissue x-ray showing invasion of the larynx and trachea. *B,* CAT scan showing erosion of the thyroid cartilage and soft tissue swelling into the laryngeal lumen.

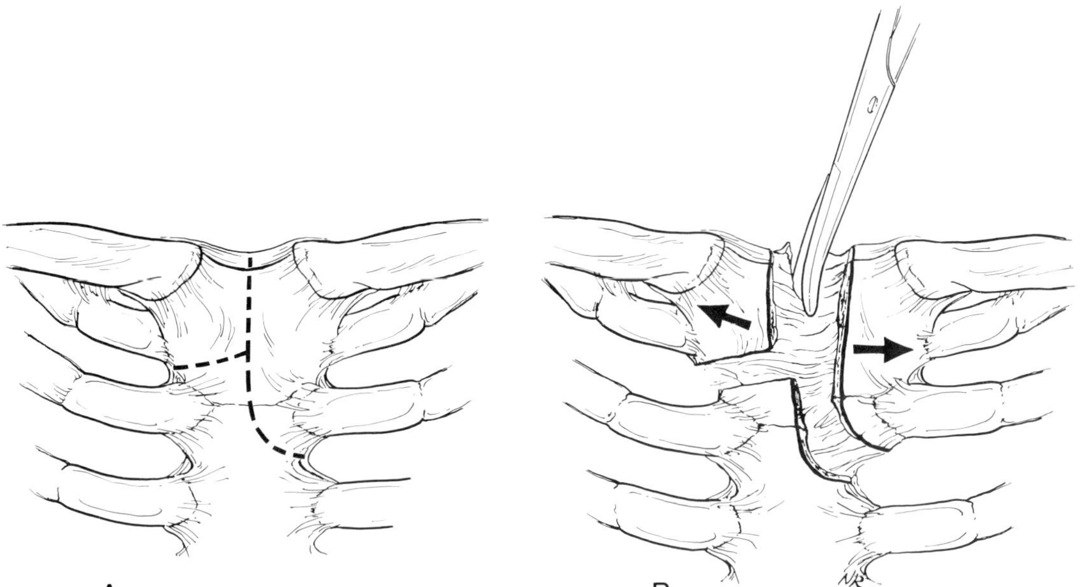

Figure 6–21. *A,* Sternal split outlined. *B,* Thick protective periosteum on the deep surface of the manubrium being incised.

who die often do so as a direct result of extensive local disease.[78]

The skin incision is in the midline, bisecting the collar incision and descending over the upper third of the sternum (Fig. 6–13*B*). Soft tissue is incised down to the sternal periosteum. The tough fibrous tissue band that stretches over the rostral surface of the manubrium and extends onto its deep surface forms a protective sheet for the underlying structures during the sternal osteotomy. Careful finger dissection between the manubrium and this fascia will permit insertion of a ribbon retractor to protect the underlying soft tissue. A periosteal elevator is used to clear a track for the sternal split as outlined in Figure 6–21. A single angled cut with a Striker saw into the second interspace may

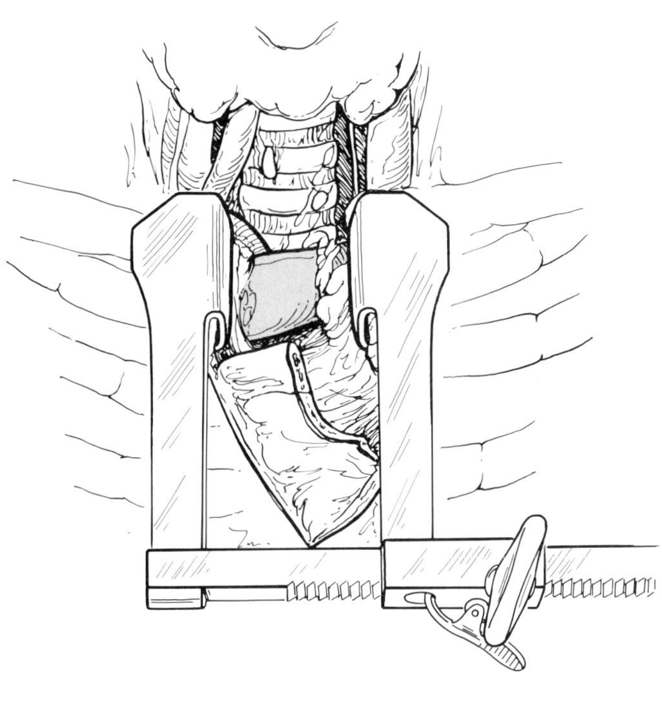

Figure 6–22. The pediatric sternal retractor is inserted and the mediastinal contents are exposed. Note how the left innominate vein obscures a complete view of the mediastinal structures.

be sufficient; however, a second relaxation osteotomy into the first interspace facilitates retraction and enhances the exposure. The heavy protective retromanubrial fascia can now be cut and the sternotomy opened with a self-retaining retractor such as a pediatric Finochietto.

The contents of the upper anterior mediastinum are now well visualized (Fig. 6–22). Care must be exercised to avoid the pleural reflections that form the lateral boundaries to the space. The principal features obvious at this juncture are direct thyroid extension of tumor, the thymus, and lymphatic and loose connective tissue. The somewhat amorphous thymus gland is dissected free of the vascular twigs that supply and drain it, with care taken to ensure hemostasis. As recommended by Loré,[67] dissection should proceed from right to left, over the superior vena cava and the left innominate vein (Fig. 6–23). The left innominate vein crosses the mediastinal space, and if tumor extensions or involved lymphatics course deep to the innominate, it may be ligated (Fig. 6–24). This also facilitates dissection around the aorta. Care must be taken to avoid damaging the recurrent laryngeal nerve at this level as it courses around the ligamentum arteriosum. The entire dissection can be done in continuity with the cervical block, and the tissue is now all removed.

After implantation of the parathyroid tissue, the sternum is closed with braided nonabsorbable suture or wire and threaded through drill holes (Fig. 6–25). A soft drain is placed in the mediastinum and the wound closed.

CASE I. Figure 6–26 shows an ^{131}I scan of the thyroid of a 25-year-old man who 6 years before had a neck node determined by biopsy to be follicular carcinoma. No further diagnostic or therapeutic steps were taken by his practitioner. On presentation the patient had multiple nodules in his right neck, including one in the right submandibular triangle. His trachea was markedly deviated to the left, and the thyroid gland itself was huge. Figure 6–27 is a computerized body scan showing mediastinal extension of tumor. Because tumor invaded the sternocleidomastoid muscle and the wall of the internal jugular vein, a radical neck dissection was done with sparing of the spinal accessory nerve (Fig. 6–28). A median sternotomy enabled the excision of a large projection of tumor (Fig. 6–29). The thymus and adjacent lymph nodes were removed (Fig. 6–30).

The patient was discharged on the seventh postoperative day. Follow-up treatment with ^{131}I was done and the patient is well 2 years after treatment.

CASE II. The elderly woman depicted radiographically in Figure 6–20 had an undifferentiated thyroid cancer that was locally very aggressive but was without symptoms, signs, or laboratory evidence of metastatic disease at the time of presentation. Extrinsic pressure on the esophageal lumen and erosion of the larynx rendered the patient severely dysphagic and caused considerable airway obstruction. Through a median sternotomy (Figs. 6–30, 6–31) complete extirpation of tumor was possible. A total laryngectomy was necessary, but lack of esophageal extension allowed sparing of

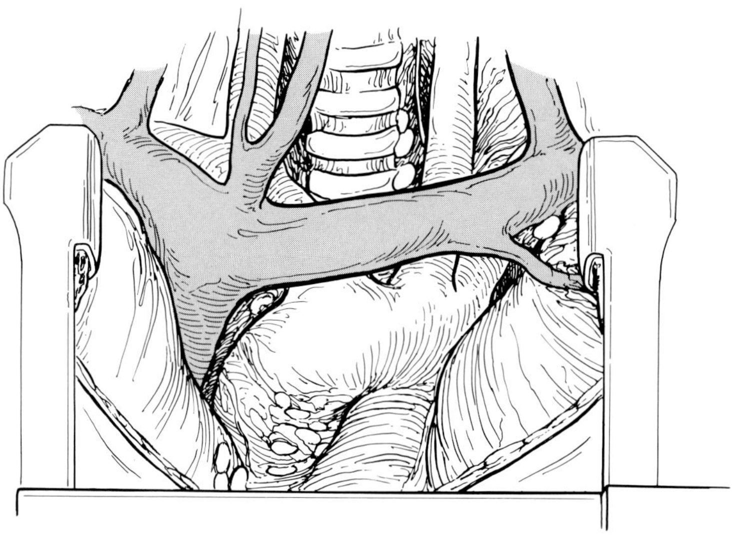

Figure 6–23. Mediastinal exposure to the level of the aorta. The left innominate vein is exposed from the superior vena cava to the takeoff of the left jugular vein. Illustration reveals more exposure than is usually apparent.

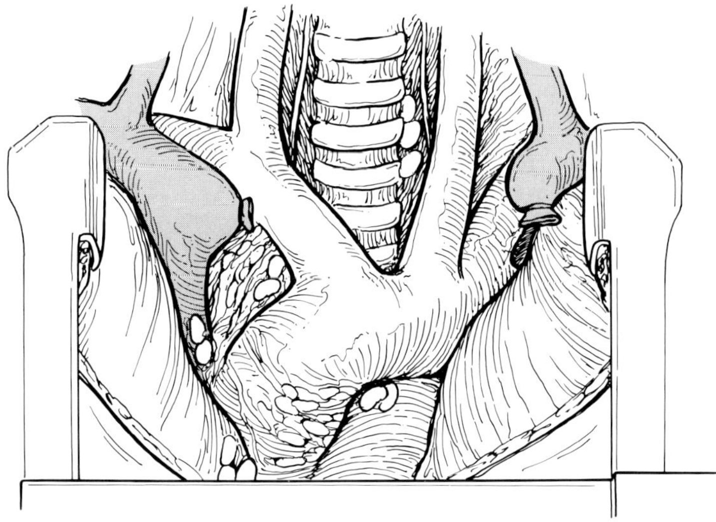

Figure 6–24. The left innominate vein is carefully ligated with silk stick-ties and incised; the rest of the anterior mediastinum is now exposed.

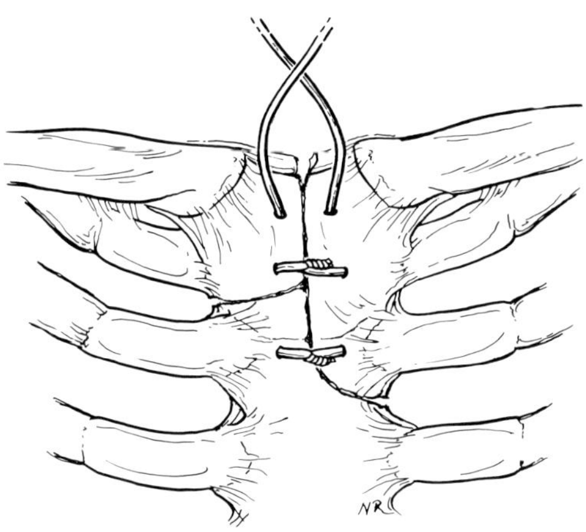

Figure 6–25. Sternotomy closed with braided wire.

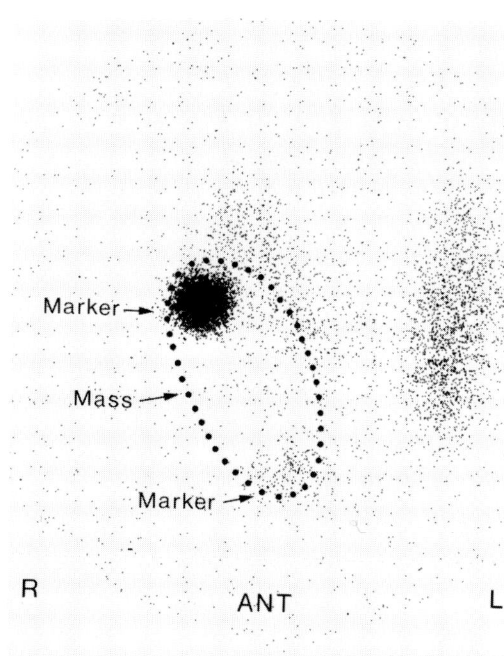

Figure 6–26. ^{131}I scan of a 25-year-old man with a large follicular carcinoma in the right lobe of the thyroid gland. Encircled area represents the tumor.

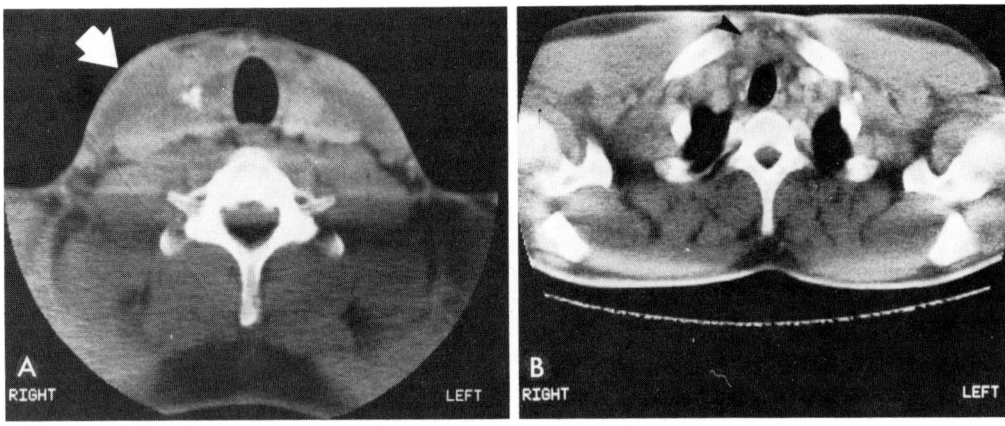

Figure 6–27. *A,* CAT scan showing large cervical metastasis *(arrow)* from thyroid carcinoma shown in Figure 6–26. *B,* CAT scan of upper mediastinum showing thyroid tumor extension into its superior aspect.

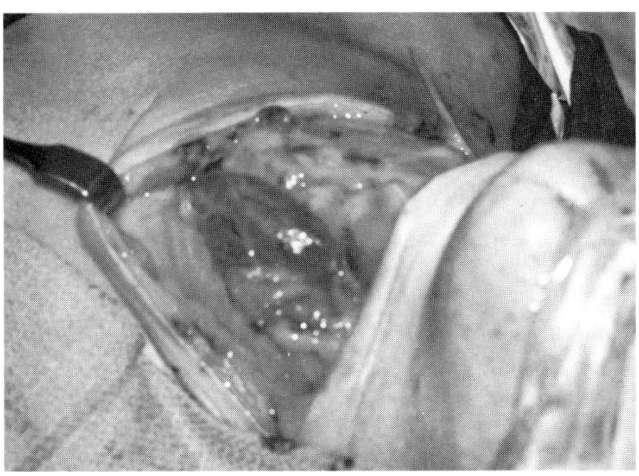

Figure 6–28. Large follicular carcinoma of patient in Figures 6–26 and 6–27.

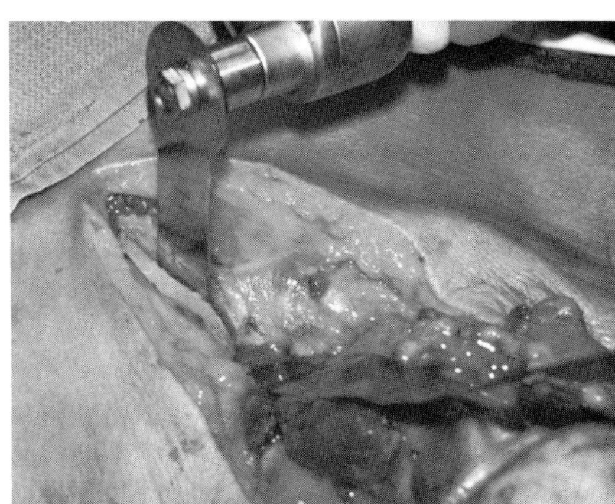

Figure 6–29. Median sternotomy done with oscillating saw. Note the large flat malleable retractor inserted between the underlying thick manubrial periosteum and the bone, protecting the underlying vessels from the saw blade. (See also Chapter 3, Fig. 3–36.)

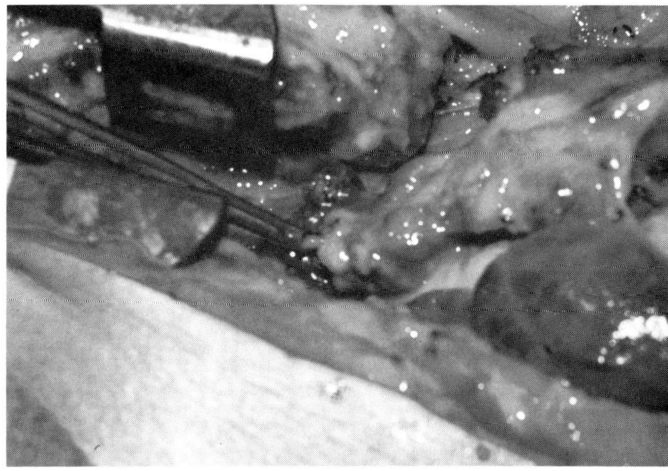

Figure 6–30. Mediastinal extension of large thyroid tumor.

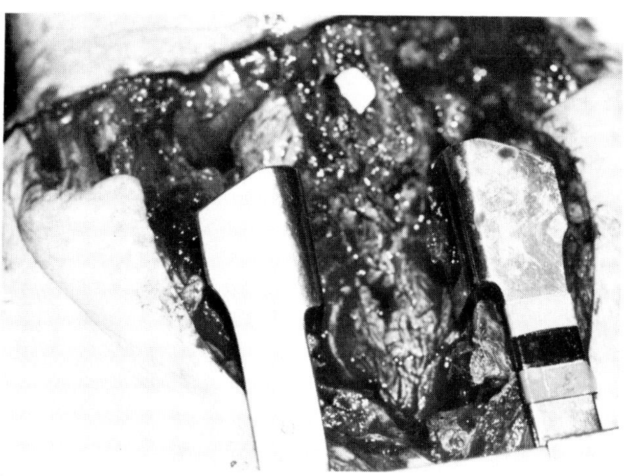

Figure 6–31. Operative photograph of woman whose tumor is depicted radiographically in Figure 6–20. Sternal split has been done, giving excellent access to tumor extension in the mediastinum.

the food conduit. She was discharged 3½ weeks postoperatively, but succumbed to pulmonary metastases 1 year later. Although a rather radical procedure was done, it provided excellent palliation, allowing her full ambulation and normal swallowing until shortly before her death.

References

1. National Cancer Institute: Information for physicians on irradiation-related thyroid cancer. Cancer 26:150, 1976.
2. Meissner WA, Warren S: Tumors of the thyroid gland. Fascicle 4, Atlas of Tumor Pathology, 2nd ed. Washington DC, Armed Forces Institute of Pathology, 1969, pp 57, 60, 72–73.
3. Lacher AB, Stucker FJ, Kirokawa RH: Management of the thyroid nodule. Otolaryngol Clin North Am 13:59, 1980.
4. Sampson RJ, Woolner LB, Rahn RC, et al: Occult thyroid carcinoma in Olmsted County, Minnesota: prevalence at autopsy compared with that in Hiroshima and Nagasaki, Japan. Cancer 34:2072, 1974.
5. Crocker DW: Thyroid carcinoma. Surgery 73:671, 1973.
6. Djalilian M, Beahrs OH, Devine KD, et al: Intraluminal involvement of the larynx and trachea by thyroid cancer. Am J Surg 128:500, 1974.
7. Geissinger WT, Horsley JS, Parker, FP, et al: Carcinoma of the thyroid. Ann Surg 179:734, 1974.
8. Ibanez ML, Russell WO, Saavedra JA, et al: Thyroid carcinoma—biological behavior and mortality. Cancer 19:1039, 1966.
9. Shelly WB, Beerman H, Enterline HT: Metastatic thyroid carcinoma. JAMA 226:173, 1973.
10. Silverberg SG, Hutler RVP, Foote FW Jr: Fatal carcinoma of the thyroid. Histology, metastases, and causes of death. Cancer 25:792, 1970.
11. Sutton JP, McSevain B, Diveley WL: Carcinoma of the thyroid. Ann Surg 167:839, 1968.
12. Carroll RE, Haddon W Jr, Handy VH, et al: Thyroid cancer: cohort analysis of increasing incidence in New York State, 1941–1962. JNCI 33:277, 1964.
13. Mazzaferri EL, Young RL, Oertel JE, et al: Papillary thyroid carcinoma: the impact of therapy in 576 patients. Medicine 56:171, 1977.
14. Favus MJ, Schneider AB, Stachura ME, et al: Thyroid cancer occurring as a late consequence of

head-and-neck irradiation. Evaluation of 1056 patients. N Engl J Med 294:1019, 1976.
15. Sommers SC: Thyroid gland. *In* Anderson WAD (ed): Pathology, Vol 2, 6th ed. St. Louis, CV Mosby, 1971, p 1431.
16. Becker SP, Skolnik EM, O'Neill JN: The nodular thyroid. Otolaryngol Clin North Am 13:53, 1980.
17. Clark LR, Cole VW, Fuller LM, et al: Thyroid. *In* Fletcher GH, McComb WS (eds): Cancer of the Head and Neck. Baltimore, Williams & Wilkins, 1967, p 293.
18. Cole WH, Slaughter DP, Rossiter LJ: Potential dangers of nontoxic nodular goiter. JAMA 127:883, 1945.
19. Veith FJ, Brooks JR, Grigsby WP, et al: The nodular thyroid gland and cancer. A practical approach to the problem. N Engl J Med 270:431, 1964.
20. Meissner WA, Adler A: Papillary carcinoma of the thyroid: a study of the pathology of 225 cases. Arch Pathol 66:518, 1958.
21. Olen E, Klinck GH: Hyperthyroidism and thyroid cancer. Arch Pathol 81:531, 1966.
22. Wegelin C: Malignant disease of the thyroid gland and its relation to goiter in man and animals. Cancer Rev, 3:297, 1928.
23. Hirabayashi RN, Lindsay S: The relation of thyroid carcinoma and chronic thyroiditis. Surg Gynecol Obstet 121:243, 1965.
24. Silverberg SG, Vidone RA: Metastatic tumors in the thyroid. Pacific Med Surg 74:175, 1966.
25. Shimaoka K, Takeuchi S, Pickren IW: Carcinoma of the thyroid associated with other primary malignant tumors. Cancer 20:1000, 1967.
26. Russell WV, Ibanez ML, Clark RL et al: Thyroid carcinoma: classification, intraglandular dissemination and clinicopathological study based upon whole organ sections of 80 glands. Cancer 16:1425, 1963.
27. Batsakis JG, Nishigama RH, Rich CR: Microlithiasis (calcospherites) and carcinoma of the thyroid gland. Arch Pathol 69:493, 1960.
28. Klinck GH, Winship T: Psammoma bodies and thyroid cancer. Cancer 12:656, 1959.
29. Block MA, Wylie JH, Patton RB, et al: Does benign thyroid tissue occur in the lateral part of the neck? Am J Surg 112:476, 1966.
30. Nicastri AD, Foote FW Jr, Frazell EL: Benign thyroid inclusions in cervical lymph nodes. JAMA 194:113, 1965.
31. Roth LM: Inclusions of non-neoplastic thyroid tissue within cervical lymph nodes. Cancer 18:105, 1965.
32. Toomey JM: Cysts and tumors of the pharynx. *In* Paparella MM, Shumrick DA (eds): Otolaryngology, Vol 3, 2nd ed. Philadelphia, WB Saunders, 1980, p 2323.
33. Sedgwick CE, Bookwalter JR: Thyroid tumors. *In* Sedgwick CE (ed): Surgery of the Thyroid Gland. Vol XV in Major Problems in Clinical Surgery. Philadelphia, WB Saunders, 1974, p 133.
34. Frazell EL, Foote FW Jr: Papillary cancer of the thyroid: a review of 25 years of experience. Cancer 11:895, 1958.
35. Warren S: The significance of invasion of blood vessels in adenomas of the thyroid gland. Arch Pathol 11:255, 1931.
36. Buckwalter JA, Thomas CG Jr: Selection of surgical treatment for well differentiated thyroid carcinomas. Ann Surg 176:565, 1972.
37. Sutton JP, McSwain B, Diveley WL: Carcinoma of the thyroid. Ann Surg 167:839, 1968.
38. Hirabayashi RN, Lindsay S: Carcinoma of the thyroid gland: a statistical study of 390 patients. J Clin Endocrinol 21:1596, 1961.
39. Beahrs OH, Pasternak BM: Cancer of the thyroid gland. Curr Probl Surg 3:1, 1967.
40. Freeman D, Lindsay S: Medullary carcinoma of the thyroid gland. Arch Pathol 80:575, 1965.
41. Hazard JB, Hawk WA, Crile G Jr: Medullary (solid) carcinoma; a clinicopathological entity. J Clin Endocrinol 19:152, 1959.
42. Williams ED, Brown CL, Doniach L: Pathological and clinical findings in a series of 67 cases of medullary carcinoma of the thyroid. J Clin Pathol 19:103, 1966.
43. Block MA, Horn RC, Miller JM, et al: Familial medullary cancer of the thyroid. Ann Surg 166:403, 1967.
43a. Ljungberg O, Cederquist E, von Studnitz W: Medullary thyroid carcinoma and pheochromocytoma: a familial chromaffinomatosis. Br Med J 1:279, 1967.
44. Potts JT: Medullary carcinoma of the thyroid and calcitonin. *In* Thorn GW, Adams RD, Braunwald E, et al (eds): Harrison's Principles of Internal Medicine, 8th ed. New York, McGraw-Hill, 1977, p 2026.
45. Wells SA Jr, Ontjes DA, Cooper CW, et al: The early diagnosis of medullary carcinoma of the thyroid gland in patients with multiple endocrine neoplasia type II. Ann Surg 182:362, 1975.
46. Woolner LB, Beahrs OH, Black BM, et al (eds): Thyroid Neoplasia: Proceedings of the Second Imperial Cancer Research Fund Symposium, London, April 1967. London/New York, Academic Press, 1968.
47. Aldinger KA, Samaan NA, Ibanez M: Anaplastic carcinoma of the thyroid. Cancer 41:2267, 1978.
48. Lore JM, Marchetta F, Conley JJ: Thyroid cancer update. Meeting of American Academy of Otolaryngology—Head and Neck Surgery, September 1982, New Orleans.
49. Hoffman GL, Thanson NW, Heffron C: The solitary thyroid nodule. Arch Surg 105:379, 1972.
50. Mustacchi P, Cutler SJ: Some observations on the incidence of thyroid cancer in the United States. N Engl J Med 255:889, 1956.
51. Winship T, Rosvall RV: A study of thyroid cancer in children. Amer J Surg 102:747, 1961.
52. Raventos A, Winship T: The latent period for thyroid cancer following irradiation. Radiology 83:501, 1964.
53. Fitzgerald PJ: I^{131} concentration and thyroid morphology in the thyroid. *In* The Thyroid. Upton (New York) Biology Department. Brookhaven National Laboratory Symposia in Biology, Number 7, 1954, p 220.
54. Becker FO, Economou PG, Schwartz TB: The occurrence of carcinoma in "hot" thyroid nodules: report of 2 cases. Ann Intern Med 58:877, 1963.
55. Dische S: The radioisotope scan applied to the detection of carcinoma in thyroid swellings. Cancer 17:473, 1964.
56. Meadows PM: Scintillation scanning in the management of the clinically single thyroid nodule. JAMA 177:229, 1961.
57. Stucker FJ, Lacher AB, Kirokawa RH: The grand biopsy for the "cold" thyroid nodule. Laryngoscope 89:1425, 1979.
58. Baim JM, Walfish PG: The assessment of thyroid function and structure. Otolaryngol Clin North Am 11:419, 1978.
59. Hill CS Jr, Ibanez ML, Samaan NA, et al: Medullary

(solid) carcinoma of the thyroid gland: an analysis of the M.D. Anderson Hospital experience with patients with the tumor, its special features and its histogenesis. Medicine 52:141, 1973.
60. Tollefsen HR, Shah JP, Huvos AG: Follicular carcinoma of the thyroid. Am J Surg 125:523, 1973.
61. Sisson GA, Feldman DE: The management of thyroid carcinoma metastatic to the neck and mediastinum. Otolaryngol Clin North Am 13:119, 1980.
62. Black BM, YaDeau RE, Wollner LB: Surgical treatment of thyroidal carcinomas. A study of 885 cases observed in a 30-year period. Arch Surg 88:610, 1964.
63. Gordon PR, Huvos AG, Strong EW: Medullary carcinoma of the thyroid gland. Cancer 31:915, 1973.
64. Millburn L, Ameen D: The place of ionizing radiation in the treatment of thyroid carcinoma. Otolaryngol Clin North Am 13:109, 1980.
65. Crile G Jr, Hawk WA: Carcinomas of the thyroid. *In* Anderson R, Hoopes JE (eds): Symposium on Malignancies of Head and Neck. St. Louis, CV Mosby, 1975, p 153.
66. Freund HR: Principles of Head and Neck Surgery, 2nd ed. New York, Appleton-Century-Crofts, 1979, p 322.
67. Loré JM Jr: An Atlas of Head and Neck Surgery, Vol II, 2nd ed. Philadelphia, WB Saunders, 1973, p 620.
68. Sedgwick CE (ed): Surgery of the Thyroid Gland. Philadelphia, WB Saunders, 1974, p 170.
69. Hunt PS: A reappraisal of the surgical anatomy of the thyroid and parathyroid glands. Br J Surg 55:63, 1968.
70. Beahrs OH: Complications of surgery of the head and neck. Surg Clin North Am 57:823, 1977.
71. Sedgwick CE: Surgical techniques. *In* Sedgwick CE (ed): Surgery of the Thyroid Gland. Philadelphia, WB Saunders, 1974, p 133.
72. Loré JM Jr, Duck JK, Elias S: Preservation of the laryngeal nerves during total thyroid lobectomy. Ann Otolaryngol 86:777, 1977.
73. Berry J: Suspensory ligaments of the thyroid gland. Proc Anat Soc Gr Brit Ireland, 1887, p 4.
74. Loré JM Jr, Surgery of the thyroid gland. Otol Clin North Am 13:69, 1980.
75. Goss CM (ed): Gray's Anatomy, 23rd ed. Philadelphia, Lea & Febiger, 1973, p 1345.
76. Tenta LT, Keyes GR: Transcervical parathyroidectomy with microsurgical autotransplantation and the viscerovertebral angle. Otolaryngol Clin North Am 13:169, 1980.
77. Beierwaltes WH: The treatment of thyroid carcinoma with radioactive iodine. Semin Nucl Med 8:79, 1978.
78. Silliphant WM, Klinik GH, Levitin MS: Thyroid carcinoma and death. Cancer 17:513, 1964.

7

EAR AND TEMPORAL BONE

Paul J. Donald, M.D.

Malignant tumors of the ear range from small lesions that can be adequately handled by desiccation and curettage to lesions involving the temporal bone proper that require a full temporal bone resection, the most formidable operative procedure that challenges the head and neck surgeon. Unfortunately, inadequate treatment of what initially seems to be an innocuous "skin tumor" of the pinna too often leads to the need for this dangerous extensive resection. In the last decade or two, there has been considerable reevaluation of what was previously considered to be optimal therapy for lesions of both the auricle and the temporal bone. Standard resection techniques for removal of basal cell and squamous cell cancers primary to the auricle have been shown to be highly ineffective in comparison with Moh's chemosurgery technique.[1, 2] Unfortunately, Moh's technique is still not widely used for lesions, principally because of the dearth of centers possessing the dermatologic and histopathologic expertise it requires. Thus in most regions, conventional surgical technique is still the standard choice of therapy.

The treatment of lesions involving the temporal bone has undergone quite a transition in the last 2 to 3 decades. Until the early 1950's the standard treatment for temporal bone cancer was irradiation therapy, radical mastoidectomy, or occasionally a combination of both. Cure rates were dismal, and a pessimism that in some quarters persists today pervaded any consideration of management. Thanks to the pioneering work of Campbell[3] and Parsons and Lewis,[4] however, the combined extracranial-intracranial approach to the temporal bone is now standard and, together with advances in anesthesia and intensive care management, has greatly enhanced patient survival.

PATHOLOGY

Basal and Squamous Cell Carcinomas. By far the most common malignant neoplasms of the periauricular area, pinna, external auditory canal, and middle ear are basal cell and squamous cell cancers (Table 7–1). In Bumstead's series of 71 auricular malignancies, 40 were basal cell and 29 were squamous cell cancers.[1] In his review of the literature describing 780 malignancies of this site, 746 were either basal or squamous cell tumors, with 40 per cent being basal cell and 55 per cent squamous cell, an almost even distribution. On the other hand, in Conley's series of 100 cancers of the external auditory canal, middle ear, and mastoid, 67 per cent were squamous cell and less than 10 per cent were basal cell tumors.[6] Of 100 patients followed for 5 years, Lewis[5] reported 86 per cent with squamous cell and only 8 per cent with basal cell carcinoma.

Later Lewis[17] in describing 150 of his own cases found that 60 per cent of these tumors originated in the auricle, 28 per cent in the external auditory canal, and 12 per cent in the middle ear and mastoid. To emphasize that he had a skewed distribution of cases he

Table 7–1. INCIDENCE AND TYPE OF EAR MALIGNANCIES*

Histologic Diagnosis	*No. of Cases (%)*
Epithelial Tumors	
Squamous cell carcinoma	
External auditory canal	24
Auricle	17
Total	41 (45)
Neuroepithelial tumors	
Paraganglioma	14
Melanocytic nevus	2
Malignant melanoma	1
Total	17 (18)
Glandular Tumors	
Adenoma	4
Pleomorphic adenoma (mixed tumor)	2
Adenoid cystic carcinoma	2
Low-grade adenocarcinoma	2
High-grade adenocarcinoma	3
Total	13 (14)
Basal cell carcinoma	
Auricle	3
External and auditory canal	1
Total	4 (4)
Mesenchymal Tumors	
Benign	
Osteoma	5
Chondroma	1
Lipoma	1
Hemangioma	1
Total	8 (9)
Malignant	
Rhabdomyosarcoma	6
Total	6 (7)
Other Tumors	
Meningioma	3
Total	3 (3)
Total	*92 (100)*

*Adapted from Chen KTR, Dehner LP: Primary tumors of the external and middle ear. Arch Otolaryngol 104:247, 1978.

quotes Broders who, drawing from a more general patient population and less of a tertiary referral setting, reported that 84 per cent of his auricular and temporal bone tumors originated in the auricle. In Conley's series,[7] 69 per cent of the tumors originated in the pinna, 22 per cent in the external auditory canal, and 9 per cent in the middle ear and mastoid (Fig. 7–1).

The basal cell tumors vary considerably in their malignant potential. The morphea-type lesions are most resistant to therapy, one of the major problems being the difficulty in achieving tumor-free margins in the surgical specimen. Recurrent lesions are similarly difficult to adequately resect. These basal cell tumors of the auricle are so often diagnosed in the early stages that they are often regarded casually. Desiccation and curettage, shave excision and other ultraconservative methods are so often successful that many physicians can hardly believe that what was formerly an innocuous appearing little "skin cancer" has now become an invasive life-threatening malignancy. Once basal cell cancers assume a more aggressive demeanor they freely invade bone and adjacent periauricular soft tissue.

Squamous cell tumors, like basal cell lesions, are usually seen in a background of solar skin damage. The surrounding pinna commonly demonstrates multiple scaling and roughened and pigmented areas in a thin atrophic skin. Squamous cancers are most commonly seen in the helix and postauricular area.[7] The lesion itself is usually ulcerated and indurated with a peripheral area of erythema. In a series by Chen & Dehner[8] of 92 malignancies of the ear, the 17 squamous cell cancers of the pinna had associated periauricular lymphadenopathy when the primary lesion was ulcerated and erythematous. The lymph node was cancerous, however, in only one instance. Histologically there is a dense chronic inflammatory response. When auricular cartilage invasion occurs, cervical lymph node metastases are much more common.[8]

Both squamous cell and basal cell cancers show a propensity to spread along the perichondrium of the auricle. Bailin et al[9] showed that pre- and postauricular cancers tend to spread toward the ear itself. They also discovered that helical tumors spread both above and below along the helix, then proceed anteriorly to the antihelix as well as posteriorly to the retroauricular area. Antihelical lesions, on the other hand, show a more concentric pattern of spread. Ceilley et al[10] have shown that these tumors tend to follow embryologic fusion lines, especially extending along the lines of fusion of the 1st and 2nd, and 1st and 6th auricular hillocks (Fig. 7–2).

Squamous cell cancers made up approximately half of the middle ear and external auditory canal malignancies in the series by Conley et al.[7]

Glandular Neoplasms. Although exceedingly uncommon, malignancies of glandular origin in the external auditory canal and middle ear make up the next largest group of otologic cancers. They represented 12 per cent of the tumors in the series described by

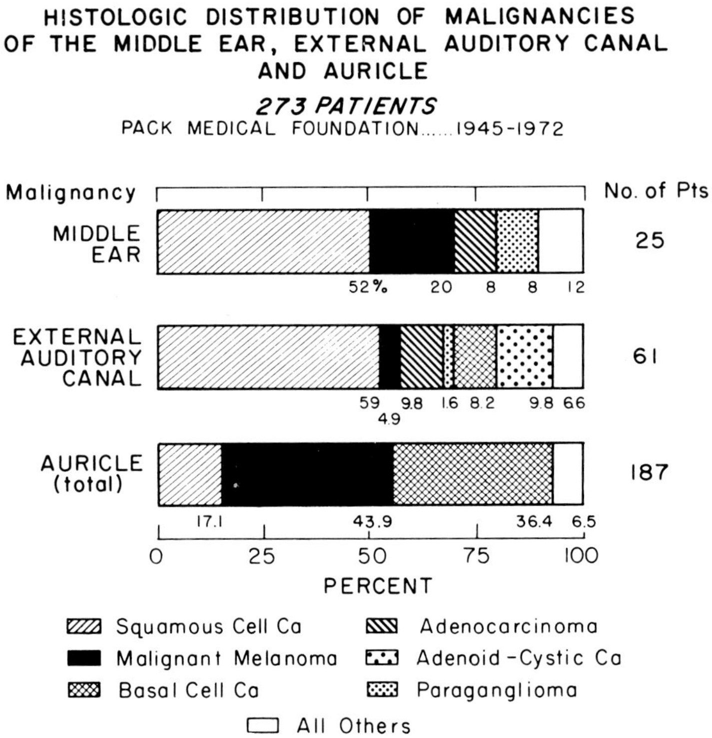

Figure 7–1. Distribution of 273 patients with malignancies of the ear and temporal bone according to histologic diagnosis. (From Conley J, Schuller DE: Malignancies of the ear. Laryngoscope 86:1147, 1976.)

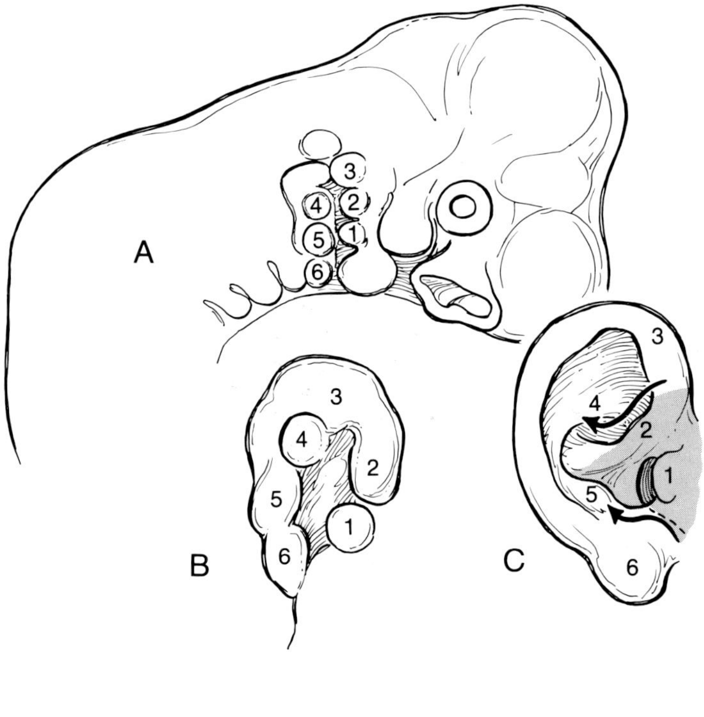

Figure 7–2. Basal cell tumors of the auricle tend to spread along the fusion lines of the 1st and 2nd and 1st and 6th embryologic hillocks.

Chen et al.[8] These neoplasms presumably originate in either the ceruminous glands of the external auditory canal or the glandular elements of the middle ear mucosa.

An excellent review by Pulec[11] divides the glandular neoplasms of the external auditory canal into four types (Table 7–2). These rare tumors are often lumped under the common appellation "ceruminoma." The adenoma is the benign variant whose cells resemble the double-layered epithelial configuration of normal ceruminous glands with an inner columnar eosinophilic layer and an outer myoepithelial layer. The adenoid cystic cancer is unfortunately the most common malignancy of these glands, but overall is distinctly rare. By 1977, only 58 cases[11] had been reported in the world literature, the old-fashioned cylindromatous type with a "Swiss cheese" histologic pattern being the most common. The tumor has the same malevolent disposition characteristic of its behavior in other body sites. Lymphatic and blood vessel spread to regional and distant sites is common. Frequently there is perineural and perivascular spread, and local recurrence following conservative resection is the rule. The conchal cartilage appears to offer some resistance to invasion, and this tumor seems to creep alongside the cartilage rather than penetrate it. The malignancy is highly radioresistant. Spread through the fissures of Santorini in the cartilaginous external canal to the adjacent parotid gland is common.

Adenocarcinoma of ceruminous gland origin is highly variable in its degree of cellular differentiation. It may be so well differentiated as to completely mimic the adjacent ceruminous glands; only its characteristic of local invasiveness distinguishes it from normal cerumen glands or a benign adenoma.[12] These tumors are very aggressive, with rapid local invasiveness being characteristic. Metastatic disease is uncommon, and patients usually succumb to cerebral extension. Adenocarcinoma of the middle ear, however, has its origin in the glandular epithelium lining the cavity rather than in the cerumen glands.

Table 7–2. HISTOLOGIC ANALYSIS OF 37 TUMORS OF GLANDULAR ORIGIN.*

Cell Type	*No. of Cases*
Adenoma	6
Mucoepidermoid carcinoma	2
Adenoid cystic carcinoma	24
Adenocarcinoma	5

*Adapted from Pulec JL: Glandular tumors of the external auditory canal. Laryngoscope 87:1601, 1977.

Mucoepidermoid tumor of the external auditory canal is the most rare, with only two cases reported in the literature. The local invasiveness of this tumor as manifested in the salivary glands is seen in the external canal. Histologically the tumor mimics the salivary lesion, although the canal tumors do not originate in salivary glandular tissue.

Melanotic Lesions. The bulk of malignant melanomas of the ear are found on the pinna; external auditory canal and middle ear lesions are decidedly rare (see Chapter 10). In the series by Conley and Schuller,[7] 9.1 per cent of the melanotic lesions had metastatic nodes in the neck and 4.6 per cent had distant metastases at the time of initial examination. Nonmelanotic lesions were present in 8.1 per cent of the cases. Most lesions in the group were less than 1 cm in size.

Glomus Body Tumors. The glomus body tumor is usually benign, although it will run a course eventuating in death if not adequately treated. These tumors arise in the parenchymal cells of the glomus bodies of the skull base, particularly of the internal jugular vein. Although the latter structure is the most common site of origin, these tumors may also arise from similar bodies on the internal carotid artery, the vagus nerve, and the tympanic plexus.[13] These organs function as chemoreceptors. Their cells are of neural crest origin, are non–chromaffin staining and non–epinephrine secreting in type. They are epithelioid in appearance and cluster around the numerous blood vessels that richly populate the tumor. Glomus tumors slowly enlarge and gradually erode the surrounding bone, which is usually that adjacent to the jugular foramen.

Arteriography reveals a characteristic flush that is caused by the rich blood supply (Fig. 7–3). Retrograde jugular venography commonly demonstrates a lack of filling of the jugular bulb (Fig. 7–4*A*). These two signs are pathognomonic of the disease. Further evaluation by CAT scanning and polytomography of the temporal bone helps to delineate the extent of the neoplasm (Fig. 7–4*B*).

Malignancy is uncommon, being found in only about 10 per cent of cases.[14] Local persistence after inadequate excision should not be construed as a sign of malignancy, but local recurrence after complete excision and/or the presence of metastases does signify malignancy. It is important to remember that

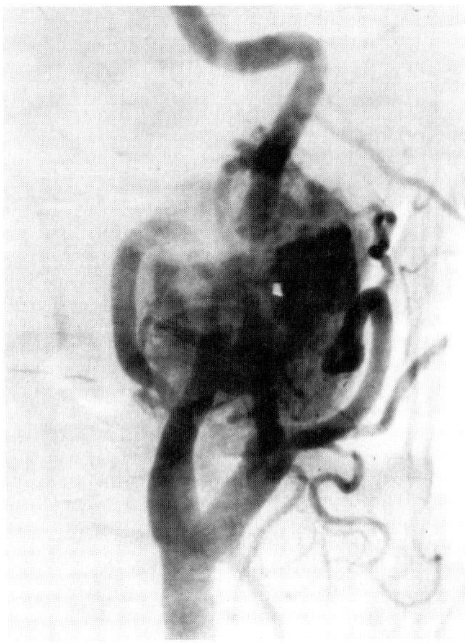

Figure 7–3. Arteriogram showing marked blush of a large glomus jugulare tumor.

the usual histologic criteria of a malignant tumor cannot be applied to these lesions. Even the most blatantly metastasizing ones may show a uniform population of cells with infrequent mitoses, and without pleomorphism or dysplasia.

Sarcomas. These malignancies are rare in the ear and temporal bone. Rhabdomyosarcoma is basically a disease of childhood, and mainly occurs in the first year of life. It begins in the middle ear and mastoid and spreads to both middle and posterior cranial fossae via the internal acoustic canal, usually along the fallopian canal.[15, 16] Local recurrences are the rule, and distant metastatic disease (especially to the lung) is common.[15] Unfortunately, the early, somewhat quiescent period in which the patient presents with only hearing loss may be the only time the tumor may remain within resectable bounds. In Myer's review[15] all patients succumbed to the disease. Lewis[17] states that the most effective treatment is combined radiotherapy and triple agent chemotherapy (see Chapters 11 and 15).

In a series of 211 sarcomas reported on by Naufal[18] in an extensive review spanning 100 years of the literature, the most common sarcoma was an undifferentiated variety composed of cells of either a spindle, round, or anaplastic configuration. The histologic distribution of the remainder is summarized in Table 7–3.

Osteogenic sarcoma may originate in a previous exostosis in a patient with multiple exostoses of the external auditory canal. Chondrosarcoma or chondromyxosarcoma may arise from cartilaginous rests within the petrous bone.

Most patients with sarcomas involving the temporal bone are not initially seen until the disease is massive, with the normal anatomic stucture already replaced by tumor. Management at this stage is difficult. Chemotherapy, especially in combination with irradiation therapy, is usually the treatment of choice.

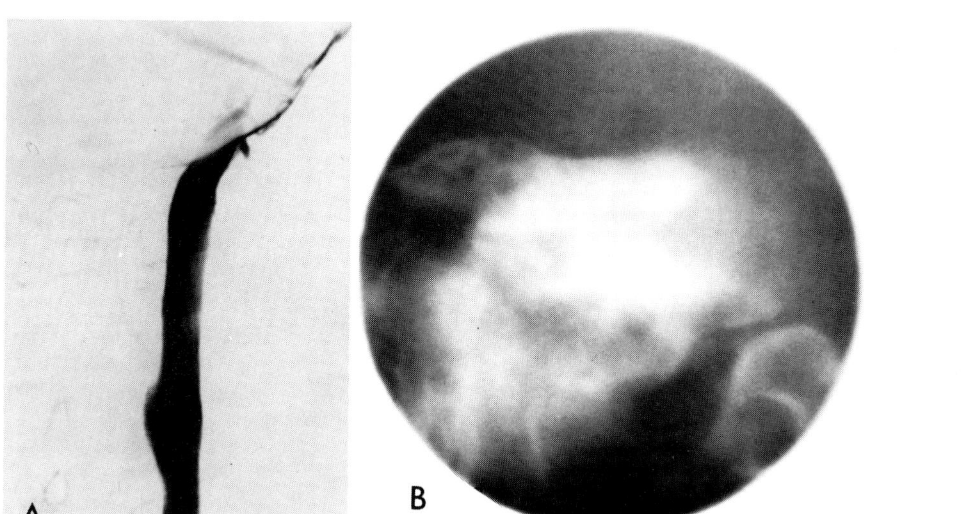

Figure 7–4. *A,* Retrograde jugular venography shows lack of fill of jugular bulb. *B,* Polytomograph showing enlargement of jugular foramen.

Table 7–3. HISTOLOGIC ANALYSIS OF 211 CASES OF PRIMARY SARCOMA OF THE TEMPORAL BONE*

Cell Type	*No. of Cases*
Undifferentiated	89
Rhabdomyosarcoma	64
Fibrosarcoma	17
Osteogenic Sarcoma	12
Ewing's Sarcoma	7
Hemangiosarcoma	8
Reticulum Cell Sarcoma	6
Myxosarcoma	5
Chondrosarcoma	1
Liposarcoma	1
Meningiosarcoma	1

*Adapted from Naufal PE: Primary sarcomas of the temporal bone. Arch Otolaryngol 98:44, 1973.

Small lesions encompassable by temporal bone resection are rarely seen.

SURGICAL MANAGEMENT

Moh's Chemosurgery

A prospective study of 71 basal and squamous cell cancers of the pinna has been done comparing projected resection using standard margins to the actual tumor-free margins using Moh's technique.[19] The standard resection margins used were as follows: for basal cell cancers less than 3 cm in diameter—8 mm; for squamous cell cancers less than 3 cm—10 mm; and for any lesion larger than 3 cm and all recurrent lesions—15 mm. Once the proposed resection was mapped out, the area was measured and then the lesion was excised using Moh's chemosurgery. Employing the histopathologic control of the margins characteristic of Moh's technique, inadequate excision would have occurred in 24 per cent of the lesions (Table 7–4) if conventional surgical resection had been employed. As would be expected, lesions that were larger than 1 cm or were recurrent in nature, or both, showed an increasingly higher incidence of positive margins with the theoretical surgery. Lesions smaller than 1 cm would have had a 13 per cent recurrence rate, and those that were recurrent and larger than 1 cm in diameter, a 33 per cent recurrence rate. On the other hand, if the proposed conventional surgery would have actually successfully removed the tumor, the amount of tissue that would have been unnecessarily excised was estimated to be 180 per cent larger on the average in primary lesions and 347 per cent larger in recurrent cancers (Table 7–5).

Table 7–4. RESULTS OF HYPOTHETICAL CONVENTIONAL EXCISION*

Lesion	*Size (cm)*	*Inadequate Excision (%)*
Primary	<1	13
Recurrent	>1	28
All	<1	13
	>1	33
All	all	24

*From Bumstead RM, Ceilley RL: Auricular malignant neoplasms. Arch Otol 108:226, 1982, Table 1.

In the judgment of those doing the study, the high-risk lesions included all tumors larger than 1 cm in diameter, all morpheaform basal cell carcinomas, and all recurrent neoplasms. The morpheaform basal cell lesion was particularly pernicious because of the high unpredictability of its extent and its propensity to recur within the scar of the initial excision.

Use of Moh's technique was justified in all the cases studied on the basis of a 4 per cent local recurrence rate with a follow-up of 3½ years or longer. All recurrences were nests of cells in discontinuity with the initial primary lesion that developed within the scar of

Table 7–5. COMPARISON OF DEFECT AREA OF MOH'S TECHNIQUE WITH CONVENTIONAL EXCISION* †

Lesion	*Size (cm)*	*% Excess Area Excised‡*	
		Average	*Range*
Primary	< 1	333	35–589
(average, 180; range, 28–589)	>1	78	28–125
Recurrent	< 1	412	79–851
(average, 347; range, 28–1051)	> 1	317	28–1051

*From Bumstead RM, Ceilley RL: Auricular malignant neoplasms. Arch Otol 108:226, 1982, Table 2.
†Only lesions successfully excised by conventional excision were included.
‡Excess area excised is percentage of the area of noninvolved tissue excised by conventional excision in relation to the area of the tissue involved with tumor (area of Moh's defect), which is equal to the area of noninvolved tissue excised divided by the area of Moh's defect.

the initial resection. This cure rate compares favorably to the projected 24 per cent theoretical recurrence rate in these lesions had they been resected by conventional surgical techniques. Recurrence rates with resections quoted in the literature are around 16 per cent.[20, 21, 22] This contrasts with a 47 to 50 per cent recurrence rate when a third and often recommended modality, radiotherapy, is used.[22, 23]

The following case report illustrates the use of the fresh frozen Moh's technique in the removal of a basal cell carcinoma of the auricular concha.

CASE I. A 45-year-old male had been treated over the years for actinic-induced basal cell carcinomas of the facial skin. He presented with a short history of a lesion of the concha with multiple small areas of breakdown (Fig. 7–5). Incisional biopsy revealed basal cell carcinoma. Because of the absence of any clear delineating margin surrounding the tumor, Moh's fresh frozen technique was elected.

In the first resection all visible tumor was excised with a very narrow margin. These margins were marked with India ink and separated into orderly fragments (Fig. 7–6). Close cooperation between surgeon and pathologist is essential at this stage. Care is taken to examine both lateral and deep margins by taking cuts close but parallel to the actual margin of resection. Those areas that were positive for cancer had a further resection done. These were again carefully marked, correctly oriented (Fig. 7–7), and sectioned. A tumor-free margin was established on the third series of resections (Fig. 7–8). The wound was then covered with a split-thickness skin graft held in place with a tie-over bolster and a mastoid dressing (Fig. 7–9). In 2 weeks, the operative site was healed, and the patient has an excellent cosmetic result by virtue of the narrow excision allowed by this technique (Fig. 7–10).

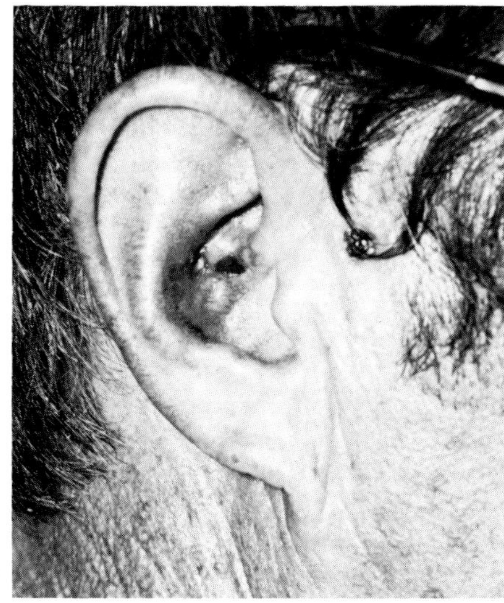

Figure 7–5. Basal cell carcinoma of the auricular concha with indistinct borders.

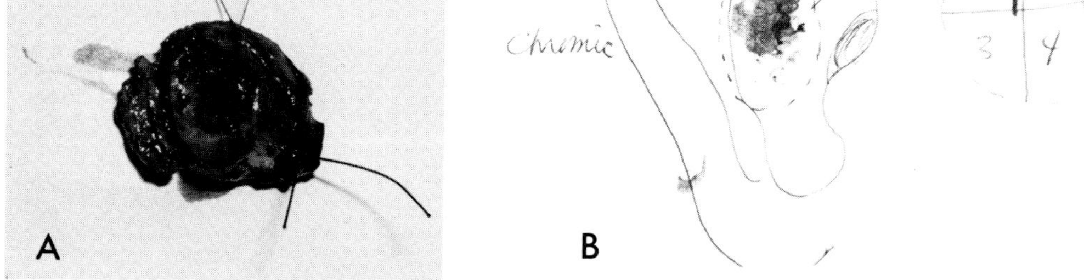

Figure 7–6. Moh's fresh frozen resection technique. *A,* Initial specimen mounted. *B,* Initial specimen with margins marked out. It is vital to transpose margin numbers to the operative site when taking next specimens.

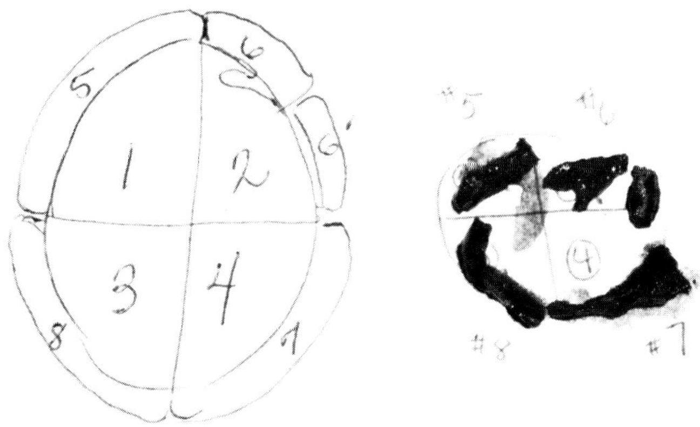

Figure 7–7. Second resection done in areas with positive margins.

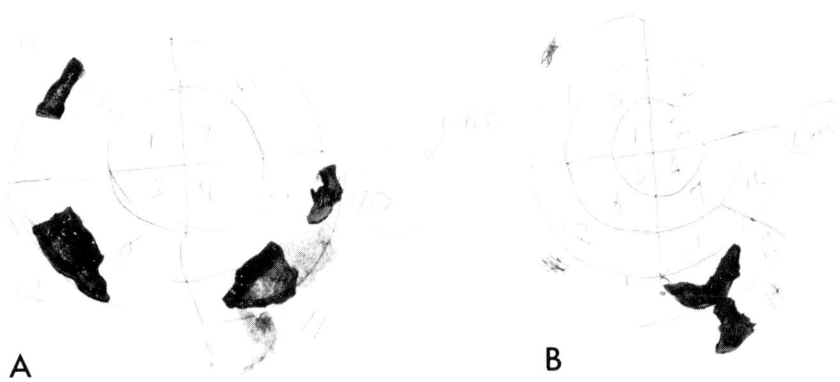

Figure 7–8. *A,* Third resection established negative margins in all but two sites. *B,* Fourth specimen yields final negative margin.

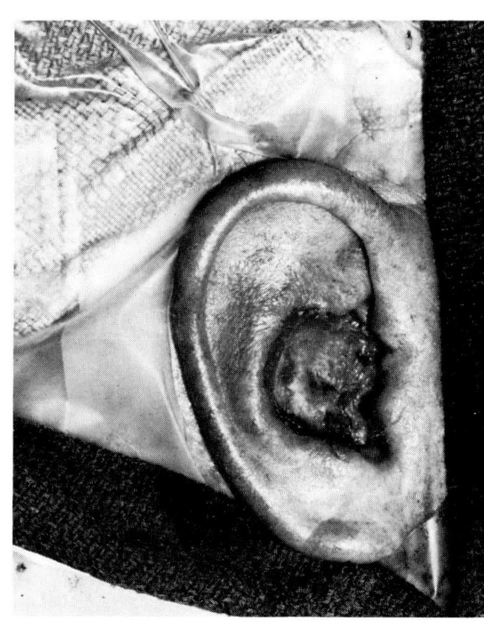

Figure 7–9. Wound prior to coverage with a split-thickness skin graft held in place with a tie-over bolster.

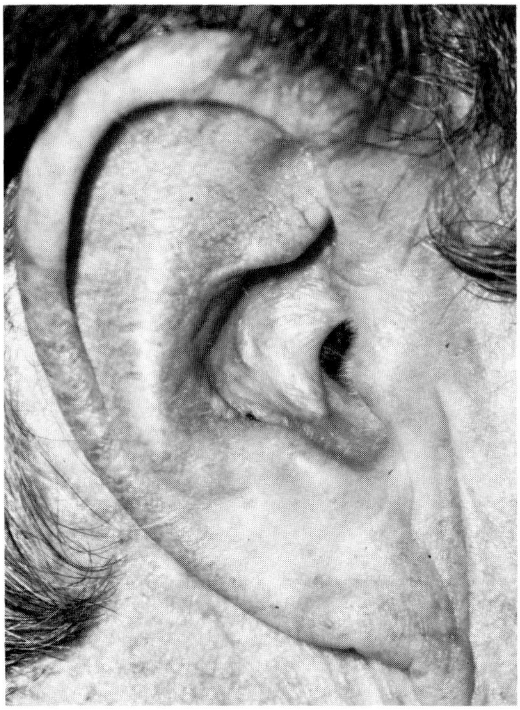

Figure 7–10. Postoperative result.

Temporal Bone Resections

One of the most frighteningly difficult operations for the head and neck surgeon is temporal bone resection. In the early years of this procedure the operative mortality rate was 10 per cent. Thanks to modern anesthesia, sophisticated monitoring equipment, innovations in surgical instrumentation, and the wisdom acquired from the experience of a number of courageous surgeons, this catastrophic figure has become considerably lower. However, the undertaking of temporal bone resection remains a substantial surgical challenge.

Because of the sensitive location of the temporal bone, under the cerebrum and anterior to the cerebellum, surrounded, as Lewis[17] describes, by an interconnecting series of blood-filled lakes, a precise anatomic understanding is essential to this operation (Fig. 7–11). Separation of the bone from these blood-containing channels and judicious protection of the cerebral contents will ensure the safe removal of temporal bone cancers, with an adequate margin yielding a reasonable prognosis for an eventual tumor-free course.

The procedures are divided into: lateral temporal bone resection, total temporal bone resection, and transcervical-transmastoid resection for removal of glomus jugulare and neurogenic tumors.

Lateral Temporal Bone Resection

This procedure is indicated for cancers in the external auditory canal that do not transgress the tympanic annulus. Lewis[17] uses a margin of 5 mm lateral to the tympanic membrane as his limit to lateral resection. Many of these tumors begin in the skin over the conchal cartilage and extend into the external canal. A number of patients have had repeated limited resections of the pinna (Fig. 7–12*A* and *B*) and even total auriculectomy (Fig. 7–13), only to later require temporal bone resection because of surgery that was too conservative.

External canal malignancies either have manifest palpable disease in the parotid gland or have highly probable microscopic extension. The fissures of Santorini in the cartilaginous portion of the canal provide free access for the passage of lymphatic disease directly into the glandular tissue that abuts it. A parotidectomy is mandatory in all cases. The facial nerve trunk and its branches are carefully dissected, sacrificing only those stuck or close to tumor. If either the zygomatic, buccal, or mandibular branches are removed, they are replaced by interposing greater auricular or sural nerve grafts.

Lesions of the conchal skin may penetrate the postauricular skin and be affixed to the periosteum of the mastoid cortex. If there is radiographic evidence of bone erosion, especially close to the middle ear space, total rather than lateral temporal bone resection may be necessary. As long as just the lateral cortex of the mastoid air cell system is involved, a lateral resection will suffice (Fig. 7–14). External auditory canal invasion may proceed anterosuperiorly into the zygomatic root (Fig. 7–15). In these instances, zygomatic resection with excision of the contents of the intratemporal fossa and even underlying skull may be necessary. With both posterior and anterior extension of tumor, often a large skin excision is necessary as well.

The patient is positioned on the table as for a mastoidectomy. The amount of postauricular skin exposure is proportional to the degree of skin involvement. The face of the

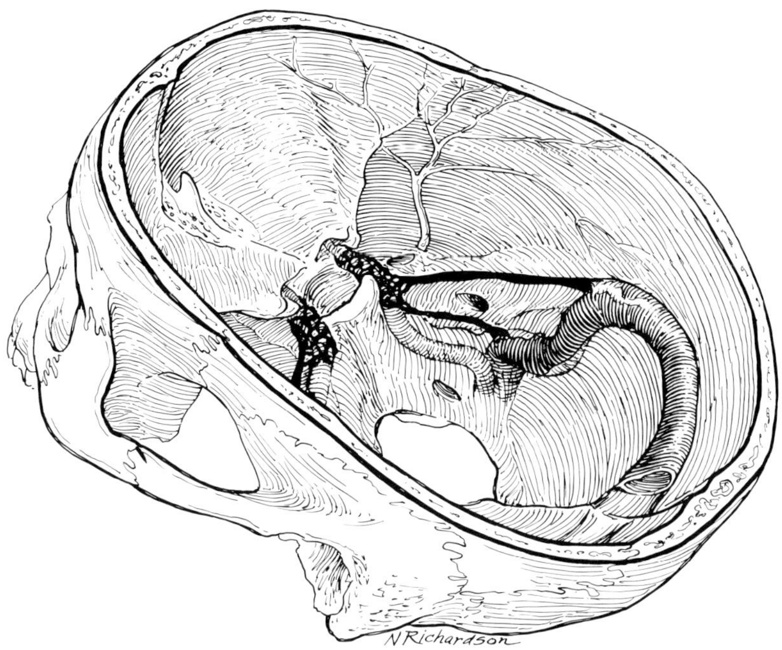

Figure 7–11. Intracranial view depicting the temporal bone encircled by blood-filled "lakes," represented by the internal carotid artery, internal jugular vein, sigmoid sinus, inferior and superior petrosal sinuses, cavernous sinus, and middle meningeal artery.

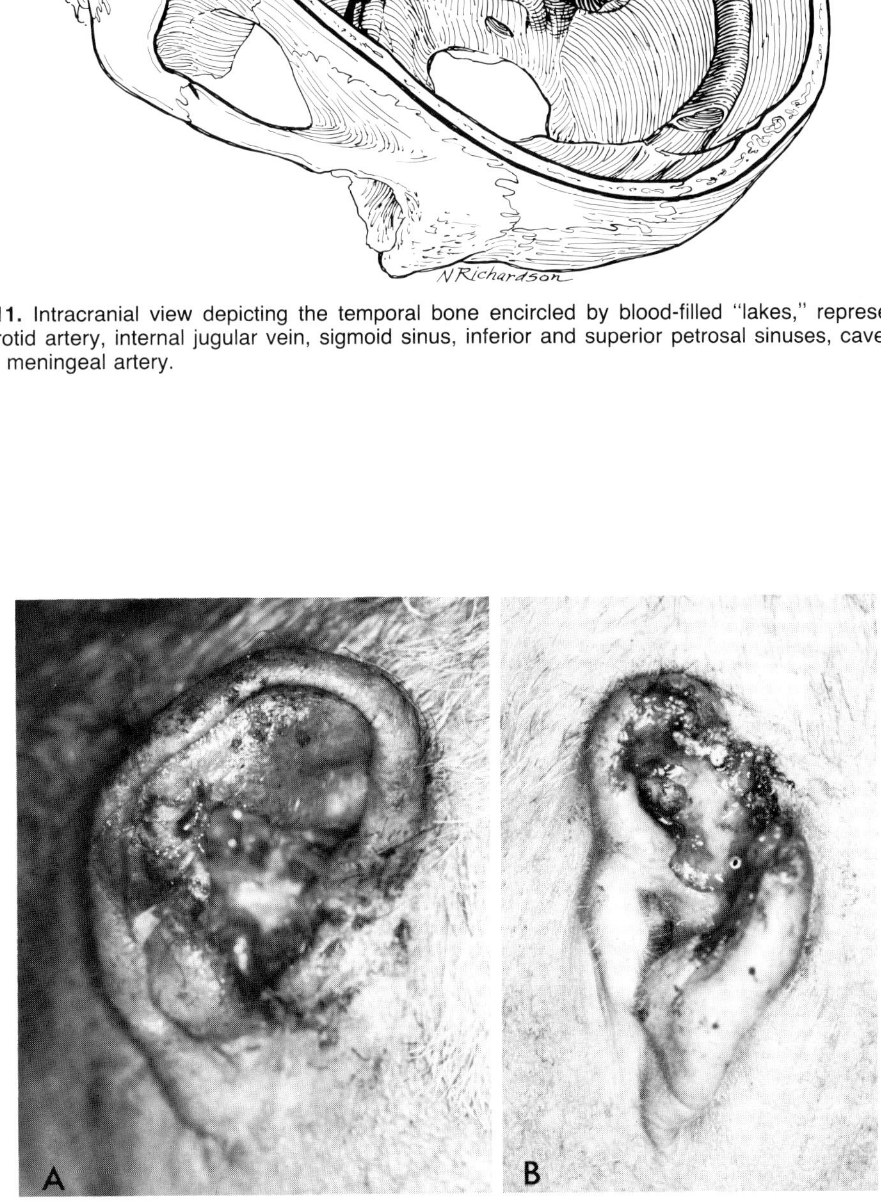

Figure 7–12. *A,* Numerous hyphercations and curettage followed by limited resections of this squamous cell carcinoma of the pinna were ineffective. *B,* Numerous limited resections plus irradiation therapy were insufficient to rid this patient of basal cell carcinoma of the pinna.

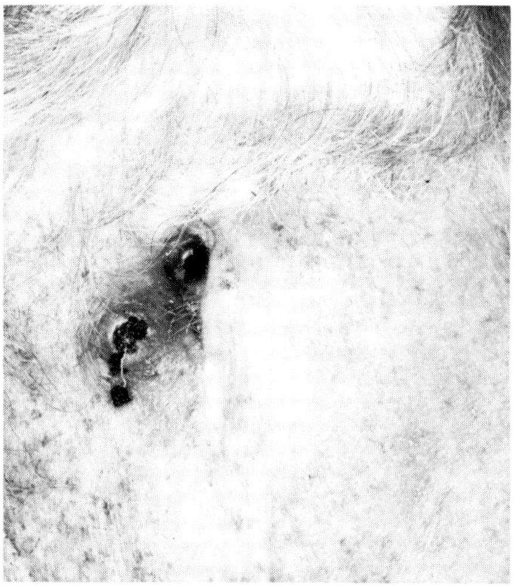

Figure 7–13. Total auriculectomy was done but with an inadequate margin that resulted in a recurrence of squamous cell carcinoma of the premastoid soft tissue.

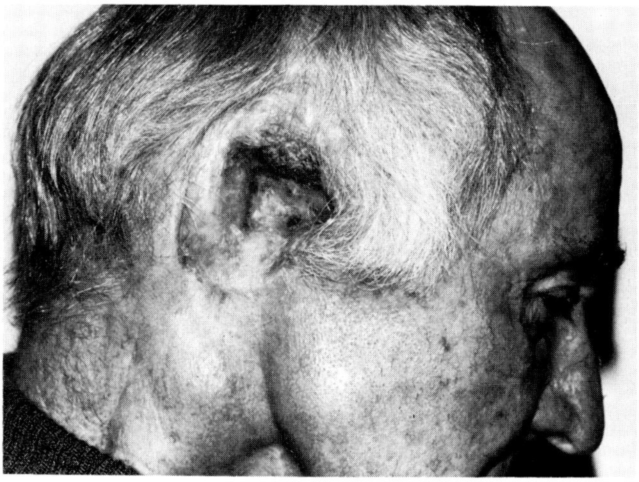

Figure 7–14. Defect following lateral temporal bone resection in patient depicted in Figure 7–12*A*. Split-thickness skin graft used to line defect in order to facilitate early detection of recurrences.

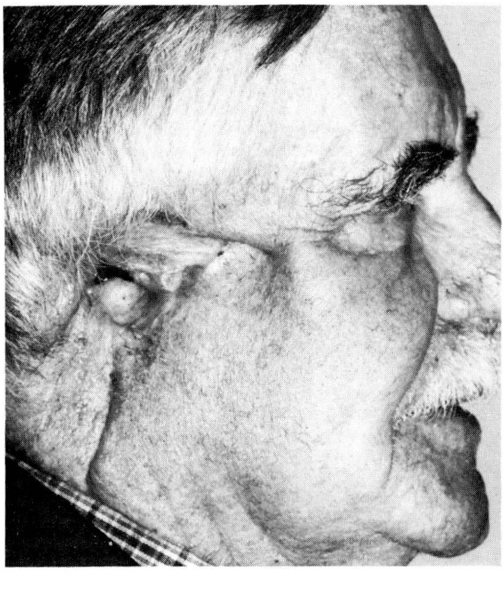

Figure 7–15. Defect following lateral temporal bone resection that included the zygomatic arch, infratemporal fossa, underlying cranium, and dura. Because of intracranial intervention the defect was lined with a scalp flap.

involved side is covered by a transparent "adherent" drape in order to permit visualization of the facial muscles. The region of the squamosal aspect of the temporal bone is sufficiently exposed to accommodate the exigencies of anterosuperior extension. If the eye branch of the facial nerve is to be sacrificed or if the nerve trunk is likely to need resection, a temporary tarsorrhaphy is done prior to the draping.

The excision is again dependent upon the soft tissue extent of the cancer. If the helical rim can be preserved, especially in conjunction with the concha, then it is included in a superiorly based flap. The basic surgical approach combines a mastoidectomy and parotidectomy type incision (Fig. 7–16). The auricular remnant is reflected superiorly. If a radical neck dissection is employed, a lazy S incision is dropped from the inferior limb of the modified Blair incision behind the carotid artery. If an extension posteriorly into the occipital scalp is required to enter the posterior fossa, it can be extended in a gentle looping arc superoposteriorly. If an anterior craniotomy or anterior access to the infratemporal fossa is mandated, an irregular loop into the anterior temporal scalp is made. The cancer itself is circumscribed by an incision that allows the neoplasm and its cutaneous margin to stay with the temporal bone. The auricular remnant can then be reflected superiorly (Fig. 7–17).

The lymph nodes adjacent to the ear are palpated for evidence of metastatic disease. If this is present, a radical neck dissection is

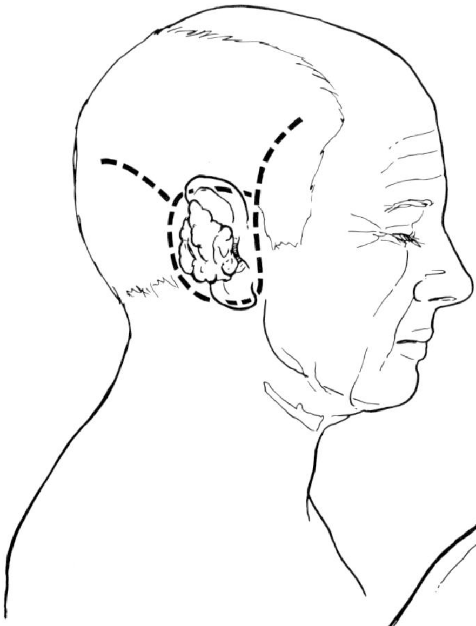

Fig. 7–16

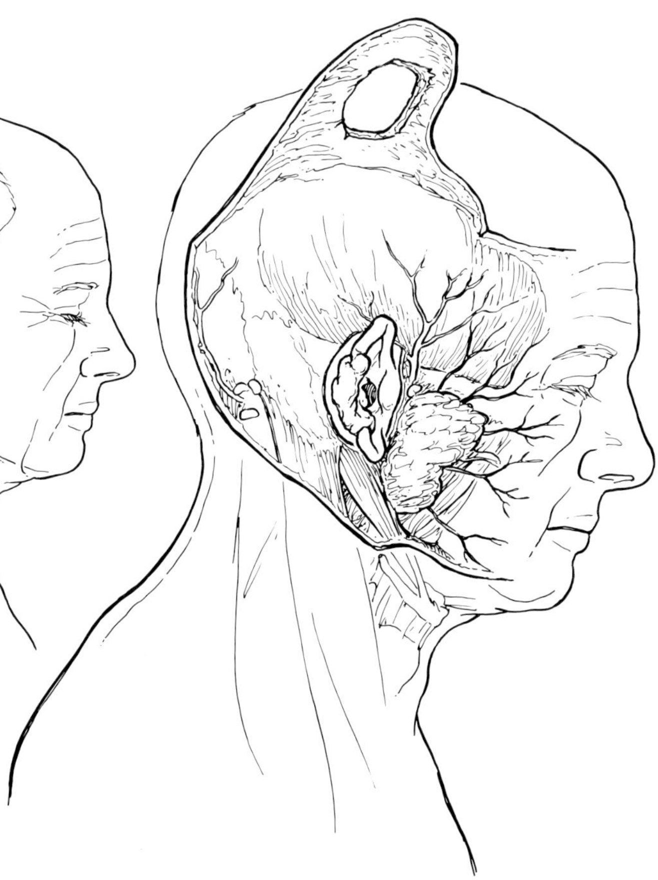

Fig. 7–17

Figure 7–16. Incision for temporal bone resection, with extensions outlined (dashed lines) for exposure of the anterior reaches of the middle cranial fossa, the posterior fossa, and inferiorly if a radical neck dissection is required. In the complete resection the superior limbs usually need to be higher and more extensive than in the lateral operation.

Figure 7–17. Lateral temporal bone resection. The flaps are retracted, and the cutaneous involvement with tumor and an adequate margin of healthy tissue remain with the temporal bone.

done. However, parotidectomy should precede the neck dissection. This sequence allows the parotid dissection to proceed unhindered by the troublesome bleeding that results when the internal jugular vein is tied as part of the radical neck dissection. If during the parotidectomy facial nerve branches are sacrificed, the ends are tagged with silk sutures or clips for nerve grafting later in the operation.

The next step is a complete mastoidectomy. The mastoid portion of the fallopian canal is skeletonized carefully throughout its length, to the stylomastoid foramen. This step is facilitated by meticulously outlining the digastric ridge. The mastoid tip is amputated, and the facial recess is developed and carried inferiorly as far as possible within the bounds of safety imposed by the facial nerve. The deep margin of resection at this point will be the nerve, and the resection skives directly over its lateral aspect. If at any point it becomes obvious that tumor has extended into the mastoid air cell system proper, or if in viewing through the facial recess it is seen to have invaded the middle ear, the lateral resection is abandoned and the operation expanded to a full temporal bone excision. As the lateral procedure continues, an atticotomy is done, with care taken to preserve the ossicular chain when possible. Drilling the lateral attic bone to a thin plate and then excising it with a stapes curette greatly aids in ossicular preservation. As the atticotomy proceeds, obvious tumor extension into the zygomatic root may be found (Fig. 7–18), in which case continued removal of the root and even the arch to the lateral orbital rim may be required (Fig. 7–16). If anything beyond a minimal amount of zygomatic extension is present, it is probably wise at this point to do a mandibular condylectomy. The condylectomy may be done either at this juncture or, if anticipated earlier, following the parotidectomy.

The mandibular condylectomy is performed as follows. The microscope is pushed to the side and an exposure of the temporomandibular joint is done. Keeping the temporal branch of the facial nerve as well as the main trunk in view, the fascia and periosteum over the zygoma is incised with a scalpel in an inverted L configuration. The horizontal portion of this incision should be only about 3 to 4 mm long, to avoid damage to the temporal branch. Further dissection forward is done with a Joseph or similar elevator. The joint capsule is incised and the joint cavity entered. The meniscus is separated from its superior attachment. A cutting bur, Gigli saw, or pneumatic-powered saw is used to cut across the condylar neck. Care is taken as the medial cortical surface is reached. The deep periosteum is not transgressed if at all possible, in order to avoid injury to the internal maxillary artery, which usually lies just deep to the mandibular neck. The condyle is grasped with bone-holding forceps, and the insertion of the lateral pterygoid muscle and the remaining attachments of the sphenomandibular and temporomandibular ligaments are cut close to the bone (Fig. 7–19). With a cutting bur, a fissure is created in the glenoid fossa that will enable the anterior aspect of the external auditory canal wall to be incised just lateral to the tympanic annulus (Fig. 7–20). It is not uncommon to expose middle fossa dura during this maneuver; that is, the dura between the zygomatic root and the tympanic bone that lies inferior to the glenoid fossa. If this occurs, a careful check is made to ensure that no damage has occurred to the middle meningeal artery. If there is extensive tumor involvement in the

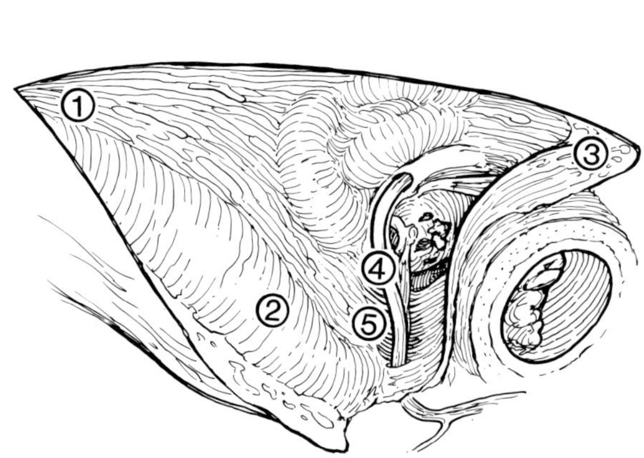

Figure 7–18. Lateral temporal bone resection: Mastoidectomy completed, the facial nerve skeletonized, and the facial recess opened. The atticotomy is proceeding. *1,* Sinodural angle sharply outlined. *2,* Sigmoid plate skeletonized. *3,* Atticotomy. *4,* Facial nerve skeletonized and facial recess opened, revealing no tumor beyond tympanic membrane. *5,* Cerebellar plate skeletonized.

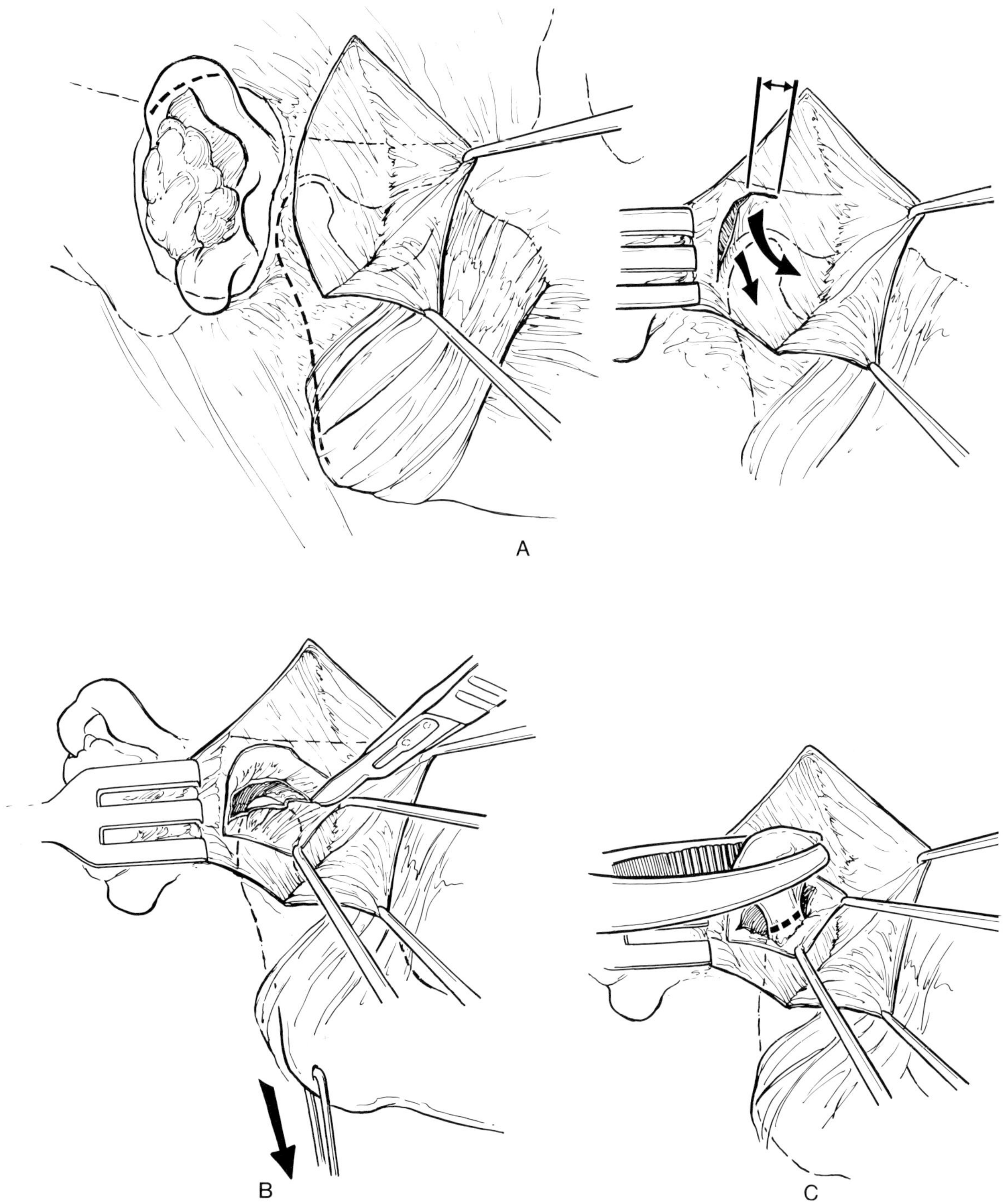

Figure 7–19. Lateral temporal bone resection: Condylectomy. *A,* A short (3 to 4 mm) incision in fascia over the zygomatic root is extended by blunt dissection with the Joseph elevator. *B,* The joint capsule is incised and the joint entered. The dissection is facilitated by downward traction exerted on the angle of the mandible. *C,* A subperiosteal excision of the condyle helps avoid injury to the internal maxillary artery.

zygomatic root, it is necessary to remove not only the zygoma up to the lateral orbital rim but the temporalis muscle and occasionally the skull deep to the infratemporal fossa as well. In the patient shown in Figure 7–15, basal cell carcinoma not only had penetrated the temporal and sphenoidal squama but had also involved the underlying dura (Fig. 7–21).

The last step in the resection is now at hand. The inferior aspect of the resection is delineated with an osteotome. An imaginary line is drawn between the most inferior aspect of the facial recess and its natural extension inferiorly, just lateral to the facial canal and the fissure previously created in the glenoid fossa with the bur. This will take the osteotome across the tympanic bone just lateral to the tympanic annulus (Fig. 7–22). The technique is to tap the osteotome until it is well seated, and then with an alternating tapping and gentle lateral torquing motion drive the instrument in an anterosuperior direction. Usually the bone will fracture just lateral to the annulus. If the break is too far laterally placed, the remaining bone can be removed with the bur. Occasionally the fracture will be too medially located. If so, a careful check is made to ensure the integrity of the facial nerve. The medial course of the osteotome will carry it to the hypotympanum. In this instance, a fascia graft must be placed under the tympanic membrane and beneath the skin graft used to line the cavity.

The specimen is removed and the cavity inspected. Because of the complexity of the specimen and the difficulty the pathologist has in establishing margins, it is vital at this point to check the specimen and relate it to the defect, ensuring the integrity of the resection margins.

The cavity should be lined with split-thickness skin (Fig. 7–14). This enables the physician to accurately follow the patient and pick up any early locally recurrent tumor. It is very tempting to fill the cavity with a flap for the sake of esthetics; however, patient safety should never be sacrificed for this cosmetically laudable but oncologically unsound practice. The exception to this is the patient with a considerable amount of exposed dura or in whom the dura or underlying brain have been resected (Fig. 7–15). A bipedicled or unipedicled flap is used because of its proximity and hair-bearing qualities. For large defects, a deltopectoral or pectoralis major musculocutaneous flap may be used.

Prior to closure, interposition of a facial nerve cable graft is done to replace any of the three critical facial nerve branches that may have been sacrificed. A greater auricular or sural nerve graft is performed under microscopic control. Approximately four to six 10–0 nylon sutures are used in the anastomosis.

The skin graft is bolstered with sponge or mechanics waste. A modified mastoid dressing is applied and changed only when the bandage is soaked. Unless the wound becomes purulent, the bolster is left in place unchanged for 10 days.

Total Temporal Bone Resection

The complete resection can be done entirely by the head and neck surgeon. However, a margin of expertise and safety is added by including a neurologic surgeon in the operative team. This is because while management of the dura and dural sinuses is easy and routine for the neurosurgeon, it often adds unnecessary anxiety to the work of the head and neck surgeon who is "going it alone." The only drawback to having the neurosurgeon along is talking him out of using a static or semifixed headrest. The mobility necessary to do the mastoid portion of the operation is severely impeded by the use of these headrests.

A stepwise plan that is devised preoperatively and followed religiously *during* the procedure is exceedingly helpful. Because the operation is so complex and done so infrequently, the dictum of "doing the operation the night before on paper" is nowhere more important than in complete temporal bone resection. Following an orderly plan will avoid the time-wasting folly of jumping from place to place throughout the large operative field during the procedure.

The operation is divided into eleven steps: (1) incision; (2) parotidectomy; (3) neck dissection (if indicated); (4) mastoidectomy; (5) condylectomy; (6) Anteroinferior exposure; (7) temporal craniotomy; (8) bony cuts; (9) cavity ablation; (10) hypoglossal to facial nerve graft; (11) closure. These are discussed in sequence in the following paragraphs.

1. Incision. The incision is similar to that for lateral temporal bone resection except that both anterior and posterior cranial limbs are carried more superiorly (Fig. 7–16). This is necessary in order to perform the small temporal craniotomy required for the medial bone cut. If the auricle is uninvolved, an incision encircling the extreme lateral aspect of the external auditory canal and the cavum

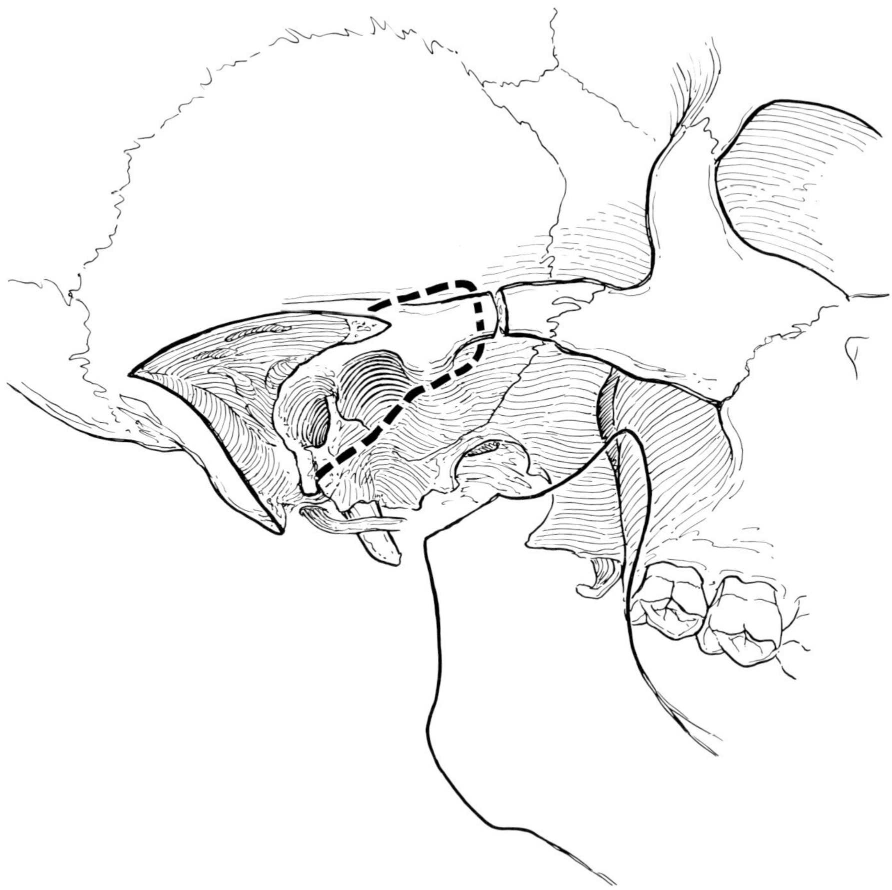

Figure 7–20. Lateral temporal bone resection. A cutting bur incises the zygomatic arch and creates a fissure in the glenoid fossa in order to create a fracture line to enable excision of the bony external auditory canal.

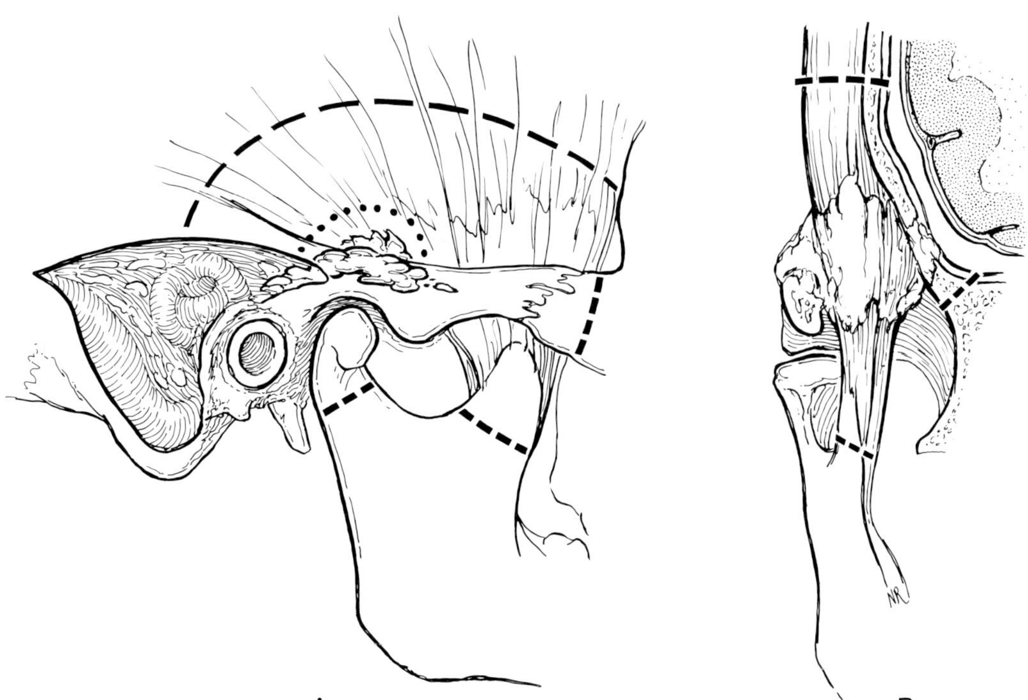

A B

Figure 7–21. Lateral temporal bone resection. *A,* Extension of tumor into the zygomatic root requires excision of the arch up to the lateral orbital rim. The temporalis muscle is excised as well in patient shown in Figure 7–15. *B,* The underlying skull and dura require resection as well.

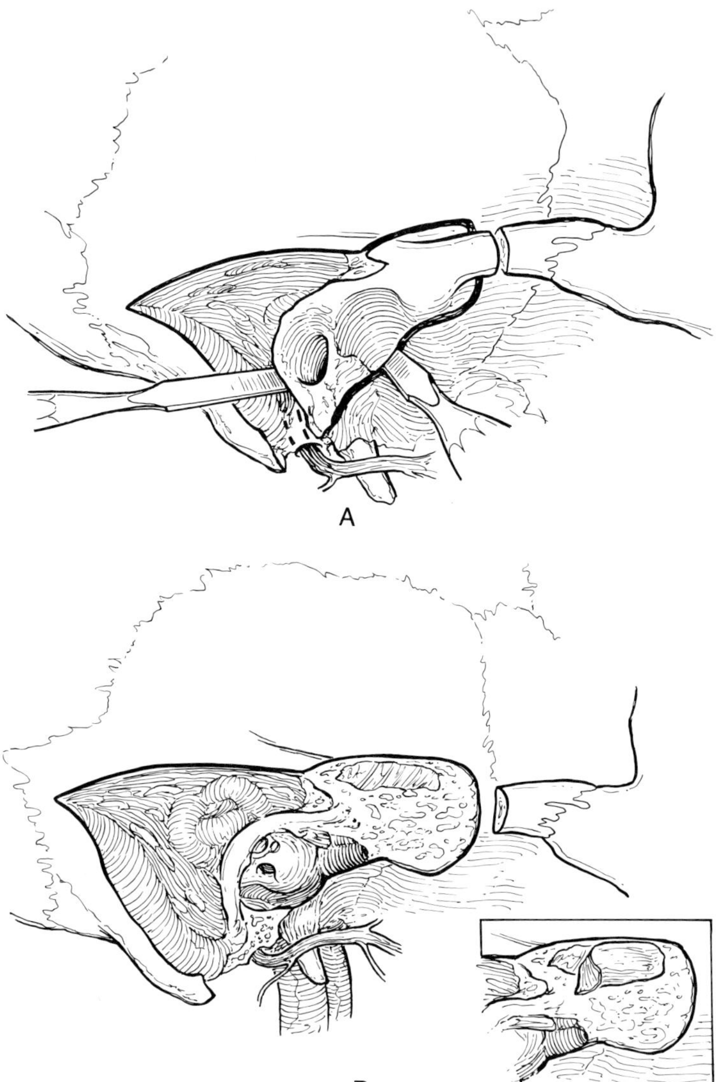

Figure 7–22. Lateral temporal bone resection. *A,* The osteotome is placed anteriorly in the fissure cut in the glenoid fossa, just medial to the tympanic bone, and posteriorly through the facial recess. A gentle tapping action with the hammer followed by a twisting of the osteotome usually results in a fracture in the desired plane. *B,* Resection completed with margin deep to the tympanic annulus. Facial nerve is intact. *Inset:* Inadvertent exposure of middle fossa dura is not uncommon and is covered with a skin graft.

concha will leave the involved part with the specimen. The auricular remnant is left attached in the superiorly based flap. The superficial temporal artery can be preserved if possible, but even with both it and the occipital artery cut, the flap will usually survive because of the wealth of collateral supply over the vertex. Rainey clips used on the incised scalp help to achieve hemostasis. Dissection of the flaps is done sufficiently wide to expose the parotid gland, the temporal squama, the temporomandibular joint, and the mastoid tip with its attached muscles.

2. Parotidectomy. The parotid gland, including both superficial and deep lobes, should be resected in all cases. The facial nerve is dissected and any tumor involvement excised with a wide margin. The main trunk or branches are clearly tagged for the hypoglossal to facial cross-over anastomosis later on. Even if cervical adenopathy is present, the parotid should be done first, because of the problems of increased hemorrhage brought about by internal jugular vein ligation.

The facial nerve branches are very gently retracted with a nerve hook as the deep lobe is separated from the nerve. This lobe can extend a long way along the undersurface of the mandibular ramus. It is often difficult to separate the last remnants of deep lobe that abut the undersurface of the temporal bone deep to the facial nerve as it exits the stylomastoid foramen.

3. Neck Dissection. Either before or after the parotidectomy, exploration of the lymphatics of the upper neck is done in search of possible metastatic disease. The preauricular, subauricular, and postauricular nodal areas are examined. Suspicious nodes are submitted for frozen section analysis; if they are found positive for cancer, a radical neck dissection is performed. If the postauricular nodes are positive for tumor, then the occipital nodes and usually a strip of underlying trapezius muscle are resected.

At this stage, control of the internal carotid artery and—if a neck dissection is not done—the internal jugular vein is secured. Umbilical tapes threaded through a length of size 16 French rubber catheter are used for control (Fig. 7–23). If a major vessel within the temporal bone is inadvertently breached during resection, instant pressure is exerted through the tapes, to prevent the rapid exsanguination that would otherwise ensue.

In cases in which the neck is not dissected, the origin of the sternocleidomastoid muscle

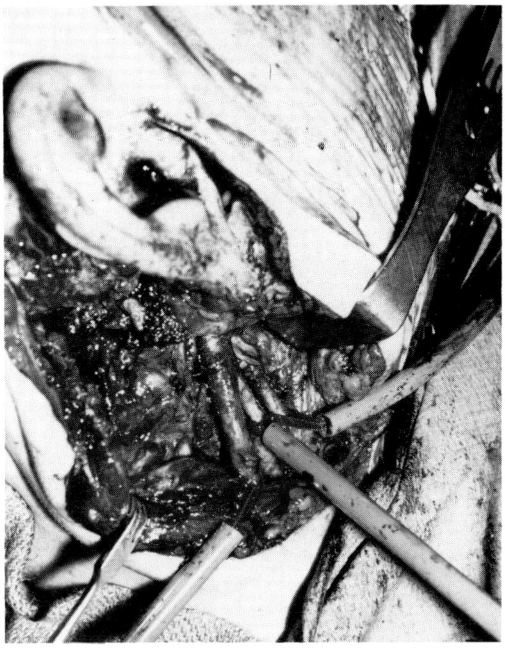

Figure 7–23. Umbilical tapes secure the internal jugular vein and the internal carotid artery in case of inadvertent massive hemorrhage.

is then severed from the mastoid tip. The posterior belly of the digastric muscle is removed from the digastric groove and dissected anteriorly. Just medial to this muscle is the groove for the occipital artery. This artery is isolated and ligated (Fig. 7–24).

The styloid process is now isolated deep to the artery and anteriorly. The inferior margin of resection is medial to the process against which lies the lateral lip of the jugular foramen. The stylopharyngeus and styloglossus muscles are dissected from the styloid to facilitate the correct placement of the osteotome.

4. Mastoidectomy. A complete mastoidectomy is done with excision of the tip and careful skeletonization of the sigmoid sinus. The cerebellar plate is skeletonized deep to it. An osteotome driven through this thin lamina will establish the posterolateral resection margin. The tegmen mastoideum and the sinodural angle are definitively outlined. The latter is a vital spot, as it is near the junction of the superior petrosal and lateral venous sinuses.

An atticotomy is done extending to the zygomatic root. Extent of disease may be now more precisely defined, as a full view of the epitympanum and mesotympanum can be obtained. A facial recess aperture may be required to facilitate the latter (Fig. 7–25).

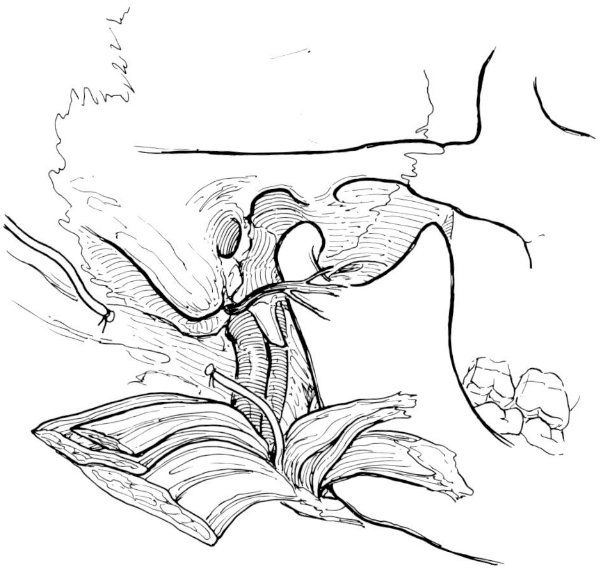

Figure 7–24. Total temporal bone resection. The mastoid tip is exposed by incision and transposition of the sternomastoid muscle. The digastric muscle is prized from its sulcus, and the occipital artery lying deep to it is tied. The vaginal process over the styloid process together with the styloid process itself is exposed by dissecting the styloid muscles from it.

5. Condylectomy. If not done at the time of parotidectomy, this step is now performed. A triangular cuff of soft tissue is raised over the proximal zygomatic arch to expose the temporomandibular joint while at the same time protecting the facial nerve (Fig. 7–19). The joint capsule is incised and the joint entered. An incision in the periosteum of the mandibular neck permits an intraperiosteal dissection of the condyle. The neck is cut across with a Gigli saw, Stryker saw, or fissure bur. Staying within the periosteum avoids injury to the internal maxillary artery. Grasping the condyle with bone-holding forceps, the remaining soft tissue connections are cut away.

This exposes the glenoid fossa, through which a connection between the craniotomy and the anteroinferior bone cut will be made in the final stages of the resection.

6. Anteroinferior Exposure. The zygomatic arch is transected just anterior to the articular eminence with a cutting bur or a Gigli or Stryker saw. As the glenoid fossa is cut inferiorly, the bony portion of the eustachian tube is transected (Fig. 7–26). It is essential to remember that the internal carotid artery is separated from the eustachian tube at this point by a thin plate of bone. The artery, because of its thin media, is particularly vulnerable to injury in its intratemporal course. As the superior aspect of this incision is made, care is taken to avoid cutting across the middle meningeal artery.

The resection line proceeds along the glenoid fossa toward the styloid process. If the styloid muscles had not been completely stripped from the process earlier, this step is now done. In this anteroinferior aspect of the resection it is important to keep in mind that

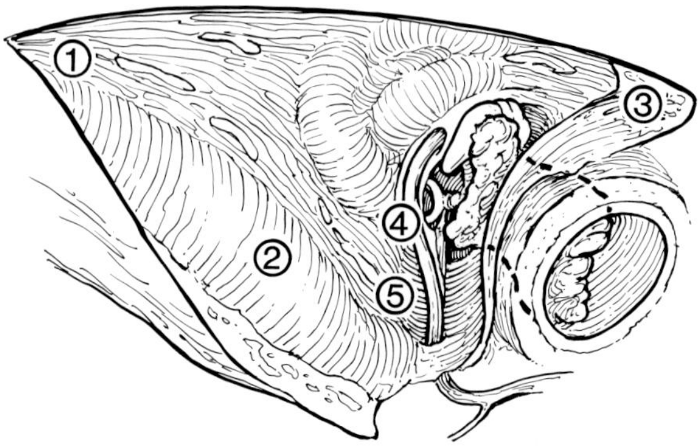

Figure 7–25. Total temporal bone resection. The mastoidectomy is completed, including (1) a clearly defined sinodural angle; (2) a well-skeletonized sigmoid plate; (3) an atticotomy extending into the zygomatic root; (4) a skeletonized facial nerve and open facial recess; and (5) a well-delineated retrofacial space.

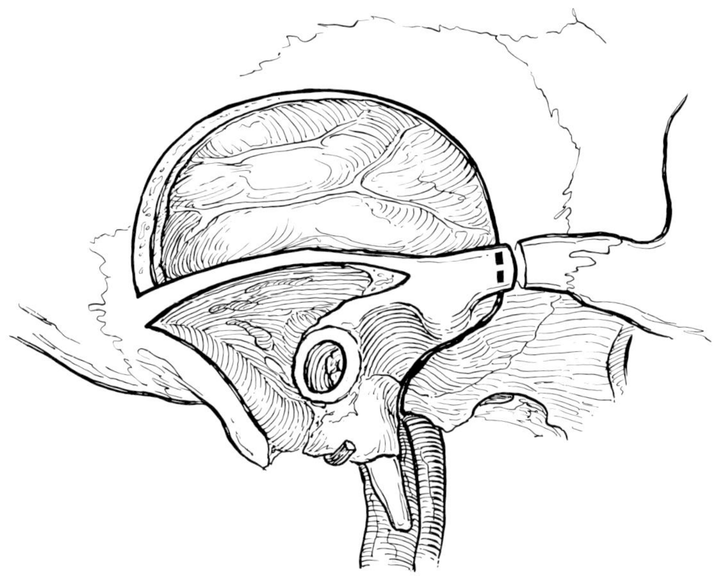

Figure 7–26. Total temporal bone resection. The glenoid fossa is cut across medially and often transects the eustachian tube and proceeds into the middle cranial fossa. This latter extension may be delayed until the completion of the craniotomy. The inferior aspect of the fissure is carried down to the level of the medial aspect of the styloid process.

the deep limit of this bony cut is the internal carotid artery as it enters the skull via the carotid canal, and the internal jugular vein as it exits the jugular foramen. The carotid canal is more anteriorly and deeply placed, located just deep to the most anterior extent of the tympanic process of the temporal bone. The jugular fossa is just behind it in a slightly lateral direction toward the more posterior part of the tympanic bone and the styloid process. The purpose of the fissure cut in the bone just lateral to these vessels is to provide a groove to safely seat the osteotome.

7. Temporal Craniotomy. The temporal craniotomy is most expeditiously outlined according to the method described by Montgomery.[24] A cutting bur is used to outline a small bony incision in the temporal squama. The incision should extend in a smooth arc from the sinodural angle to a point 4 cm above the external auditory canal, and then arch forward to the cut in the zygomatic arch (Fig. 7–27). Before extending the cut to the dura, the intracranial fluid volume is diminished by extracting cerebrospinal fluid either from a previously placed lumbar drain, through a lumbar puncture, or by use of an osmotic diuretic such as mannitol.

Next the inner table of skull is carefully cut through and the bone flap carefully dissected from the underlying dura. This is usually fairly easy to do, except in the elderly, in whom the dura is brittle and adherent to the skull. This part of the procedure may be done by either the neurosurgeon or the head and neck surgeon. I prefer to cut the bone flap myself and leave the rest to the neurosurgeons, as they seem to think that a bigger craniotomy is desirable. The purpose of this operative step is to control the superior petrosal sinus and the middle meningeal artery, detect and resect any dural invasion or temporal lobe extension if possible, and establish the medial margin of resection. As the temporal lobe dura is elevated from the floor of the middle fossa and retracted with a Teflon-coated retractor, the superior petrosal sinus is prized from its fissure in the posterosuperior extremity of the temporal bone (Fig. 7–27). This elevation proceeds toward the cavernous sinus and Meckel's cave, judiciously avoiding both.

Exposure of the middle fossa floor to the portion of temporal bone medial to the arcuate eminence is done with the dural elevator.

All aspects of the circumference of the temporal bone are now outlined, and final bony cuts may now be made.

8. Final Bony Cuts. This critical part of the resection is where most surgical disasters occur. The problem is that the internal cuts that will sever the temporal bone from the skull run adjacent to the course of the internal carotid artery and the jugular bulb. Injury to the latter structures is no great problem, since bleeding can be controlled from below by the umbilical tape and from above through tamponade of the sigmoid or lateral sinuses. However, hemorrhage from a rent in the internal carotid can be life-threatening, since bleeding can be only partially controlled in

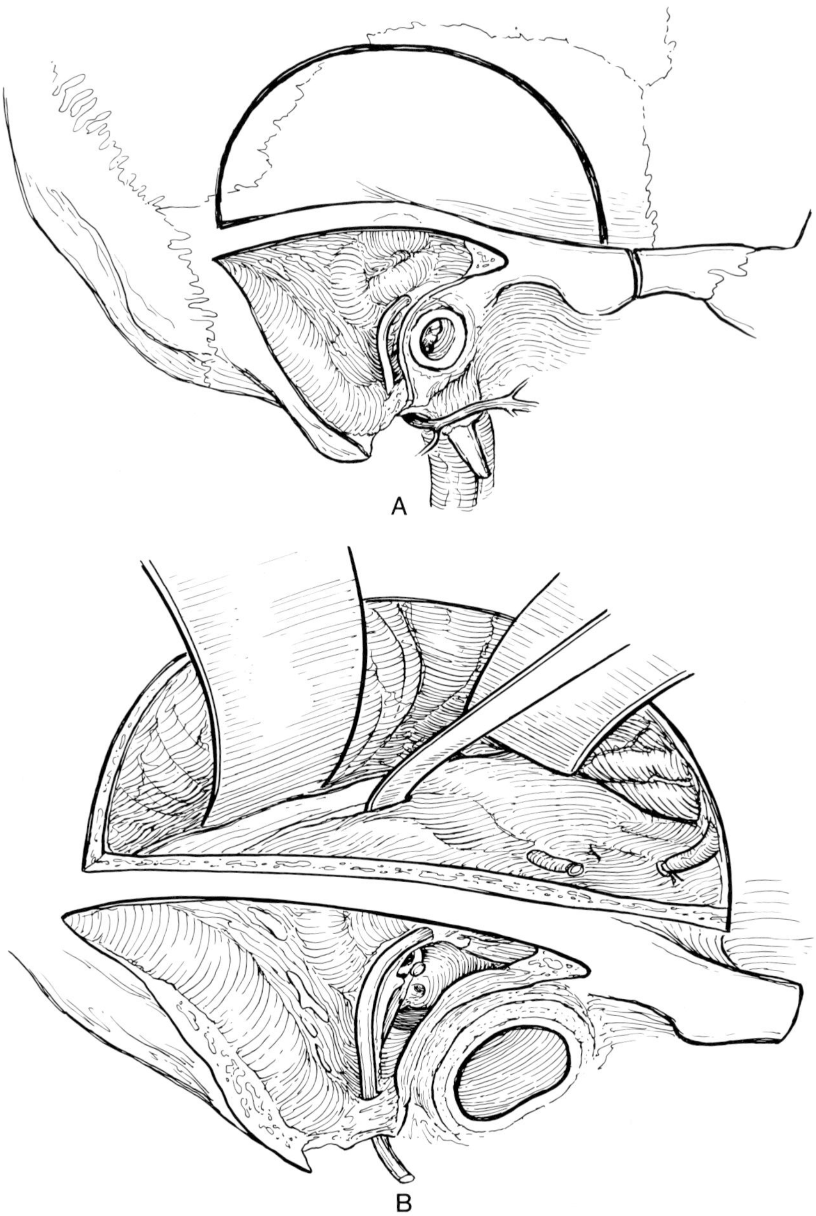

Figure 7–27. Total temporal bone resection. *A,* The temporal craniotomy is outlined with the cutting bur. *B,* The temporal lobe is elevated and the superior petrosal sinus elevated from its sulcus.

the neck. Moreover, occlusion of the vessel may result in stroke and even death.

Osteotome cuts are initiated at the following sites:

1. Posteriorly through the back surface of the bone at its most medial aspect, through the most medial limit of cerebellar plate skeletonization.

2. From cut #1 a superolaterally directed bony incision is made to the sindodural angle. A cut through the tegmen mastoideum connects this to the craniotomy and is carried medially.

3. Inferiorly just medial to the styloid process and directly lateral to the jugular bulb. This cut is directed superiorly and slightly medially.

4. Anteroinferiorly through the fissure in the glenoid fossa.

5. The "coup de grâce": Superiorly through the floor of the middle fossa just medial to the arcuate eminence (Fig. 7–28).

These bony incisions are best made with an osteotome. The instrument is guided toward the theoretical center of the temporal bone near the internal acoustic meatus by

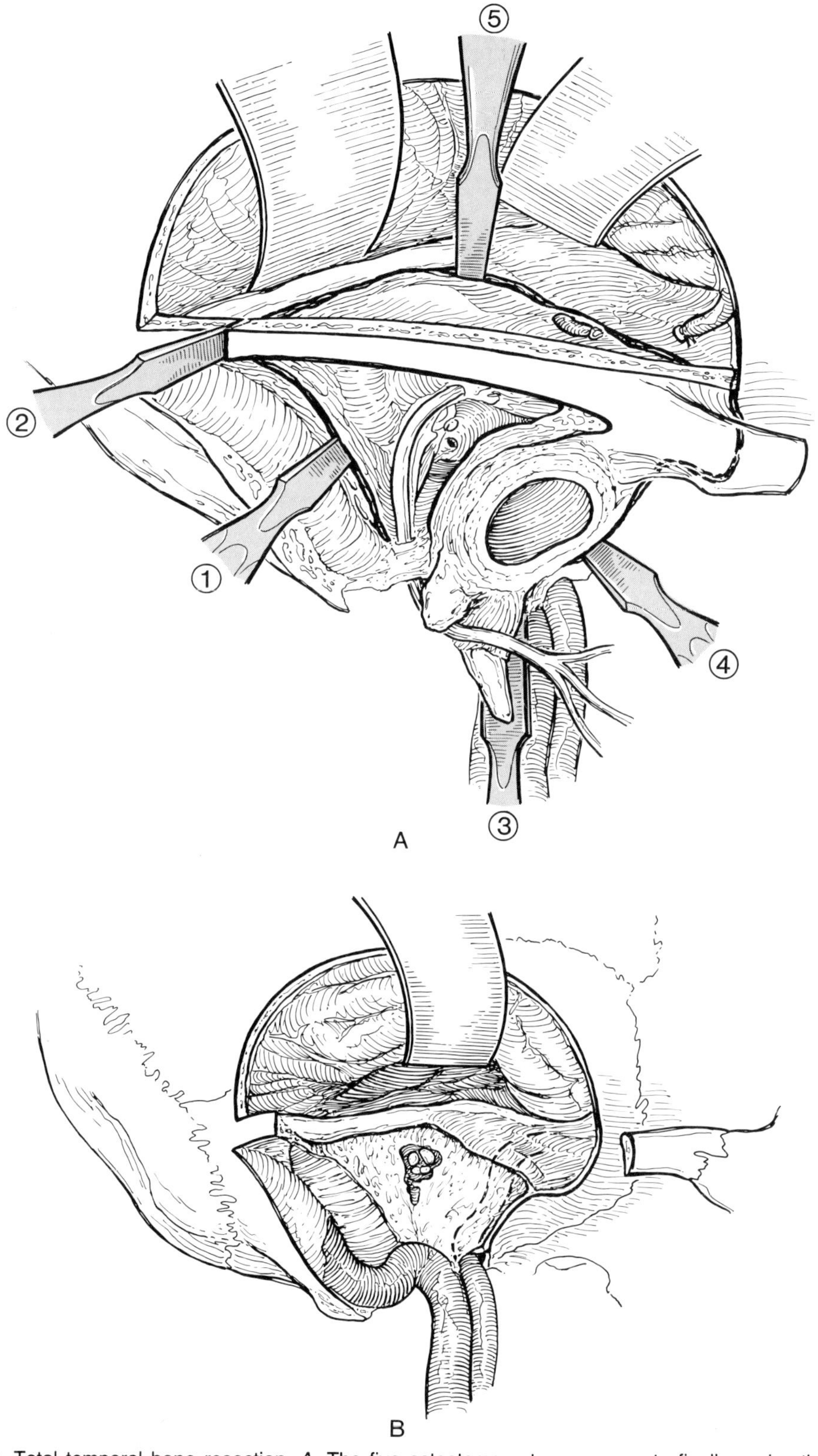

Figure 7–28. Total temporal bone resection. *A,* The five osteotome cuts necessary to finally excise the bone are outlined. (The numbers correspond to those in the text.) *B,* Defect following excision.

being angled slightly medially. A gentle tapping with the mallet is followed by a slight twisting of the osteotome. This results in a more controlled type of incision. The cut made medial to the arcuate eminence has to penetrate the otic capsule and thus requires a more brisk blow with the hammer.

Anteroinferiorly the cutting and twisting motion of the osteotome usually results in the bone splitting along the plane of the initial ascending portion of the internal carotid artery. The bone is most commonly transected through either the cochlea or the internal auditory canal.

9. Cavity Ablation. If the bone transection is quite medial in the internal auditory canal, a cerebrospinal fluid leak may result. A fat graft taken from the subcutaneous area of the abdomen and placed at the site of the leak is usually an effective plug.

Temporalis muscle flaps may be used to ablate the cavity. However, the cavity should not be so effaced that possible tumor recurrences might be obscured in their early stages.

The most important aspect of closure is the careful replacement of any resected dura with fascia together with the securing of a watertight closure of any rents.

10. Hypoglossal to Facial Nerve. Full temporal bone resection always necessitates transection of the facial nerve. Although some thought may be given to cable grafting the nerve, this connection must extend from the proximal internal acoustic canal to the transected main trunk near the resected parotid bed. This is a difficult maneuver, and I have elected in most cases to do a hypoglossal to facial nerve cross-over anastomosis.

The hypoglossal nerve is cut as far down in the neck as possible so the anastomosis will be tension free. The approximation is made under microscopic control using 10-0 nylon sutures. About 10 sutures are placed through the epineurium of these nerves (Fig. 7–29).

11. Closure. When a portion of the auricle remains, the flap is returned and the gap created by the conchal and external canal skin excision is bridged with a split-thickness skin graft. The graft is inverted into the cavity and packed with iodoform or antibiotic-impregnated gauze packing. The graft is sutured to the auricular cut edges, and the remaining wound in the neck and scalp is closed with interrupted sutures.

The neck is drained and a large pressure dressing applied or suction drains are used. Excision of the entire auricle occasionally presents a problem in closure. Since most

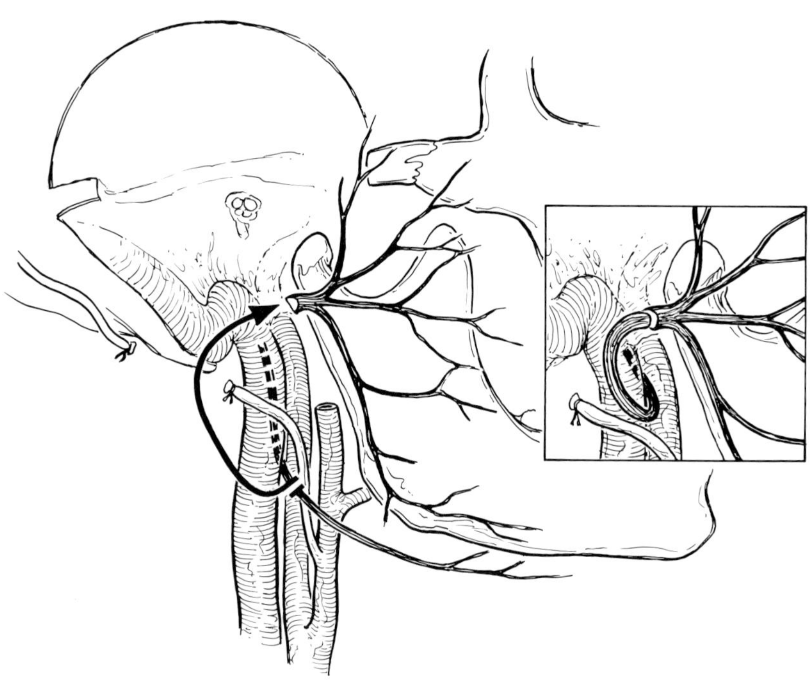

Figure 7–29. Total temporal bone resection. Hypoglossal nerve to facial nerve cross-over anastomosis.

patients who are afflicted with temporal bone carcinoma are elderly, an elevation of the facial skin similar to that of a face lift will enhance flap advancement. When this is not enough, a relaxation incision can be done and a bipedicled scalp flap advanced into the wound. The donor site on the skull is skin-grafted and the wound closed and drained.

Transcervical-Transmastoid Resection

Management of acoustic neuroma is beyond the scope of this book. However, some vasoformative and neurogenic tumors originate within the temporal bone and extend into the neck, or have a cervical origin and spread superiorly, usually through the neural or vascular foramina of the bone.

Non–chromaffin staining paragangliomas arise most commonly on the jugular vein (glomus jugulare), at the carotid bifurcation (carotid body tumor), or on the vagus nerve (glomus vagale). The large tumors that present simultaneously in the neck and ear require a combined transcervical and transtemporal approach. If the tumor extends to the posterior or middle fossa, this approach may need to be augmented by a transcranial exposure.

Most procedures described for the removal of these tumors require either mobilization and transposition of the facial nerve or its transection and later reconstruction. A trans-occipital, retrofacial approach described by Mischke and Balkany[25] provides an excellent exposure between the occiput and the transverse process of C1 without mobilization of the facial nerve and often with preservation of hearing. A small occipital craniotomy in continuity with the mastoid defect provides the necessary exposure of the posterior fossa contents so that the continuity of the tumor can be adequately visualized and the neoplasm easily removed.

The head is placed in the lateral position and flexed acutely forward. The usual post-auricular incision for mastoidectomy is made about 2 cm posterior to the postauricular crease and extended into the neck, similar to the inferior limb of the modified Blair parotidectomy incision. A superiorly placed limb arching posteriorly over the occiput gives excellent access for an occipital craniotomy (Fig. 7–30). The incision is placed through

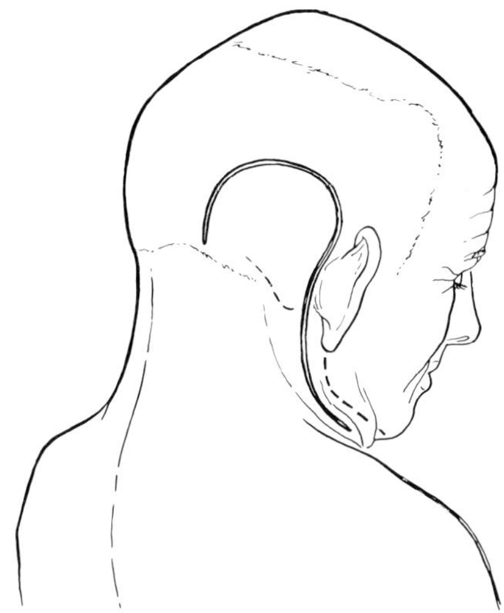

Figure 7–30. Patient's head is flexed acutely forward, and a postauricular incision is directed posterosuperiorly over the occipital scalp and anteroinferiorly toward the hyoid bone.

skin and mastoid periosteum and the auricle dissected anteriorly.

The inferior limb of the incision exposes the contents of the upper neck. The sternocleidomastoid, lateral trapezius, and posterior belly of the digastric muscle are dissected from the mastoid tip and occipital bone. In addition, some of the laterally placed deep cervical muscles inserting on the occiput are dissected from the calvarium; specifically the splenius capitis, longissimus capitis and even the obliquus capitis superior. This opens a space up between the undersurface of the temporal bone and the transverse process of C1 (Fig. 7–31).

A complete mastoidectomy is performed, with emphasis on careful skeletonization of the sigmoid sinus and the facial canal. The mastoid tip is completely removed with a Lempert rongeur, and at least 180 degrees of the sigmoid sinus is skeletonized. It becomes readily apparent that as the inferior aspect of the sigmoid approaches the region of the facial canal it begins to sharply deviate medially, moving deeply into the substance of the temporal bone. As the facial nerve is skeletonized, it is important to preserve a surrounding thin shell of bone to protect it during the subsequent resection. The stylomastoid foramen is also skeletonized, and that part of the nerve that exits the foramen is exposed for a short distance. The subsequent dissection is carried out deep to the nerve both in its mastoid and upper cervical parts.

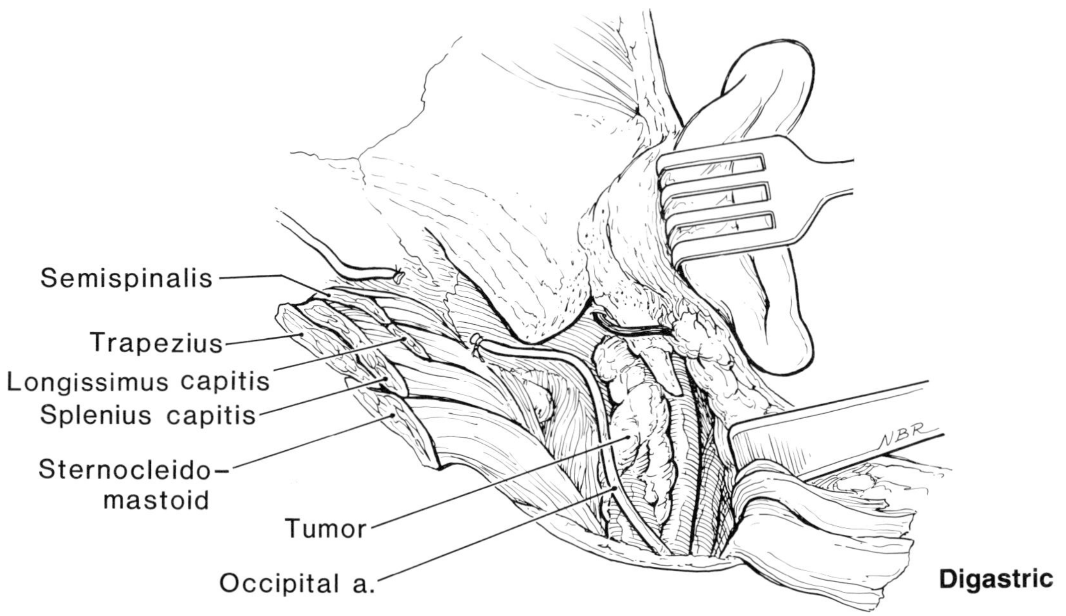

Figure 7–31. Incision of the sternocleidomastoid, trapezius, posterior belly of digastric, splenius capitis, and longissimus capitis opens up a space between the mastoid tip and C1.

At this point attention is turned to the neck. The internal jugular vein and internal carotid artery are identified below the cervical extent of tumor. An umbilical tape is placed around each in case of sudden hemorrhage. Preoperative embolization of any feeding vessels as well as nitroprusside-induced hypotension during the part of the operation in which the tumor is being dissected helps immensely in reducing blood loss. As dissection proceeds, meticulous care must be exercised to preserve the vagus, hypoglossal, and spinal accessory nerves as well as the sympathetic plexus. Unfortunately, in the case of large tumors, impairment of these nerves may have already occurred preoperatively as a result of tumor encroachment in the jugular foramen.

Dissection of the tumor at the carotid bifurcation may produce wide fluctuations in pulse rate. Deposition of lidocaine in this region is advised prior to tumor manipulation. The space between the proximal internal and external carotids and the skull base is very narrow. This is the parapharyngeal or pharyngomaxillary space. Strong lateral traction on the angle of the mandible with a large bone hook opens it up. This is often sufficient, but if not, a transverse osteotomy of the mandibular ramus provides excellent exposure. The osteotomy is done between the insertions of the lateral and medial pterygoid muscles. If the transection is high enough, transection of the inferior alveolar neurovascular bundle may be avoided. A stair-step osteotomy is done to facilitate approximation later (Fig. 7–32). Sectioning of the stylomandibular ligament as it inserts on the medial aspect of the mandibular angle facilitates retraction of the fragments and enhances the exposure of the great vessels all along their course to the skull base. The internal jugular vein is ligated just below the tumor and the vessel transected (Fig. 7–33).

The tumor is now approached from both above and below the jugular foramen. Returning to the ear, the sigmoid sinus is dissected deep to the facial nerve until the point

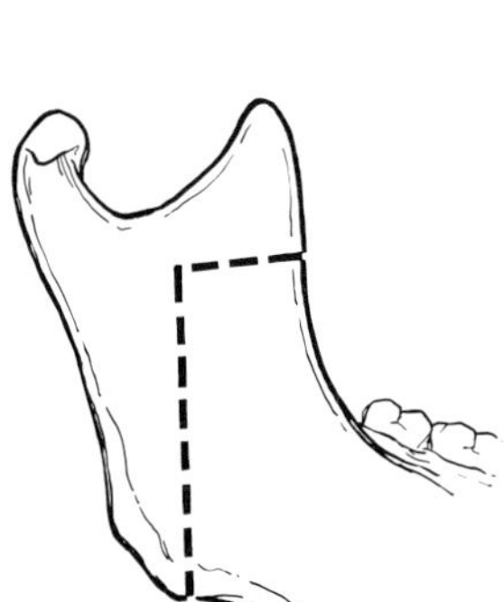

Figure 7–32. A stair-step osteotomy is done in the mandibular ramus and the bone reflected to improve visualization of the skull base.

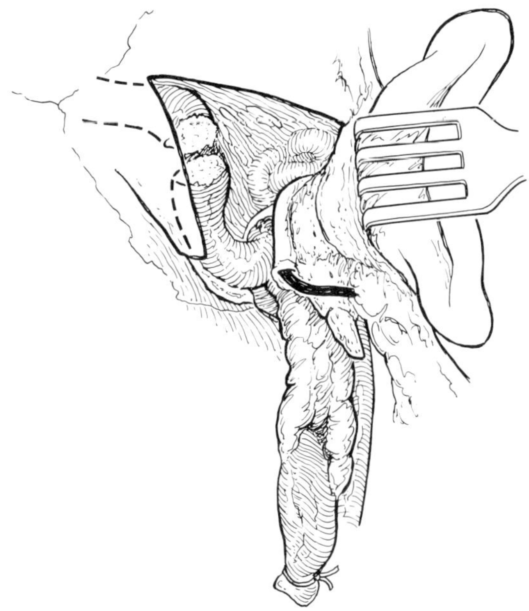

Figure 7–33. The internal jugular vein is tied below the skull base, and the sigmoid sinus is controlled with a hemostatic absorbable cotton plug.

where it becomes the jugular bulb. The jugular bulb and attached tumor are exposed as much as possible by finally removing a portion of the posterolateral rim of the jugular foramen (Fig. 7–34).

Bleeding from the lateral venous sinus is controlled either by circumferential ligation or by venorrhaphy and stuffing the lumen with Oxycel cotton. The sigmoid sinus is transected and with contained tumor is dissected toward the foramen. Near the jugular bulb the inferior petrosal sinus is identified, transected, and plugged with Oxycel (Fig. 7–35). This site is the most troublesome area for bleeding during the procedure.

The intratemporal portion of the tumor is delivered into the neck and the specimen removed. In the case of intracranial extension, which is usually into the posterior fossa, an occipital craniotomy is done in continuity with the mastoid defect. Dura is reflected and tumor removed (Fig. 7–36). The mandible is wired together, a suction drain placed, and the wound closed.

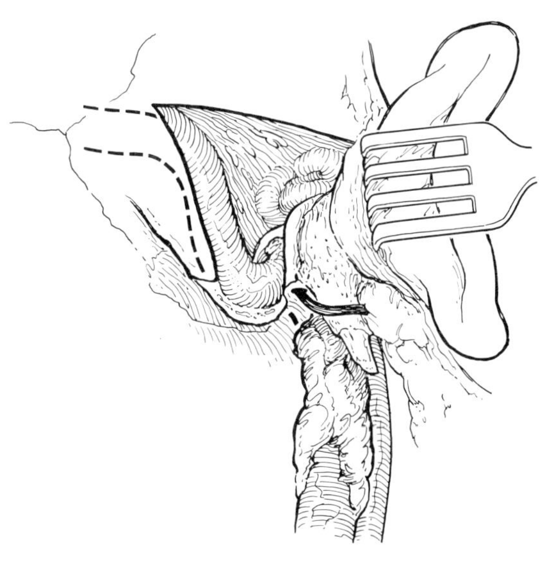

Figure 7–34. The final portion of the tumor is exposed by removing the remaining bone lateral to the sigmoid sinus and the lateral lip of the jugular foramen.

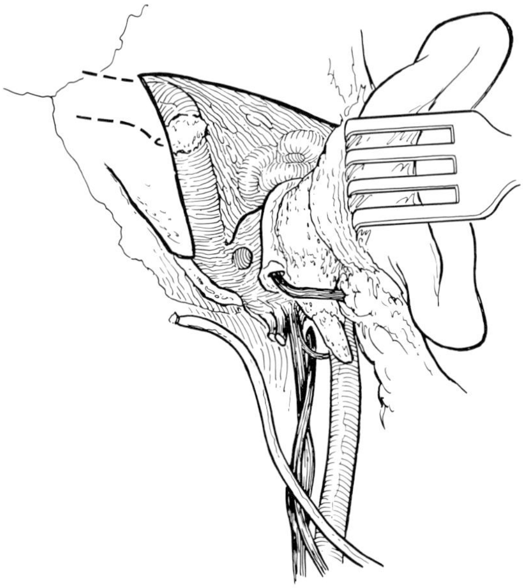

Figure 7–35. Bleeding from the inferior petrosal sinus is controlled with a hemostatic cotton plug.

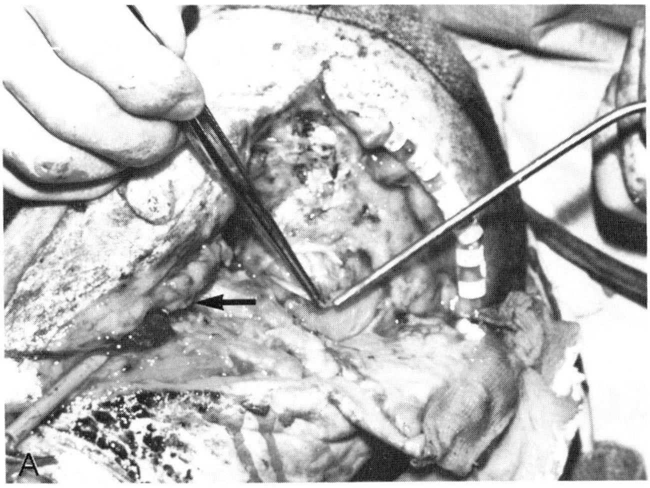

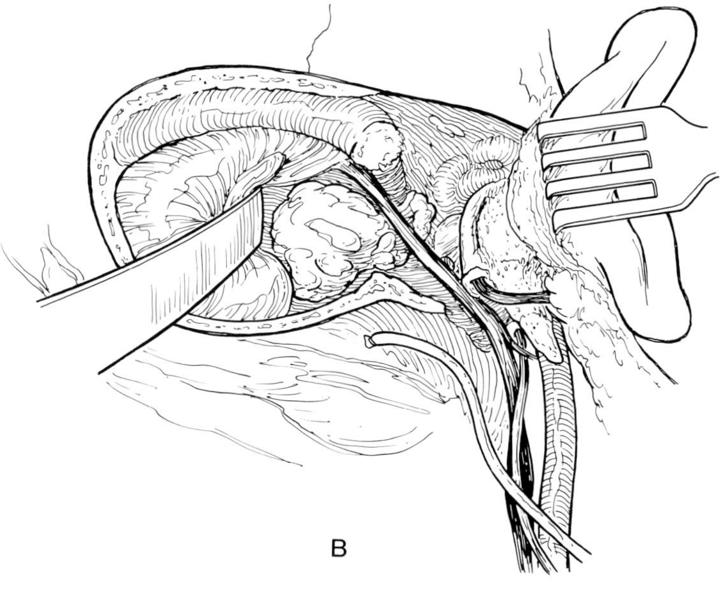

Figure 7–36. *A,* Massive glossopharyngeal schwannoma, with tissue forceps shown grasping cerebellar dura. Arrow indicates tumor in the mastoid extending into the posterior cranial fossa. *B,* Drawing of lesion in *A.* Extensions into the posterior fossa are exposed by occipital craniotomy and reflection of cerebellar dura.

References

1. Bumstead RM, Ceilley RI, Panje WR, et al: Auricular malignant neoplasms: When is chemotherapy (Moh's technique) necessary? Arch Otolaryngol 101:721, 1981.
2. Bumstead RM, Ceilley RI: Auricular malignant neoplasms. Arch Otolaryngol:225, 1982.
3. Campbell E, Volk BM, Burkland CW: Total resection of the temporal bone for malignancy of the middle ear. Ann Surg 134:397, 1951.
4. Parsons H, Lewis JS: Subtotal resection of the temporal bone for cancer of the ear. Cancer 7:995, 1954.
5. Lewis JS: Temporal bone resection. Arch Otolaryngol 101:23, 1975.
6. Conley J: Concepts in Head and Neck Surgery. New York, Grune & Stratton, 1970, p 69.
7. Conley J, Schuller DE: Malignancies of the ear. Laryngoscope 86:1147, 1976.
8. Chen KTR, Dehner LP: Primary tumors of the external and middle ear. Arch Otolaryngol 104:247, 1978.
9. Bailin PL, Levine HL, Wood BG, et al: Cutaneous carcinoma of the auricular and periauricular region. Arch Otolaryngol 106:692, 1980.
10. Ceilley RI, Bumstead RM, Smith WH: Malignancies on the external ear: Methods of ablation and reconstruction of defects. J Dermatol Surg Oncol 5:762, 1979.
11. Pulec JL: Glandular tumors of the external auditory canal. Laryngoscope 87:1601, 1977.
12. Wetli CV, Pardo V, Millard M, et al: Tumors of ceruminous glands. Cancer 29:1169, 1972.
13. Schuknecht HE: Neoplastic growth. *In* Pathology of the Ear. Cambridge, MA, Harvard University Press, 1974, p 420.
14. McCabe B: Personal communications, 1973.
15. Myers EM, Stool S, Weltschew MA: Rhabdomyosarcoma of the middle ear. Ann Otol Rhinol Laryngol 77:949, 1968.
16. Karaty S: Rhabdomyosarcoma of the middle ear. Arch Otolaryngol 50:330, 1949.
17. Lewis JS: Tumors of the external ear and temporal bone in otolaryngology. *In* English GM (ed): Otolaryngology, Vol 2. Hagerstown, MD, Harper & Row, 1979, Chapter 26.
18. Naufal PE: Primary sarcomas of the temporal bone. Arch Otolaryngol 98:44, 1973.
19. Moh FE: Chemosurgery for skin cancer: fixed tissues and fresh tissue techniques. Arch Dermatol 112:211, 1976.
20. Fredericks S: External ear malignancy. Br J Plast Surg 9:136, 1969.
21. Pless J: Carcinoma of the external ear. Scand J Plast Reconstr Surg 10:147, 1976.
22. Blake GB, Wilson JSP: Malignant tumors of the ear and their treatment. Plast Surg 27:67, 1974.
23. Conway H, Howell J: Carcinoma of the external ear. Plast Reconstr Surg 20:45, 1957.
24. Montgomery WW: Surgery of the Upper Respiratory Tract, Vol I. Philadelphia, Lea & Febiger, 1971, p 471.
25. Mischke RE, Balkany TJ: Skull base approach to glomus jugulare. Laryngoscope 90:89, 1980.

8

SALIVARY GLANDS

Paul J. Donald, M.D.

Tumors of the salivary glands are unique among head and neck tumors in that their cell type may be of epithelial or glandular origin or a mixture of both. Each specific gland appears to have a peculiar predisposition to develop a particular variety of tumor with a greater frequency than its neighbor. This is true both of the quality of benignity vs. malignancy and of the specific cell type. The salivary glands are classified as major or minor and are principally ringed in a roughly U-shaped pattern around the oral cavity. The parotid, submandibular, and sublingual are the major glands, while the small submucosal glands of the oral cavity make up the minor glands. Other minor salivary glands are found throughout the upper air and food passageway, but these appear to be firmly resistant to the development of neoplasms. The oral cavity is the site of 95 per cent of the tumors of minor salivary gland origin.[1]

ANATOMY

A thorough knowledge of the anatomy of these glands aids in the anticipation of the pathophysiology of malignancies that may arise therein.

The paired parotid glands are wrapped around the vertical rami of the mandible. The superficial lobe is lateral to the ramus and overlies the masseter muscle, while the deep lobe lies against the periosteum of the bone's medial surface and the medial pterygoid muscle (Fig. 8–1). The facial nerve splits the gland into these two lobes. Although there is still some debate concerning the existence of an anatomic separation between them, dissection during surgery on the gland consistently reveals a fascial plane at the level of the nerve (Fig. 8–2). The tail of the gland lies over the mastoid tip and may be of considerable size (Fig. 8–3). The gland abuts the anterior aspect of the external auditory canal and occasionally the undersurface of the temporal bone. It may extend superiorly to overlie the temporomandibular joint and the root of the zygomatic arch. The close relationship of the parotid to the mandible and external auditory canal requires their frequent inclusion in the resection of large tumors afflicting the gland. The deep lobe of the gland is intimately related to the external carotid artery. It may, especially if involved with tumor, involve both the internal jugular vein laterally and the internal carotid artery medially (Fig. 8–4). A third small accessory lobe is often found along the course of Stensen's duct. In one series of 96 consecutive cadaver dissections it was found in 21 instances.[2]

As the parotid wraps around the mandible, the submandibular gland wraps around the posterior edge of the mylohyoid muscle (Fig. 8–1). The amount of gland on the superior surface of the mylohyoid is highly variable. The superior portion of the gland is covered by oral mucosa, while the inframylohyoid part is wedged between the anterior belly of the digastric and the mylohyoid muscle. As the patient ages, the mylohyoid muscle relaxes and the gland becomes more of an upper cervical structure than a paramandibular one. This allows the gland to be more easily palpated by both physician and patient,

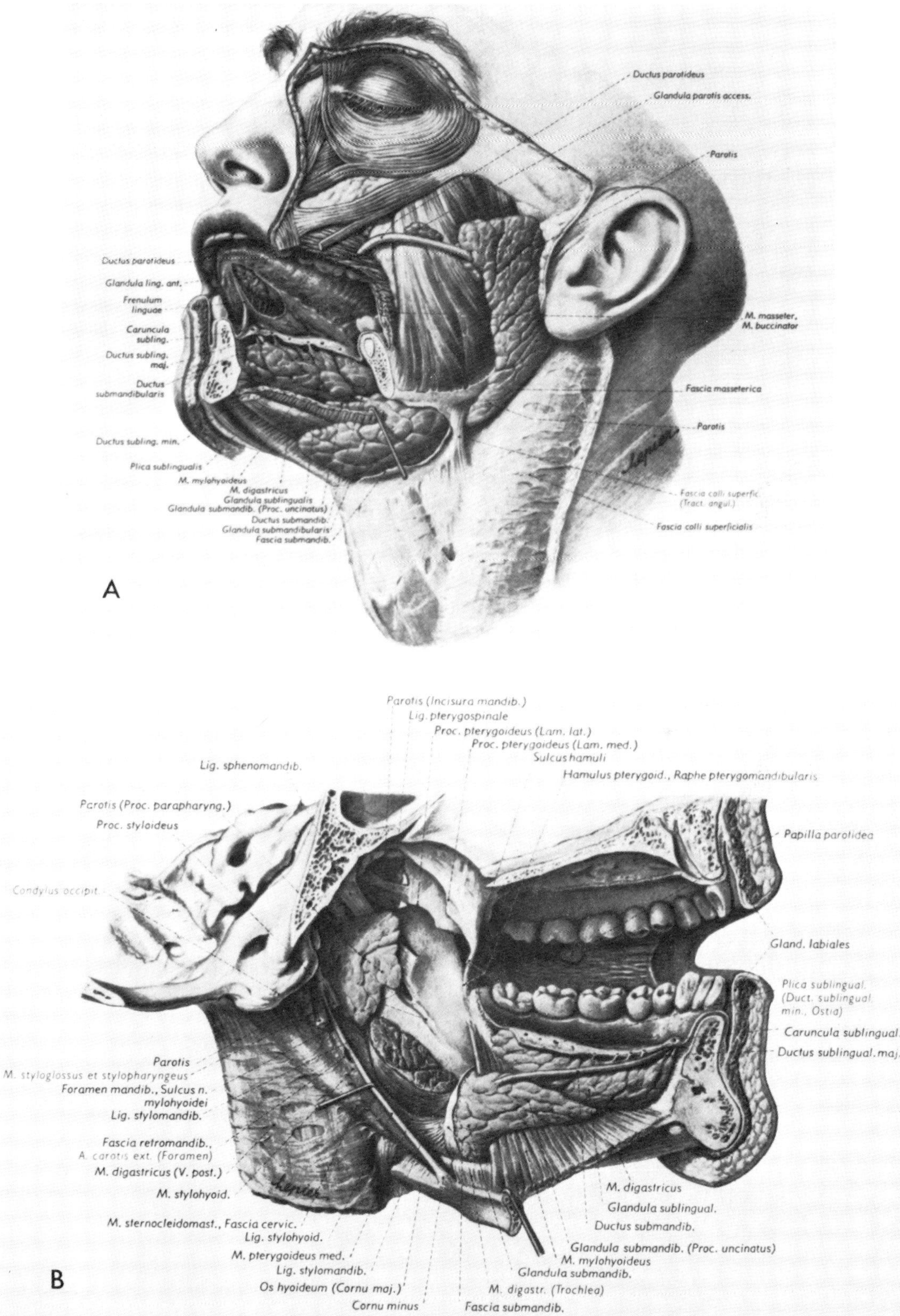

Figure 8–1. The major salivary glands and their anatomic relations. *A,* Lateral view with a portion of the body of the mandible removed to expose the sublingual gland. *B,* Medial view of the salivary glands of the left side. (From Pernkopf E: Atlas of Topographical and Applied Anatomy. Vol 1: Head and Neck. Philadelphia, WB Saunders, 1980.)

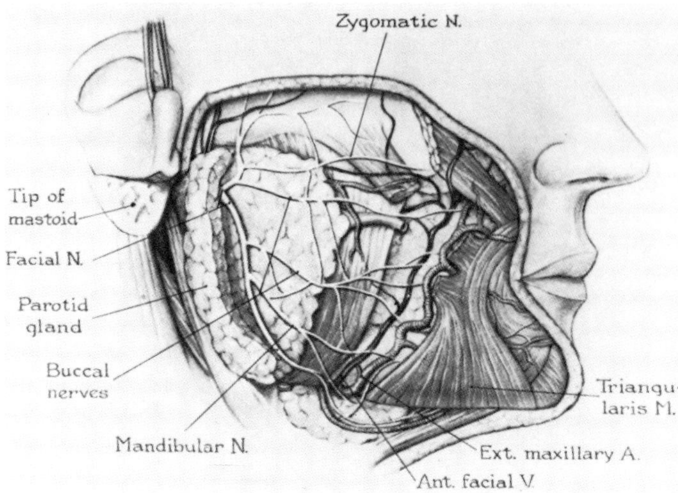

Figure 8–2. The facial nerve branches separate the parotid gland at its superficial and deep lobes. (From Conley J: Salivary Glands and the Facial Nerve. New York, Grune & Stratton, 1975.)

occasionally frightening the patient into thinking he may have cancer. The ramus mandibularis of the facial nerve frequently courses across the gland superficial to the investing fascia. The hypoglossal and lingual nerves have a close relationship to the submandibular gland; the hypoglossal in the neck and the lingual to Wharton's duct in the floor of the mouth.

The sublingual gland is about one-half the size of the submandibular gland, lying in the middle third of the floor of the mouth and related to the mylohyoid inferoposteriorly and to the inferior longitudinal portion of the hyoglossus medially. It may partially overlap the submandibular gland and at times appears almost in continuity with it. The gland abuts the lingual plate of the parasymphyseal aspect of the mandible. Anteromedially the gland is related to the genioglossus. The lingual nerve courses between this muscle and the gland. Numerous small short ducts lead from the gland and open directly into the floor of the mouth along the sublingual fold adjacent to Wharton's duct of the submandibular gland.[3, 4]

The minor salivary glands are scattered throughout the oral mucosa and vary somewhat in form and function with their site of origin. The labial and buccal glands are situated in the submucosa of the lips and cheek. They may be extensive enough to penetrate through the fibers of the orbicularis oris and buccinator muscles. Although they are classically described as mixed serous and mucus-secreting glands similar in histologic structure to the submandibular and sublingual glands, recent ultrastructural studies reveal evidence of mucous elements only. The glossopalatine glands extend along the palatal-glossal fold. The palatine glands are richly distributed throughout the soft palate, making up half of its bulk. Both are of the pure mucous variety. The lingual minor salivary glands are anteriorly and posteriorly located. The anterior glands (Nuhn's glands, or the glands of Blandin) are located in the undersurface of the tip of the tongue and are mixed in type. The posterior glands are of two types. Those of the mucous variety are lateral to the circumvallate papillae and related to the lingual tonsil. The more numerous serous glands (Von Ebner's glands) are entwined by lingual

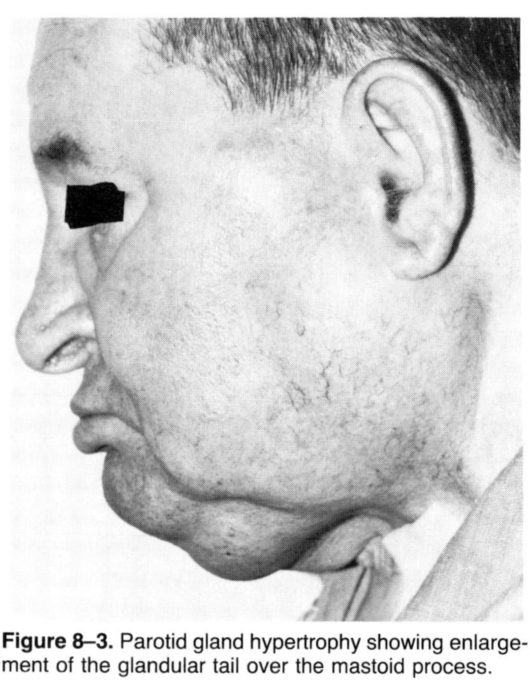

Figure 8–3. Parotid gland hypertrophy showing enlargement of the glandular tail over the mastoid process.

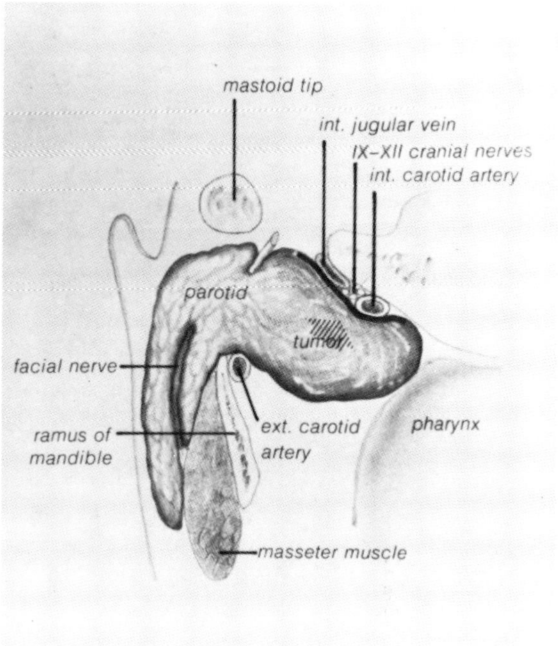

Figure 8–4. Relationship of the deep lobe of the parotid gland to the external carotid artery. There is encroachment on the internal jugular vein and the internal carotid artery when the deep lobe of the gland is involved with tumor. (From Rankow RM, Polayes IM: Diseases of the Salivary Glands. Philadelphia, WB Saunders, 1976.)

muscle in the posterior third of the tongue, lying under the circumvallate papillae and emptying into their troughs. They are also related to the foliate papillae on the posterolateral tongue surface.

PATHOLOGY

In an attempt to sort out the most appropriate treatment of salivary gland cancer, one of the greatest dilemmas is to unravel the complexity of nomenclature that surrounds this protean group of tumors. A variety of classifications have emerged over the years, but considerable order was restored by the excellent work of Foote and Frazell in 1953.[5] Since then a number of investigators have contributed to the understanding of these lesions.[6-8] Kleinsasser, through an extensive investigation of the light- and electron-microscopic appearance of a large number of tumors, which he then correlated with operative findings and personal clinical follow-up of the patients involved, has developed a most meaningful classification.[9]

Pleomorphic Adenoma and Carcinoma

Pleomorphic adenoma is considered by most authorities to be a benign lesion with only a rare malignant variant. Benign mixed tumors, as they are also called, occur in the parotid gland 84 per cent of the time[10] and represent 60 to 65 per cent of all parotid tumors.[11] The malignant variant makes up only 2 to 5 per cent of all mixed tumors (Table 8–1), and these are limited almost exclusively to the parotid gland. This neoplasm in its benign form has an unusual pathophysiologic characteristic that distinguishes it from most other benign tumors. Without wide excision it has a marked propensity for local recurrence. This was initially thought to be due to the phenomenon of satellitosis or multicentricity. Using histologic serial sectioning, Eneroth[12] established that the peculiar character of multiple tumor bosellations or outgrowths on the tumor's surface is responsible for the frequent recurrences following "lumpectomy" of benign mixed tumors.

Kleinsasser established that pleomorphic adenomas originate from two stem cells of the ectodermal layer: the ductal epithelial cell and the myoepithelial cell.[13] He conceptualizes that the malignant mixed tumor is a "new" cancer that arises within the substance of usually a longstanding benign pleomorphic adenoma. Its cell type is often mixed epidermoid and adenomatous. A focus of anarchistic cancer cells is seen to have developed in an otherwise perfectly unremarkable, benign-appearing pleomorphic adenoma. It is not

Table 8–1. FREQUENCY OF MALIGNANT MIXED TUMORS*

Authors	*No. of Salivary Gland Tumors*	*No. of Malignant Mixed Tumors*	*Percentage of Malignant Mixed Tumors*
Foote and Frazell	877	57	7
Eneroth	802	16	2
Morgan and Makenzie	151	14	9.3
Moberger and Eneroth	2211	34	1.8
Skolnik et al	116	2	1.7
Brown et al	286	12	4.2
Mustard and Anderson	287	16	5.5
Wheelock et al	209	15	5.3
Freeman et al	545	5	0.9
Chaudhry et al	1414	29	2.0

*Except for the data from the study by Chaudhry et al, all other information is from a series dealing with the major salivary glands (predominantly the parotid gland).

thought of as a "degenerative process," as the lesion begins unifocally, without signs of such malignant transformation appearing elsewhere within the tumor.

The histologic picture of pleomorphic adenoma is characteristic (Fig. 8–5). Cell lines of both epithelial and mesenchymal origin must be present in order to make the diagnosis. The appearance of stellate mesenchymal cells, islands of cartilage with chondrocytes, mucinous deposits, and structures resembling glandular acini provoked the name of "mixed tumor." Occasionally a more spindle shaped cell may predominate, in which case the lesion is called a monomorphic adenoma. The malignant variant is characterized by a partial or complete replacement of the usual cellular make-up of pleomorphic adenoma by a "malignification" of one or more of its cellular components (Fig. 8–6).

A painless hard lump that is often irregular in outline is the usual clinical presentation of pleomorphic adenoma. The tumor may attain considerable size and is occasionally cystic (Fig. 8–7). Malignant mixed tumors may be indistinguishable from the benign variety but may present with the common stigmata of malignancy—pain, fixation, and facial nerve paralysis.

Adenocarcinoma

Most neoplasms of benign or malignant type originate in the cells of the ductal elements of the gland. Adenocarcinomas by definition ought to include all those lesions that take their origin in the glandular elements of the parenchyma. Strictly speaking, these cancers would be primarily from the serous or mucous acinar cells. Complicating the picture are those malignancies that are obviously glandular but for which no definitive stem cell can be identified, as well as others in the class of mucoepidermoid cancers that form mucin-secreting acini. Finally,

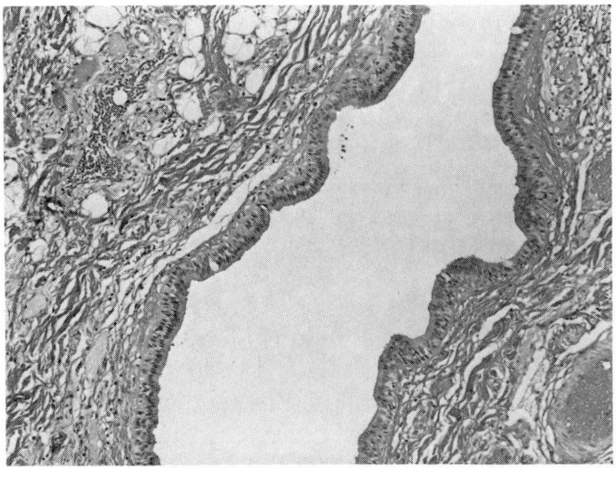

Figure 8–5. Photomicrograph of patient with pleomorphic adenoma. Note large epithelium-lined cyst. Some chondroid and myxoid material is dispensed in loosely arranged connective tissue. (H & E × 100)

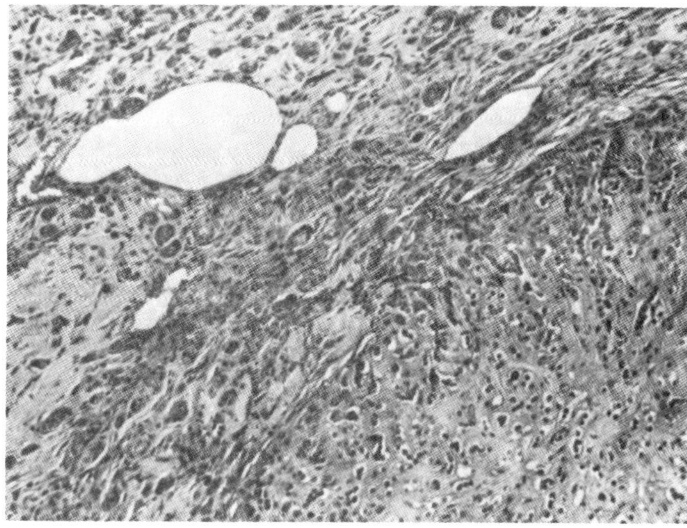

Figure 8–6. Photomicrograph of patient with malignant mixed tumor. (H & E × 90) (From Thackray AC, Lucas RB: Tumors in the major salivary glands. Fascicle 10, Atlas of Tumor Pathology, 2nd ed. Washington, DC, Armed Forces Institute of Pathology, 1974, p 111.)

many authorities, beginning with Foote and Frazell,[5] have included adenoid cystic carcinoma under the heading of adenocarcinoma.

Kleinsasser[9] used the term adenocarcinoma to comprise those lesions that could not be clearly identified as either acinic cell, adenoid cystic, mucoepidermoid, or mixed cancers. As Batsakis[14] has clearly outlined, many of the salivary adenocarcinomas are papillary or cystic, or both, in type, and closely resemble adenocarcinomas of the gastrointestinal tract (Fig. 8–8). However, many are rather undifferentiated, albeit glandular in type. Their biologic behavior is variable, ranging from highly malignant to relatively benign depending on histologic invasiveness rather than on any particular cellular structure.

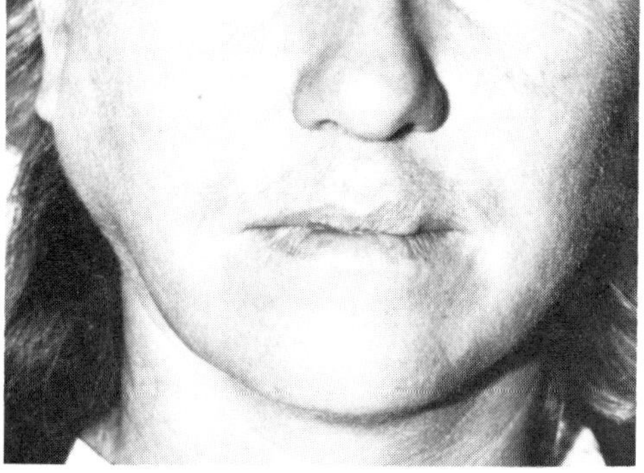

Figure 8–7. Young woman with moderately sized pleomorphic adenoma containing a large cystic area.

Adenocarcinomas probably make up about 20 per cent of less of the malignancies in the salivary glands and are found in both the major and minor glands. The highly invasive type are extremely malignant and are characterized by frequent regional and distant metastases.[15] They present as hard, firm, mixed masses. They are rapid-growing and frequently invade the mandible and temporal bone (Fig. 8–9). They may ulcerate through the overlying skin of these structures or that of the external auditory canal. Invasion of the adjacent masseter muscle may produce trismus.

Acinic Cell Cancer

Acini of the salivary glands are serous, mucous, or mixed seromucinous in type. Tumors of the acinic type are almost exclusively serous (Fig. 8–10).[16,17] This has been proved not only by light microscopy (by which the zymogen granules of the tumor are seen to be identical to those of the normal serous acinar cell) but by ultrastructural and histochemical analysis as well. These acinic tumors are found almost exclusively in the superficial lobe and tail of the parotid gland and make up 2 per cent of all tumors and 17 to 19 per cent of all malignancies there. They are rarely found in the submandibular and sublingual glands. Only seven acinous tumors of intraoral minor salivary gland origin have been identified.[18]

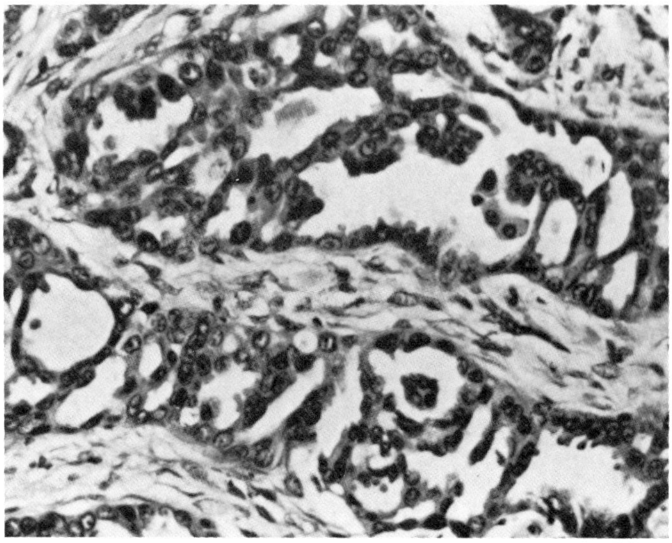

Figure 8–8. Photomicrograph of a patient with adenocarcinoma of the parotid gland. Note similarity to gastrointestinal malignancy. (× 250) (From Thackray AC, Lucas RB: Tumors in the major salivary glands. Fascicle 10, Atlas of Tumor Pathology, 2nd ed. Washington, DC, Armed Forces Institute of Pathology, 1974, p 101.)

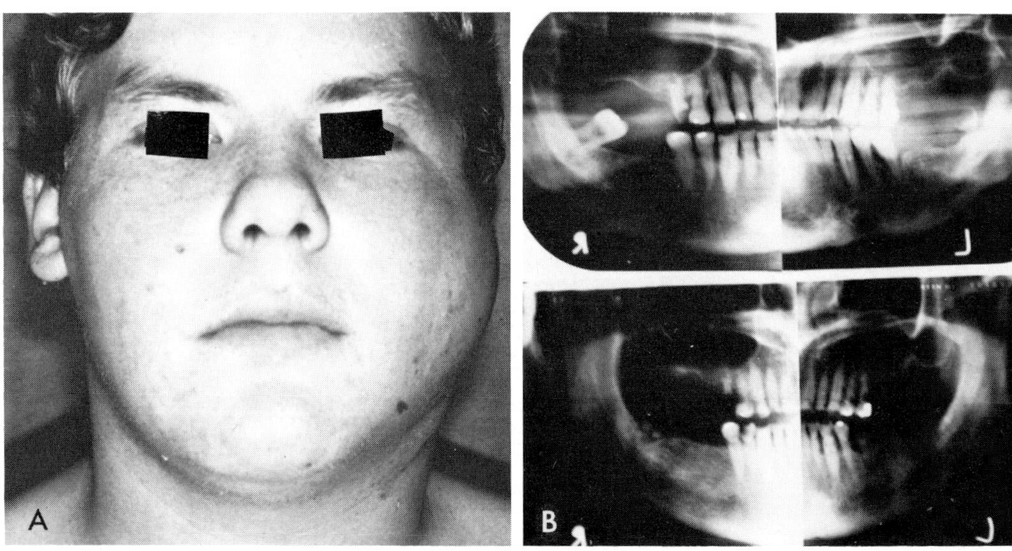

Figure 8–9. *A,* A 19-year-old male with a large adenocarcinoma of the parotid gland. *B,* Orthopantomograph showing extensive erosion of the left mandibular ramus from tumor in *A.*

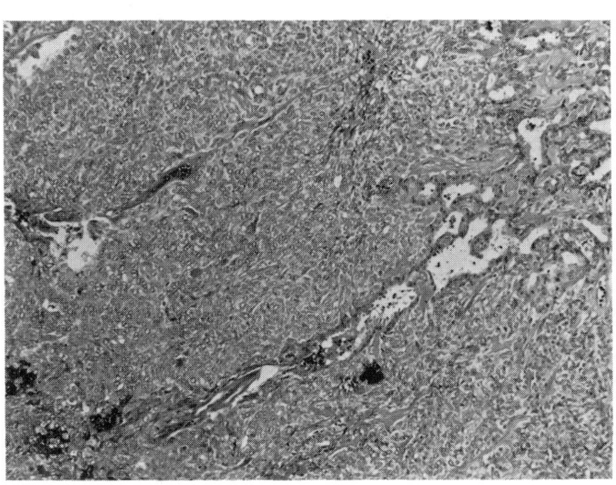

Figure 8–10. Photomicrograph of acinic cell tumor of the minor salivary glands of the buccal mucosa. (H & E × 100)

Histologically the tumors appear benign. It is impossible to differentiate those that will undertake a malignant course from the benign lesions. Fortunately, the benign variety is the most frequently encountered type; however, it is important to bear in mind that the pathologist cannot make a judgment concerning the malignancy or benignity of the tumor's eventual course on the basis of histology. Only the biologic activity exhibited in each individual case can determine this. Two cellular variants of the serous cell exist—the granular and the clear cell. The clear cell type is very uncommon, and its ultrastructural appearance suggests that it originates from ductal epithelial rather than acinar cells.

Acinic cell tumors are slow-growing, and local recurrences are seen many years after primary excision. Eneroth et al[19] quote a 90 per cent 5-year survival and a 50 per cent 25-year survival rate for patients with acinic cell cancer of the parotid gland. A compendium of cases involving 296 patients revealed a local recurrence rate of 27 per cent, a metastatic rate of 10.8 per cent, and a mortality rate of 14 per cent.[14]

Adenoid Cystic Cancer

Adenoid cystic carcinoma is an enigmatic tumor with an unpredictable course. It is locally invasive with a peculiar propensity to invade nerve sheaths. This invasiveness can extend in discontinuity a considerable distance from the primary lesion. A not uncommon finding is that of nests of tumor cells along an involved nerve an unexpectedly long way from the main lesion, sometimes even as far as the cranial foramina. Metastases are both lymphatic- and blood-borne. A tragic but more than occasional scenario in the treatment of these tumors is to have achieved local control only to be thwarted by a pulmonary nodule presenting 5 or 10 years after the initial resection. Because such a course is seen so often, an air of pessimism tends to pervade any consideration of management of these tumors.

The cell of origin is thought to be derived from the epithelium of the intercalated ducts. These basiloid cells often form a cribrose or lacy pattern and have a tendency to form glandular or cystlike structures. However, the cystic spaces may be missing and, because of its stromal component, made up of an eosinophilic hyaline or mucinous element, the tumor is occasionally confused with mucoepidermoid or mixed tumors. The other two histologic patterns are the solid and so-called tubular configurations. The solid type consists of a monotonous sheet of cells. The tubular configurations are represented by numerous small rounded structures, the result of cutting across closely packed thin tubules of cells (Fig. 8–11).[20]

Perzin et al[21] have shown an interesting correlation between survival and the predominant histologic type of the tumor. Tumors with a 30 per cent or greater solid pattern have the worst prognosis, while those with a predominantly tubular pattern have the best, with intermediate survival rates seen with tumors of the cribrose variety.

In an extensive review of the literature by Batsakis,[14] the parotid gland was found to be the site of origin of only 17.3 per cent of all adenoid cystic tumors of head and neck origin. The submandibular and sublingual glands are much more common sites, and adenoid cystic tumors are the most prevalent type found in the minor salivary glands. In Conley's series, 58 per cent of all adenoid cystic cancers were in these glands.[22] Conley's review of his experience with 134 adenoid cystic carcinomas graphically illustrates the metastatic potential of these tumors.[23] Pulmonary metastases occurred in 41 per cent of his patients, 22 per cent had secondaries in the brain, 16 per cent in lymph nodes, 13 per cent in bone, and 4 per cent in other body organs. A fascinating aspect of these tumors is the ability of the patient to live for prolonged periods of time, even 5 years or longer, often asymptomatically, with obvious metastatic disease (Fig. 8–12). In Conley's series, 42 per cent of the patients had at least one local recurrence, and most had more.

There were a number of patients in Conley's series[23] who had repeated local recurrences that were controlled by repeated resection. Their survival ranged from 11 to 30 years. However, in my more limited experience, local recurrence in most instances heralded a demise from the disease within 1 to 2 years.

Adenoid cystic carcinoma is commonly painful and locally tender. The lesion may be present for a long time before the patient seeks medical attention. In the parotid gland, the lesion commonly causes a facial paralysis, which may be the presenting symptom in the absence of a palpable mass.[21] Because the tumor is the most important malignancy of the minor salivary glands, pain, ulceration, bleeding, and a local mass are symptoms in

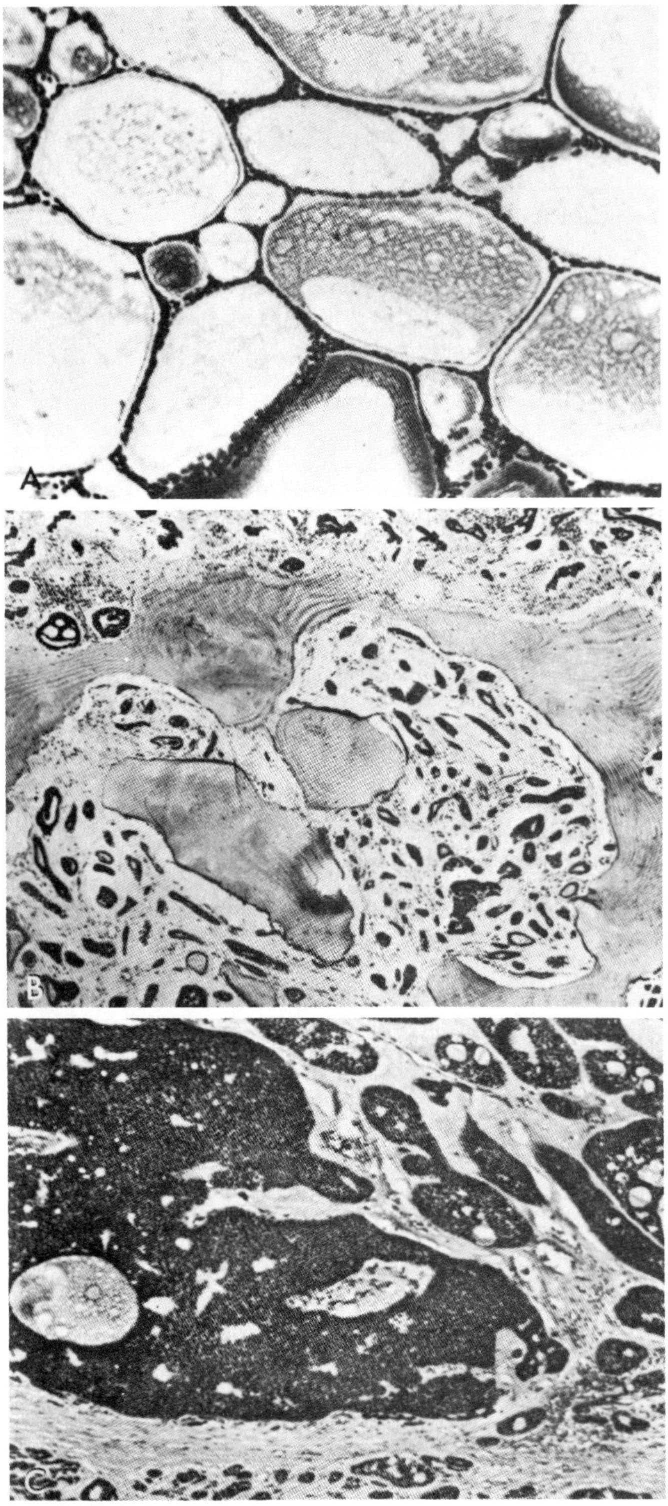

Figure 8–11. Three histologic configurations assumed by adenoid cystic carcinoma. *A,* Cribrose variety. Note large cystic spaces filled with mucoid material and lined by cells only one or two layers thick. (× 50). *B,* Tubular variety. A small ductlike or tubular pattern is seen in this adenoid cystic tumor invading the bone of the hard palate. (× 50) *C,* Solid configuration. This type is the most malignant in behavior (× 60) (From Thackray AC, Lucas RB: Tumors of the major salivary glands. Fascicle 10, Atlas of Tumor Pathology, 2nd ed. Washington, DC, Armed Forces Institute of Pathology, 1974, p 74.)

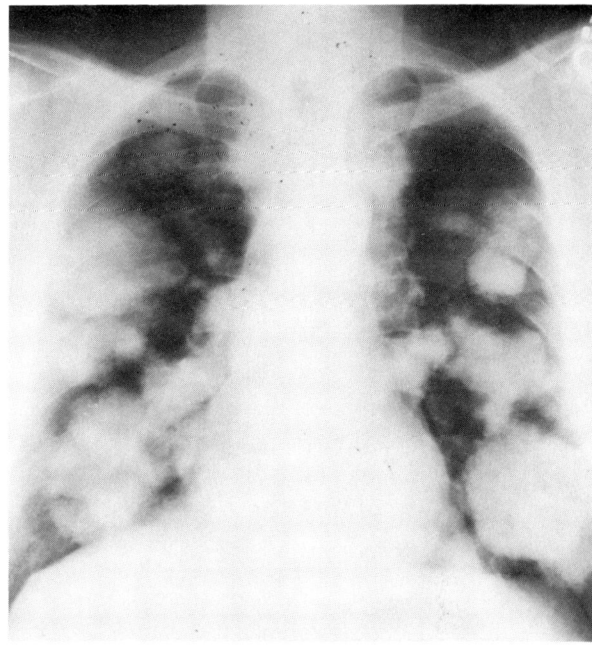

Figure 8–12. Chest x-ray of a patient with extensive metastatic adenoid cystic carcinoma to the lung. The patient had no lower respiratory tract symptoms at the time this x-ray was taken.

these sites. Nasal, paranasal sinus, and nasopharyngeal tumors present with airway obstruction and epistaxis; those of the soft palate and pharynx with dysphagia and ulceration.

Mucoepidermoid Tumor

Mucoepidermoid tumor is a highly variable neoplasm whose most innocuous form has been classified by some as "benign." The lesions form 6 to 9 per cent of all primary salivary gland tumors. About 60 per cent of them occur in the parotid gland.[14, 16] With some exceptions there appears to be a fairly close correlation between the cellular composition of the tumor and its biologic behavior. There are six morphologic types of cells found in these tumors: "maternal cells," intermediate, epidermoid, clear, columnar, and mucous (Table 8–2). A predominance of intermediate and epidermoid cells (especially plemorphic forms of the latter) signifies malignancy (Fig. 8–13). These more invasive tumors are characterized by relatively rapid growth, local invasion of skin and facial nerve, and regional as well as distant metastases. The more benign forms display glandular structures with formation of mucin, well-differentiated epidermoid cells, and a dearth of intermediate cells (Fig. 8–14). The problem is that despite a completely benign histologic appearance an occasional low-grade mucoepidermoid tumor will metastasize. These lesions thus are all potentially

Table 8–2. CELLULAR CHARACTERISTICS OF MUCOEPIDERMOID TUMORS

Cell Type	*Description*	*Type of Cytoplasm*	*Characteristic*
Maternal	Small; round or oval	Scant basophilic	Progenitor of other cell types
Intermediate	Oval; larger than maternal	Pale eosinophilic; scant	Characteristic of malignancy
Epidermoid	Squamous cell appearance; may form keratin	Eosinophilic	Characteristic of malignancy
Clear	Variable size; central nucleus	Water-clear	Characteristic of benignity
Columnar	Similar to secretory cells of ducts	Granular to foamy	None diagnostic
Mucous	Large, swollen, balloon-shaped; small eccentric nucleus	Foamy or reticular	Characteristic of benignity

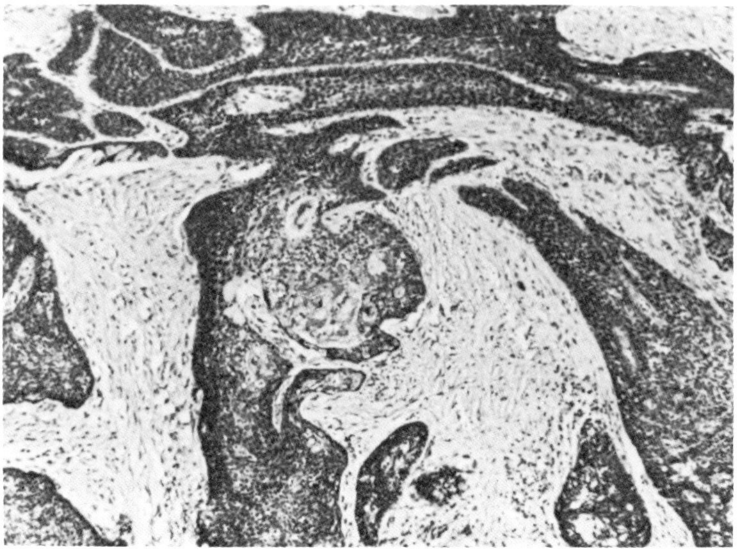

Figure 8–13. Photomicrograph of a malignant mucoepidermoid tumor. (× 60) (From Thackray AC, Lucas RB: Tumors of the major salivary glands. Fascicle 10, Atlas of Tumor Pathology, 2nd ed. Washington, DC, Armed Forces Institute of Pathology, 1974, p 74.)

malignant and must be treated accordingly. Fortunately, if local recurrences or metastases do occur, they do so within 5 years.[24] Another favorable factor is that the bulk of the tumors are of the more benign variety.[22]

These neoplasms present most commonly as a firm, painless, slow-growing mass in the superficial lobe of the parotid. Facial nerve involvement, cutaneous fixation, and pain are common in only the most malignant types. The more benign are indistinguishable clinically from a benign mixed tumor. The lesion has a pseudocapsule, and the cut surface may be solid or cystic. The cysts, which are variable in size, contain clear but usually viscid material.

Squamous Cell Carcinoma

Squamous cell carcinoma is an uncommon malignancy of the salivary glands, being mainly limited to the parotid and the submaxillary. This tumor makes up 0.1 to 3.4 per cent of all parotid neoplasms and 12 per cent of those in the submaxillary gland.[14] It is often difficult to determine whether a squamous cell cancer is primary in the parotid or is a metastatic lymph node from a primary in the skin or elsewhere in the upper aerodigestive tract. The skin primaries that produce the metastases are usually 2 cm or greater in diameter.

Clincally these malignancies are usually

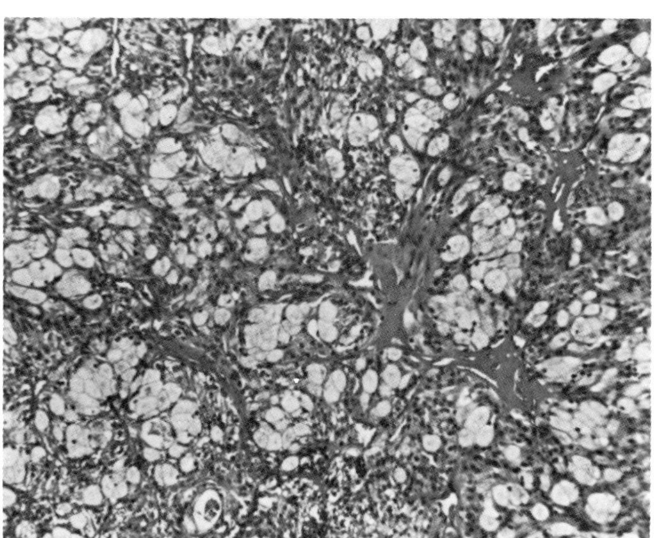

Figure 8–14. Photomicrograph of a benign mucoepidermoid tumor. Note the number of mucous cells with scant squamous or intermediate cells. (× 75) (From Thackray AC, Lucas RB: Tumors of the major salivary glands. Fascicle 10, Atlas of Tumor Pathology, 2nd ed. Washington, DC, Armed Forces Institute of Pathology, 1974, p 74.)

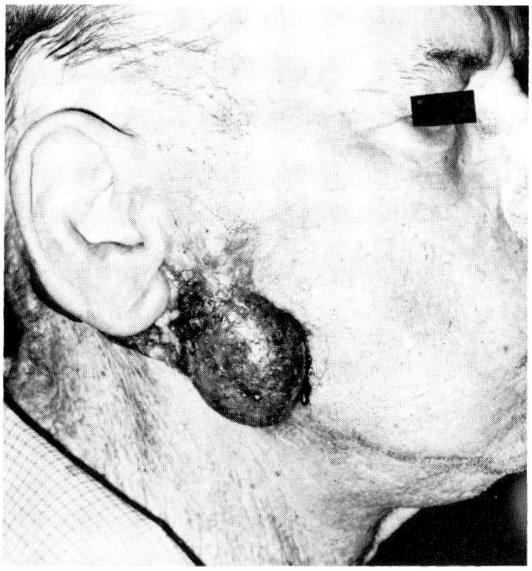

Figure 8–15. Extensive squamous cell carcinoma of the parotid gland that has eroded through the skin.

very obvious. They are rock hard and are often fixed to the underlying structures or overlying skin, even eroding through the latter, producing an ugly suppurating ulcer (Fig. 8–15). The lesion is painful, tender, and rapid-growing. Facial nerve paralysis is found in about 30 per cent of patients. Neck metastases are present about 25 per cent of the time.

Histologically the tumors are composed of keratin-producing cells with intercellular bridges. There is no mucin production. If the cancer is the result of metastasis to the lymph node from a cutaneous lesion, some residuum of the node may be seen. However, these metastases are often substantial prior to resection, and the lymphatic architecture may be entirely replaced by tumor.

DIAGNOSIS

Unfortunately, the clinical differentiation between benign and malignant lesions may be determined only when the signs of malignancy become evident. Pain, ulceration, facial nerve paralysis, fixation to surrounding structures, and metastases are the hallmarks of cancer, although notable exceptions to this rule occur. Many salivary gland cancers, for instance, are painless and do not produce paralysis, while on the other hand, it is not uncommon to find a benign pleomorphic adenoma arising in the minor salivary glands of the palate that ulcerates (Fig. 8–16). Recurrent pleomorphic adenomas are commonly fixed to deep structures and even the adjacent skin, despite their benign histology. Facial nerve paralysis is almost a sure sign of malignancy, but there are rare exceptions to even this rule (Fig. 8–17).

Contrast sialography is sometimes helpful. Cavitary sialectasis is a strong presumptive sign of malignancy (Fig. 8–18). Erosion of ducts, giving a rough irregular pattern, is further suggestive of this diagnosis, whereas ductal displacement is more characteristic of a benign lesion. The use of CAT scanning combined with positive contrast sialography helps in differentiating between intra- and extraglandular lesions. This is especially helpful in determining the nature of lesions of the

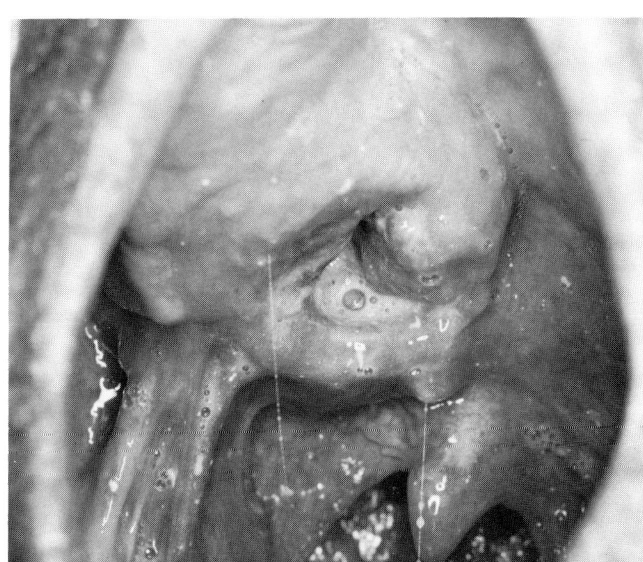

Figure 8–16. Large pleomorphic adenoma of the hard palate with ulceration.

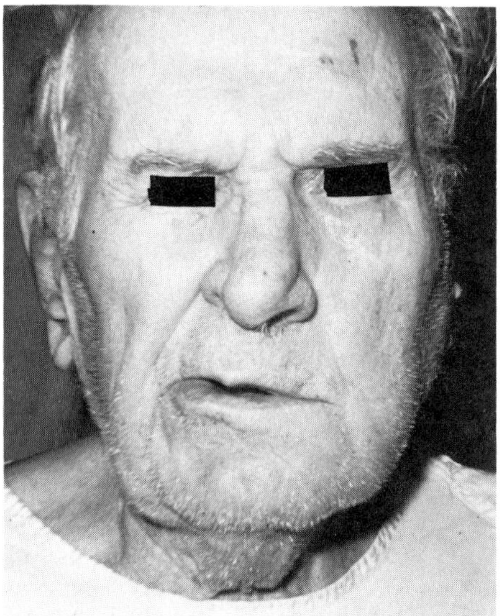

Figure 8–17. Elderly man with a swelling of the parotid gland and a facial palsy, raising a high index of suspicion for malignancy of the gland. The patient in actuality had an abscess.

deep lobe, where a hard mass is palpable deep in the neck and diagnosis is uncertain.

Standard radiography of the facial skeleton helps reveal bone erosion. A panoramic x-ray (Panorex film) of the mandible may demonstrate mandibular invasion of the ramus (Fig. 8–9*B*) in the case of parotid cancers, whereas lucency of the mandibular body would indicate submaxillary or sublingual gland malignancy. Tomography may be of further assistance in this delineation.

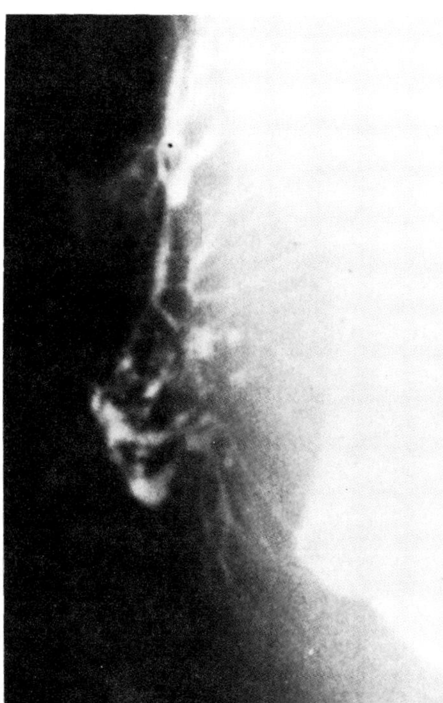

Figure 8–18. Contrast sialography revealing cavitory sialectosis in a patient with adenoid cystic carcinoma of the parotid gland. (From Lizmor J, Noyek AM: An Atlas of Otolaryngologic Radiology. Philadelphia, WB Saunders, 1978.)

Needle biopsy and fine needle aspiration have risen in popularity as contemporary diagnostic tools. Needle biopsy as developed by Eneroth[25] and others is the definitive diagnostic test in Sweden and other European countries. However, Conley[26] has seriously questioned the validity of this approach, and with considerable justification. Considering the difficulty in establishing a definitive diagnosis even on the basis of the large tissue volume produced by resection, it is hard to conceive of making this diagnosis from the minute specimen produced by needle biopsy. The wisdom of predicating therapy on the basis of this small portion of tumor from a limited area is therefore open to question. Fine needle aspiration biopsy is an exciting new technique that requires special training and substantial experience on the part of the pathologist. It holds considerable promise but has yet to stand the test of time in terms of diagnostic utility in salivary gland neoplasms.

Tumors of the minor salivary glands are amenable to incisional biopsy, as they present in the oral cavity, pharynx, or nasal cavities. Lesions of the major glands, however, do not lend themselves to this diagnostic exercise, and excisional biopsy is the method of choice. This is particularly true with regard to parotid gland tumors.

Parotidectomy with facial nerve preservation has become the definitive procedure for excisional biopsy of a parotid neoplasm. The recurrence rate of benign tumors is exceptionally small following this procedure, especially when compared to recurrence rates seen with the fortunately discarded procedure of "lumpectomy," or worse, incisional biopsy. The unfortunate results of these latter procedures are still with us and provide a considerable therapeutic challenge.

SURGICAL CONSIDERATIONS

Recurrent Pleomorphic Adenoma

Once a pleomorphic adenoma recurs, it acquires a tenacious hold on adjacent tissue. It assumes an almost malignant demeanor with numerous extensions and tumor excrescences in seeming discontinuity. In the truly benign form, however, metastases never occur. The surgical problem is that of encompassing local tumor extension, which can be accomplished only by a radical attack on the tumor. Even with an aggressive excision, if tumor-free margins are not obtained, the lesion will recur (Fig. 8–19).

One of the most difficult facts to accept is that occasionally portions of the facial nerve will need to be excised in order to achieve an adequate resection. Work[11] established this as a basic principle in these cases as recently as 1976. A fruitless attempt to dissect through a mass of fibrous tissue and tumor to preserve the nerve will produce not only further recurrence but neural injury as well.

The patient in Figure 8–27 presented 8 years previously with a history spanning 20 years of 14 prior attempts at eliminating a pleomorphic adenoma. The tumor had been initially diagnosed by incisional biopsy and then locally excised. The surgeon when faced with repeated recurrence had, in a desperate attempt at removing the lesion, even resorted to a radical neck dissection. In light of the benign form of this tumor, this was unnecessary, as nodal metastases never occur. However, the tumor may locally invade muscle, bone, and skin. Resection of this recurrent lesion required partial mandibulectomy, mastoid tip excision, and removal of the posterior belly of the digastric muscle, part of the trapezius, splenius capitis, and masseter muscles, the main trunk of the facial nerve, and substantial neck skin.

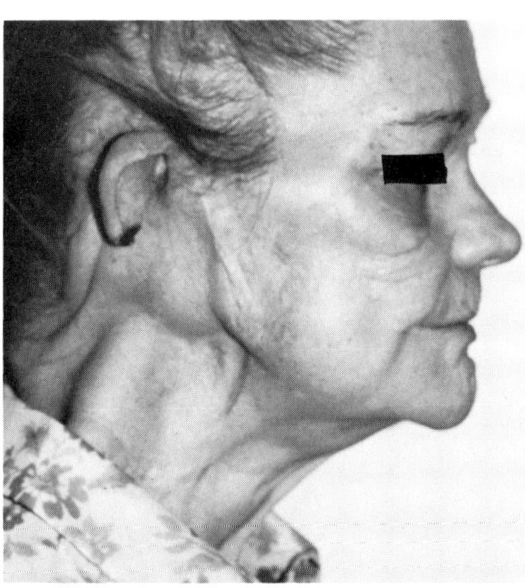

Figure 8–19. Middle-aged woman following 16 attempts at resecting a pleomorphic adenoma. The original operation was an incisional biopsy. Radical neck dissection, mandibulectomy, and temporal bone excision were fraught with recurrence.

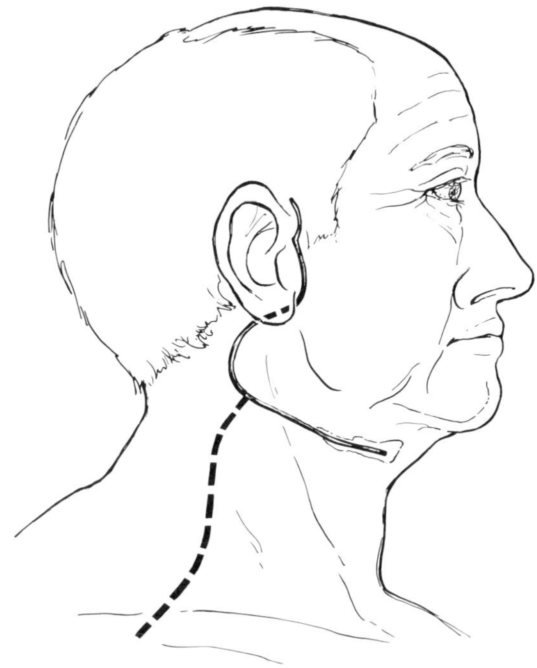

Figure 8–20. Modified Blair incision. Dotted line represents extension if radical neck dissection is required.

A modified Blair incision[27] (Fig. 8–20) yields excellent access to the gland. It was modified in this instance to include a large portion of postauricular and superior neck skin in order to circumscribe the area of cutaneous involvement (Fig. 8–21). Skin flaps

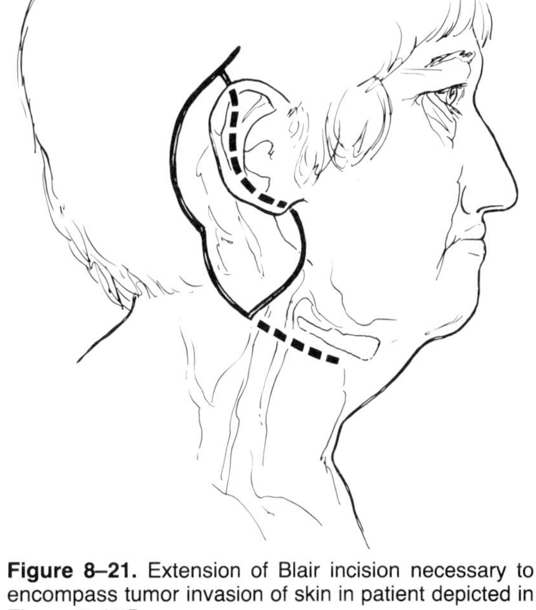

Figure 8–21. Extension of Blair incision necessary to encompass tumor invasion of skin in patient depicted in Figure 8–27*B*.

are developed to expose the tumor and the peripheral branches of the facial nerve. In the previously operated patient, much fibrosis between the facial skin and the underlying tissue is encountered, and frequent use of the facial nerve stimulator helps to localize the various branches. Also in such cases the elevation of the facial flap over the parotid bed and the site of tumor recurrence is extremely tedious, in marked contrast to the easy, quick dissection that is the norm in the previously unoperated case. Pleomorphic adenomas tend to push the various branches of the facial nerve in front of them. In the recurrent cases, however, the tumor has more of a tendency to envelop the nerves. In addition, fibrosis secondary to past surgical intervention also envelops and further binds the branches into the bed.

Once the flaps are elevated, the main trunk of the facial nerve is located. The key to all parotid gland surgery is the isolation of this nerve, and for a detailed account of this step, the beautifully exact description of facial nerve localization by McCabe and Work[27] is unsurpassed in the literature. The most consistent landmark is the tragal "pointer" on the cartilaginous external auditory canal. The trunk of the nerve is usually found approximately 1 cm deep to it (Fig. 8–22). In the case of the patient in Figure 8–27, the nerve could not be identified because of tumor envelopment. A simple mastoidectomy with skeletonization of the fallopian canal was done. Parchment-thin layers of the bone of the canal were chipped away, unroofing the nerve, and tumor was seen invading the stylomastoid foramen. The nerve was sectioned about half the distance up the mastoid portion of the facial canal. The nerve stump and tumor excrescences were dissected from the canal into the upper neck. Attempts to isolate the upper and lower main divisions were thwarted by the presence of tumor and fibrosis. The distal branches of the nerve were then identified, tagged, and severed.

Posteriorly and superiorly an incision was made outside of tumor involvement and carried through the underlying trapezius and splenius capitis muscles to the skull. Because the deeper muscles were not involved, the dissection stopped at this level. Sweeping the dissection inferiorly, the digastric and stylohyoid muscles were excised, with care taken to ligate the occipital artery, which sits in its own groove deep to the digastric muscle. The mastoid tip was excised at this point and the bloc carried forward (Fig. 8–23).

Pleomorphic adenomas are usually attached to the masseter muscle, and a generous portion surrounding the tumor is resected. The deep margin anteriorly may be either the ramus of the mandible or the medial pterygoid muscle. If there is bone

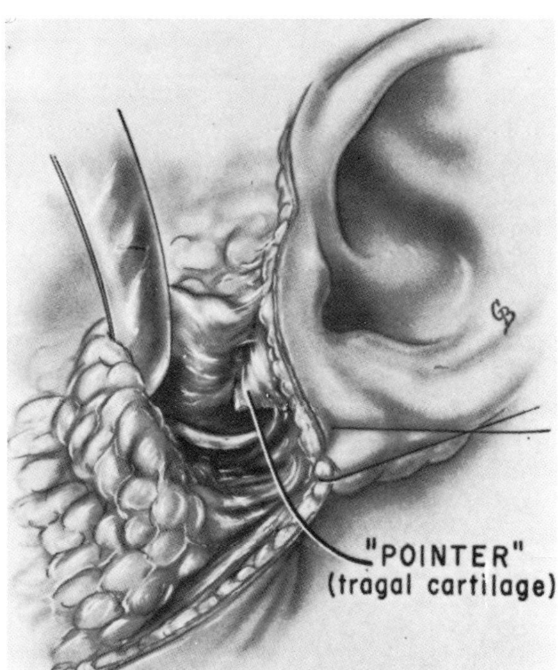

Figure 8–22. Dissection of the facial nerve showing relationship to the tragal pointer. (From McCabe BF, Work PW: Parotidectomy with special preference in the facial nerve. *In* English GM (ed): Otolaryngology, Vol. 4. Hagerstown, MD, Harper & Row, 1967, p 43.)

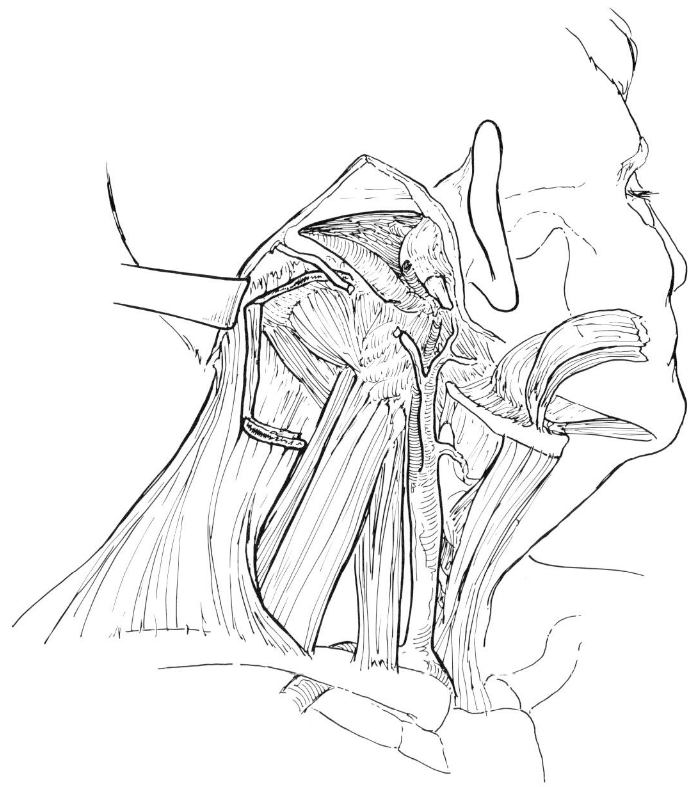

Figure 8–23. Resection of the upper aspects of the trapezius and splenius capitis muscles as well as of the digastric and stylohyoid is required to achieve a tumor-free margin on the superior and deep aspects. The sternomastoid muscle was resected in a prior operation. The mastoid tip is amputated. The facial nerve is resected within the fallopian canal.

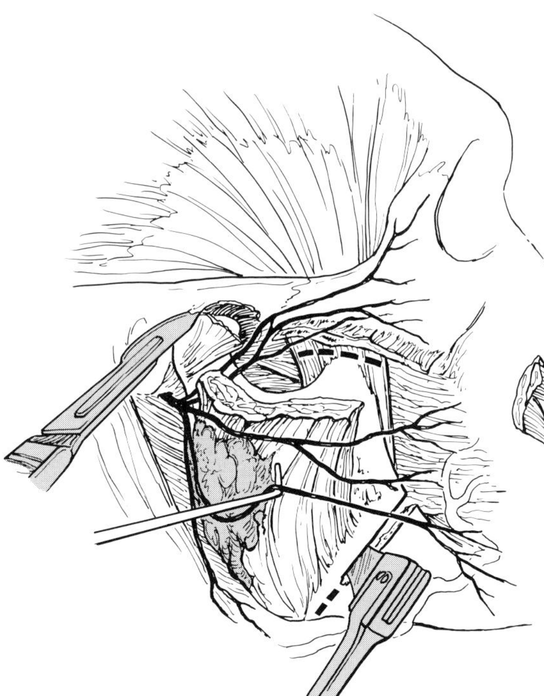

Fig. 8–24

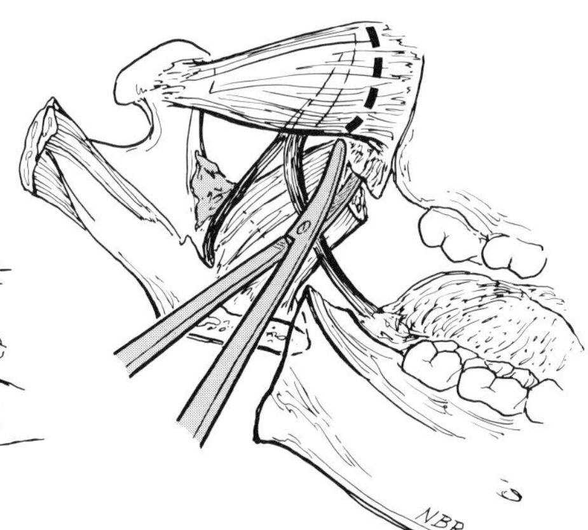

Fig. 8–25

Figure 8–24. When the tumor is stuck to mandible, the condylar head, neck, and a portion of the ramus are resected, as well as overlying masseter muscle.

Figure 8–25. If the deep lobe of the parotid gland is involved with tumor, the medial and lateral pterygoid muscles are excised.

involvement, however, the ramus must be sacrificed (Fig. 8–24). If the tumor wraps around its medial surface or if the deep lobe remnant is infiltrated, not only the mandibular ramus but the pterygoid muscles as well are taken (Fig. 8–25). Bleeding from the internal maxillary artery on the medial surface of the mandibular neck, as well as from the pterygoid venous plexus, can be somewhat troublesome. Stick ties of 3–0 vascular silk may be necessary to ensure hemostasis in the pterygoid plexus. Sometimes bleeding is so persistent that only a pack of hemostatic cotton or gauze such as Oxycel or Surgicel will stop it. Tumor invasion of the pterygoid musculature renders complete excision difficult. The internal carotid artery presents in the bed as further deep progression is made along the skull base. Superior invasion of the external auditory canal may require lateral temporal bone resection (see Chapter 7). The bloc is removed and suspicious margins checked by frozen section.

The head is turned and excision of the greater auricular nerve is done from the opposing side. In revision cases, the ipsilateral nerve has invariably been sacrificed previously. The nerve graft is approximated to the facial trunk in the fallopian canal. Although it is not essential to have a suture at this site, if one or two sutures can be placed, this is done. The distal branches are sutured to the other end of the graft with 8–0 or 10–0 nylon under microscopic control (Fig. 8–26). Closure of the wound is by skin grafting or a local rotation flap (Fig. 8–27). Thick regional skin flaps or musculocutaneous flaps are initially avoided, to prevent obscuring early local recurrences. If resection margins are found to be positive on permanent pathologic section, immediate revision is advised in the hope of getting ahead of the disease. This was necessary on two occasions in my experience and was successful in ablating the tumor in each instance. Radiation therapy is not an effective means of dealing with residual tumor.[6]

Mucoepidermoid Tumor

The treatment of this lesion is problematic. If the surgeon could be assured that all histologically benign tumors would pursue a benign course, they could be safely excised with a narrow margin. However, the protean nature of mucoepidermoid tumors is such that resection with adequate margins is mandatory. The issue of the facial nerve is a tricky one. Direct tumor invasion or the presence of tumor close to a branch or to the main trunk of the nerve necessitates its sacrifice. In the cases of a very well differentiated tumor, some tempering of this harsh dictum may be in order, since local recurrences are very uncommon and their reexcision is not necessarily associated with a poor prognosis.[22]

The more histologically malignant types

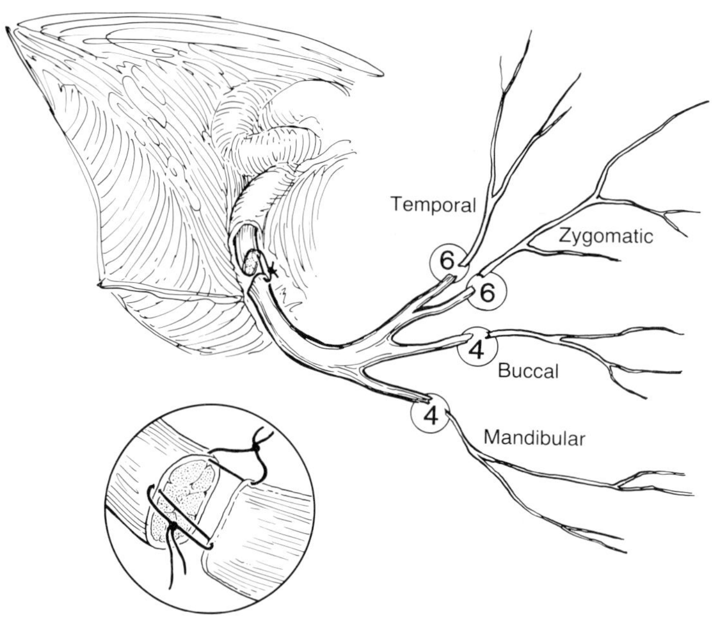

Figure 8–26. A greater auricular nerve graft is placed, with the thickest end of the graft within the fallopian canal secured to the main trunk by one or two sutures when possible. The distal arborization of the graft is sutured to at least the three most functionally important facial nerve branches; the zygomatic, buccal, and mandibular.

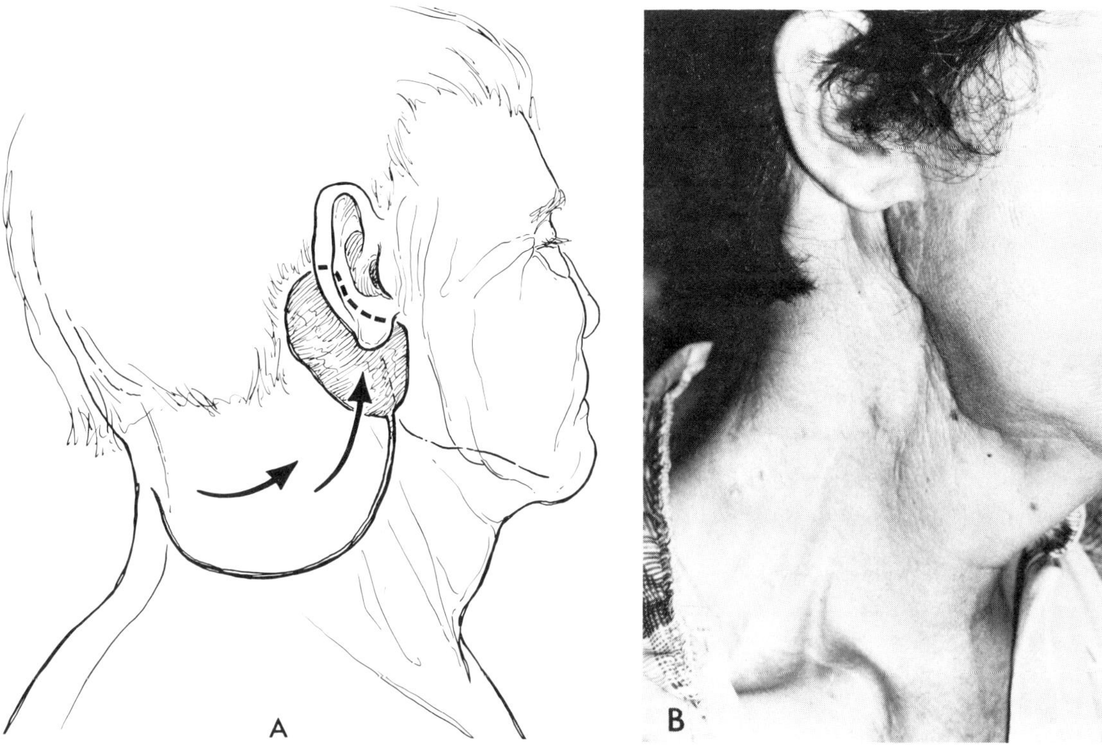

Figure 8–27. *A,* Wound closure is effected by using a rotation flap from the nape of the neck. *B,* Appearance of patient postoperatively.

have a marked tendency to metastasize with rates quoted as high as 66 per cent.[5, 22] On the other hand, the low-grade tumors rarely spread. Distant metastases are again a feature of the more poorly differentiated tumors and are much more common in patients with cervical adenopathy.[5, 22, 24]

The overall 5-year survival rate of patients with mucoepidermoid tumor is between 80 and 90 per cent.[16, 22, 24] Those with the most highly differentiated tumors have a rate close to 100 per cent. However, the more malignant, poorly differentiated mucoepidermoid carcinomas have a much different clinical course and eventual prognosis. In Conley's series of 278 patients with cancer of the parotid gland, 27 per cent had mucoepidermoid tumors, and of these only 30 were of the poorly differentiated type.[22] Of those with this poor differentiation who were initially treated by Conley, the 5-year survival rate was 56 per cent. These patients all had radical excisions as the primary attack. The ones who presented with recurrent disease and had their initial management elsewhere did not do nearly as well. The surgical technique for the more malignant forms of mucoepidermoid tumor is the same as that for squamous cell cancer (see below).

Squamous Cell Cancer

The best treatment of squamous cell carcinoma is radical excision. Postoperative irradiation should be added if significant spread beyond the gland has occurred or when there are neck metastases. Even though the prognosis of poorly differentiated mucoepidermoid carcinoma is better than that of squamous cell, the surgical management should be just as aggressive.

One of the few violations of the en bloc technique of cancer removal in head and neck surgery is the isolation of the facial nerve in parotid gland tumor resection. As dissection of the main trunk and its branches proceeds, constant vigilance must be kept in keeping track of the tumor margins. Branches of the nerve are preserved whenever possible, the most important functionally being the zygomatic or eye branch.

In planning the excision, any skin fixation or penetration must be skirted by a wide margin of at least 4 cm, since skin recurrences are common when narrower margins are employed. Conley's principle of the first attack being by far the most successful is epitomized in salivary gland cancer surgery. Anticipation of the possible adjacent structures that will

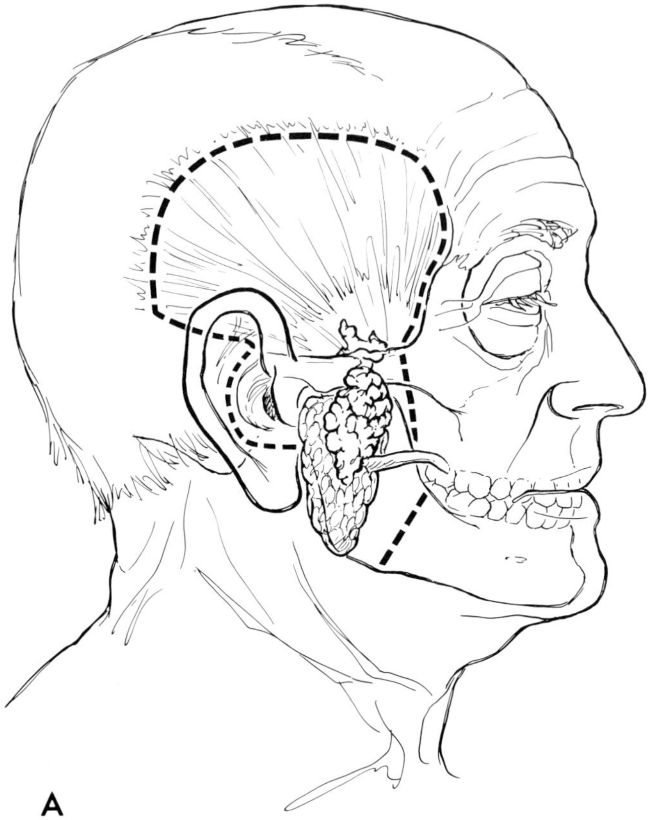

A

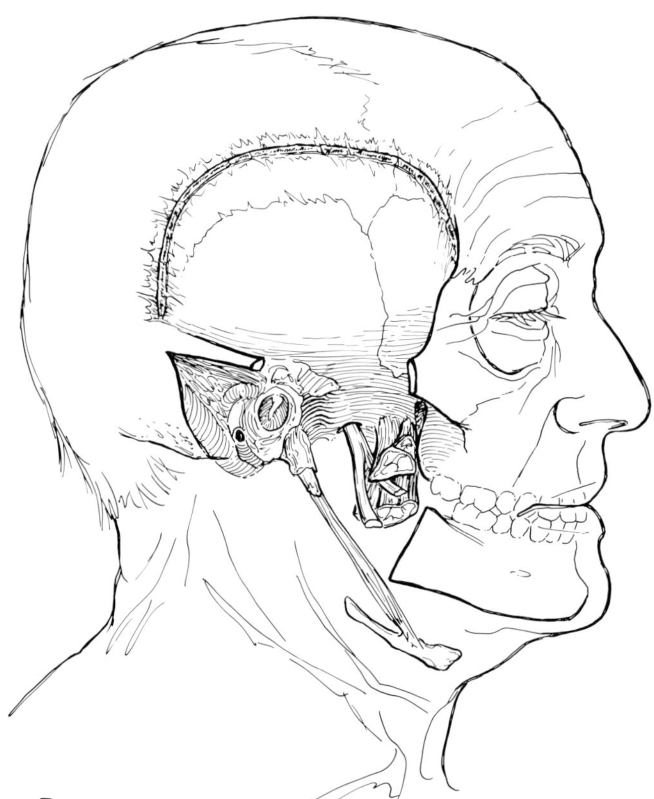

B

Figure 8–28. *A,* When a malignancy approximates the zygomatic arch or temporalis muscle, resection includes the temporalis, the arch, neck, and condyle of the mandible, and usually the ramus. *B,* Often a lateral temporal bone resection is necessary because of the proximity of the tumor to the external auditory canal.

require resection also helps in planning the excision. Provision must be made for exposing the mastoid tip if a portion of the temporal bone requires resection. Extending the incision into the scalp allows excellent exposure of the temporomandibular joint and zygomatic roots. If a radical neck dissection is required, a lazy S excision can be dropped from the inferior limb of the modified Blair incision (Fig. 8–20). The neck dissection is done only in the presence of manifest cervical metastases, since these occur in only 25 per cent of patients. However, if the parotid lesion is itself secondary to a tumor elsewhere in the upper aerodigestive tract, a neck dissection is indicated.

Tumor stuck to the cartilaginous portion of the external auditory canal requires removal of the portion of the canal and a generous margin of conchal cartilage. Often some bony canal must be removed as well. When the neoplasm is fixed to the osseous external canal, a lateral temporal bone resection must be done (Fig. 8–28*B*) (see Chapter 7).

In squamous cell cancer of the parotid gland, often the tumor has extended beyond the deep margin of the superficial lobe. This area is often neglected by many surgeons who pay more attention to the esthetic implications of the proximity of the tumor to the facial nerve and skin. The masseter muscle lies in the parotid bed and should always be included in resections of malignancies of the superficial lobe. Deep lobe involvement automatically dictates inclusion of portions of the medial and even lateral pterygoid muscles in the resection. Fixation of tumor to the paraspinal muscles indicates nonresectability, and one can hope for only palliation as the primary therapeutic goal. Tumor invasion of the internal carotid, except in a few rare cases (see Chapter 9), is a dire prognostic sign. "Mopping up" with postoperative irradiation in these cases does little to improve survival, although it may prolong temporary local control. Gross residual disease, even though scant in amount, almost invariably dooms the patient to death from the cancer.

Both superficial and deep lobe involvement usually necessitates partial mandibulectomy. Whereas in resections involving the oropharynx the mandibular condyle is usually preserved, here the condyle must be included in the resection of the mandibular ramus (Fig. 8–24). Vigilance for the internal maxillary artery during this phase will prevent the problem of troublesome bleeding. If tumor extends beyond the mandibular ramus, it may be necessary to remove the glenoid fossa itself and the posterior aspect of the zygomatic arch. Temporalis muscle excision and removal of the contents of the infratemporal fossa (Fig. 8–28) may also be required to achieve a safe margin (Fig. 8–29). The resection of bone in this region (with the exception of the condyle) is most easily achieved with a cutting bur. Care must be taken to get well beyond the tumor, even if it means exposing middle fossa dura.

Those branches of the facial nerve sacrificed during resection are replaced with nerve grafts. When the main trunk is taken, the sural or the greater auricular nerve can be used as a cable graft. The branching network of the greater auricular may be employed to graft in various severed branches of the facial nerve. If sufficient graft arborization is not available, the graft can be split longitudinally. The nerve is sutured with 10-0 monofilament nylon, using 8 to 10 sutures in the trunk, 6 to 8 in a main division, and 4 to 6 in a named branch. The operating microscope, especially if fitted with a zoom lens, greatly facilitates this part of the surgery.

Lost skin is replaced by a flap. A myocutaneous flap improves the cosmetic appearance by virtue of the bulk supplied by the muscular portion. The only problem with these flaps is that they will obscure any local recurrence. The trapezius or pectoralis flaps are the most commonly used, although a

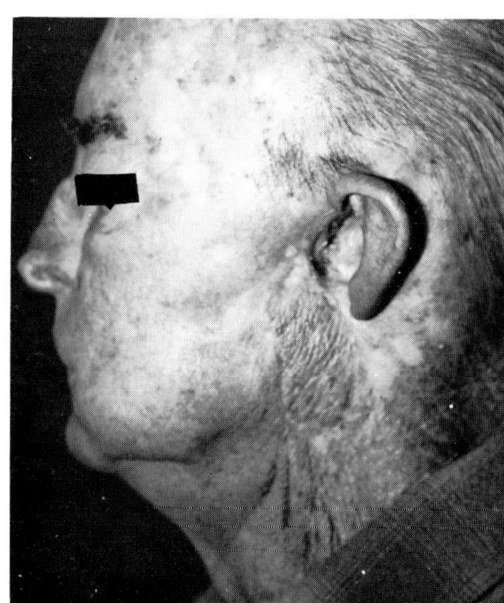

Figure 8–29. Patient following the resection illustrated in Figure 8–28.

deltopectoral flap may be done if an axial pattern skin flap is preferred. If a large defect is to be produced, this latter flap should be delayed ahead of time. A good rule of thumb is to delay the flap when the width of the pedicle is less than half the length of the deltoid portion (that portion from the delto-pectoral groove to its most lateral extent). However, lining the surgical defect with a split-thickness skin graft, although unsightly, is the safest method for early detection of local recurrences.

Adenoid Cystic Carcinoma

A philosophy of therapy directed at these pernicious, aggressive, and unpredictable tumors must bring to bear a host of considerations relative to the patient's age and general state of health, the presence of regional or distant metastases, and the local extent of tumor. The basic foundation of effective long-term local control is aggressive surgical resection.[20, 28, 29] Although distant metastases are not uncommon, the sooner the entire primary tumor is removed, the less vulnerable the patient will be to the risk of metastasis. The local "recurrence" of cancer is in reality local persistence. As long as tumor persists at the primary site, there is an increasing likelihood that the patient may have tumor emboli that are continually breaking away from the lesion to lodge elsewhere in the body. This is especially important to remember in the management of adenoid cystic cancer, in which locally persistent disease often remains occult for prolonged periods of time before finally becoming manifest. During these extended periods when tumor is present but obscured at the primary site, the patient is at continuous risk for metastases. Thus the importance of complete surgical removal cannot be overemphasized. In a series of 58 patients with adenoid cystic carcinoma reported by Smith et al,[29] with one exception, all of those patients clinically free of disease 10 years or longer had negative surgical margins. No patient with a negative margin had metastatic disease. On the other hand, when surgical margins were inadequate, 79 per cent developed metastatic disease, and only 8.8 per cent of these patients were alive and clinically free of disease at 10 years. In Conley's series of 40 patients followed longer than 10 years, 11 (27.5 per cent) were alive and tumor free.[23] An analysis relative to margins was not made, but Conley's impression of an association between aggressive surgery and increased longevity has guided our management philosophy.

In a young person, an aggressive operation is done that includes total parotidectomy, resection of all involved or adjacent facial nerve branches, mastoidectomy, excision of the infratemporal fossa, possible mandibulectomy, and often radical neck dissection.

Both the deep and superficial lobes of the gland are removed. Facial nerve branches that are anywhere near the tumor are excised. If no perineural invasion is evident and no facial paralysis was present preoperatively, all branches outside a 2 to 3 cm perimeter are spared. When neural invasion is evident, the safest procedure is to excise the nerve as far as the region of the stylomastoid foramen or even into the fallopian canal. A cable graft is interposed, or if this is not feasible, a hypoglossal to facial cross-over anastomosis is done. Mastoidectomy and resection of the external auditory canal, including both its cartilaginous and bony portions, must be performed in most cases, because of the proximity of the gland to these structures. The need for masseter and temporalis muscle as well as mandibular and zygomatic arch resection is determined on an individual basis, depending on tumor proximity. If the external auditory canal needs resection, the mandibular condyle is removed. Access to the glenoid fossa and hence the bony wall is thus affected. Often the root of the zygomatic bone is excised as well. A substantial resection margin must be maintained in all planes. The issue of radical neck dissection is a difficult one to resolve. Because lymph node metastases occur infrequently,[23, 30] the absence of clinically involved nodes militates against radical neck dissection. However, a neck dissection should be done when any suspicion of nodal disease is encountered. I do a radical neck dissection in most cases.

The older or infirm patient, and all patients with distant metastases, should be treated by a lesser procedure. Because of the slowly progressive nature of the disease and its sensitivity, albeit limited, to irradiation therapy, local control can be maintained for a reasonable time. Extensive resections resulting in profound esthetic and functional compromise should be limited to the younger patients.

The extreme arduousness of these decisions makes management of adenoid cystic carcinoma difficult. Evaluation of each case on an individual basis is absolutely essential to determining the best possible treatment plan. The prognosis for survival is better when the disease is in the major salivary

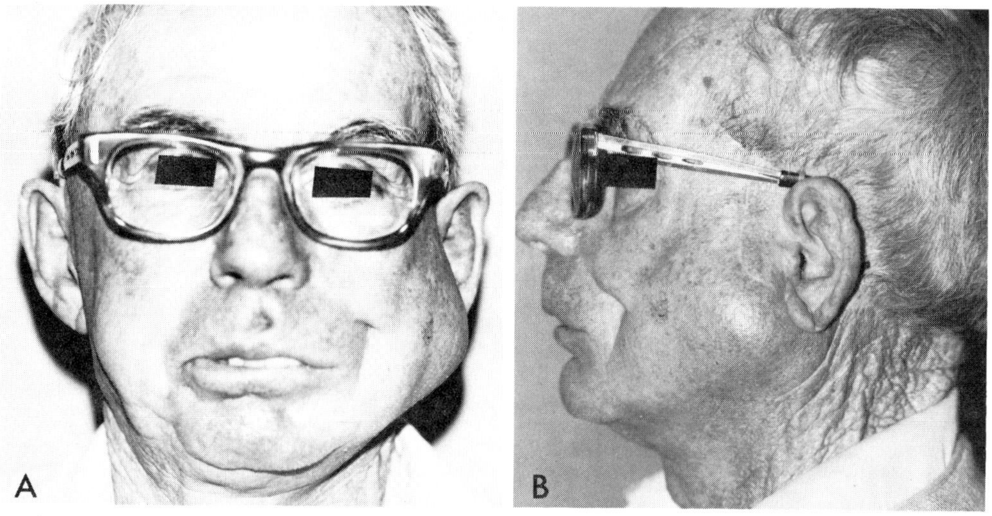

Figure 8–30. Patient with a large deep lobe parotid gland malignancy extending under the skull base, presenting with findings of compromise of the maxillary division of the trigeminal nerve. Tumor had eroded through the floor of the middle cranial fossa. *A,* Frontal view. *B,* Side view.

glands, especially the parotid, than in the minor glands. Conley's disease-free survival rate was 75 per cent at 5 years, 30 per cent at 10 years, and 20 per cent at 15 years for all sites.[23]

Adenocarcinomas and Acinic Cell Tumor

Resection for these tumors is similar to that for squamous cell and poorly differentiated mucoepidermoid carcinoma. The limits of excision are dictated by tumor extent. Lymph node metastases are uncommon, and therefore neck dissection is rarely performed. Mandibular and lateral temporal bone resections are usually necessary, and often even the zygomatic arch and the muscles deep in the parotid bed have to be removed. Deep lobe involvement may extend under the skull base, almost to the nasopharynx. In some cases, tumor may extend beyond these confines into the middle fossa (Fig. 8–30). At this point, a combined neurosurgical–head and neck procedure through a temporoparietal craniotomy and the infratemporal fossa may completely expose the tumor in its intracranial and extracranial extents. Details of this procedure are given in Chapter 9.

Submandibular and Sublingual Gland Tumors

Whereas most parotid neoplasms are benign, the submandibular and sublingual gland tumors are more often malignant. In Conley's series[22] 47 per cent of submandibular gland tumors and 90 per cent of sublingual glands were carcinomatous. Neoplasms of the sublingual glands are unusual. Although some mucoepidermoid, squamous cell, and acinic cell tumors are seen, most are adenoid cystic carcinoma. The same philosophy of radical excision applied to this tumor in the parotid gland is followed when it arises in the submaxillary and sublingual glands. The excision includes partial glossectomy, resection of the floor of the mouth and adjacent mandible, and radical neck dissection. The lingual and hypoglossal nerves as well as the ramus mandibularis of the facial nerve will need to be resected because of the propensity of adenoid cystic carcinoma to invade the nerve sheath. Excision of these nerves as close to their origin as possible is important to ensure completeness of tumor removal.

The mandibulectomy is necessary because of the proximity of bone to both glands. A more posterior excision can be done with submandibular primaries (Fig. 8–31), but sublingual gland tumors require excisions that include the arch (Fig. 8–32). These are segmental resections. The submandibular gland excisions should encompass mandible from the angle to the region of the mental foramen or just anterior to it. If there is numbness of the lip, denoting inferior alveolar nerve involvement, much wider resection must be done. The tumor in these instances must be considered to have extended into the marrow cavity along the sheath of the nerve. In order to get above possible tumor, the mandibu-

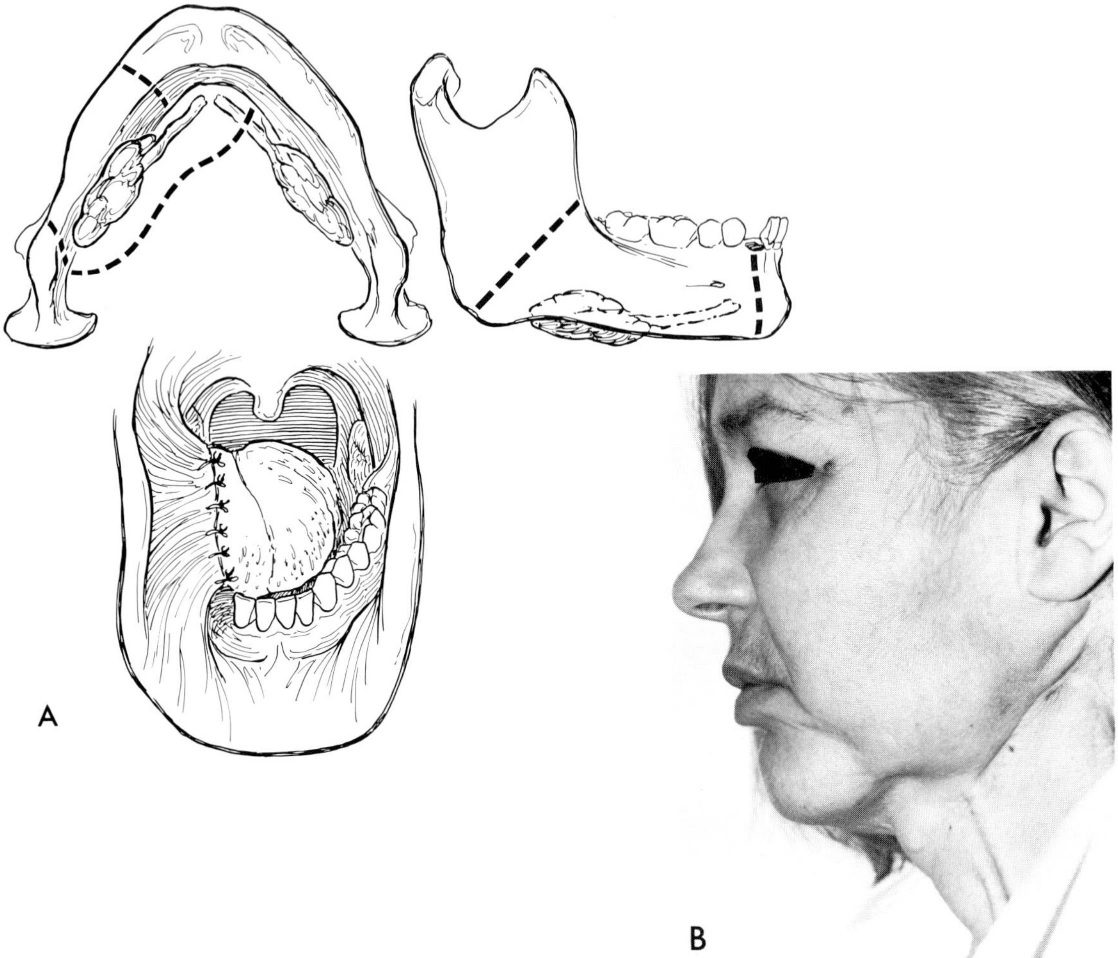

Figure 8–31. *A,* Mandibulectomy for adenoid cystic carcinoma of the submandibular salivary gland includes the ramus angle and part of the mandibular body. *B,* Appearance of patient 8 years after resection and 1 year after reconstruction of the defect with a fat-dermis graft.

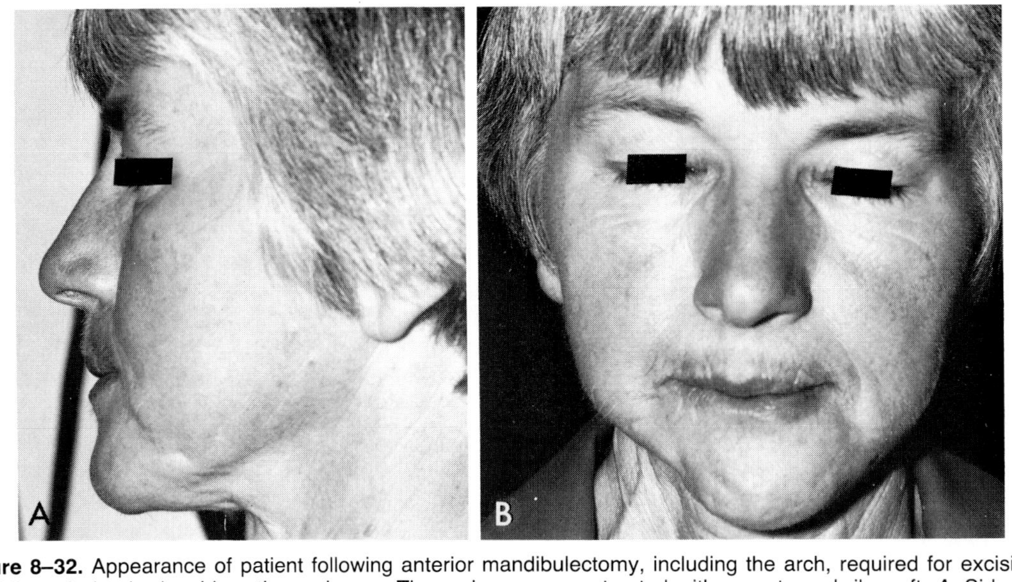

Figure 8–32. Appearance of patient following anterior mandibulectomy, including the arch, required for excision of a sublingual gland adenoid cystic carcinoma. The arch was reconstructed with a contoured rib graft. *A,* Side view. *B,* Frontal view.

lectomy incision must be through the neck above the coronoid notch. The anterior incision is curved through the parasymphyseal area well in front of the mental foramen. The inferior alveolar nerve should be cut as closely as possible to its emergence from the submandibular division of the trigeminal nerve near the foramen ovale. Similarly, the lingual, buccal, and hypoglossal nerves should be excised if they show clinical evidence of tumor involvement. Cranial nerve invasion is a poor prognostic sign.

Resection of the parasymphyseal area is necessary with adenoid cystic tumors of the sublingual gland. The usual extent is from midbody on the side of involvement to the region of the mental foramen of the opposing side. This is a more difficult area to reconstruct, and effective replacement by either autogenous rib grafts, skewered by a Kirschner wire, that have been shaped into an arch configuration or the use of a metal tray with cancellous bone chips will be required to rebuild this essential support to the anterior floor of the mouth. (The details of mandibular and oral cavity reconstruction are in Chapter 1.) The defect resulting from the more limited submandibular gland resection can be replaced with a piece of rib or iliac crest. The recent review of mandibular reconstruction by Lawson et al[31] illustrates the increased reliability of delayed osseous reconstruction using rib over other methods.

Sublingual primaries involve the undersurface of the tongue. The patient in Figure 8–32 had the tongue sectioned horizontally through much of its width, with preservation if its upper half and attendant blood supply from the lingual arteries (Fig. 8–33). The primary reconstruction of the defect created from the tongue to the buccal and labial mucosa may leave the patient "tongue-tied" and require a sulcoplasty later on. If there is further invasion of tumor requiring more

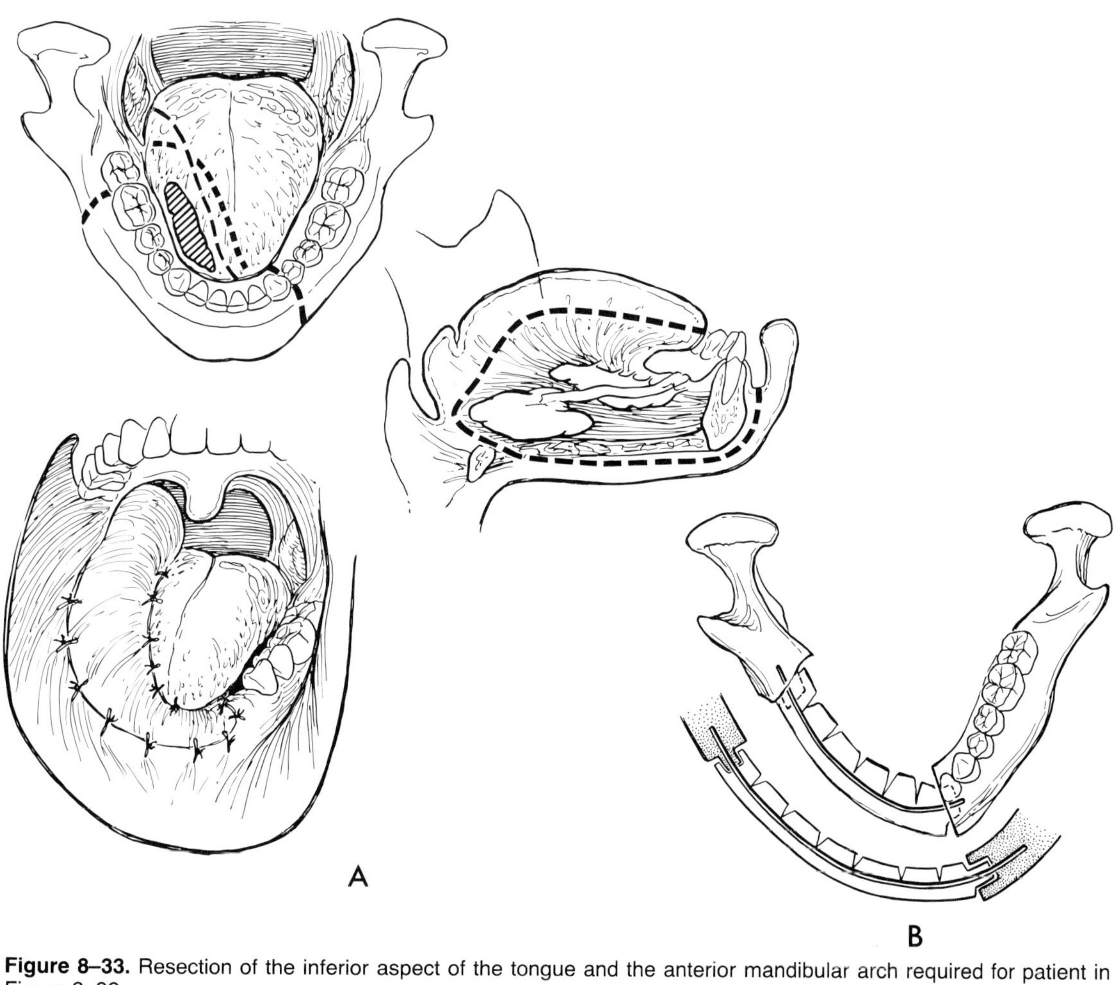

Figure 8–33. Resection of the inferior aspect of the tongue and the anterior mandibular arch required for patient in Figure 8–32.

extensive resection, reconstruction with a trapezius or sternomastoid myocutaneous flap may be necessary. The now somewhat obsolete forehead flap was ideal for this site and still may be considered in selected cases.

For low-grade malignant tumors of these glands, a more conservative resection that includes adjacent muscles and mandibular periosteum is appropriate. If tumor proximity to mandible presents any doubts as to its preservation, an excision employing a lingual splitting procedure can be done.

Minor Salivary Gland Tumors

Considering that there are 400 to 500 minor salivary glands in the oral cavity alone, it is remarkable that the incidence of neoplasm is only one-fifth that of the major glands.[32] In Conley's series[22] of 200 minor salivary gland tumors, 65 per cent were malignant. Adenoid cystic carcinoma accounts for the biggest percentage of tumor types, comprising 35 to 50 per cent of all malignancies.[22, 32, 33] Mucoepidermoid, malignant mixed, adenocarcinoma (mainly of the poorly differentiated type), and finally the rare acinic cell tumors make up the remaining varieties in descending order of frequency.

The palate is a common site for the benign mixed tumor (Fig. 8–34), which often attains significant size before the sufferer seeks help. Careful histologic examination is important to ensure that the lesion is neither a malignant mixed tumor nor an adenoid cystic carcinoma. Unlike squamous cell tumors of the same site, intraoral tumors of minor gland origin, either benign or malignant, are usually nonulcerating.

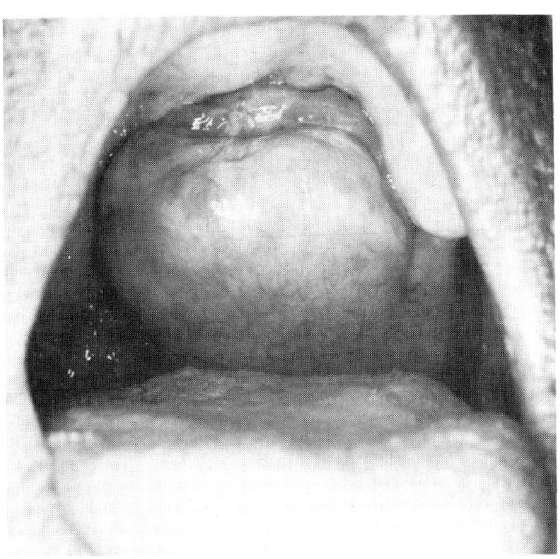

Figure 8–34. Benign mixed tumor of the palate.

Extraoral sites may be involved but less commonly so. However, in Conley and Dingman's[23] series of 78 adenoid cystic carcinomas, 19 of the lesions involving the minor salivary glands were located in the nose or paranasal sinuses. This site is extremely unfortunate both because of the long delay to diagnosis that is characteristic of sinus malignancy and because of the affinity of the tumor for adjacent nerves that are so close to the cranial foramen from which they emerge.

The trachea, larynx, and even bronchi can harbor adenoid cystic tumor. The responsiveness of small squamous cell cancers of the larynx to irradiation therapy should not delude one into thinking that this modality is equally applicable to adenoid cystic cancers in this site. Conservation laryngeal surgery and irradiation are *not* adequate for cure. Rather, the same wide field resection principles used for treating this tumor in the major salivary glands should be applied to the laryngeal lesion as well (Fig. 8–35).

Salivary gland lesions of the oral cavity are resected according to the same criteria imposed by the various tumor types in the major salivary glands. Mucoepidermoid tumors of the minor salivary glands tend to be of low malignancy, and conservatism in resection is generally justifiable (Fig. 8–36). However, limited resection of mucoepidermoid tumors of minor glands is not always successful, and these patients suffer disastrous results. Careful attention must be paid to the histologic grade of the tumor, histologically negative margins must be ensured at the time of resection. In the poorly differentiated varieties this inevitably requires the excision of bone.[34]

Adenoid cystic tumors are resected with a wide margin, which for buccal mucosal or lip tumors often requires through-and-through excision and replacement with a flap. Adenocarcinomas require a similar approach. Figure 8–37 illustrates a patient with an acinic cell tumor of the labial mucosa that, because of its proximity to skin, required resection from the skin to mucosa in the labial sulcus as well as removal of the underlying bone of the anterior wall of the maxillary sinus. The malignant potential of the acinic cell tumor is very hard to predict on the basis of histologic appearance. Therefore it is better to be overcautious in order to assure a sufficiently radical excision. The fact that for adenoid cystic cancer the local recurrence rate was 50 per cent in Conley's series, compared with

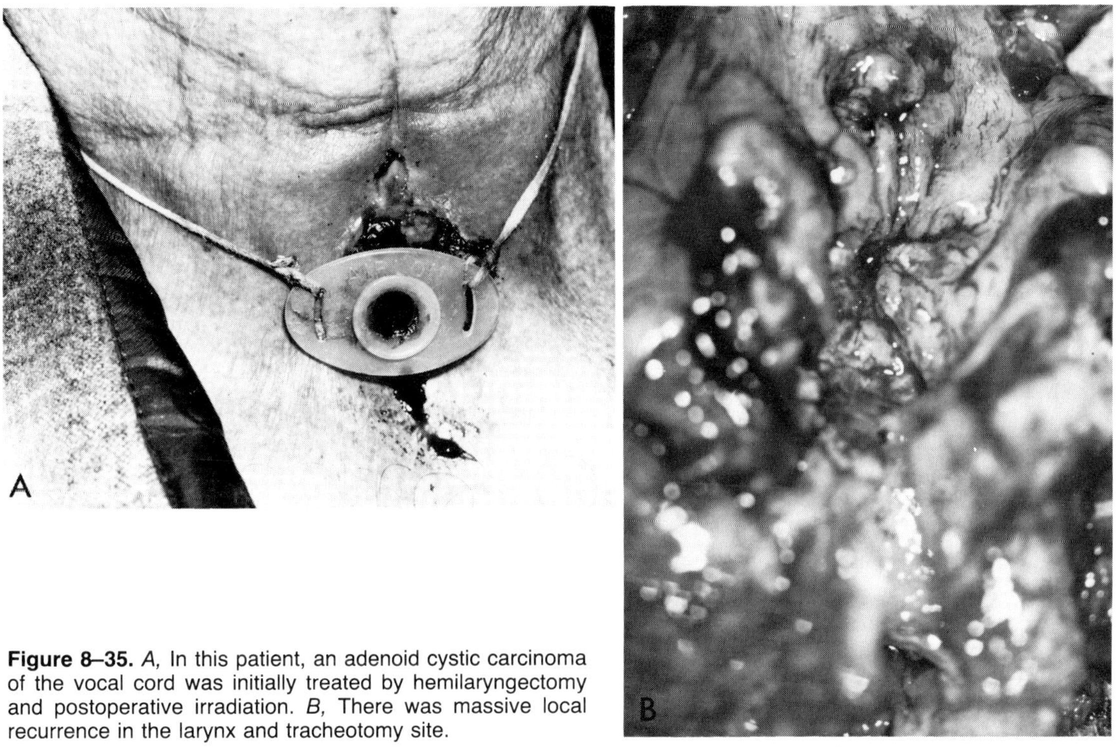

Figure 8–35. *A,* In this patient, an adenoid cystic carcinoma of the vocal cord was initially treated by hemilaryngectomy and postoperative irradiation. *B,* There was massive local recurrence in the larynx and tracheotomy site.

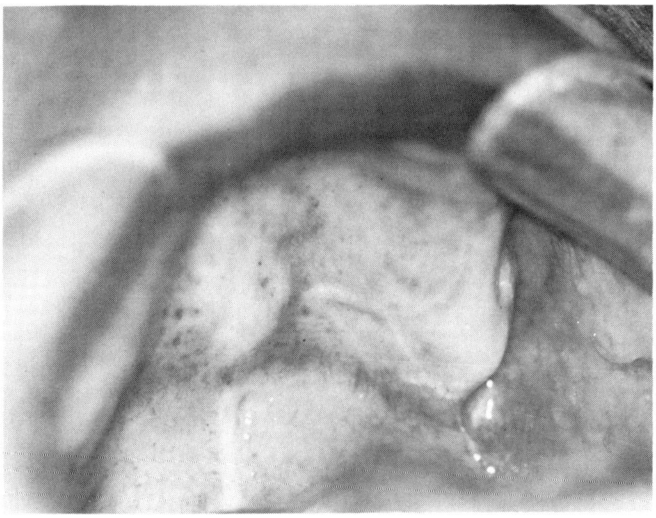

Figure 8–36. Minor defect in the hard palate seen 7 years following local excision for a low-grade mucoepidermoid carcinoma.

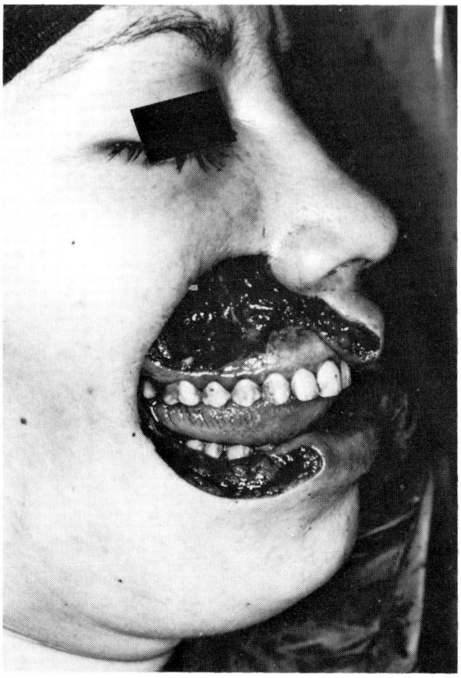

Figure 8–37. Defect following excision of an acinic cell carcinoma of the right upper buccal and labial mucosa.

30 to 47 per cent for the other tumor types,[22] emphasizes this point. Repeated resection is often needed, and even histopathologic evidence of clear surgical margins is no guarantee of success.

References

1. Conley J: Concepts in Head and Neck Surgery. New York, Grune & Stratton, 1970, pp 255–260.
2. McFarland J: Adenoma of the salivary gland with report of a possible case. Am J Med Sci 174:362, 1927.
3. Polayes IM, Rankow RM: Cysts, masses and tumors of the accessory parotid gland. Plast Reconstr Surg 64:17, 1979.
4. Rankow RM, Polayes IM: Diseases of the Salivary Glands. Philadelphia, WB Saunders, 1976, pp 162–163.
5. Foote FW, Frazell EL: Tumors of the major salivary glands. Cancer 6:1065, 1953.
6. Conley J: Salivary Glands and the Facial Nerve. New York, Grune & Stratton, 1975, p 151
7. Eneroth CM: Histological and clinical aspects of parotid tumors. Acta Oto-Laryngol (Stockholm) 191 (suppl):111, 1964.
8. Evansweather RW, Cruickshank AH: Epithelial Tumors of the Salivary Glands. Philadelphia, WB Saunders, 1970.
9. Kleinsasser O: Behavior and adequate treatment of epithelial tumors of the parotid gland. *In* Conley J: Salivary Glands and the Facial Nerve. New York, Grune & Stratton, 1975, pp 15–33.
10. Rauch S, Seifert G, Gorlin RJ: Disease of the salivary glands: tumors. *In* Gorlin RJ, Goldman HM (eds): Thomas' Oral Pathology, 6th ed. St. Louis, CV Mosby, 1970, p 1013.
11. Work WP, Hecht DW: Tumors and cysts of major salivary glands. *In* Shumrick DA, Paparella MM (eds): Otolaryngology, 2nd ed, Vol 3. Philadelphia, WB Saunders, 1980, p 2244.
12. Eneroth CM: Mixed tumors of major salivary glands: prognostic role of capsular structure. Ann Otol Rhinol Laryngol 74:944, 1965.
13. Hubner G, Klein HJ, Kleinsasser O, et al: The role of the myoepithelial cells in the development of salivary gland tumors. Cancer 27:1255, 1971.
14. Batsakis JG: Tumors of the major salivary glands. *In* Tumors of the Head and Neck—Clinical and Pathological Considerations. Baltimore, Williams & Wilkins, 1974, pp 1–37.
15. Blanck C, Eneroth CM, Jakobsson PA: Mucus-producing adenopapillary (nonepidermoid) carcinoma of the parotid gland. Cancer 28:676, 1971.
16. Rankow RM, Polayes IM: Diseases of the Salivary Glands. Philadelphia, WB Saunders, 1976, pp 119–123.
17. Seifert G: Mundspeicheldrusen Tonsillen und Rachen. *In* Doerr-Seifert-Vehlinger: Spezielle Pathol. Anatomie Bd 1. Berlin, Springer, 1966.
18. Wertheimer FW, Georgen GJ: Intraoral acinic cell adenocarcinoma. Oral Surg 32:923, 1971.
19. Eneroth CM, Jakobsson PA, Blanck C: Acinic cell carcinoma of the parotid gland. Cancer 19:1761, 1966.
20. Thackray AC, Lucas RB: Tumors in the major salivary glands. *In* Atlas of Tumor Pathology, 2nd ed, Fascicle 10. Washington, DC, Armed Forces Institute of Pathology, 1974.
21. Perzin KH, Gullane P, Clairmont AC: Adenoid cystic carcinomas arising in salivary glands. Cancer 43:265, 1978.
22. Conley J: Salivary Glands and the Facial Nerve. New York, Grune & Stratton, 1975, pp 153–154.
23. Conley J, Dingman DL: Adenoid cystic carcinoma in the head and neck (cylindroma). Arch Otolaryngol 100:81, 1974.
24. Jakobsson PA, Blanck C, Eneroth CM: Muco-epidermoid carcinoma of the parotid gland. Cancer 22:111, 1968.
25. Lajicek J, Eneroth CM: Cytological diagnosis of salivary gland carcinomata from aspiration biopsy smears. Acta Otolaryngol 263:183, 1970.
26. Conley J: Salivary Glands and the Facial Nerve. New York, Grune & Stratton, 1975, p 81.
27. McCabe BF, Work PW: Parotidectomy with special preference in the facial nerve. *In* English GM (ed): Otolaryngology, Vol 4. Hagerstown, MD, Harper & Row, 1967, p 39.
28. Conley J: Salivary Glands and the Facial Nerve. New York, Grune & Stratton, 1975, p 183.
29. Smith LC, Lane N, Rankow RM: Cylindroma (adenoid cystic carcinoma): a report of fifty-eight cases. Am J Surg 110:519, 1965.
30. Rankow RM, Polayes IM: Disease of the Salivary Glands. Philadelphia, WB Saunders, 1976, pp 38–51.
31. Lawson W, Lascalzo L, Baek, S, et al: Experience with immediate and delayed mandibular reconstruction. Laryngoscope 92:5, 1982.
32. Del Balso AM: Malignant disease of the minor oral salivary glands. Otolaryngol Clin North Am 12:135, 1979.
33. Rafla-Demetrious S: Mucous and Salivary Gland Tumours. Springfield, IL, Charles C Thomas, 1970.
34. Smitheringale A, Hoyek AM, Chapnik JS, et al: Mucoepidermoid carcinoma of the palate. J Otolaryngol 10:261, 1981.

9

INFRATEMPORAL FOSSA AND SKULL BASE

Paul J. Donald, M.D.

Possibly the most challenging area in head and neck surgery is the region of the skull base. It was only a short time ago that neoplasms, especially malignancies, close or adherent to the undersurface of the cranium were considered inoperable. Once the barrier had been breached and tumor had spread intracranially, the patient's prognosis became entirely hopeless. This pessimistic situation has radically changed in recent years, however, thanks to the concurrence of three major developments: the advent of microvascular surgery, the emergence of the era of combined craniofacial surgery, and the advances in modern anesthesia in both the areas of pharmacologic manipulation and monitoring.

In 1972, McLean and Buncke[1] first transplanted omentum to the cranium using a microvascular anastomosis. During the past decade, the work of such pioneers as O'Brien, Acland, Taylor, and Harii established this technique as a viable clinical tool. The application of these principles to the revascularization of compromised cerebral circulation was one of the major breakthroughs in expanding the scope and safety of skull base surgery.[2] One of the principal stumbling blocks in this area has always been the inviolability of the internal carotid artery. If this vessel was compromised, the viability of the ipsilateral cerebral hemisphere became severely jeopardized. Despite the assurance of numerous investigative procedures indicating collateral supply, this viability could not be guaranteed. The development of the superficial temporal-to-middle cerebral artery vascular anastomosis has made internal carotid artery sacrifice possible.[3] This then permits en bloc resection of neoplastic processes in the area of the base of the skull that were formerly treated by, at best, compromised piecemeal procedures.

In recent years, much has been made of the so-called "team approach," in which paramedical and medical personnel coordinate their efforts in the management of patients. The impetus for this has largely come from the paramedical disciplines. It is curious that this most laudable concept had somewhat slow acceptance among some of the surgical disciplines when it concerned intercooperation between certain surgical specialties. Cooperation between head and neck surgeons, especially otorhinolaryngologists, and neurologic surgeons was initially halting and with good reason. The training of many ear, nose, and throat physicians 25 and 30 years ago ill prepared them for the rigors of major head and neck surgery. Some individuals had little or no background training in general surgery, and many training programs were only 2 or 3 years long. However, the neurosurgeons' reluctance to cooperate was based not only on a lack of trust in their counterparts' ability to handle the cervicofacial end of the surgery but also on a deep concern that the carefully guarded, sterile cranial cavity would be exposed to the profusion of microorganisms inhabiting the environs of the upper aerodigestive tract. The pioneering work of such men as Dean Lierle,

John Loré, Sr., Max Som, and John Conley laid the foundation to equip the modern otorhinolaryngologist with the necessary training to become a complete head and neck surgeon. The work of Paul Tessier, probably more than anyone, clearly demonstrated that a substantial surgical communication could be temporarily created between the cranial cavity and the upper aerodigestive system without undue hazard to the patient. The experiences of Ketcham et al[4, 5] and of Sisson et al[6] in the resection of extensive paranasal sinus tumors proved that combined craniofacial surgery can be done safely and with a low infection rate.

The cooperation between the neurologic surgeon and the head and neck surgeon should be "a natural," since their respective skills are complementary with regard to the skull base region. The areas that hold a morbid fear for the head and neck surgeon—the contents of the cranial cavity—are regions of easy familiarity for the neurosurgeon. Those areas beneath the skull base and deep in the face that for the neurosurgeon are an anatomic and physiologic mystery are common ground for his cohort in the head and neck.

The advances of modern anesthesia are largely responsible for the safety of the technical manipulations of the surgical team. Air embolism is a constant threat, especially if the patient is operated upon in the sitting position. In general, most of the procedures done by the author are done in the supine position. However, despite this, air embolism via the dural venous sinuses or the large veins in the neck, although less frequently a problem, is still a constant threat. Considerable evidence has been accumulated to show that the Doppler ultrasound can monitor the emergence of an air embolus much more precisely than any other monitoring system.[7] Its sensitivity compared to other methods is illustrated in Table 9–1. In the dog, a volume of air as scant as 0.12 to 0.25 ml can be detected. The characteristic murmur of an air embolus heard over the precordium is not heard until at least 15 to 30 ml of air is present.[8]

The profusion of blood vessels in the region of the skull base, as well as in the equivalent area intracranially, creates a problem of significant blood loss. Controlled hypotension using nitroprusside or similar agents reduces hemorrhage markedly. A mean circulating blood pressure of 60 to 70 mm Hg adequately perfuses vital organs while markedly facilitating dissection, thus reducing both blood loss and operating time. Central venous and arterial pressure monitoring devices are essential in the safe application of this technique. A continuous digital readout displaying these parameters, as well as pulse and respiratory rates, greatly facilitates observation of the patient's intraoperative course.

Table 9–1. DETECTABLE LEVELS OF EMBOLI IN DOGS*

Method	*Embolus Volume per Body Weight (ml/kg)*
Doppler	0.01–0.02
	0.10
Decreased end-tidal CO_2	0.25–0.50
	0.50–1.00
Elevated pulmonary artery pressure	0.25–0.50
Decreased blood pressure	4.00–8.00
Electrocardiography	4.00–8.00

*From Hybels R: Venous air embolism in head and neck surgery. Laryngoscope 90:950, 1980.

Monitoring of intracranial pressure with a catheter in the third ventricle permits an indirect assessment of intracranial volume. A clear understanding of the relationship between intracranial volume and intracranial pressure is vital. Diminution of intracranial volume is an essential step in promoting optimal conditions for the neurosurgical part of the operation. A number of measurements are involved in determining this critical factor. As cerebral blood flow increases, so does the cerebral volume (Fig. 9–1). A mean cir-

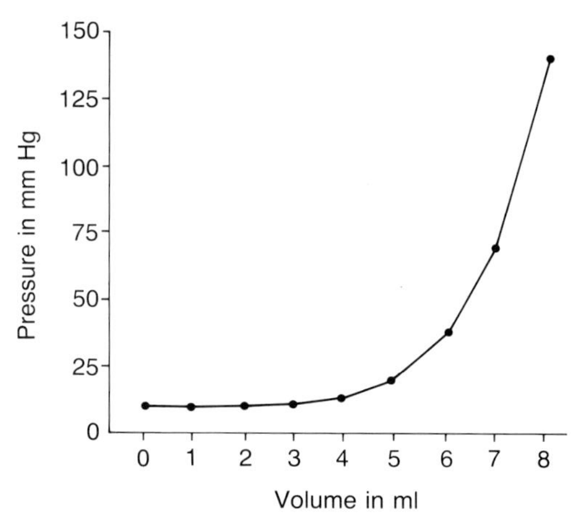

Figure 9–1. A pressure-volume curve relating rises of intracranial pressure to increases in intracerebral volume. Pressure is in millimeters of Hg and volume is in cubic cm. This curve was extrapolated from an experiment relating intracranial volume and pressure using an inflatable balloon in the cranium of a Rhesus monkey. (From Youmans JR: Neurological Surgery, Vol II, 2nd ed. Philadelphia, WB Saunders, 1982, p 854.)

culating blood pressure of between 60 and 100 mm Hg has little effect on blood flow to the brain. However, once 100 mm Hg is exceeded, cerebral blood flow and, concomitantly, intracranial volume increase. Cerebral vascular tone is exquisitely sensitive to concentrations of PCO_2. An elevation of PCO_2 of 1 mm Hg will increase the cerebral blood flow by 2 per cent. Although intracranial blood flow, and hence intracranial volume, is highly sensitive to PCO_2, there is no change in cerebral blood flow when the PaO_2 is between 40 and 300 mm Hg. Therefore it is essential to maintain a low PCO_2 during the intracranial part of the procedure. The insertion of a Dean tube, a catheter inserted into the endotracheal tube and connected to a CO_2 analyzer, records end tidal CO_2, providing a continuous precise monitoring of this vital parameter. Care must be taken to maintain the airway pressure on the respirator below 25 cm H_2O. Pressures in excess of this will raise intracranial pressure.

Anesthetic agents may have an effect on cerebral blood flow as well. Inducting agents such as Althesin and thiopental (Pentothal) bring about a decrease in cerebral flow, and hence a fall in intracranial pressure. On the other hand, halothane causes an increase in pressure. Although methoxyflurane (Penthrane) appears to be the agent of choice at some institutions,[9] the best anesthetic for minimizing cerebral flow is a combination of nitrous oxide and narcotics (Table 9–2).

Table 9–2. PHYSIOLOGIC FACTORS AND DRUGS AFFECTING CEREBRAL BLOOD FLOW

Factors During Anesthesia Causing an Increase in Intracranial Pressure
Straining during induction
Increased blood flow
Increased intrathoracic or intra-abdominal pressure
Agents
Halothane
Methoxyflurane
Trichlorethylene
Enflurane
Ketamine
Factors During Anesthesia Causing a Decrease in Intracranial Pressure
Hyperventilation
Osmotic diuretics
Nitroprusside
Atropine
Agents
Innover
Nitrous oxide
Barbiturates

Successful craniofacial surgery depends not only on the smooth coordination of the surgical team but on expert nursing care as well. Diligent postoperative observation and rapid intervention in the event of an alteration in the patient's status is vital in the care of these patients. Following a technically successful procedure, the loss of life or the development of permanent morbid sequelae as a result of inadequate, inattentive postoperative care is an execrable tragedy. A therapeutic dilemma that occasionally follows extensive craniofacial procedures is the problem of poor systemic perfusion in a hypotensive patient in whom restoration of an adequate blood pressure with intravascular volume augmentation will result in an intolerable increase in cerebral volume. Early intervention by an experienced skilled medical team for the delicate management of volume replacement and pharmacologic regulation of systemic pressure is the only hope of saving the patient from the ravages of profound cerebral edema. Monitoring of the patient's hemodynamics, blood gases, and cerebrospinal fluid pressure must be continuous and compulsively exercised pursuits.

ANATOMY

Skull base anatomy is complex, requiring the head and neck surgeon who endeavors to perform surgical procedures on it to have a meticulous three-dimensional conception of the topography and contents of the region. Moreover, it is mandatory to comprehend the structures that lie on the opposing cranial surfaces of the plates and buttresses on which one is working. Much like acquiring an appreciation of the anatomy of the temporal bone during dissections prior to performing ear surgery, the central anatomy must be studied "from the outside in." Preparation for surgery is done in the dissecting laboratory or the autopsy room where, with the aid of anatomic texts, a spacial conception of this region can be formulated. Surgery in the skull base area is very demanding but is not outside the scope of any well-trained head and neck surgeon who is willing to do a little homework and acquire the necessary team members.

Nasopharyngeal carcinoma has been generally considered and still remains essentially a nonsurgical disease. The mucosa of this region suffers the disadvantage of being adherent and adjacent to a number of vital structures. It is tightly affixed to the bone of the clivus, precluding a clean plane of dissection, as is usually found throughout the rest of the pharynx. In addition, the internal carotid artery in the lateral recesses is separated from the nasopharynx by a mere plug of cartilage in the inferior aspect of the foramen lacerum, and the brain stem is located on the deep surface of the clivus (Fig. 9–2).

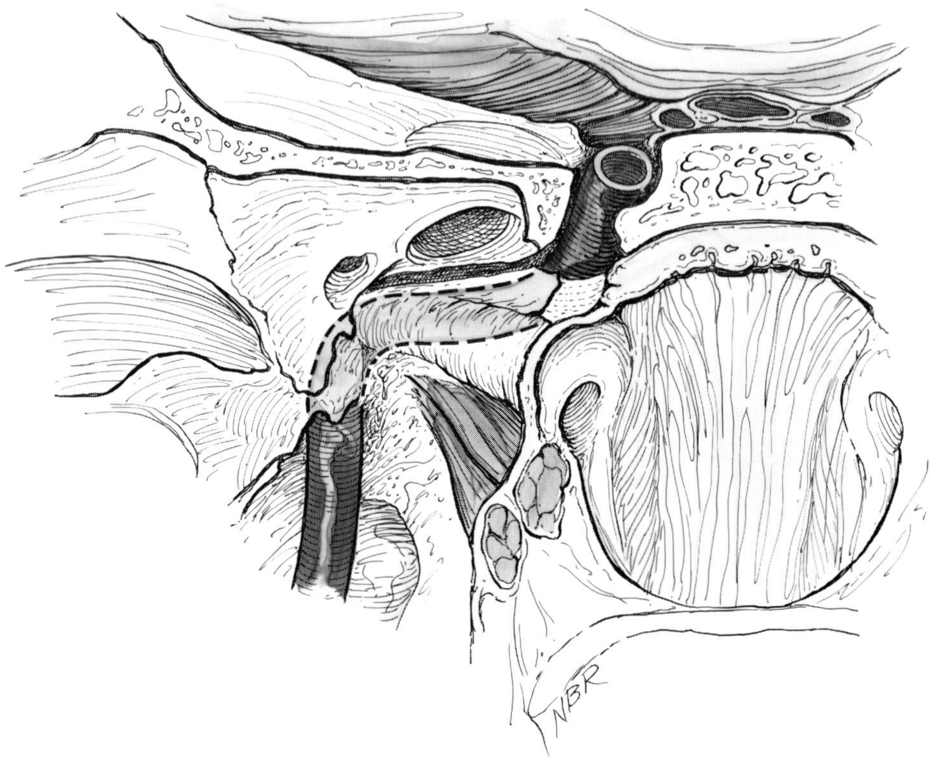

A

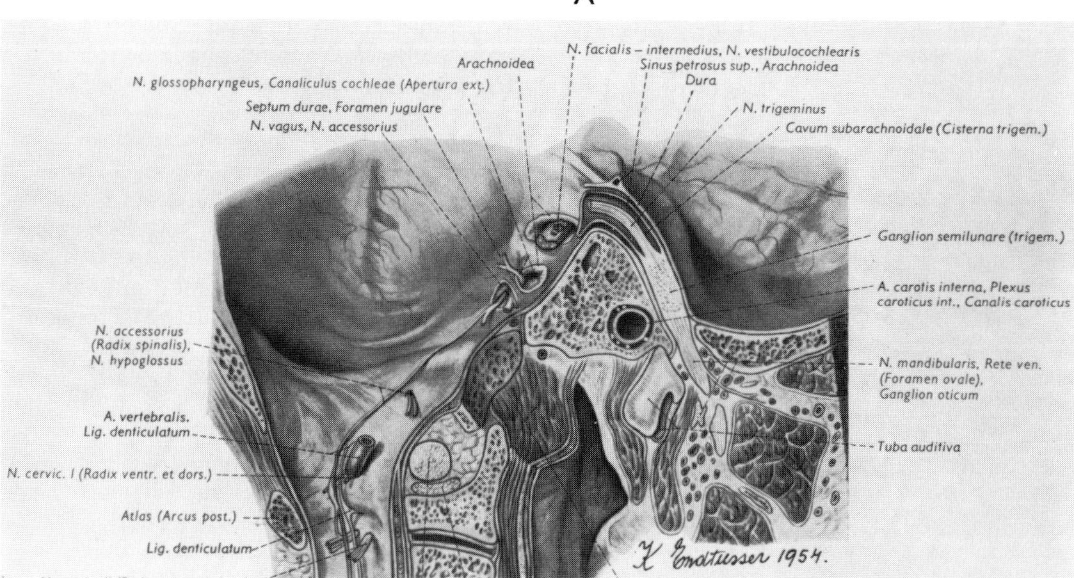

B

Figure 9–2. *B,* Coronal section through the nasopharynx and overlying brain at the level of the foramen lacerum. *B,* Parasaggital cut through the nasopharynx and clivus through the petrous apex. (*B* from Pernkoff E: Atlas of Topographical and Applied Human Anatomy, Vol I. Philadelphia, WB Saunders, 1963.)

However, despite these complicating factors, recent surgical advances have permitted nasopharyngeal resections in highly selected cases.

Soon after the pharyngeal tube enters the region of the nasopharynx, the superior constrictor muscle of the nasopharynx becomes attached to its origin, the pharyngeal tubercles of the basiocciput. This area is the origin of both the pharyngobasilar and the buccopharyngeal fascial sheaths that encase the superior constrictor muscle in its anterior and posterior aspects respectively (Fig. 9–3). The remainder of the clivus is covered by a thick layer of mucosa that overlies a very heavy layer of periosteum. The lateral walls of the nasopharynx are made up mainly of the structures in the foramen of Morgagni—that gap which extends between the clivus and the superior border of the superior constrictor. The eustachian tube and its pharyngeal elaboration, the torus tubarius, along with the tensor and levator muscles of the palate, are the principal structures occupying this gap (Fig. 9–4). They are leashed together by the pharyngobasilar fascia. At the anterior aspect of the lateral extent of the nasopharyngeal roof, just medial to the region of the pterygoid plates, is the foramen lacerum. The inferior portion of the foramen is obliterated by a cartilage plug, but the superior part harbors the internal carotid artery as it sweeps out of the petrous apex into the cavernous sinus. The proximity of the internal carotid artery and cavernous sinus, and the presence of the brain stem on the intracranial side of the clivus, had until recently precluded the use of surgery for lesions in the nasopharynx. In 1972, for example, Hsu[10a] attempted to devise a nasopharyngeal resection that would encompass a nasopharyngeal carcinoma, but numerous attempts in the dog proved unsuccessful and the animals invariably died. Within the last 5 years, however, Fang and Ong,[42] Menezes et al,[51] Panje and McCabe[54] and others have outlined relatively safe approaches to some neoplasms of this area in highly selected cases.

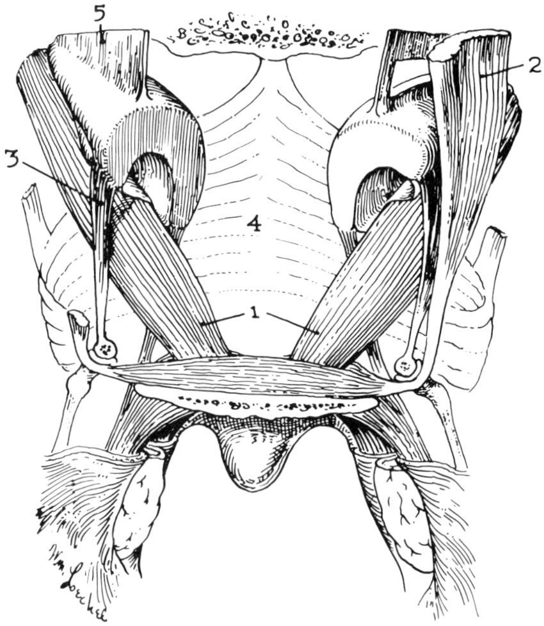

Figure 9–4. Schema showing the position of the levator muscle (1) with respect to the eustachian tube, superior tubal ligament (5), and two components of the tensor veli palatini muscle—one that tenses the palate (2) and another that pulls the hook of the eustachian cartilage downward (3). The superior pharyngeal constrictor muscle (4) is also shown.

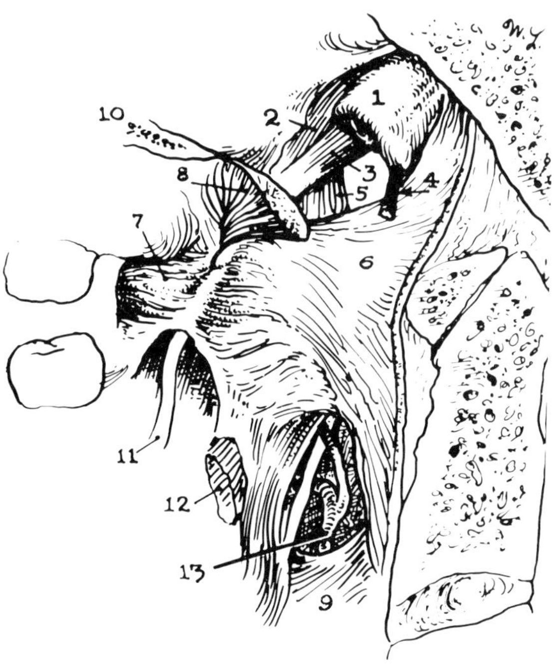

Figure 9–3. Lateral view of the nasopharynx and oropharynx to show superior constrictor of the pharynx (6), which is shown attaching to the hamulus and pterygomandibular raphe and continuing on as the buccinator (7). The levator muscle (3) and the tubal cartilage (1) are shown passing through the sinus of Morgagni. The tensor muscle (2) is shown descending and passing around the hamulus (8). Other structures shown are: medial pterygoid muscle (5); salpingopharyngeal muscle (4); hard palate (10); middle constrictor muscle (9); lingual nerve (11); palatoglossus (12); and facial artery (13). (From Proctor B: Anatomy of the eustachian tube. Arch Otolaryngol 97:6, 1973.)

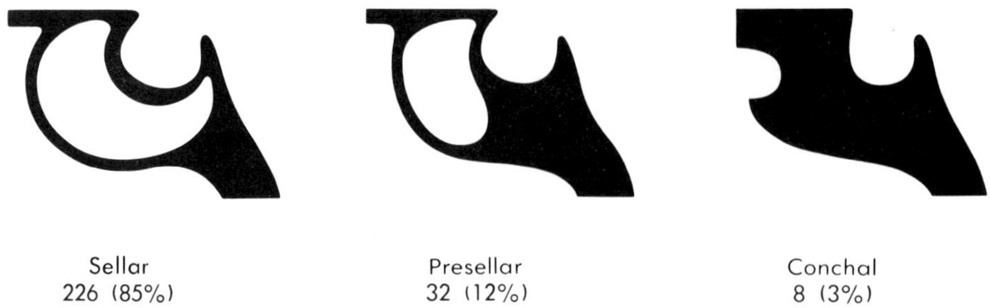

Figure 9–5. Varieties of sphenoid sinus pneumatization. (From Hardy J, Maina G: Microsurgical anatomy in transsphenoidal hypophysectomy. J Neurol Sci 21:151, 1977.)

Sphenoid Sinus

The sphenoid sinus resides in a unique area in the head, occupying its anatomic center. Lying above it, suspended from the region of the hypothalamus, in the sella turcica, is the grand orchestrator of bodily hormonal function, the pituitary gland. It is related laterally to the cavernous sinus and its contents. (A more complete discussion of the anatomy of the sphenoid sinus is found in Chapter 5.)

Posterior to the sphenoid sinus is the posterior extent of the basisphenoid and its articulation with the basiocciput; these latter two bones are commonly called collectively the clivus. The anterior surface of the sinus contains its ostium, emptying into the sphenoethmoidal recess in the posterior vault of the nasal chamber. The sphenopalatine artery runs under the sinus ostium and may be a source of troublesome bleeding if not adequately coagulated prior to severance. In cases of marked pneumatization, the thick floor of the sinus may form a small part of the anterior roof of the nasopharynx. The inferior aspect of the anterior sinus wall forms the sphenoid rostrum, which is at the posteriormost extremity of the roof of the nasal cavity.

The sphenoid sinus may be highly variable in its extent (Fig. 9–5). It is described in relation to the sella turcica, which is a vital consideration in the trans-sphenoidal approach to the pituitary. Pneumatization may consist merely of a dimple on the anterior surface of the basiocciput. Presellar and especially postsellar pneumatization will permit a satisfactory approach to the gland. Although the optic nerve is usually related to the sphenoid sinus high on its lateral wall (see Chapter 5, Fig. 5–3), in certain individuals the sinus actually wraps around the optic nerve (Fig. 9–6). Before extensive surgery in this area, a careful study of base-view radiographs is mandatory to establish the nature of this anatomic relationship.

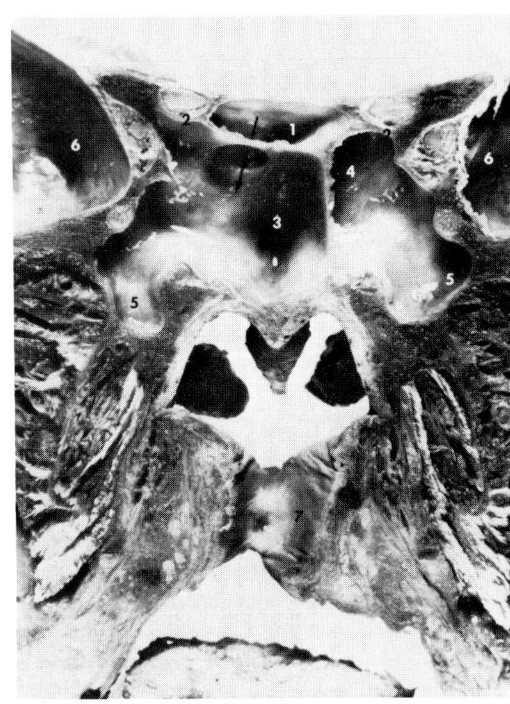

Figure 9–6. Anatomic specimen cut in coronal section through the sphenoid sinus, illustrating the sinus surrounding about 200° of the left optic nerve. Posterior facing surface. (1) Superior compartment in the sphenoid sinus; arrow demonstrates foramen communicating with the main body of the sinus. (2) Optic nerves separated by a thin plate of bone from the sphenoid sinus, which wraps around it on the left side for 280°. (3) Left sphenoid sinus larger than the right. (4) Right sphenoid sinus. (5) Pterygoid extensions of the sphenoid sinuses. (6) Greater wings of the sphenoid bone. (7) Cleft palate defect. (Adapted from Ritter FN: The Paranasal Sinuses: Anatomy and Surgical Techniques, 2nd ed. St Louis, CV Mosby, 1976, p 83.)

Cavernous Sinus and Clivus

The cavernous sinus lies directly against the bone making up the lateral wall of the sphenoid sinus (Fig. 9–7). The dura that forms each sinus is derived from the sphenoidal periosteum. Each cavernous sinus extends from the orbital apex anteriorly to the petrous ridge posteriorly. The petrous apex terminates in the floor of the sinus. A plethora of veins drain into it, making it vulnerable to a variety of sources of infection. The cavernous sinus connects to both the superior and inferior petrosal sinuses, the former emerging from the transverse sinus and the latter draining the cavernous sinus inferiorly into the jugular bulb. Further anteriorly, connections to the superior and inferior orbital veins establish a direct connection to the veins of the face. The neurovascular foramina in the floor of the cavernous sinus establish routes to the paranasal sinuses, the principal vein being the connection to the pterygoid plexus through the foramen of Vesalius. The foramen lacerum, the conduit for the internal carotid artery, is also in the sinus floor.

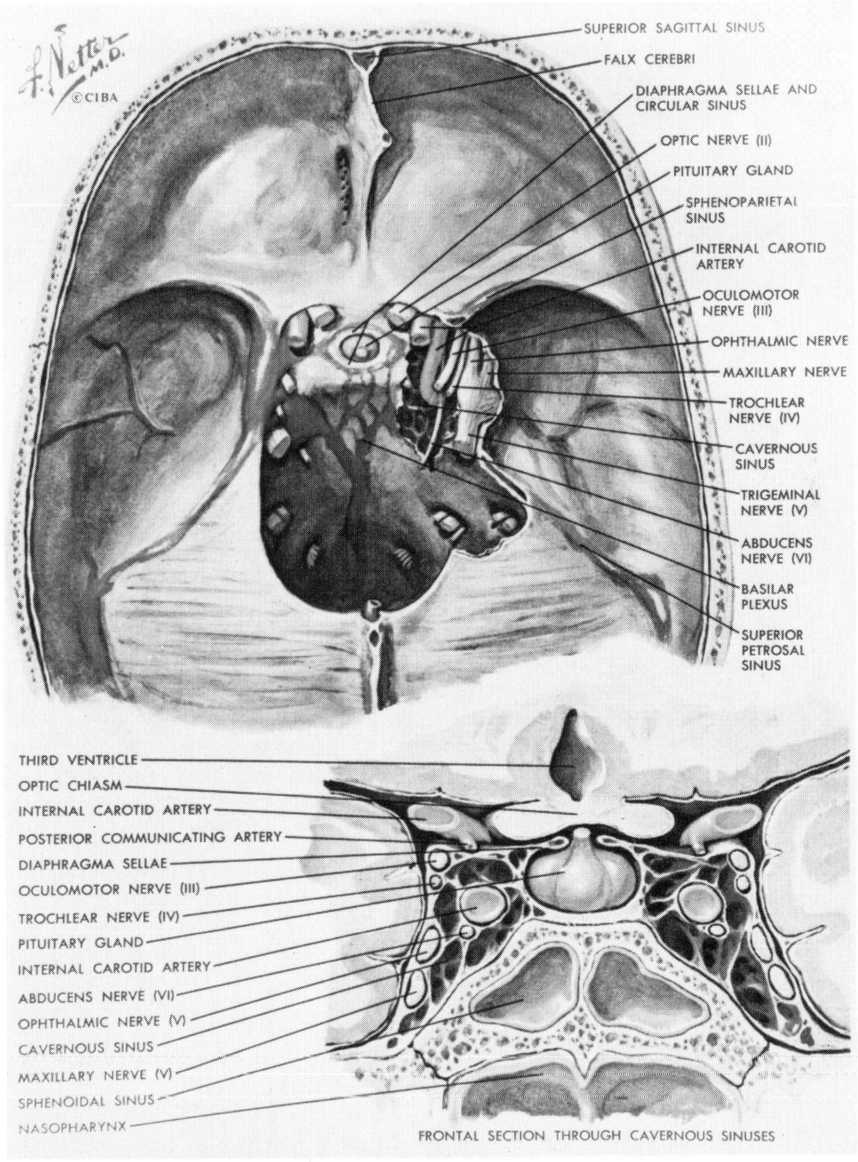

Figure 9–7. The relationships of the pituitary gland to the sphenoid sinus and cavernous sinus. (From the CIBA Collection of Medical Illustrations by Frank N. Netter, M.D.)

Each of the dural venous cavernous sinuses is commonly connected to its fellow on the opposite side of the sphenoid sinus by the circular sinus. The circular sinus, although it encircles the pituitary stalk, is in reality a labyrinth of blood-filled channels and spaces rather than a single venous conduit (Fig. 9–8). Running through the cavernous sinus are the optic nerve, the third, fourth, and sixth cranial nerves, the first, second, and occasionally the third branches of the trigeminal nerve, and the internal carotid artery (Fig. 9–6). The artery may indent the posterolateral wall of the sphenoid sinus and appear as a bulge.

The clivus is composed of the basisphenoid bone anteriorly and the basiocciput posteriorly. The two bones are connected by a synostosis. Much of the basisphenoid is often occupied by the sphenoid sinus.

Undersurface of the Temporal Bone

To most otorhinolaryngologists, the anatomy of the temporal bone is well understood. However, unless they are engaged in considerable inner ear surgery, most practitioners find that their comprehension of the inferior surface of the bone (Fig. 9–9) dims with time.

Although the temporal bone itself is shaped roughly like a triangle, with the base situated laterally and the apex at the petrous tip medially, it may be helpful to envision its site as a rectangular space canted at roughly 45 degrees to the side of the skull (Fig. 9–10). The lateral corners are bounded by the articular eminence anteriorly and the anterior lip of the occipital condyle posteriorly. Although the inferior surface of the temporal bone makes up 90 per cent of this area, small contributions are made by the sphenoid anteromedially and the occiput posteromedially.

Deep to the mastoid tip, the posterior belly of the digastric muscle takes its origin and receives its innervation directly from the main trunk of the facial nerve. A notch medial to the muscle houses the occipital artery. This artery can be responsible for considerable hemorrhage during surgery if not well controlled. As further progress anteromedially is made, the styloid process is seen with the origin of the styloid muscles and ligament. Just deep and posterior to it are the stylomastoid foramen and the emergence of the facial nerve.

Directly medial to the styloid process is the jugular foramen, and just deep and anterior to it, separated by a thin ridge of bone, the carotid canal. Posteromedial to the carotid is the occipital condyle and its articulation with C1. Posteromedial to the carotid canal and under the lip of the occipital condyle is the foramen of the hypoglossal canal, the iter of the hypoglossal nerve. The vagus, glossopharyngeal, and spinal accessory nerves exit the skull adjacent to the medial surface of the jugular vein, through the incisura between the temporal and occipital bones.

Returning more laterally to the anterolateral corner of the skull base rectangle, and proceeding from the articular eminence medially, the remaining anatomy of this complex region is revealed. Just posterior to the eminence is the condyle of the mandible in the glenoid fossa. The glenoid fossa lies directly underneath the lateral aspect of the middle cranial fossa. Its medial extent lies anteromedial to the foramina for the great vessels. A fissure cut coronally, directly through the center of the glenoid fossa plate, will expose the eustachian tube. Surgical removal of the condylar head is essential to the complete exposure of the skull base.

With the condylar head removed and sighting from lateral to medial, the undersurface of the temporal bone appears to be a steep triangle. Anteriorly, the lateral pterygoid muscular insertions retract into the infratemporal fossa, and these, as well as the temporal muscle, form the anterior wall. The posterior wall is formed by the tympanic bone and its vaginal process. At the blunted apex of the triangle, the beginning of the cartilaginous eustachian tube, the tensor palatini anteriorly and the levator platini posteriorly are located. At the anteriormost aspect of this apex is the sphenoid spine.

Adjacent to the medial surface of the sphenoid spine is the foramen spinosum, which contains the middle meningeal artery. The sphenoid spine is also one of the points of origin for the tensor muscle of the soft palate, which courses along and takes further origin on the lateral plate of the cartilaginous portion of the eustachian tube on its way to the nasopharynx.

The Infratemporal Fossa and Pterygomaxillary Space

The infratemporal fossa is a space on the side of the head that lies deep to the zygomatic arch and just in front of the "skull base

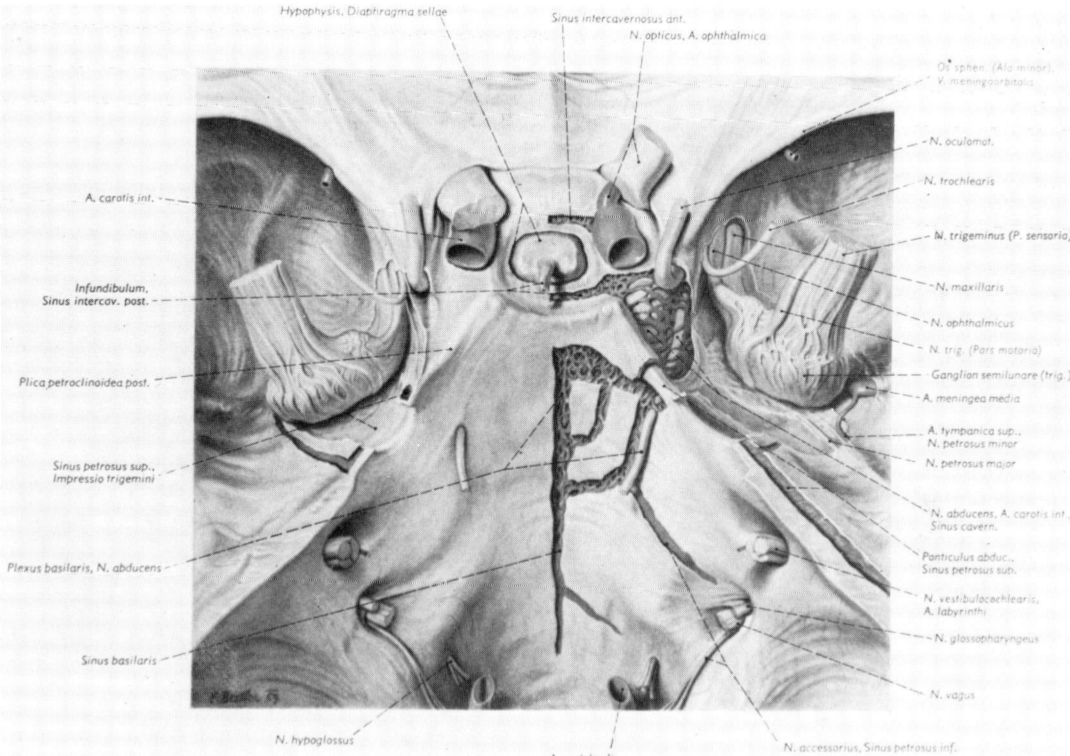

Figure 9–8. The circular sinus. (From Pernkoff E: Atlas of Topographical and Applied Human Anatomy, Vol. I. Philadelphia, WB Saunders, 1963.)

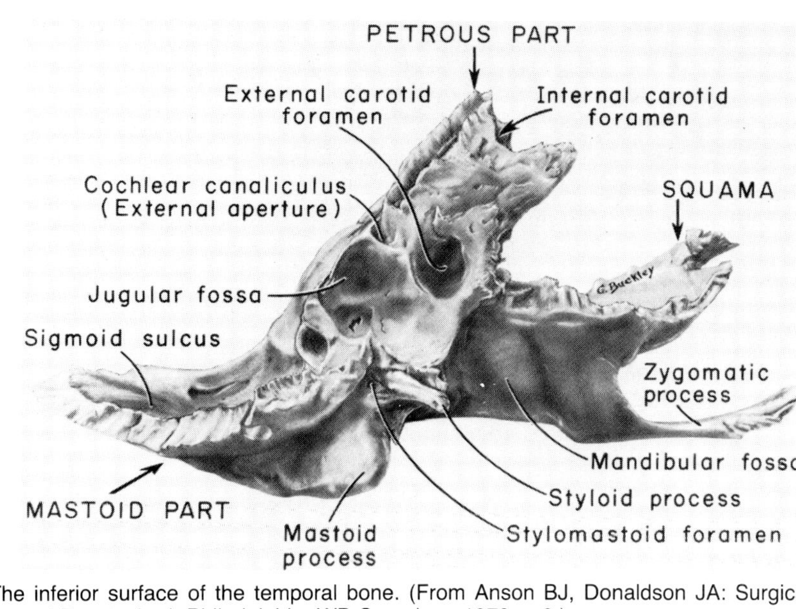

Figure 9–9. The inferior surface of the temporal bone. (From Anson BJ, Donaldson JA: Surgical Anatomy of the Temporal Bone and Ear, 2nd ed. Philadelphia, WB Saunders, 1973, p 9.)

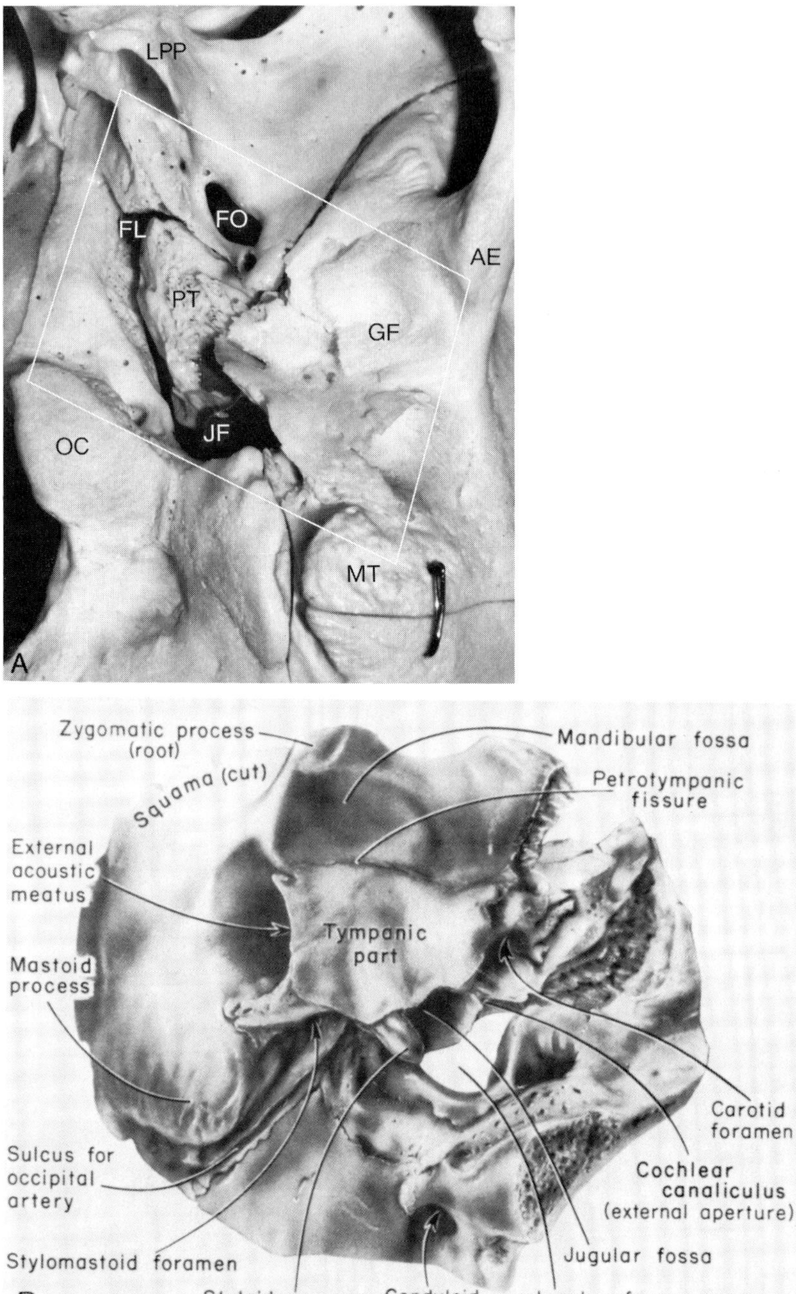

Figure 9–10. *A,* The undersurface of the skull base. This area is roughly rectangular and is canted anteromedially at 45°. (LPP = lateral pterygoid plate; AE = articular eminence; FL = foramen lacerum; FO = foramen ovale; PT = petrous tip; GF = glenoid fossa; JF = jugular foramen; OC = occipital condyle; MT = mastoid tip.) *B,* Anteroinferior view of temporal bone. (*B* from Anson BJ, Donaldson JA: Surgical Anatomy of the Temporal Bone and Ear, 2nd ed. Philadelphia, WB Saunders, 1973, p 11.)

rectangle." It houses the temporalis and pterygoid muscles and the internal maxillary artery (Fig. 9–11). The medial wall of the fossa is the squamosal portion of the skull superiorly and the lateral maxillary sinus wall and lateral pterygoid plate inferiorly. The fossa leads into the pterygomaxillary space through the fissure of the same name in the middle of this medial wall.

The pterygomaxillary space (Fig. 9–12) is directly behind the maxillary sinus, just under the medial aspect of the skull base and just

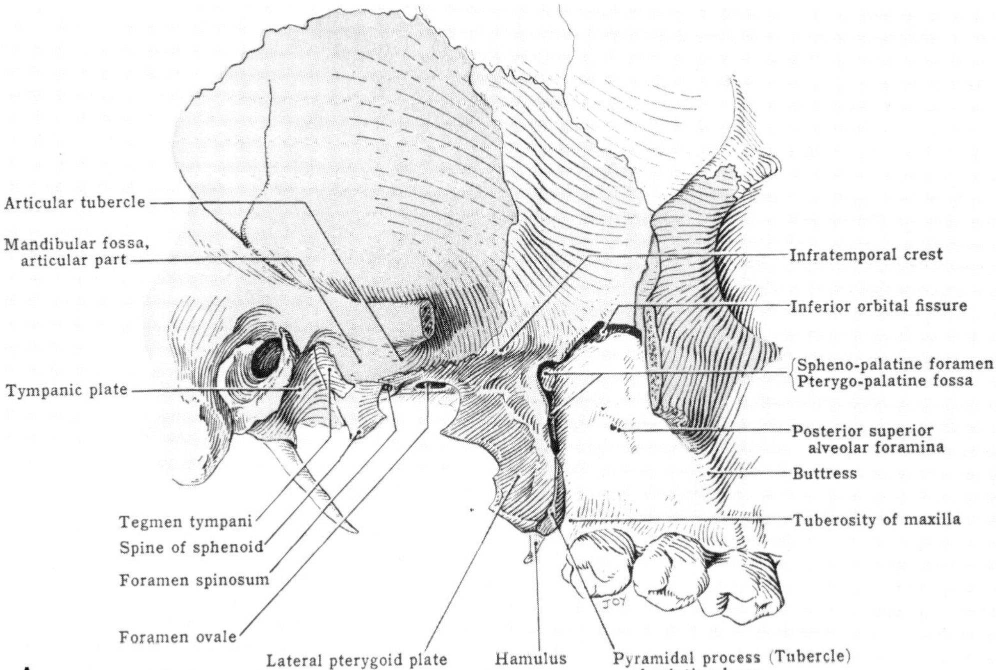

A

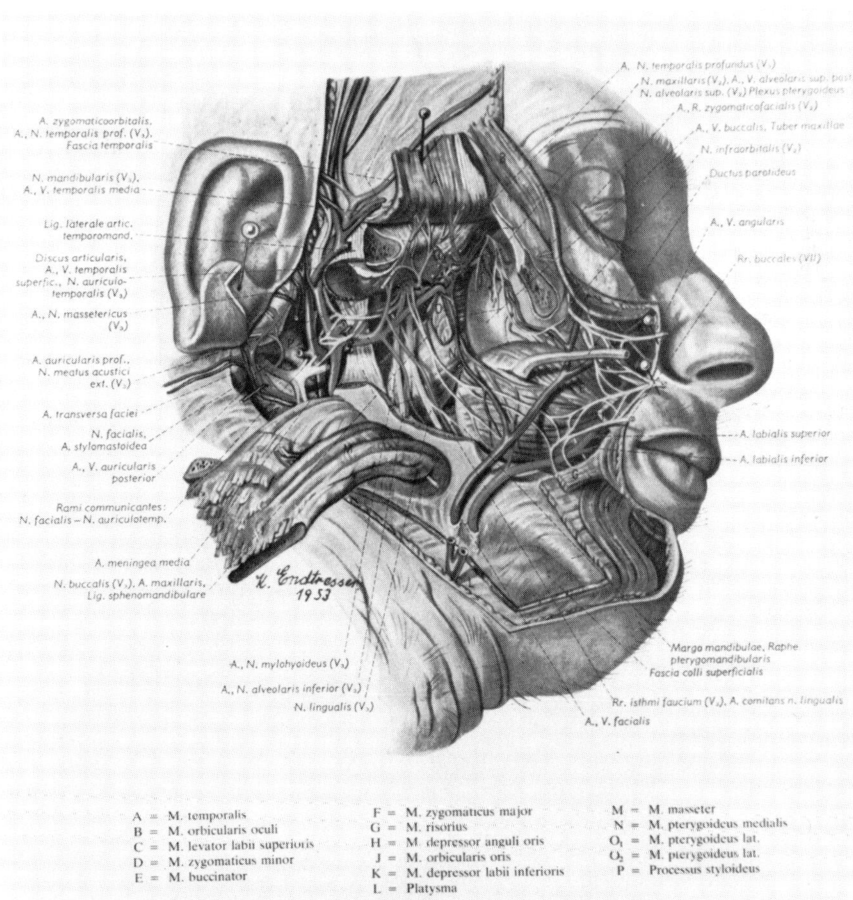

B

Figure 9–11. The infratemporal fossa. *A,* Bony landmarks. *B,* The infratemporal fossa contents. (*A* from Grant JCB: Grant's Atlas of Anatomy, 6th ed. Baltimore, Williams & Wilkins, 1972. *B* from Pernkoff E: Atlas of Topographical and Applied Human Anatomy, Vol I. Philadelphia, WB Saunders, 1963.)

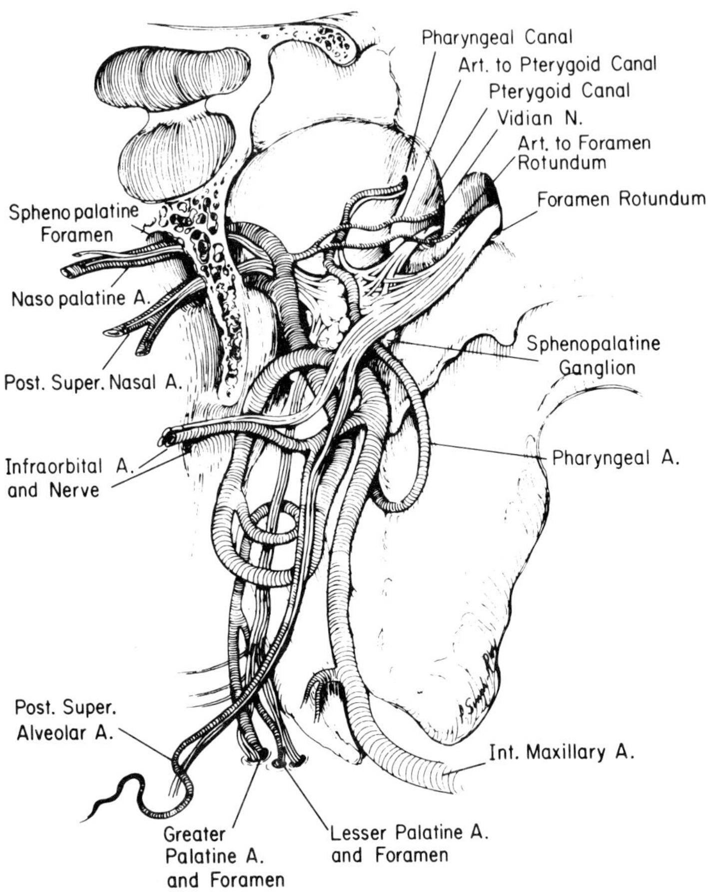

Figure 9–12. The pterygomaxillary space. (From Morgenstein RM: Surgery of the pterygopalatine fossa. *In* English GM (ed): Otolaryngology. Hagerstown, MD, Harper & Row, 1976, p 3.)

above the pterygoid plates. The internal maxillary artery enters the space following its passage between the two heads of the internal pterygoid muscle. Upon reaching the space, it ramifies into its terminal branches. The maxillary nerve, gaining entrance via the foramen rotundum, traverses the space while arborizing into branches that pass together with their accompanying vessels through the various exiting foramina. The vidian canal enters the pterygomaxillary space posteriorly, carrying the amalgamation of the deep petrosal and greater superficial petrosal nerves. Although tumors rarely take origin in this space, neoplasms originating in the nasopharynx, buccal space, maxillary sinus, and infratemporal fossa often find their way to this site. The foramen ovale with its contained nerve, the mandibular branch of the trigeminal, is situated slightly anterior and medial to the middle meningeal artery. The medialmost limit of the foramen approximates the beginning of the lateral pterygoid plate. Now the anteromedial apex of the skull base rectangle has been reached. An imaginary line subtended from the medial pterygoid plate to the anterior limit of the occipital condyle marks the lateral wall of the nasopharynx.

PATHOLOGY

Although this book is intended to deal mainly with malignancies, some benign tumors, because of their location and biologic behavior, are considered malignant by position and proclivity. This is particularly true of tumors located at the skull base. For instance, *juvenile nasopharyngeal angiofibroma,* a vasoformative tumor of vascular channels and spaces and intervening fibrous connective tissue (Fig. 9–13), has a predilection for prepubertal males, often is hormonally dependent, and can remain occult for some time until presenting with nasal obstruction or epistaxis (Figs. 9–14, 9–15). The tumor arises in the clivus, possibly from vestig-

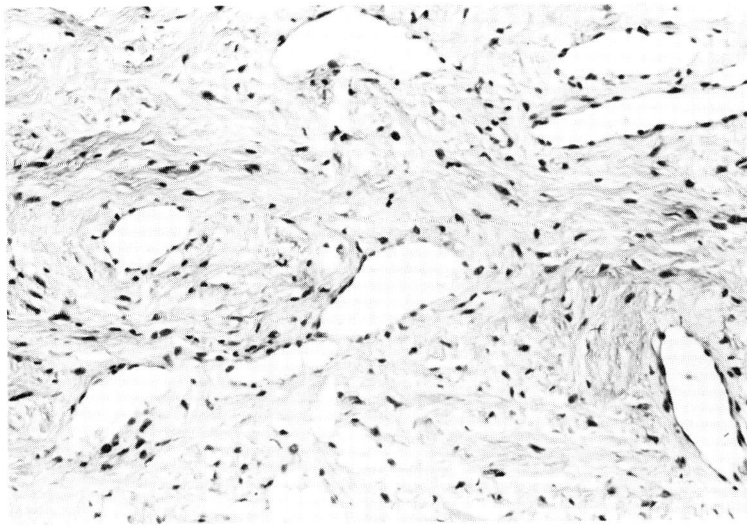

Figure 9–13. Photomicrograph of juvenile angiofibroma showing numerous vascular spaces in a fibrous tissue stroma (H & E × 220). (From Donald PJ: Sarcomatous degeneration in a nasopharyngeal angiofibroma. Otolaryngol Head Neck Surg 87:42, 1979.)

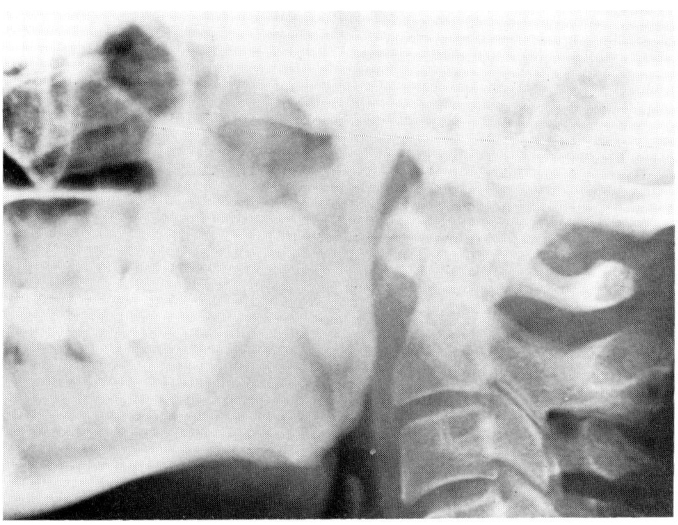

Figure 9–14. Lateral radiograph of skull showing soft tissue mass in the nasopharynx of a 52-year-old man who presented with a 35-year history of nasal obstruction. Diagnosis was nasopharyngeal angiofibroma.

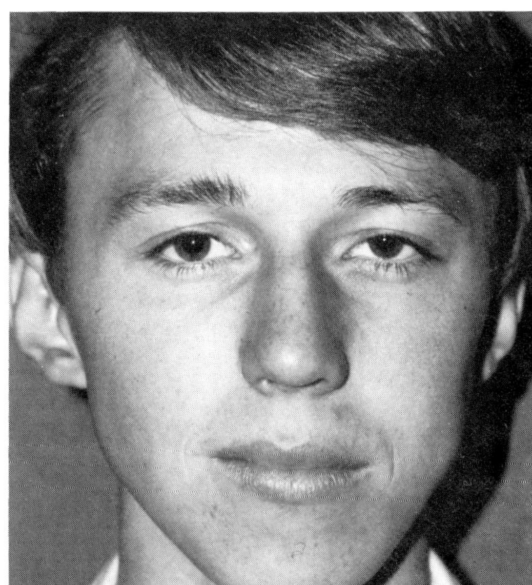

Figure 9–15. Twenty-year-old man presenting with a massive nasopharyngeal angiofibroma that produced nasal obstruction, proptosis, and epistaxis. The lesion extended into the cheek, middle cranial fossa, infratemporal fossa, and pterygomaxillar space. It caused bulging of the eye, cheek, and soft palate.

ial embryonic occipital plate remnants. It slowly expands into the nasopharynx and then extends into the paranasal sinuses, infratemporal fossa, skull base, and even the anterior and middle cranial fossae. The bony erosion produced by the tumor is probably a pressure phenomenon, and large protrusions often occur through the osseous barriers in its path. The characteristic presenting symptom of profuse epistaxis may be absent or of reduced intensity, masquerading as a routine "nuisance type" nosebleed. Such tumors may assume considerable size, as in the patient shown in Figure 9–15, who presented with total nasal obstruction, a mass in the cheek and palate, and proptosis. As intracranial involvement occurs, contributions to an already abundant blood supply are made by the cerebral vasculature.

Chordoma, a locally malignant but rarely metastasizing tumor of notochordal origin, is one of the tumors that can be best managed by partial clivectomy. It arises from cells that are remnants of the embryologic notochord. The nasopharyngeal variety accounts for about one third of these tumors, which in the main take origin in the clivus at the suture line between the basisphenoid and the basiocciput. According to Binkhorst et al[11] chordomas can also arise from the dorsum sellae, the retropharyngeal area, the apical ligament of the odontoid, and the nucleus pulposus of the cervical vertebrae. Because of their slow growth they often do not present until they have compromised cranial nerves either in the optic or otic systems.[12, 13] Histologically they are composed of trabeculations of polygonal cells containing eosinophilic granular or homogeneous cytoplasm. Cytoplasmic vacuolations are present in foci throughout the tumor and are thought to represent cellular aging.[13] This pathognomonic vacuolated cell—the so-called physaliphorous cell—is characteristic of chordoma. These grossly lobulated tumors have a tendency to erode bone and invade soft tissue structures. Envelopment of cranial nerves and the internal carotid artery, together with aggressive invasion of the dura, renders complete resection of these lesions extremely difficult. Until recently, total excision was considered impossible, and palliative surgery and radiotherapy were often the only choices of therapy. Refinements in craniofacial surgery and the advent of transclival resection with rerouting of the cerebral circulation have made possible total resection in heretofore hopeless cases.

Connective tissue tumors such as fibromas, schwannomas, lipomas, and their malignant counterparts can inhabit the skull base region. Both benign and malignant forms can erode bone and extend intracranially. Moreover, neither type can be differentiated on the basis of local behavior alone. Sarcomas of the nasopharynx or those invading the skull base from adjacent regions have a uniformly dismal prognosis because of local recurrence. On the other hand, the benign forms, if totally removed, have an excellent prognosis. Although the major problem with sarcomas is local recurrence, occasionally regional lymphatic, but especially distant blood-borne, metastases pose a significant problem.

The erosion of bone is not the only route of spread. The neural and vascular foramina of the middle fossa floor also provide portals of tumor intrusion. Often these tumors remain occult until compromise of the nerves traversing these foramina produces symptoms suggesting their presence. The patient whose x-ray appears in Figure 9–16 had symptoms of hoarseness and aspiration secondary to vocal cord paralysis from vagus nerve compromise for 1 year. It was not until the remaining nerves in the jugular foramen (IX and XI), as well as the hypoglossal, became paralyzed that the diagnosis of an invasive schwannoma extending from the upper neck into the posterior fossa was made. The tumor was managed by a transcervicomastoid-occipital approach, described in Chapter 7 (p. 245). Schwannomas of the nerves of the jugular foramen, when high in the neck, may be mistaken for neoplasms in the tail of the parotid. Sialography combined with a simultaneous CAT scan of the upper neck will make the differentiation.[14]

Malignant connective tissue tumors are rare. Leiomyosarcoma, fibrosarcoma, liposarcoma, myxoma, malignant histiocytoma, rhabdomyosarcoma, and malignant schwannomas have all been reported and commonly occur in the recesses near the skull base. Malignancies of blood vessel origin, such as hemangiopericytoma and malignant glomus jugulare tumor, are also seen. *Hemangiopericytomas,* originating in the pericytes of Zimmerman, have a dismal prognosis when intracranial spread occurs, since local invasion to this extent usually means that there are concomitant distant metastases. The orbit and nasopharynx are the most common sites of origin in the head and neck.[15] The skin and muscle account for the majority of tissues

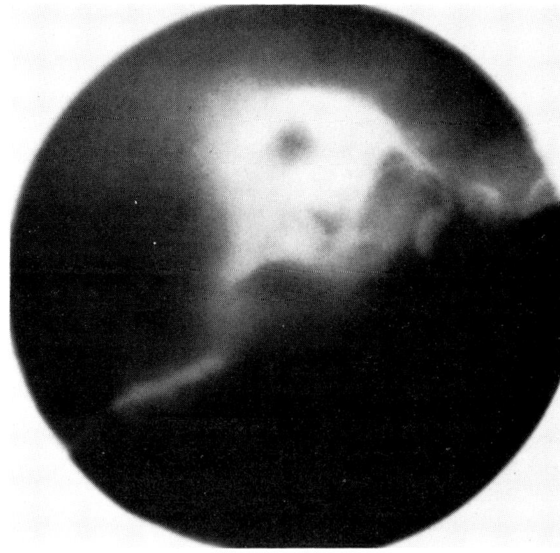

Figure 9–16. Polytomography of a patient with a massive schwannoma eroding the jugular foramen. (See Chapter 7, Fig. 7–36.)

primarily involved, and about 25 per cent of all such lesions occur in the head and neck. Hemangiopericytoma is a rapidly growing, locally aggressive tumor with a high local recurrence rate. Regional lymph node metastases are uncommon. The histologic diagnosis is sometimes difficult. The tumor cells are located between the flattened endothelial cells of the numerous capillaries of the tumor and the investing reticulin layer.[16] Reticulin stains are often necessary to clarify this relationship. Curiously there is some electron-microscopic evidence indicating a similar origin of hemangiopericytoma and subungual glomus tumors.[17] Malignancy is difficult to determine histologically. Mitotic figures and anaplasia are features common to both benign and malignant varieties and are inaccurate predictors of biologic activity. Disturbance of the relationship between the tumor cells to the reticulin layer has been reputed to be a sign of malignancy.[18]

Leiomyosarcoma is very uncommon and is rarely seen in the head and neck. Most of these tumors arise in the subcutis, probably from the erector pili muscles, but occasionally lesions will develop from the wall of the internal jugular vein. *Rhabdomyosarcoma* is most commonly seen in the orbit in children, with the next most frequent site being the nasopharynx.

It is not the purpose of this chapter to present an exhaustive treatise on soft tissue tumors, since this confusing group of neoplasms is expertly dealt with by a number of other recognized authorities.[19, 20, 21] However, some attention should be given to the *fibrous neoplasms,* as they are a confusing melange of tumors and proliferations. Not all types are common problems in the region of the skull base, but an understanding of the natural history of these tumors as a group is necessary to have a clear picture of them as a pathologic entity.

In describing tumors of connective tissue cell origin, Conley eloquently states, "Although these specific tissue entities lend themselves to an arbitrary academic classification, their dynamism for capricious primitive cellular development, functionalism, and partial mutation seems to create critical obstacles to their accurate microscopic classification."[22] Batsakis[19] roughly classifies fibrous lesions as benign, malignant, or indeterminate. Of the last group he explains, "Classifications of this group of tumors (proliferations and neoplasms) have often been rambling monstrosities with terms such as fasciitis, nodular fasciitis, infiltrative fasciitis, pseudosarcomatous fibromatosis, aggressive fibromatosis, cellular keloid, differentiated or Grade I fibrosarcoma, and non-metastasizing fibrosarcoma, either lumped together or sharply defined by ill-defined and often intangible criteria." The differentiation of fibroma from fibrosarcoma on a histologic basis is often extremely difficult, since the usual criteria of mitotic activity, cellular pleomorphism, nuclear hyperchromatism, and extracapsular invasion cannot be reliably used to make this distinction. The presence of metastases, of course, definitively designates the

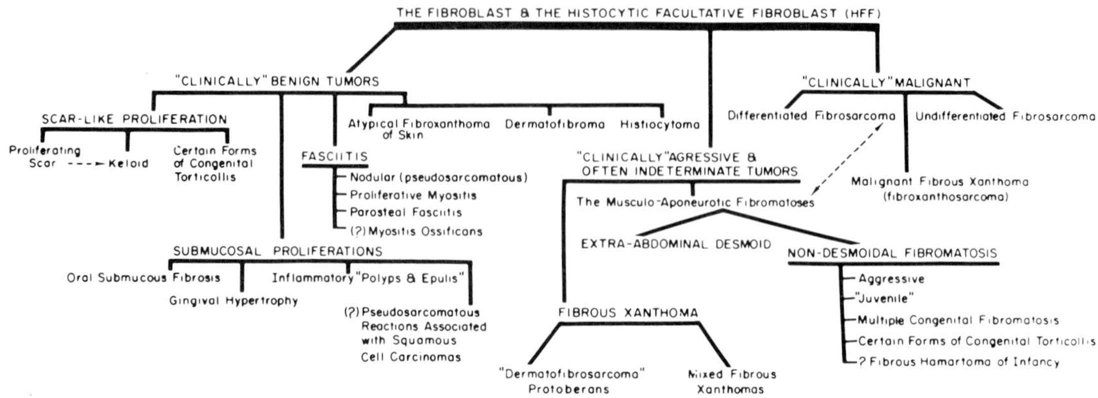

Figure 9–17. Schematic attempt to classify fibrous tumors and fibroproliferative diseases of the head and neck. (From Batsakis JG: Tumors of the Head and Neck—Clinical and Pathological Considerations. Baltimore, Williams & Wilkins, 1974, p 180.)

lesion as malignant, but this is an uncommon occurrence in fibrosarcoma. Very often the differentiation has to be made on the basis of biologic activity. The pathologic diagnosis then emerges from a composite of clues derived from historic, radiographic, and histologic data. Very often the definitive diagnosis must be made by the surgeon who is managing the case, since he alone is cognizant of the aggressiveness of the specific tumor he is treating.

Figure 9–17 portrays even more graphically the confusion that exists over the classification of fibrous tumors, although it does in some way provide a framework to work by. *Fibromas* are difficult to diagnose and are quite uncommon. Many of the tumors formerly bearing this appellation were in fact histiocytomas. Most of these tumors occur in skin and are rarely seen in the region of the skull base.

Fibrosarcoma was formerly one of the most commonly diagnosed soft tissue malignancies, often in error. In recent times, they have been determined to make up approximately 0.5 to 5.5 per cent of all soft tissue malignancies.[23] The degree of histologic differentiation usually determines the biologic activity. The well-differentiated tumor rarely metastasizes and tends to be less locally aggressive. Regional and distant metastases, as well as aggressive local spread, characterize the poorly differentiated form. The well-differentiated variety demonstrates an admixture of fibers and cells. The cells are fairly uniform, mitoses are infrequent, and nuclear hyperchromatism is occasionally seen. Varying degrees of cellular anaplasia designate the malignancy of the undifferentiated forms. The metastatic rate in the latter is around 20 to 25 per cent[19, 20] and is usually hematogenous.

A much more common tumor in the skull base area is the *schwannoma.* Electron-microscopic and histochemical evidence definitely points to the Schwann cell as the origin of both schwannomas (also called neurolemmomas) and neurofibromas.[24] Clinically and grossly, the two have characteristic differences. One of the most important, from the surgical standpoint, is that the neurofibroma has neural elements that traverse the tumor, whereas the schwannoma, although attached to a nerve, has no actual nerve fibers traversing it. *Neurofibromas* are characteristic of von Recklinghausen's disease and carry a significant potential for malignant degeneration. Histologically, the Antoni A and B configuration and the presence of Verocay bodies are characteristic (Fig. 9–18). Although the configuration of a central cytoplasmic mass encircled by pallisaded nuclei that together comprise the Verocay body is occasionally seen in neurofibromas, the usual picture is of an unencapsulated tumor composed of fibers and spindle cells insinuated within the nerve substance. The fibrous component is commonly randomly distributed, and the cellular nuclei take on a serpiginous configuration.

Batsakis[19] prefers to designate malignancies of nerve cell sheath origin as neurogenous sarcomas. Malignant schwannoma would appear to be a misnomer, as clear evidence of malignant degeneration in a schwannoma is wanting. The appearance of some cellular pleomorphism—an occasional mitotic figure or multinucleated cells—must be recognized

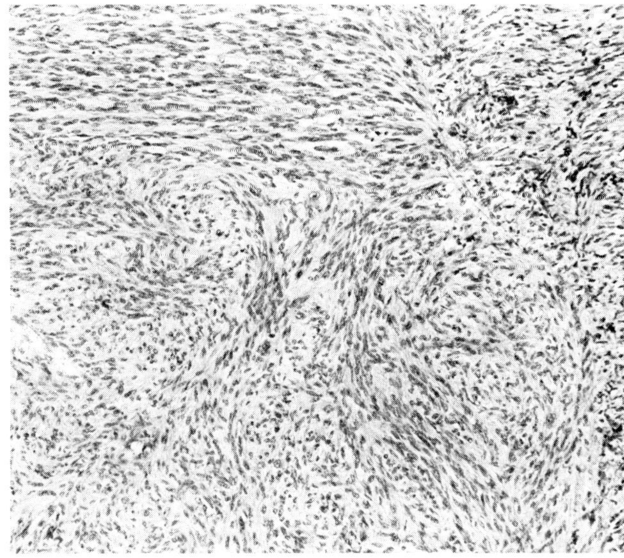

Figure 9–18. Photomicrograph of a schwannoma. (× 130)

as a regressive step and not as a sign of malignancy.

Neurofibromas appear to be the principal source of malignancy among neural tumors of the head and neck. Histologically, the differentiation of neurogenous sarcoma from fibrosarcoma is almost impossible. The origin of the tumor in a nerve is the prime distinguishing feature. These malignancies frequently metastasize and have rapid local spread. Only wide radical local excision provides any hope of salvage.

Sarcomas are rare in the nasopharynx, and *squamous cell carcinoma* is by far the most common malignancy seen, usually of a poorly differentiated cellular type or as a lymphoepithelioma. For some time controversy over the precise categorization of lymphoepithelioma and transitional cell cancer raged. The electron-microscopic findings of keratin granules and desmosomes[25, 26] have definitively classified these tumors as variants of epidermoid carcinoma. Their biologic behavior is similar to that of poorly differentiated squamous cell cancers, and, like them, they are more radiosensitive than their more differentiated relatives. Both lymphoepithelioma and transitional cell cancer may be grossly exophytic, ulcerative, or infiltrative. The occult infiltrative type is the most common (Fig. 9–19).

Following the palatine tonsil the nasophar-

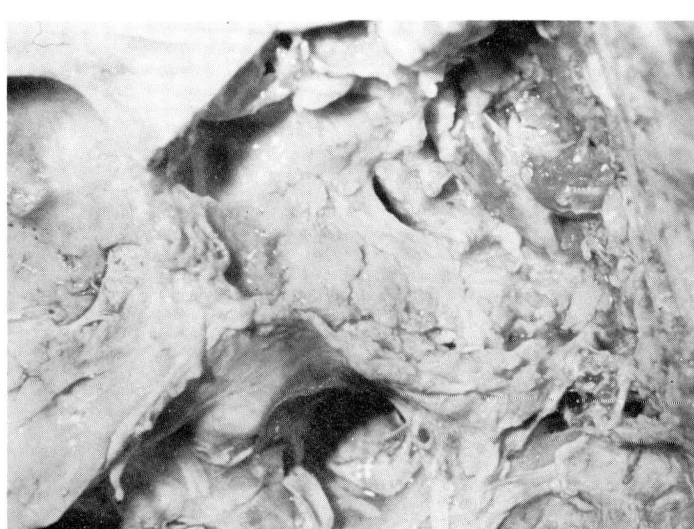

Figure 9–19. Autopsy specimen showing massive intracranial extent of an infiltrating nasopharyngeal carcinoma arising in the fossa of Rosenmeuller.

ynx is the most common site of lymphoma. It is frequently accompanied by cervical lymphadenopathy.

Nasopharyngeal malignancies in general are uncommon, making up only 0.25 per cent or so of all cancers. In the population at large this is an overall incidence of only about 0.0005 per cent.[27] A notable exception is the high incidence of nasopharyngeal cancer in China, where it is responsible for about 15 per cent of all deaths due to malignant disease.[25] This is not true for Chinese born in other countries. Although this incidence of nasopharyngeal malignancy is still high, it diminishes among each successive generation of Chinese born outside their native country. The role of the Epstein-Barr virus in the etiology of this disease continues to remain obscure, although a common association between elevated titres of Epstein-Barr antibody commonly coexist with the disease. Further, Coates et al showed a decrease in antibody titres in those cured of their disease.[28]

The most common presenting sign in nasopharyngeal carcinoma is a lump in the neck. Conversely, one of the most common of the unknown primaries in patients who present initially with a lump in the neck is nasopharyngeal carcinoma.[29] Fletcher and Million[30] found only 16 cases out of a total of 112 (14.3 per cent) that had no metastasis to the neck. Vilar[31] reported 21/24 (87.5 per cent) of patients with nodal involvement, and another authority[32] quotes 90 per cent of patients with unilateral and 50 per cent with bilateral disease.

The lymphatic drainage system of the nasopharynx offers a number of different routes of metastatic spread. There are from one to three high laterally placed retropharyngeal lymph nodes that are the principal filtering stations of the lymphatic channels draining the nasopharynx. The lymph proceeds from these to the upper internal jugular nodal group or to the nodes of the posterior cervical triangle. In some instances, the high nodes are bypassed and the first manifestation of nasopharyngeal tumor is an enlarged node in the posterior triangle or, less commonly, in the upper internal jugular chain.[33] The original study done by Rouvière[34] over 40 years ago clearly delineating the lymphatic system in the head and neck has not been improved upon since.

SURGICAL PROCEDURES

Preoperative Planning

One of the most important steps in the performance of procedures in the infratemporal fossa and skull base areas is preoperative planning. Because of the exigencies of each case, there will be considerable variation in the approach and extent of the surgery. Once a comprehensive examination and investigation has been conducted by both the head and neck surgeon and neurosurgeon, a presurgical conference should be scheduled, at which time the two surgeons together should establish the sequence of operative steps, including the incisions, the temporal order of intracranial and transfacial dissections, the method of tumor delivery, and finally the stages of reconstruction and closure.

With careful planning, often the cranial and facial incisions can complement one another. Care must be taken not to compromise the cutaneous blood supply by poor flap design. In many instances, a single incision can afford a perfectly adequate exposure for both facets of the procedure. The use of curved incisions not only is more cosmetic but also enhances exposure. Determining the sequence of the steps of dissection often requires considerable deliberation. This should not take the form of a power struggle but should be a process of deciding how best the dissection should proceed.

Reconstructive efforts have as a first priority a watertight dural closure and separation of the cranial cavity from the upper aerodigestive system. Dural grafting is often required. The experience of Ketcham et al[35] of improved results with use of temporalis fascia over fascia lata as dural replacement is borne out by my own. Considerable time is often required to ensure precise dural integrity. This is time well spent, as it is the key to the prevention of cerebrospinal fluid leakage and subsequent meningitis. Isolation of the cranial cavity from the air and food stream may not be a problem. Sufficient soft tissue in the upper neck or around the skull base may exist to reinforce the dural repair. If not, the interposition of a flap or the application of a skin graft may be necessary to seal off the defect. Neurosurgeons commonly employ alloplastic materials for re-establishing cranial continuity. However, the use of these materials has no place in the correction of cranial base defects secondary to tumor excision. Adequately vascularized tissue is essential for the take of both dural and skin grafts.

A good general principle is for both surgeons to be present during most of the operation. As the partnership matures, substantial assistance can be rendered between participants. Anticipation of problems can be better predicted and more efficient dispatch of the operative process can be effected. Sudden unexpected hemorrhage may be best handled by the complementary team member; when both are present, the success of this cooperative venture will be maximized.

Superficial Temporal–to–Middle Cerebral Arterial Anastomosis

The performance of this technique will be dealt with in a superficial manner only, while providing enough information for the head and neck surgeon to understand what has to be done. Comprehension of the details regarding incisions, cranial bone removal, and interruption of distal external carotid arterial supply is essential in order to plan the definitive surgical excision and reconstruction. The surgical procedure for revascularizing the cerebrum should be done by the neurosurgeon, who in turn must be familiar with microvascular surgical techniques.

A large frontoparietal scalp flap is elevated, with great care taken to preserve both branches of the superficial temporal artery. The parietal branch is dissected free. Directly beneath it, a 4-cm diameter craniotomy is done at a point approximately 6 cm superior to the external auditory canal (Fig. 9–20). The superficial temporal artery branch should measure between 1.5 and 2.5 mm in diameter in order to best accommodate the recipient cortical vessel. A dural incision exposes a large cortical arterial branch of the middle cerebral artery. An end-to-side anastomosis is done, with the excised stump of the parietal branch sutured into a recipient site created in the wall of the cerebral vessel (Fig. 9–21). The anastomosis is made with from 10 to 12 size 10-0 nylon sutures. Systemic anticoagulation is unnccessary since the local instillation of heparin during the vessel approximation is sufficient to prevent thrombosis. Flow

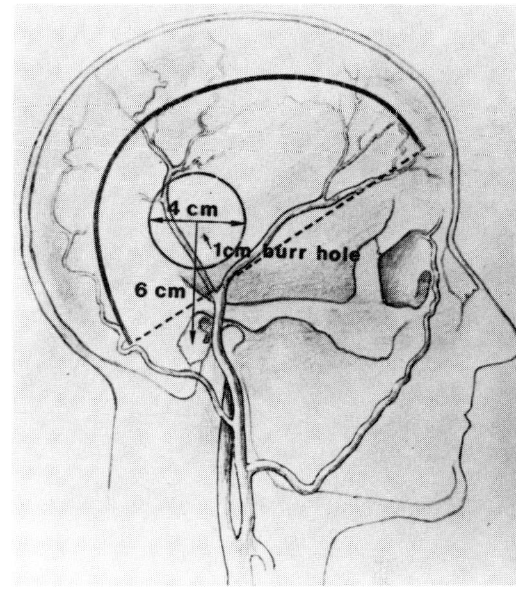

Figure 9–20. Temporoparietal scalp flap elevated to expose the posterior branch of the superficial temporal artery (STA) for an STA to middle cerebral artery microvascular anastomosis. The temporoparietal bur hole, 4 cm in diameter, is marked out and is located 6 cm directly superior to the external auditory meatus. (From Silber SJ: Microsurgery. Baltimore, Williams & Wilkins, 1979, p 426.)

rates of 30 to 75 cc per minute have been measured at these anastomotic sites intraoperatively.[36] The superficial temporal artery has a capacity for expansion with time, and patency rates are reported to be 90 per cent at 1 year in most series.[37, 38] If the superficial temporal artery is not suitable for grafting, the occipital artery can be used as an alternative.

In the subsequent tumor resection, it is most important to preserve the external carotid artery. The sites at which it is in most jeopardy are deep in the parotid gland and behind the neck of the mandible. If the internal maxillary artery is cut during subsequent tumor extirpation, great care must be exercised to control the bleeding distal to the vessel's emergence from the carotid. Although a small amount of collateral flow can traverse across the scalp to maintain the patency of the superficial temporal artery in the event that the ipsilateral carotid is ligated, the flow is usually insufficient to maintain adequate cerebral nutrition.

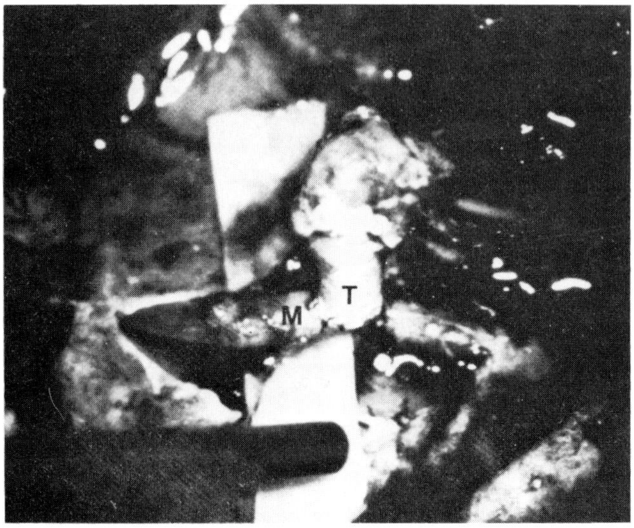

Figure 9–21. Photograph taken through the surgical microscope of a superficial temporal to middle cerebral artery anastomosis (× 10). (From Silber SJ: Microsurgery. Baltimore, Williams & Wilkins, 1979, p 427.)

Lateral Approach to the Skull Base

The undersurface of the skull base, specifically the inferior surface of the temporal bone, can be adequately exposed through a lateral approach. Visualization is enhanced not only by mandibulotomy but by osteotomy and mobilization of the zygoma.[39] Mandibulotomy or condylectomy improves exposure through the parotid bed or with the parotid retracted anteriorly. The gland is more often retracted when it is small or atrophic. The zygomatic osteotomy approach was developed by Fisch[39] for enhancing the exposure of large acoustic neuromas and glomus jugulare tumors with extensive intracranial and upper cervical involvement. His primary motivation was to eradicate extensive otologic disease. We have found this approach useful also for deep-seated lesions such as extensive deep lobe parotid tumors and extensive schwannomas originating from the nerves of the jugular foramen, as well as tumors that reach to or extend from the nasopharynx, sphenoid sinus, and even the pituitary fossa.

Since most of Fisch's cases were primarily otologic, the procedure begins with a radical mastoidectomy and anterior transposition of the facial nerve. The management of otologic tumors is discussed in Chapter 7. In this section, we will concern ourselves primarily with lesions in which transtemporal exposure of the internal carotid artery or internal jugular vein is not necessary. Transtemporal exposure of the internal carotid artery requires violating the eustachian tube, which then necessitates either the marsupialization or obliteration of the middle ear cleft. In the cases to be dealt with here, internal carotid control is achieved both intracranially and transcervically without violation of the temporal bone, since in its petrous part, only very small branches of the carotid are given off (corticotympanic, vidian, hypophyseal, and cavernous).

The incision is an adaptation of the modified Blair incision for parotidectomy (Fig. 9–22). The anterior limb is extended into the temporal scalp anteriorly, while a posterior limb extends postauricularly, arching into the occipital region. If a superficial temporal–to–middle cerebral anastomosis has been done to bypass the internal carotid, extreme care must be exercised to preserve the superficial temporal artery and to avoid the anastomotic site at the time of incision and during subsequent flap elevation. The extent of the pre- and postauricular limbs of the incision is dependent on the amount of exposure needed and on whether or not mastoidectomy is required. The external auditory canal is transected and the auricle retracted superiorly, if the latter is to be retained. The cervical extension of the incision is used not only for access to the parotid tail but also as a means of exposing the great vessels from the carotid bifurcation to the skull base. If a radical neck dissection is required, a lazy S extension is made at right angles to the cervical aspect of the incision inferiorly. As always, the junction is made behind the carotid sheath.

If a radical neck dissection is required, it

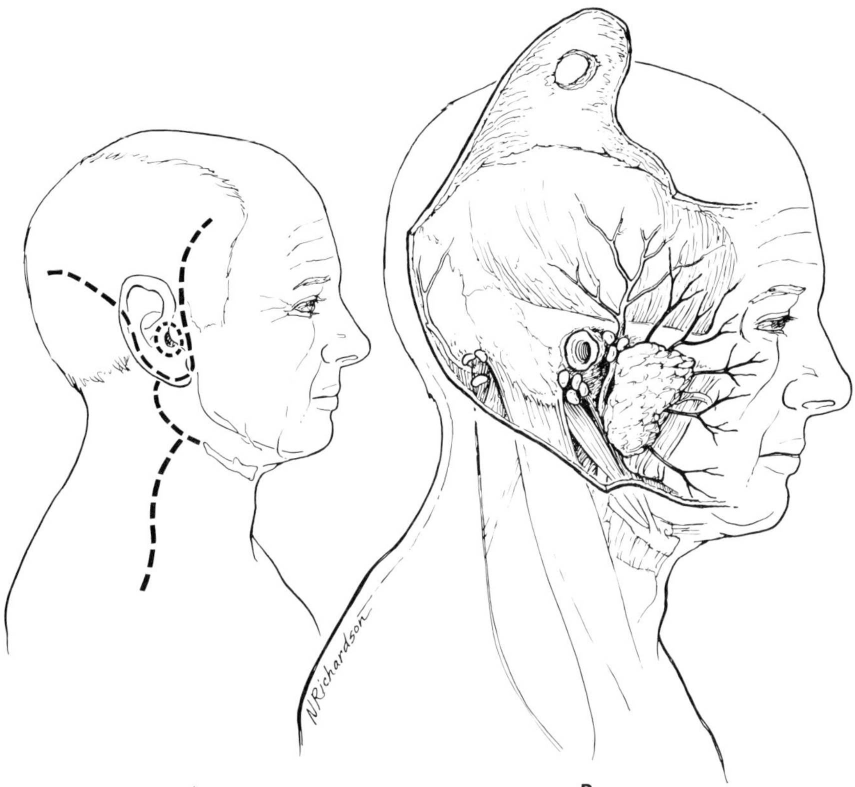

Figure 9–22. *A,* Incision for exposure of the skull base through the infratemporal fossa. Dashed line represents extension if a radical neck dissection is required. *B,* Flaps are dissected. Auricle is reflected superiorly on the flap after transection of the external auditory canal at the bony-cartilaginous junction.

is done after a parotidectomy, when the latter is necessary. Often both the superficial and deep lobes are removed. The facial nerve is carefully dissected in the manner described by McCabe and Work[40] (see Chapter 6). In resecting the deep lobe, the nerve is gently retracted with a Zimmer hook (Fig. 9–23). During the rest of the dissection, the continuity of the nerve is preserved up to the point where further retraction puts it in danger of severe neuropraxia or avulsion. At this point, severance just beyond the point of main branching is done so that when continuity is restored (near the termination of the operation), subsequent reinnervation will result in differential function. A radical neck dissection is done at this point, if required by the exigencies of the tumor. If not, the inferior aspect of the apex of the temporal bone is now approached in a stepwise manner from lateral to medial.

The initial exposure is gained by excising the origin of the sternocleidomastoid muscle from the mastoid tip. A slicing motion with a scalpel blade against the mastoid cortex is often quicker than the standard dissection with the mastoid elevator. Deep to this muscle is the posterior belly of the digastric. This is elevated from its fossa with a Joseph elevator, with care taken anteriorly not to traumatize the facial nerve (Fig. 9–24). The occipital artery in its groove is dissected free and ligated. It is wise to control this vessel with a ligature or suture-ligature at the outset, since failure to do so leads to annoying hemorrhage.

As one proceeds medioanteriorly, the styloid process comes into view. The stylohyoid, stylopharyngeus, and styloglossus muscles are removed and dissected anteriorly, with the facial nerve always kept in clear view. Care is taken while dissecting the stylopharyngeus muscle not to damage the glossopharyngeal nerve. The pharyngeal anesthesia and the even minor motor disturbance that may result from damage to cranial nerve IX may render the patient dysphagic, an especially troublesome consequence in elderly patients.

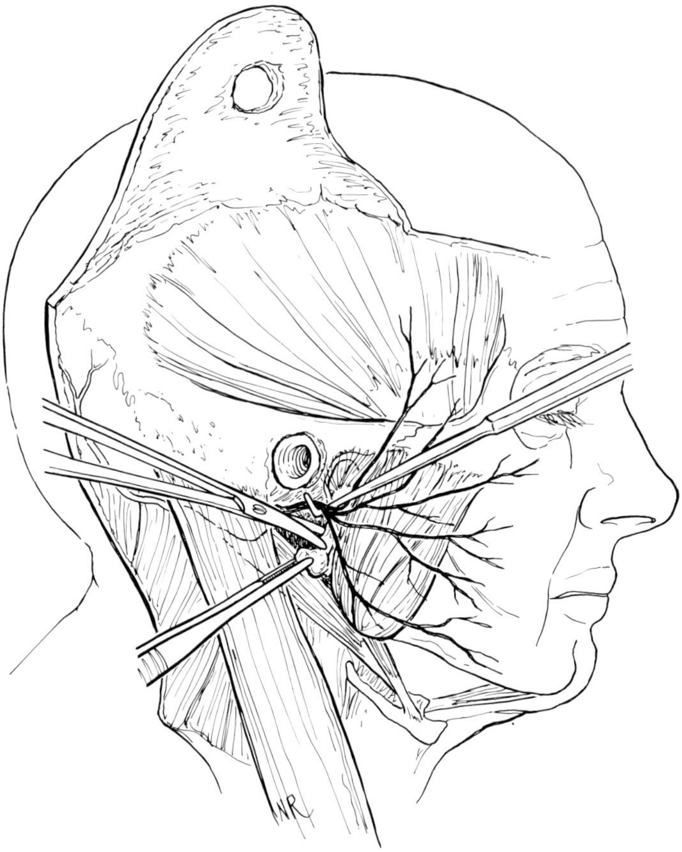

Figure 9–23. A superficial lobe parotidectomy is done. A nerve hook retracts the facial nerve (VII) while the deep lobe is being removed.

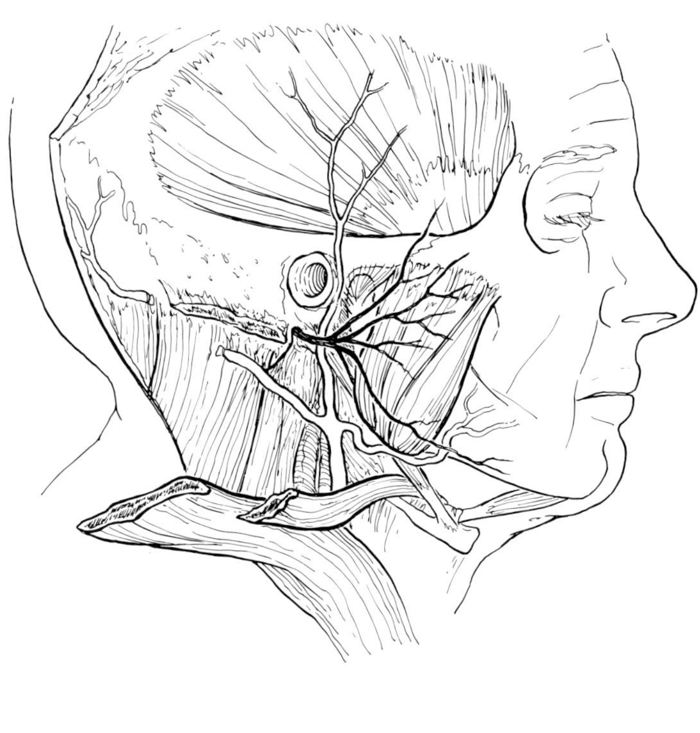

Figure 9–24. The sternocleidomastoid muscle is cut from its origin on the mastoid process. The posterior belly of the digastric muscle is dissected from its groove, and the occipital artery is exposed and ligated.

Progress beyond the styloid becomes difficult because of the mandibular condyle and neck. The triangle gets tighter as the dissection proceeds more deeply. If the lesion is no deeper than the jugular vein, firm retraction at the mandibular angle with a stout bone hook, in addition to the previously mentioned dissection, will sometimes provide adequate exposure. Most often, however, this is insufficient, and condylectomy or mandibulotomy is necessary. Because the former procedure is preferred by the author, it will be described first.

The anterior limb of the incision assists in the exposure of the temporomandibular joint and the zygoma up to its orbital process. The frontal branch of the facial nerve must be handled with great care, as it is extremely sensitive to trauma by traction and susceptible to injury by virtue of its position. The temporomandibular ligament forms much of the stout lateral component of the joint capsule. More posteriorly, the capsule is less substantial, albeit still tough. The capsule is incised, the joint entered, and the condyle cut from its attachments medially. Great care must be taken when freeing soft tissue from the neck of the mandible, because of the proximity of the internal maxillary artery deep to it. Avulsion of this vessel can produce significant hemorrhage that will prolong operating time substantially, a pitfall that can be avoided by maintaining a subperiosteal plane of dissection and exercising caution when removing the insertion of the lateral pterygoid muscle on the anteromedial surface of the condylar neck. The condyle is grasped with a Dingman bone clamp and is excised using a Striker or Gigli saw (Fig. 9–25). Following its removal, the meniscus is excised as well. An alternative is to do a stair-step osteotomy, as illustrated in Figure 9–26.

Just medial to the glenoid fossa is the sphenoid spine. The foramen spinosum adjacent to it harbors the middle meningeal artery. The artery is carefully ligated, and dissection proceeds medially. Very close to the artery is the large trunk of the manidublar branch of the trigeminal nerve as it exits the skull through the foramen ovale. Just anteromedial to this is the origin of the tensor veli palatini muscle in the shallow fossa at the base of the pterygoid plates.

Further medial dissection will now approach the foramen lacerum and the lateral wall of the nasopharynx. An improved exposure of this region as well as of the area more anteriorly—the infratemporal fossa—is made possible by a zygomatic osteotomy. The malar bone is cut with a Striker saw posteriorly through the arch, superiorly through the orbital process, and anteriorly through the body (Fig. 9–27). It is important to stair-step the osteotomy in the body for ease of reapproximation at closure. The zygoma is now reflected inferiorly, exposing the infratemporal fossa. The temporalis muscle is incised superiorly and reflected with the zygoma in order to reach the floor of the fossa, made up of the lateral maxillary wall and the lateral pterygoid plate. The pterygoid muscles, especially the lateral, also occupy the

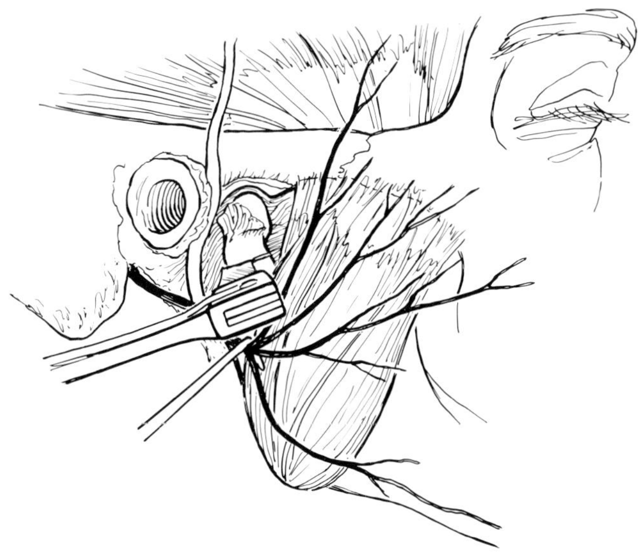

Figure 9–25. The temporomandibular joint capsule is incised, the condyle grasped with a bone clasp, and the mandibular neck incised with a bone saw.

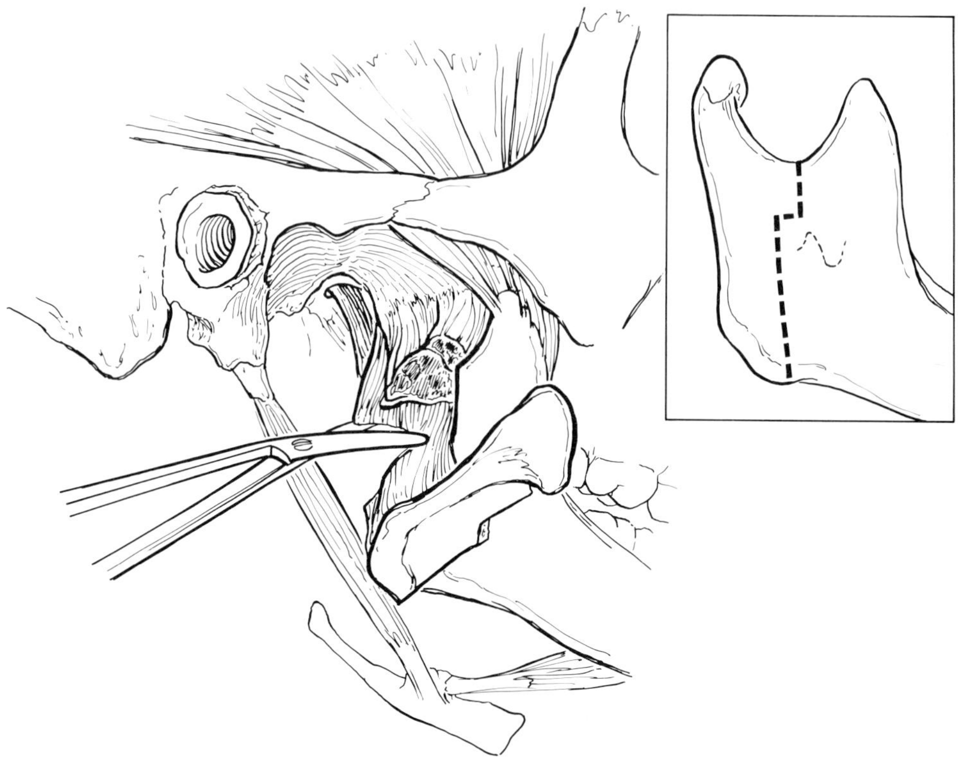

Figure 9–26. Alternative method of mandibular osteotomy to approach the skull base or infratemporal fossa. A stair-step osteotomy is done, with care taken to avoid the inferior alveolar nerve. A medial view of the mandible is shown, with the osteotomy outlined. The masseter muscle and overlying facial nerve are retracted in a subperiosteal plane. The stair-step osteotomy is outlined. The pterygoid muscles are cut and the mandibular segments retracted.

fossa. The internal maxillary artery passes between the two heads of the lateral pterygoid muscle and must be controlled. Considerable hemorrhage often is incurred by disruption of the pterygoid venous plexus. Even numerous suture ligatures may be insufficient, and oxidized cellulose gauze or cotton packs may be necessary to achieve hemostasis.

Just beyond the inlet to the temporal bone for the internal carotid artery is the emergence of the cartilaginous portion of the eustachian tube. A thin bony plate, which may be incomplete, is all that separates the bony portion of the tube from the lateral wall of the artery. The cartilaginous continuation of the tube is nestled in a groove between the sphenoid bone and the undersurface and anterior wall of the petrous tip. It is flanked by the tensor veli and levator veli palatini muscles. If tumor involves the tube and resection is required, excision should be followed by tubal obliteration, done according to the method described by Fisch.[39] The tubal mucosa is stripped toward the nasopharynx and the lumen occluded with bone paste and a fascial graft.

If the tumor transgresses the cranial cavity into the middle fossa, the subpetrous approach is coupled with a temporal-parietal craniotomy. The area of the cavernous sinus may be infiltrated by tumor, but with control of the internal carotid artery in the neck and in the cranial cavity this sinus can be transgressed and tumor removed. Despite the sinus being a low-pressure system, hemorrhage is vigorous. Attempts at hemostasis by the application of clips or suture ligatures are usually fruitless, and oxidized cellulose packs must generally be used to arrest bleeding. At this point in the resection, both the head and neck surgeon and the neurologic surgeon must be present, since a combined effort is needed to deliver the tumor and control hemorrhage.

Surgery in the region of the cavernous sinus must be undertaken with a full understanding of its difficulties. The optic nerve is in jeop-

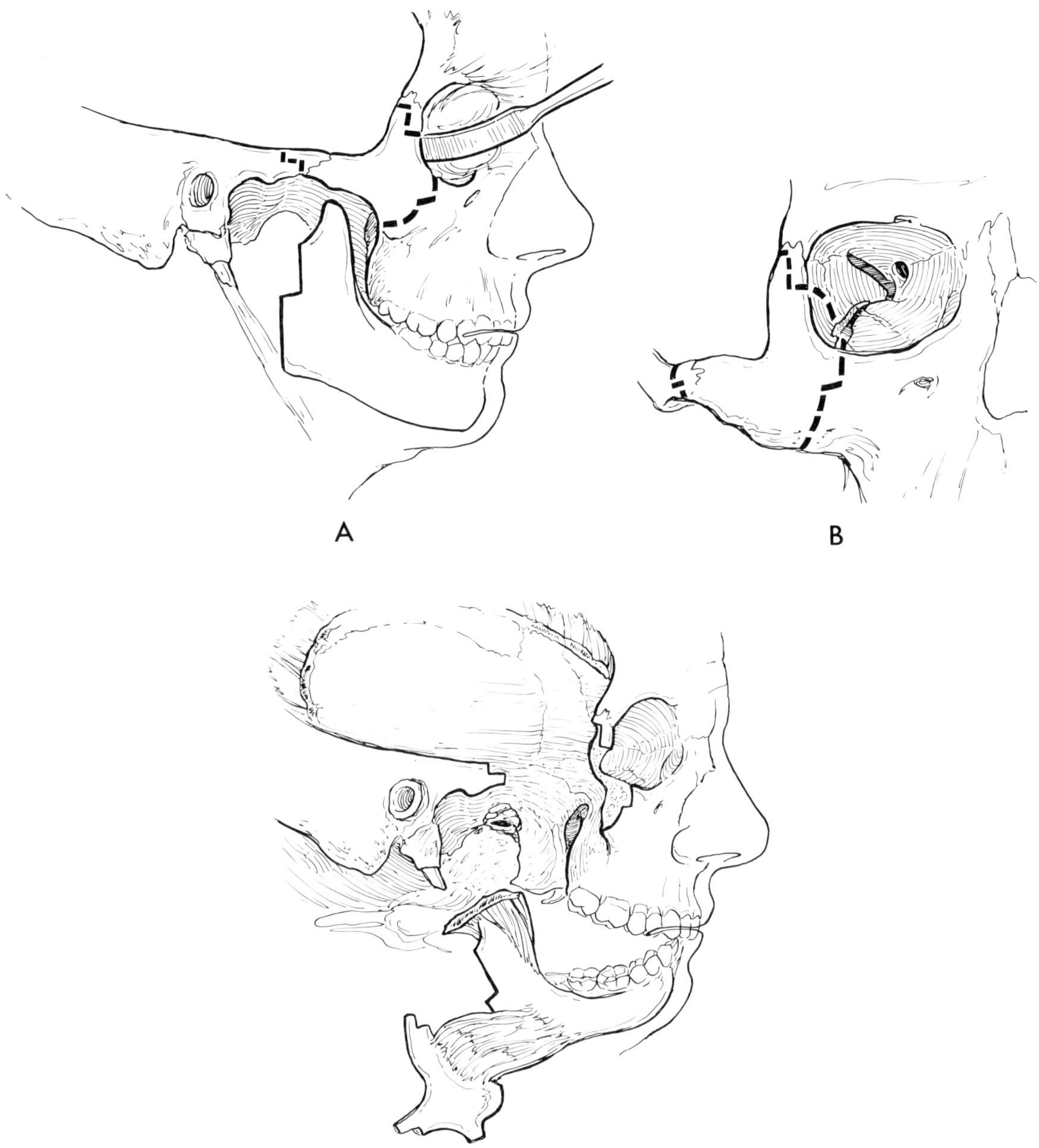

A

B

C

Figure 9–27. *A,* Osteotomy incisions outlined. The periorbita must be elevated to the region of the infraorbital fissure. The osteotomy goes through the lateral orbital rim and the inferolateral orbital wall to the fissure. The floor is cut back to the infraorbital rim, and a stair-step osteotomy is done in the zygomatic body. *B,* Intraorbital view. *C,* The zygoma is retracted, the temporalis muscle reflected, and the infratemporal fossa exposed.

Illustration continued on following page

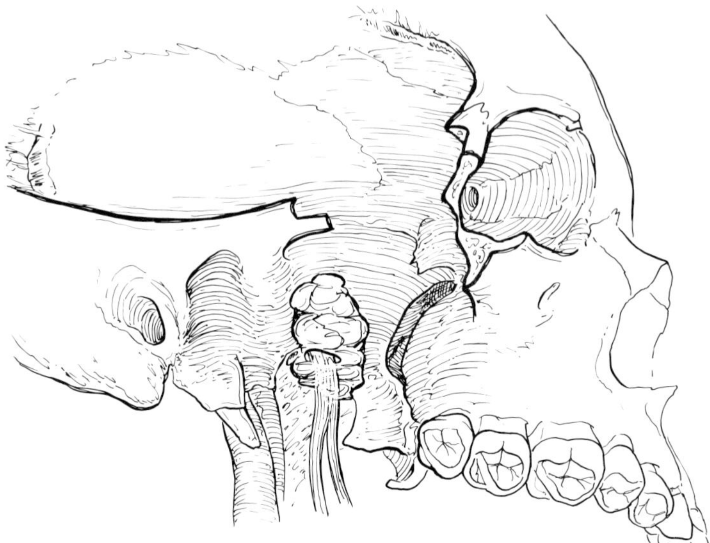

D

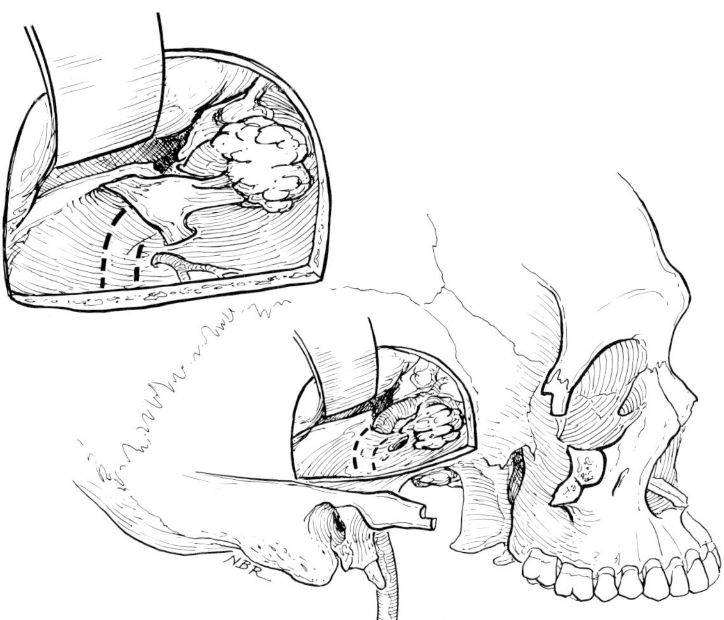

E

Figure 9–27 *Continued. D,* With the zygoma and mandible removed for illustration purposes, the tumor is exposed at the base of the skull, near the foramen ovale. *E,* Transcranial and infratemporal view of the tumor, which has intracranial extension into the cavernous sinus, requiring internal carotid ligation.

Illustration continued on opposite page

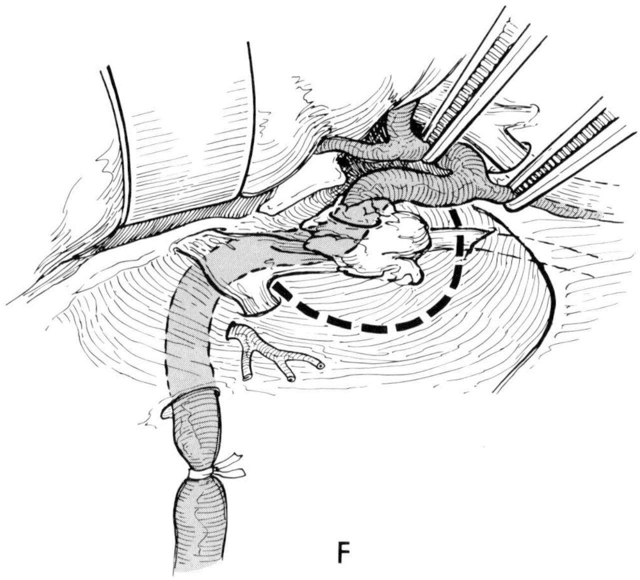

F

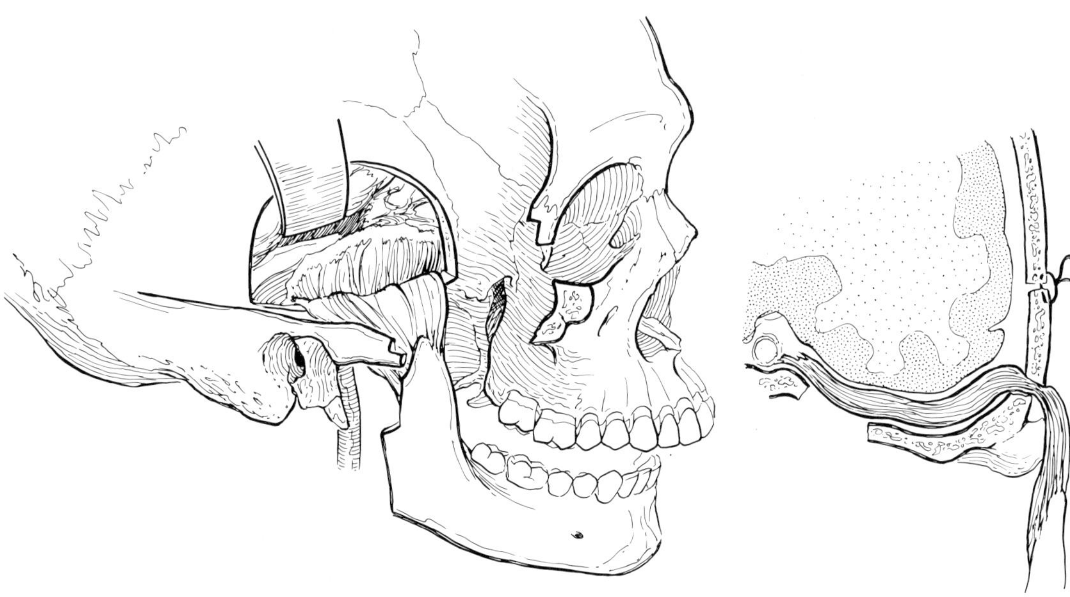

G

Figure 9–27 *Continued. F,* Ligation and clipping of the internal carotid artery. *G,* Closure of the defect, with temporalis muscle used to relnforce the cranial floor.

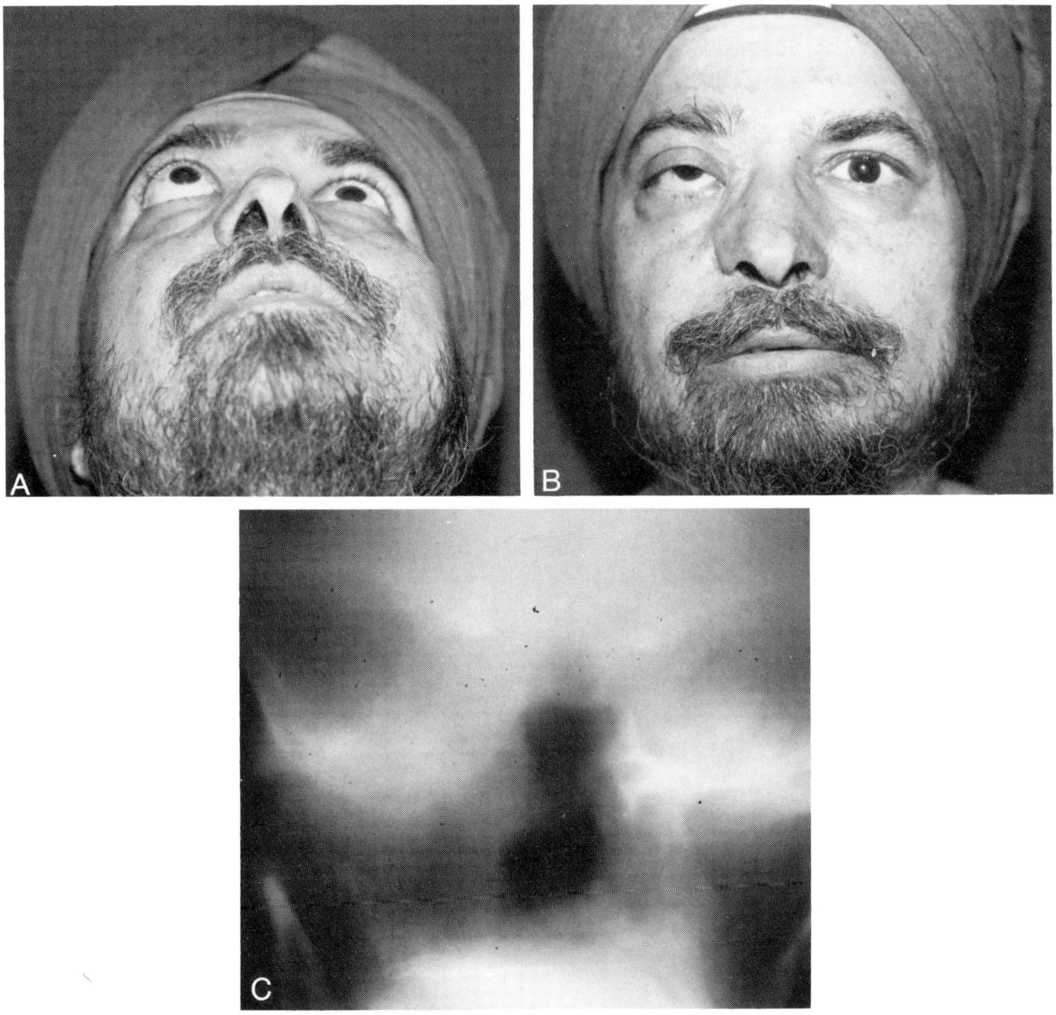

Figure 9–28. A 57-year-old patient with a large fibrosarcoma that originated in the nasopharynx and extensively invaded the middle cranial fossa. *A,* Tumor protruding from nose. *B,* Disturbance of ocular motility from invasion of the cavernous sinus and involvement of cranial nerves III, IV, and VI. *C,* Coronal tomography demonstrating intracranial extension into both the anterior and middle cranial fossae. *D,* Intraoperative photo at the beginning of maxillectomy, demonstrating massive tumor extension in the maxillary sinus. The ethmoid sinuses, orbit, nasal cavity, pterygomaxillary space, and infratemporal fossa were also involved. *E,* Intraoperative photo of postresection appearance of anterior and middle cranial fossa resection. *F,* Line drawing of *E.*

Illustration continued on oposite page

ardy, as is the ophthalmic artery. If carotid control is necessary proximal to the latter, blindness is inevitable; therefore, preoperative apprisal of the patient in this regard is essential. Any degree of dissection in the cavernous sinus will, at the least, result in disturbed ocular motility. Figure 9–28 shows a patient with a large fibrosarcoma from the nasopharynx invading the middle cranial fossa. The cavernous sinus involvement produced interference with ocular motility. Unfortunately, the patient delayed permission for surgery until the point at which the optic nerve was compromised by tumor and blindness occurred.

Closure is initially directed at achieving a watertight dural seal. If sufficient local soft tissue is present, then no further support is required. However, if there is a dearth of soft tissue, a temporalis muscle flap can be swung into the defect. Cutaneous tumor involvement may necessitate the placement of a pectoralis major or trapezius musculocutaneous flap. The zygoma is closed by interosseous wires (Fig. 9–29).

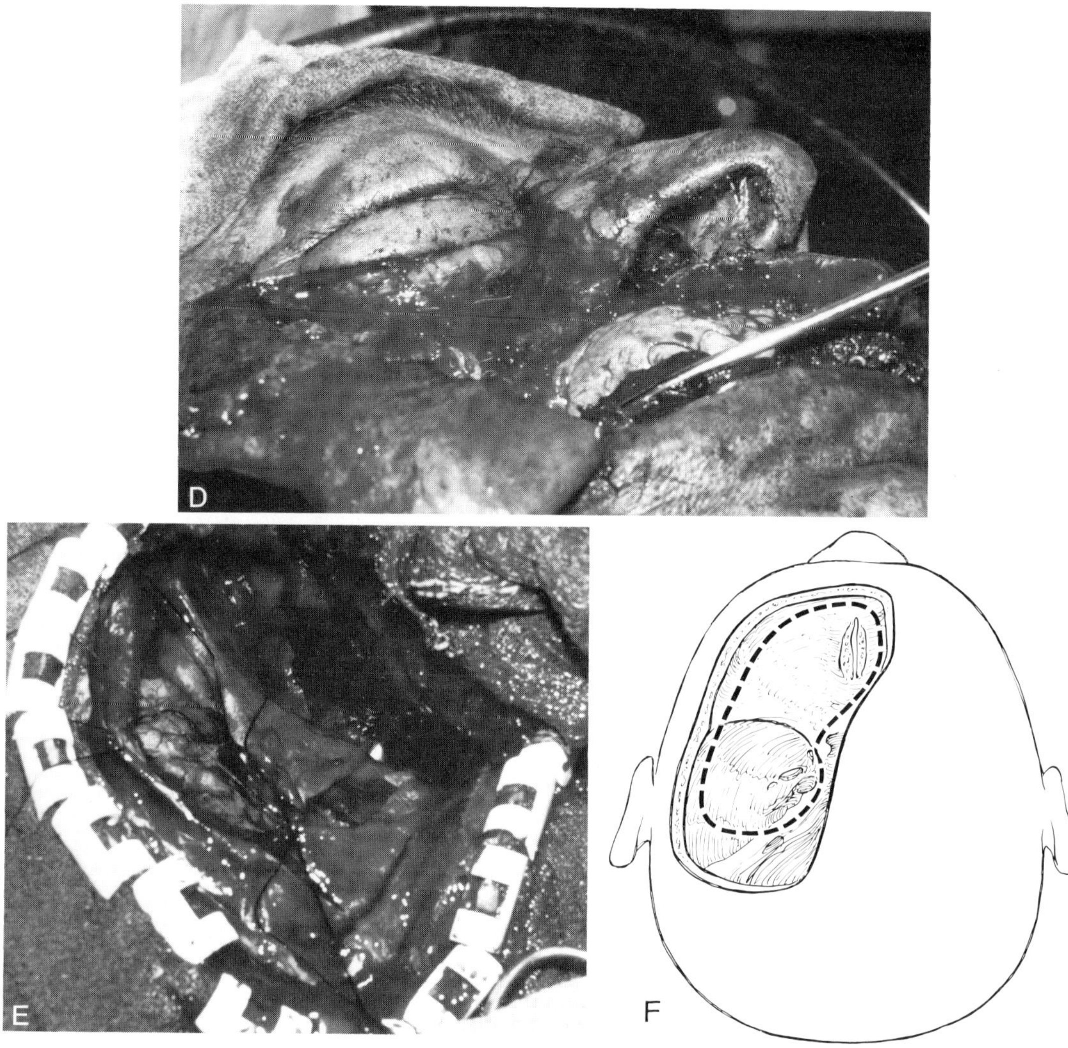

Figure 9–28 *Continued. D, E* and *F.*

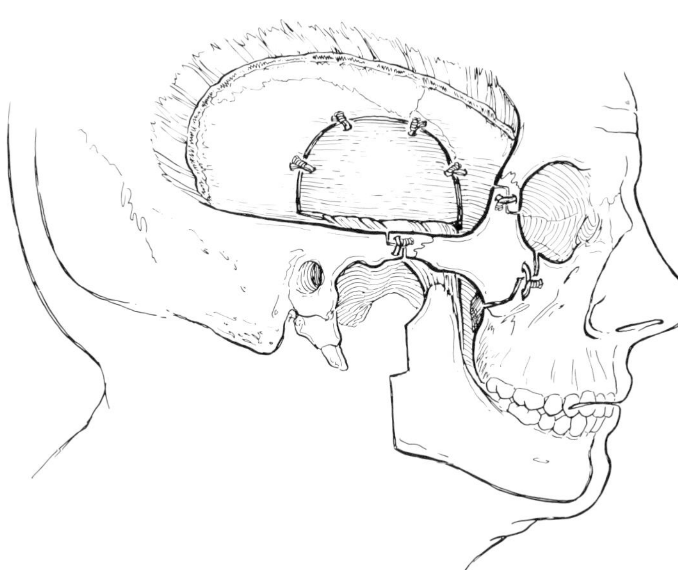

Figure 9–29. Zygoma reapproximated with interosseous wires.

Clivectomy

The pioneering surgery in this somewhat frightening area was done initially by neurosurgeons and orthopedic surgeons in attempts to manage fracture dislocations at the atlantoaxial and atlanto-occipital joints.

A transoropharyngeal approach was employed by Southwick et al[41] in 1957 to excise a bony tumor in the body of C2. They based their technique on that of their otolaryngologic colleagues, who routinely opened the retropharyngeal space for drainage of retropharyngeal abscesses, usually without incident. The absence of intercurrent infection and the rapidity of closure by secondary intention encouraged them to use this approach.

These injuries were difficult, if not impossible, to adequately reduce and fix through a posterior approach. The most logical access to this region would be through the oral cavity, but a natural reluctance existed because of the fear of contamination by oral flora. Moreover, the transoral approach was unfamiliar to these surgeons, who were used to a more direct access and extensive exposure.

Fang and Ong[42] in 1962 were the first to describe an anterior approach to the top end of the spine through the transoral transpalatal route. Four years later, De Rougement and Barge[43] reported on their experience with this procedure. The same year, Mullan et al[44] described a slightly more rostral incursion into the skull base. They executed a partial removal of a tumor in the region of the foramen magnum. Stevenson et al,[45] also in 1966, described a resection of the clivus. By using a transcervical route, they excised a chordoma that had invaded both the clivus and upper cervical spine. In the following year, based on this procedure, both Fox[46] and Wissinger[47] produced large enough openings in the clivus to control the hemorrhage from basilar arterial aneurysms. Both used the transcervical approach. The disadvantage of this transcervical route is that the extensiveness of the dissection required compromise of many cranial nerves. Yassargil[48] in 1969 reported his experience with two patients in whom the transoral route was used. Both patients suffered postoperative neurologic deficits and eventually died. Successful control of a basilar aneurysm was done by transoral clivectomy and reported by Haselden and Brice.[49] This approach has been used by the authors and others for clivectomy and odontoidectomy in patients with basilar impression syndrome.[50–52] As resections progress superiorly beyond the body of C1, simple soft palate retraction becomes ineffective in exposing the field. Soft palatal splitting, as well as vomerine and hard palate resection, permits extension of operative intervention up to the sphenoid sinus.

Technique

Anesthesia is induced through an oroendotracheal tube or a tracheostomy. (The latter is preferable because of exclusion of the delivery of anesthesia from the field and postoperative airway control.) The head is dropped into the Rose position, similar to that for tonsillectomy. The mouth is propped open with a mouth gag such as the Dingman or Crowe-Davis types. The posterior pharyngeal wall is injected with 0.5 per cent lidocaine with 1:200,000 epinephrine. Similar injections are made in the hard and soft palates. The nose is cocainized with a 5 per cent aqueous cocaine solution on pledgets or cotton-tipped applicators.

A linear midline incision is made in the soft palate with either a scalpel or a cutting cautery. This incision is carried directly through the nasopharyngeal mucosa up to the junction of the hard and soft palates. The tensor and levator veli palatini muscles are dissected from their insertions into the posterior surface of the hard palate with a blunt elevator. If further exposure is required, the incision in the mucosa is extended laterally to the point where the maxillary tuberosity emerges (Fig. 9–30) and is then carried around the palate anteriorly, staying posterior to the foramen incisivum. The palatal mucoperiosteal flap is elevated and pedicled on the opposing greater palatine artery. The ipsilateral neurovascular flap is elevated and pedicled on the opposing greater palatine artery. The ipsilateral neurovascular bundle should be identified at its emergence from the greater palatine foramen, isolated, and ligated (Fig. 9–31). With the mucosal flap retracted with self-retaining retractors, the bony palate is drilled away with a cutting bur. The posterior nasal septum is exposed, and its mucosal leaves are dissected on either side and then split along the back surface (Fig. 9–32). This cut is continued over the vault of the nasopharynx, being carried down through the entire thickness of mucoperios-

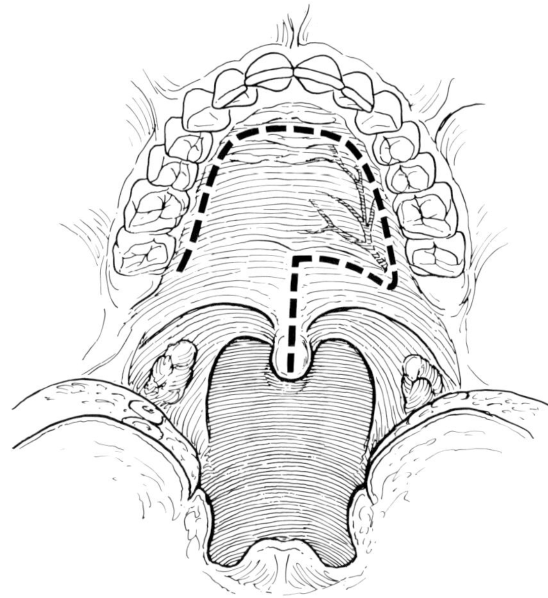

Figure 9–30. Palatal splitting procedure to expose the undersurface of the clivus in the nasopharynx and the arch of C1 in its more posterior reaches.

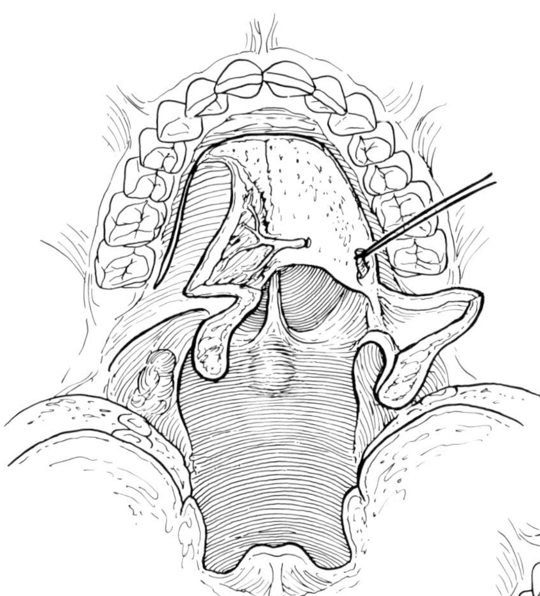

Figure 9–31. Ligation of the greater palatine neurovascular bundle and dissection of the palatal flap to the opposing side, with care taken to stay posterior to the foramen incisivum. A dissection is used to separate the aponeurotic insertions on the posterior aspect of the bony palate on the right side.

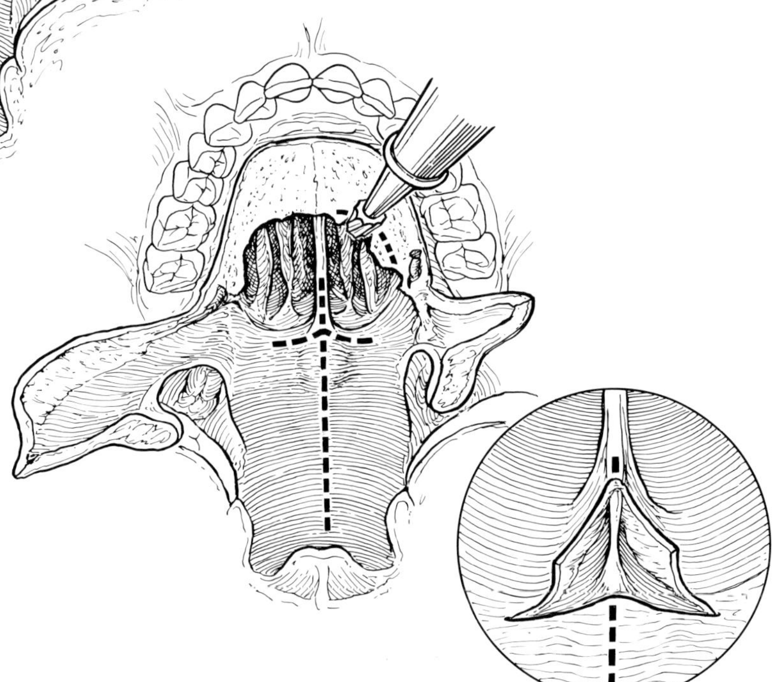

Figure 9–32. The hard palate is removed as far as necessary with the cutting bur, exposing the interior of the nose. The nasal septal mucosa is split up the posterior surface of the vomer.

teum to bone. As much nasal septum is taken as necessary to achieve adequate exposure. The bony septum is removed in pieces as large as possible, so that they may be used later in the reconstruction of the clival defect. The septal resection is best accomplished by making a vertical cut with a small osteotome, and then fracturing the bone and removing it with Luc or Takahashi forceps (Fig. 9–33). Exposure to the level of the sphenoid sinus can be accomplished in this manner. If the oral cavity or oropharynx is too small to achieve adequate exposure, a median labial mandibuloglossoptomy is done (Fig. 9–34). This vastly improves exposure and provides more room in which to maneuver.

A linear incision is made in the midline of the posterior pharyngeal wall as far inferiorly as is required. This connects with the incision in the posterior septal mucosa. The mucoperiosteum is dissected laterally with the Joseph or Dean or even a Langenbeck periosteal elevator, the fibrous connective tissue over the clivus being particularly dense. The periosteum is intimately bound with the pharyngobasilar fascia and is somewhat resistant to dissection. A self-retaining retractor is again used to hold the incison apart.

At any time during this procedure the tumor may be encountered. A chordoma may invade or simply bulge the mucosa. A squamous cell tumor in or invading the nasopharynx will be mucosal in origin and require peripheral incision to a degree necessary to

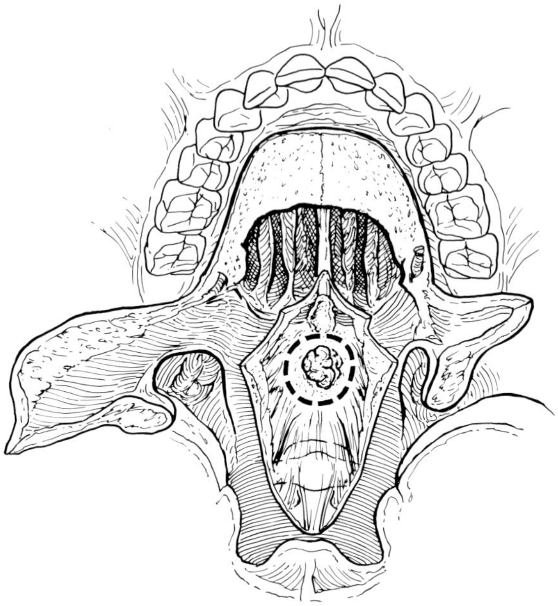

Figure 9–33. The posterior septum is resected as much as possible to expose the sphenoidal contribution to the clivus. The mucoperiosteum in the vault of the nasopharynx is incised in the midline. Soft tissue is dissected laterally, and clivus is exposed, demonstrating tumor.

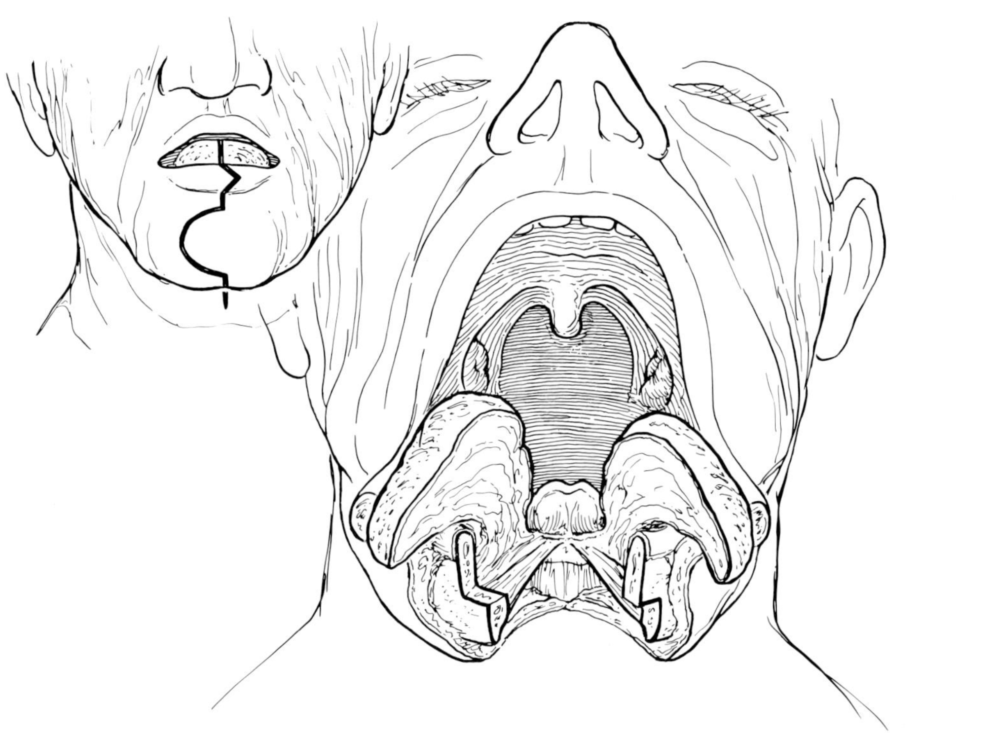

Figure 9–34. Median labial mandibuloglossoptomy improves exposure and provides more room for surgical manipulation.

ensure a tumor-free margin. This squamous cell type of tumor, especially if it is exophytic, may obscure any attempt at underlying bony resection. The en bloc principle will then need to be violated to permit adequate exposure of the tumor bed. Tumor is then removed with bone, the latter by use of the cutting bur. The headlight in this situation is indispensable. The dissecting microscope may be needed for accurate tumor control. Bony removal proceeds until the pontine and medullary dura is encountered. The basilar artery is on the opposite side and often casts a shadow on the dura overlying it (Fig. 9–35). If dural invasion is encountered, the neurosurgeon is required for this part of the resection. The basilar arterial supply must not be interrupted. Brain-stem involvement by tumor renders it unresectable.

Lateral extensions of tumor may encroach on the cavernous sinus and the internal carotid artery as it emerges from the foramen lacerum. This is an extremely hazardous area, incursions into which frequently are fraught with serious complications. Such tumors have a totally hopeless prognosis unless resected, and the surgeon must carefully weigh all the factors in each case prior to venturing into this region. Tumors of this magnitude have been successfully extricated from this region by Yassargil,[48] Panje,[54] and the author. The author's patient died 48 hours postoperatively because of cerebral edema, which was secondarily induced by the fluid volume that was required to elevate the blood pressure sufficiently to restore renal function. The other two surgeons' patients recovered and are alive and well at this time.

The internal carotid artery, as previously discussed, must be controlled both intracranially and transcervically. A prior revascularization procedure is essential. The cavernous sinus is controlled principally by pressure and oxidized cellulose. The patient must be advised preoperatively that vision in the eye on that side will be lost.

Resection of "pushing tumors" such as angiofibromas, chordomas, and fibrosarcomas is more feasible than of more invasive neoplasms, such as those of epithelial origin.

Once any chance of tumor incursion into the intracranial cavity presents itself, a temporal-parietal craniotomy must be done. This is the only way any degree of safety can be assured. Figure 9–15 illustrates a 20-year-old man who presented with proptosis, total nasal obstruction, and a mass that bulged his cheek, soft palate, and lateral pharyngeal wall. An arteriogram demonstrated neoplastic invasion of the middle cranial fossa and a nutrient vessel from the cavernous sinus branch of the internal carotid artery (Fig. 9–36). The presumptive diagnosis of juvenile nasopharyngeal angiofibroma was made. Following tumor-shrinking medication with diethylstilbestrol, a craniofacial resection was done. Substantial reduction in tumor volume resulted in minimal tumor in the region of the floor of the middle fossa and retraction of tumor from the orbital apex. The rather meager blood supply from the internal carotid system was easily controlled. Complete resection of a tumor close to 800 grams in weight was then done through a transpalatal-transmaxillary approach. The patient had a full, uneventful recovery and is still free of tumor 5 years later. In retrospect, the craniotomy may well have been unnecessary. However, the safety of the patient was ensured by the excellent control from above.

Additional exposure can be obtained by a lateral approach through the parotid bed. The beginning of this extension may already have been affected by virtue of the clivectomy's being but the superior extension of a pharyngectomy for a cancer extending across the boundary from meso- to epipharynx. The concomitant radical neck dissection commonly done, as well as the mandibulectomy portion of the pharyngectomy, provides access. The patient's head position may have to be frequently altered to facilitate exposure, and it is important to bear in mind and prepare for it at the start of the procedure. During subsequent manipulation, exposed brain-stem dura must be carefully protected.

Bilateral disease that jeopardizes the contralateral internal carotid artery renders the tumor unresectable. Under these circumstances, only attempts at reasonable palliation should be taken.

Tumor extension from the maxillary or ethmoidal sinuses may be the reason for this approach. Similarly, tumors arising in the nasopharynx, notably the angiofibroma, have a tendency to invade the paranasal sinuses. The transpalatal–trans-sinal excision of this and other tumors as well as management of the pterygomaxillary space are dealt with in Chapter 5.

Reconstruction of the clival defect is begun by fascia lata or temporalis fascia grafting of any dural defects. The bony defect is plugged with septal bony fragments and Gelfoam (Fig. 9–35*B*). If the mucosa has not been sacrificed, approximation with absorbable sutures is done in one layer. If mucosal excision has been done, replacement with a flap is

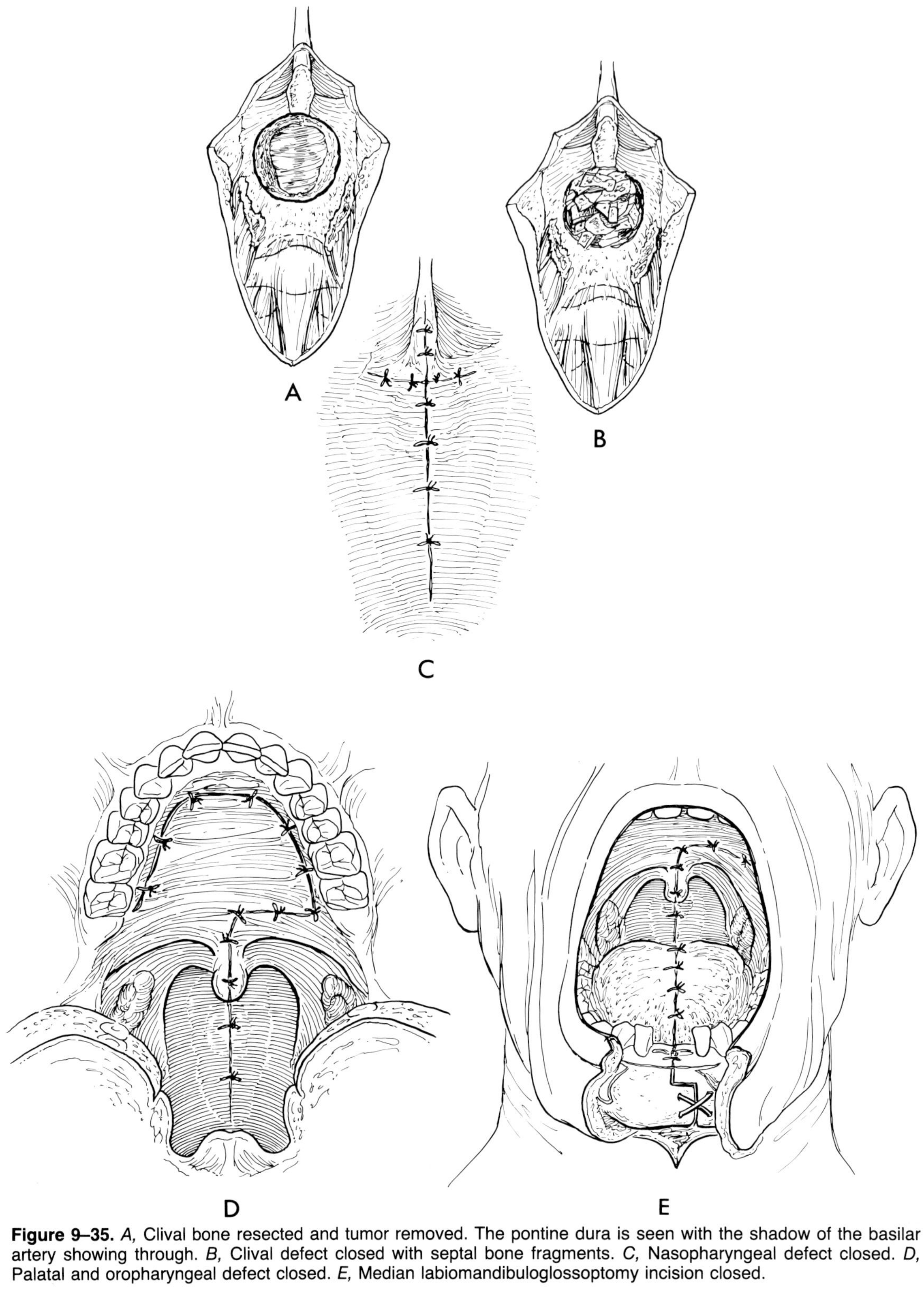

Figure 9–35. *A,* Clival bone resected and tumor removed. The pontine dura is seen with the shadow of the basilar artery showing through. *B,* Clival defect closed with septal bone fragments. *C,* Nasopharyngeal defect closed. *D,* Palatal and oropharyngeal defect closed. *E,* Median labiomandibuloglossoptomy incision closed.

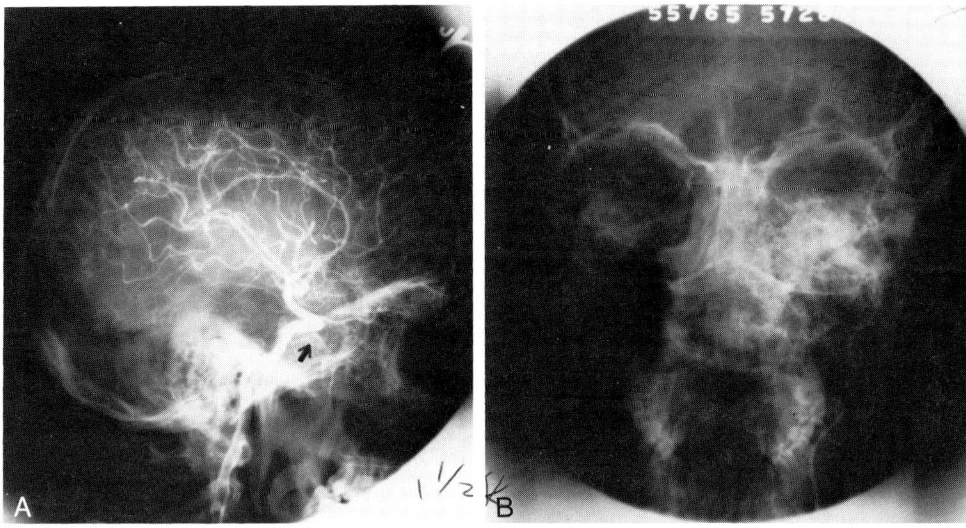

Figure 9–36. *A,* Arteriogram demonstrating the intracranial extent of tumor in the patient seen in Figure 9–15. The arrow indicates the cavernous sinus arterial branch contribution to the tumor's blood supply. *B,* Tumor blush in delayed phase of arteriogram, showing tumor extent. Caldwell view.

essential. The pectoralis major and trapezius musculocutaneous flaps are prime candidates for this. Their rich blood supply, copious soft tissue, and durable cutaneous surfaces are ideal for resurfacing this area. The palate is sutured with interrupted absorbable suture (Fig. 9–35*C*). Alimentation is best administered through a pyriform sinus or esophagostomy tube.

Antibiotic coverage is begun 24 hours preoperatively, continued intraoperatively, and terminated 48 hours postoperatively. The patient is nursed in the semi-Fowler position. Care is taken to maintain a low CSF pressure by means of fluid restriction and a subarachnoid drain. The patient is strongly discouraged from straining. The importance of sneezing through an open mouth, the use of laxatives, and the avoidance of bending over must be carefully emphasized to the patient and nursing staff in these early postoperative days.

References

1. McLean DH, Buncke HJ Jr.: Autotransplant of omentum to a large scalp defect with microvascular revascularization. Plast Reconstr Surg 49:268, 1972.
2. Yassargil MG: Reconstructive operations on the cerebral blood vessels in microsurgery applied to the neurosurgery. Stuttgart, Thieme, 1969, pp 96–114.
3. Chater N, Popp J: Microsurgical vascular bypass for occlusive cerebrovascular disease: review of 100 cases. Surg Neurol 6:115, 1976.
4. Ketcham AS, Wilkins RN, Van Beuren JM, et al: A combined intracranial facial approach to the paranasal sinuses. Am J Surg 106:698, 1963.
5. Ketcham AS, Chretien PB, Schour L, et al: Surgical treatment of patients with advanced cancer of the paranasal sinuses in neoplasia of the head and neck. *In* MD Anderson Hospital: Neoplasia of the Head and Neck. Chicago, Year Book Medical Publications, 1974, p 187.
6. Sisson GA, Bytell DF, Becker SP, et al: Carcinoma of the paranasal sinuses and craniofacial resection. J Laryngol Otol 90:59, 1976.
7. Hybels LR: Venous embolism in head and neck surgery. Laryngoscope 90:946, 1980.
8. Maroon JC, Goodman JM, Horner TG, et al: Detection of minute venous air emboli with ultrasound. Surg Gynecol Obstet 127:1236, 1968.
9. Broderson BR, Barky N: Acoustic tumor surgery: anesthetic considerations. *In* House WF, Luetje CM (eds): Acoustic Tumors, Vol 2. Baltimore, University Park Press, 1979, p 3.
10. Schiff M: Juvenile nasopharyngeal angiofibroma. A theory of pathogenesis. Laryngoscope 69:981, 1961.
10a. Hsu MM: Personal communication, 1972.
11. Binkhorst CD, Schierbeck P, Petten GHW: Neoplasms of the notochord: report of a case of basilar chordoma and bilateral orbital involvement. Acta Otolaryngol 47:10, 1957.
12. Conley J: Concepts in Head and Neck Surgery. New York, Grune & Stratton, 1970, p 202.
13. Batsakis JH: Soft tissue tumors of the head and neck: unusual forms. *In* Tumors of the Head and Neck—Clinical and Pathological Considerations. Baltimore, Williams & Wilkins, 1974, p 264.
14. Rice DH, Manusco A, Hanafee WN: Computed tomography with simultaneous contrast sialography. West J Med 133:321, 1980.
15. Stenhouse D, Mason DK: Oral hemangiopericytoma: a case report. Br J Oral Surg 6:114, 1968.
16. Stout AP, Murray MR: Hemangiopericytoma: vascular tumor featuring Zimmerman's pericytes. Ann Surg 116:26, 1942.

17. Murad TM, von Haam E, Murthy MSN: Ultrastructure of a hemangiopericytoma and a glomus tumor. Cancer 22:1239, 1968.
18. Batsakis JG: Tumors of the Head and Neck—Clinical and Pathological Considerations. Baltimore, Williams & Wilkins, 1974, p 213.
19. Batsakis JG: Tumors of the Head and Neck—Clinical and Pathological Considerations. Baltimore, Williams & Wilkins, 1974, p 178.
20. Stout AP, Lattes R: Tumors of the soft tissues. Fascicle 1, Atlas of Tumor Pathology, 2nd ed. Washington, DC, Armed Forces Institute of Pathology, 1967.
21. Stout AP: Fibrous tumors of the soft tissues. Minn Med 43:455, 1960.
22. Conley J: Concepts in Head and Neck Surgery. New York, Grune & Stratton, 1970, p 199.
23. Thompson DE, Forest HM, Hendrick JW, et al: Soft tissue sarcomas involving the extremities and the limb girdles. South Med J 64:33, 1971.
24. Fisher ER, Vuzevski VD: Cytogenesis of schwannoma (neurilemmona), neurofibroma, dermatofibroma, and dermatofibrosarcoma as revealed by electron microscopy. Am J Clin Pathol 49:141, 1968.
25. Laing D: Nasopharyngeal carcinoma. Otolaryngol Clin North Am 2:703, 1969.
26. Batsakis JG: Carcinomas of the nasopharynx. *In* Tumors of the Head and Neck—Clinical and Pathological Considerations. Baltimore, Williams & Wilkins, 1974, p 123.
27. Toomey JM: Cysts and tumors of the pharynx. *In* Paparella MM, Shumrick DA (eds): Otolaryngology, Vol 3, 2nd ed. Philadelphia, WB Saunders, 1980, p 2323.
28. Coates HL, Pearson GR, Neel HB, et al: Epstein-Barr virus—associated antigens in nasopharyngeal carcinoma. Arch Otolaryngol 104:427, 1978.
29. Loke YW: Lymphoepitheliomas of the cervical lymph nodes. Br J Cancer 19:482, 1965.
30. Fletcher GH, Million RR: Malignant tumors of the nasopharynx. Am J Roentgenol 93:44, 1965.
31. Vilar P: Nasopharyngeal carcinoma: a report on 24 patients seen over six years. Scot Med J 11:315, 1966.
32. Raventos A, Davis LW: Cancer of the nasal cavity, paranasal sinuses, and nasopharynx: radiotherapeutic management. *In* English GM (ed): Otolaryngology, Vol 3. Hagerstown, MD, Harper & Row, 1979, pp 1–13.
33. Jing GS: Tumors of the nasopharynx. Radiol Clin North Am 8:323, 1970.
34. Rouvière H: Anatomy of the Human Lymphatic System. Translated by MJ Tobias. Ann Arbor, JW Edwards, 1938.
35. Ketcham AS, Chretien PB, Schour L, et al: Surgical treatment of patients with advanced cancer of the paranasal sinuses. *In* M.D. Anderson Hospital: Neoplasms of the Head and Neck. Chicago, Year Book Medical Publications, 1974, pp 187–202.
36. Weinstein PR: Microsurgical techniques in neurosurgery. *In* Silber SJ (ed): Microsurgery. Baltimore, Williams & Wilkins, 1979, pp 424–428.
37. Chater N, Popp J: Microsurgical vascular bypass for occlusive cerebral vascular disease: review of 100 cases. Surg Neurol 6:115, 1976.
38. Tew JM: Reconstructive intracranial vascular surgery for prevention of stroke. Clin Neurosurg 23:264, 1975.
39. Fisch V, Pillsbury HC: Infratemporal fossa approach to lesions in the temporal bone and base of the skull. Arch Otolaryngol 105:99, 1979.
40. McCabe FB, Work WP: Parotidectomy with special reference to the facial nerve. *In* English GM (ed): Otolaryngology, Vol 4. Hagerstown, MD, Harper & Row, 1967, p 37.
41. Southwick WO, Robinson RA: Surgical approaches to the vertebral bodies in the cervical and lumbar regions. J Bone Joint Surg (Am) 39:631, 1957.
42. Fang HS, Ong GB: Direct anterior approach to the upper cervical spine. J Bone Joint Surg (Am) 44-A:1588, 1962.
43. De Rougemont J, Abada M, Barge M: Les possibilités de la voie d'abord antérieure dans les lésions des trois premières vertèbres cervicales. *Neurochirurgie* 12:323, 1966.
44. Mullan S, Naunton R, Hekmatpanah J, et al: The use of the anterior approach to ventrally placed tumors in the foramen magnum and vertebral column. J Neurosurg 24:536, 1966.
45. Stevenson GC, Stoney RJ, Perkins RK, et al: A transcervical transclival approach to the ventral surface of the brainstem for removal of clivus chordoma. J Neurosurg 24:544, 1966.
46. Fox JC: Obliteration of midline vertebral artery aneurysm via basilar craniectomy. J Neurosurg 26:406, 1967.
47. Wissinger JP, Danoff D, Wisial ES: Repair of an aneurysm of the basilar artery by a transclival approach. J Neurosurg 26:417, 1967.
48. Yassargil MC: Reconstructive operations on the cerebral blood vessels. *In* Microsurgery Applied to the Neurosurgery. Stuttgart, Thieme, 1969. (Also published by Academic Press, New York, 1969.)
49. Haselden FG, Brice JG: Transoral clivectomy. J Maxillofac Surg 6:32, 1978.
50. Donald PJ, Bernstein LB: Transpalatal excision of the odontoid process. Trans Am Acad Otolaryngol 86:729, 1978.
51. Menezes AH, Van Gilder JC, Graf CS, et al: Craniocervical abnormalities; a comprehensive surgical approach. J Neurosurg 53:444, 1980.
52. Apuzzo MLJ, Weiss MH, Heiden J: Transoral exposure of the atlantoaxial region. Neurosurgery 3:201, 1978.
53. Corkill G: Personal communication, 1980.
54. Panje WR, McCabe BF: Transparotid approach to the infratemporal fossa and base of the skull. Presented at the Yale Symposium on Skull Base Surgery, June 1980.

10

MELANOMA

Paul J. Donald, M.D.

Melanoma of the head and neck is a terrifying but fortunately uncommon malignancy. Its propensity for rapid local spread and distant metastases often precludes adequate control.

The tumor arises when a melanocyte becomes autonomous in its growth pattern, rapidly replicating itself in the manner that hallmarks malignancy. The melanocyte is a cell that resides in the dermal-epidermal junction and in the matrix of hair follicles. Its dendritic processes intrude themselves between the cells of the malpighian layer of the epidermis. Melanin, a brown pigment produced in the melanocyte by the metabolism of L-tyrosine, collects in these processes in the form of granules. These are extruded into the intracellular spaces by a "pinching-off" process known as clasmatosis.[1] The granules are phagocytosed by adjacent nonpigmented cells, thereby becoming the main contributor to skin pigmentation. The concentration of melanocytes in the skin of the head and neck is double that of the trunk and extremities.

Nevi are aggregations of melanocytes that are present from birth and often do not make their appearance until puberty. According to Pack,[2] each individual has an average of 15 nevi. These benign lesions are generally classified according to the histologic location of the melanocytes. The junctional nevus is found at the dermal-epidermal interface and is the most common variety to undergo malignant degeneration. The compound nevus has concentrations of melanocytes both in the junctional zone and in the dermal layer. As puberty progresses, the junctional component occasionally regresses and the intradermal portion hypertrophies, thus transforming the compound nevus to a purely intradermal one. The intradermal nevus is usually small and like the compound nevus has a very low malignant potential. A rare form of nevus that is only rarely seen in the head and neck, but which has a frighteningly high incidence of malignant degeneration of 10 per cent, is the giant hairy nevus. Histologically it may be either compound or intradermal. Exquisite judgment must be exercised in the management of this lesion. It is important to remember that total prophylactic excision, which is often advised, may result in extensive scarring and deformity. Careful frequent observation is essential to detect any change indicating focal malignant degeneration.

Most malignant melanomas arise in a preexisting nevus. NcNeer and Das Gupta[3] reported a series of 557 patients in which 27 per cent of the melanomas occurred in a nevus present since birth and 39 per cent in a pigmented lesion that had been present for longer than 5 years. Therefore only 34 per cent of their patients had a melanoma develop de novo. Malignant transformation can occur in any form of nevus but develops most commonly in the junctional and giant varieties. However, the chance of a pigmented lesion becoming malignant is approximately one in a million. This statistic, coupled with the fact that it would take 10,000 surgeons excising a nevus every 15 minutes for 8 hours a day approximately 25 years to excise all the nevi in the population,[4] has consoled many a cancerphobic patient with regard to the probable lack of necessity for excision.

EPIDEMIOLOGY AND ETIOLOGY

According to Silverberg,[5] melanoma represents 2 per cent of all cancers in the United

States. The incidence is much higher in populations exposed to high-intensity sunlight. MacDonald[6] in 1948 reported a melanoma incidence of 1.6 per 100,000 population in males and 2 per 100,000 population in females recorded in the Connecticut Tumor Registry. This contrasts with a 6.9 per 100,000 white population found in six counties surveyed in Texas in 1975[7] and 16.4 per 100,000 in Queensland, Australia, in 1966.[8]

Sex incidence in most series is equal. Because melanomas rarely appear before puberty, theories have developed centering on the notion that they are hormone-dependent. Additional evidence for this relationship was thought to be found in the once prevalent idea that pregnant women with melanoma had a poorer prognosis.[9] However, more recent work[10, 11] has cast doubt on this belief, leaving obscure the implication of hormones in the disease. There is evidence to indicate a familial tendency in some melanomas.[12] In those patients who have a positive family history, Anderson[13] found a younger median age of presentation of the disease and a higher incidence of multiple pigmented tumors. He postulated that the genetic location involved multiple chromosomes and that the carrier was female.

Although Caucasians have the highest incidence of malignant melanoma, the lesion is also found in the pigmented races. Afro-Americans commonly have nevi but have a lower frequency of melanoma than Caucasians. Curiously, however, melanoma on the sole of the foot is relatively common among African Negroes. This may be explained by the fact that nevi in blacks generally tend to occur much more frequently in the less pigmented parts of the body. In addition, in the African, the sole of the foot is frequently exposed to trauma. This tends to support the still popular notion of the role of frequent irritation of a mole in the genesis of malignant melanoma. Melanoma is rare in Japanese and uncommon in Sri Lankans and Javanese. Among those of Indian-Spanish descent in Texas and in Cali, Colombia, it is as common as in the Caucasian race.[7]

The implication of sunlight as an etiologic factor has already been alluded to. The mechanism of action is unclear, but it is thought that in addition to the alteration in melanocyte metabolism resulting in malignant behavior, continued actinic exposure also causes the production of a melanoma-stimulating factor.[1] This would explain the frequent occurrence of melanoma in non–sun exposed areas of individuals in high sunshine density geographic regions. The protection of the skin by increased melanin pigment seems indisputable. This is evidenced by the predominance of melanomas in those with blond or red hair, blue or hazel eyes, and a fair complexion.[7]

Polychlorinated biphenyls, hydrazine, dimethylsulphate, DDT,[14, 15] and the by-products of the steel and nonferrous[6, 7] metal industries have all been implicated as etiologic agents in malignant melanoma. The epidemiologic studies of Morton and Starr[18] lend further support to these findings. They showed an increased incidence of melanoma in some counties in Oregon in which there was high environmental exposure to malathion, fenthion, and DDT and little exposure to comparatively dense sunlight.

PATHOLOGY

Once a melanocyte becomes autonomous, replicates rapidly, and breaks through the host's immune barrier, it may assume a variety of growth patterns and hence a highly variable clinical course. The most common case reports of spontaneous tumor regression involve melanoma patients. On the other hand, a lesion may remain relatively static for years and then suddenly enlarge and metastasize. In some cases, the primary lesion has spontaneously resolved in the presence of manifest metastasis. Furthermore, spontaneous regression of metastases has occurred coincidentally with the development of new lesions. These facts coupled with the discovery that melanoma will often regress following inoculation with the bacillus Calmette-Guérin (BCG) strongly implicate the activity of the immune system in this disease. Further, a membrane-associated tumor-specific antigen has been identified in a large number of patients with melanoma. Antibodies to these antigens have been detected in the sera of most of the melanoma patients studied and in 20 per cent of normal individuals.[19]

The approach to the management of malignant melanoma has been greatly facilitated in the past decade by the work of Clark.[20] By relating the morphologic pattern of the disease to its natural history, he classified these lesions on the basis of gross appearance into three types: lentigo maligna melanoma (the melanotic freckle of Hutchinson); the superficial spreading type; and the nodular variety.

The lentigo maligna is a superficial, pigmented lesion found primarily in the elderly; it is 2 to 3 times more common in females. It is found on the cheek and temporal skin and has irregular borders and a smooth surface. Malignant degeneration is slow to develop and then gradually progressive, but never metastatic. Nodular thickening or ulceration in lentigo maligna melanoma denotes malignant transformation.

The superficial spreading type is smaller and more circumscribed than the lentigo maligna variety. It may demonstrate a wide spectrum of colors ranging from black through various hues of brown to the pinkish cast of amelanotic melanoma. The lesions seldom reach a size greater than 2 cm in diameter without ulcerating or bleeding. These signs denote dermal penetration. Histologically, the malignant melanocytes assume a pagetoid appearance and initially penetrate the epidermis. As the lesion progresses, dermal invasion occurs. The head and neck area is the most common site for this form of melanoma.[22]

Nodular melanoma comprises 10 to 15 per cent of all melanomas and is the principal form of the mucosal lesion. It invades dermis immediately and frequently metastasizes. Pre-existing nevi are less commonly associated with its development, and there is a positive association with actinic exposure. It is papular in type and shows no "staining" of the surrounding skin. Goldsmith[21] points out that it usually assumes various shades of blue, from blue-black through bluish-gray to blue-red. The amelanotic variety is often very difficult to diagnose and escapes detection until a high index of suspicion is aroused. The presence of melanotic spots near its base is an important diagnostic clue. Because of early dermal invasion, frequent ulceration is common in nodular lesions, even when they are still quite small. Cellular anaplasia is more marked in this type than in the others. Clark et al[20] established the diagnostic criterion that if junctional activity does not extend more than three rete pegs beyond the epidermal extent of the lesion, the lesion may be classified as nodular.

Smith[23] makes a cogent point that there are a number of intermediate types of melanoma that cannot be pigeonholed into one or another of these categories. For instance, a nodular excrescence may develop in a superficial melanoma, have deep dermal invasion, yet spread at the junctional zone beyond three rete pegs. Thus, the disease process must be recognized as a continuum with varieties that cross the boundaries of definitive classification.

Clark's histologic classification,[20] based upon the depth of invasion, has greatly aided the surgeon in planning the width of excision and determining the necessity for neck dissection. Figure 10–1 illustrates the five levels of penetration that he describes. He discovered that the incidence of metastases increases and survival rates diminish with increasing depths of tumor penetration. In most series, Level I is associated with almost no metastases, and in Level II they are infrequent. However, Levels IV and V are associated with frequent regional and distant secondaries and a high mortality rate. Fortner et al[24] reported only 1 patient with lymph node metastasis among 22 patients with Clark Level II penetration. Das Gupta[25] found no lymph node metastasis in 10 patients with this level of invasion, and Wanebo et al[26] had only 1 patient with secondaries in 28 such patients. But with Level V involvement, these 3 groups of investigators found a 71, 100, and 70 per cent incidence of metastatic disease respectively. Curiously Gumport and Harris,[27] as well as Conley and Pack,[28] had a small number of patients with lentigo maligna melanoma who developed metastases. These idiosyncratic secondaries had a pathognomonic histologic pattern characterized by a marked desmoplastic reaction similar to that of fibrosarcoma.

Breslow and Macht[29] have presented some recent data that bring into question the accuracy of the Clark histologic staging system. They quote McGovern's experience of a 48 per cent 10-year survival rate in each of two groups of melanoma patients, one group having Level II involvement and the other group, Level IV. The fact that these levels of invasion had equivalent survival rates, coupled with the difficulty in determining the anatomic cut-off point between the two levels, encouraged Breslow and Macht to investigate an alternative method of classification. They correlated the measured depth of penetration of melanoma cells, mitotic activity, and inflammatory response to prognosis, and found that the only consistently significant factor was the measured depth of tumor extension. They had a total of 62 patients in their series whose excised tumors had penetrated less

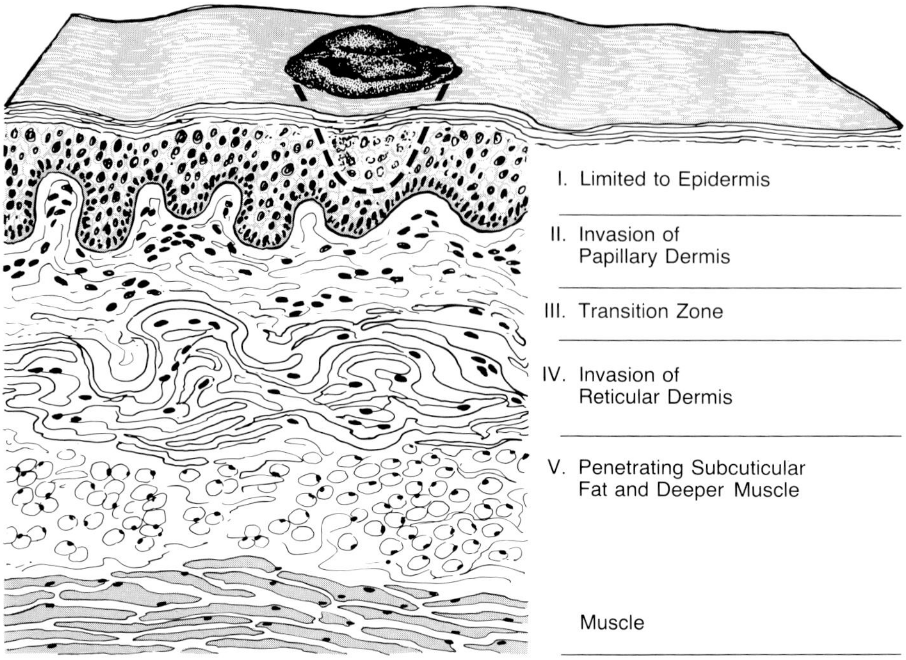

Figure 10–1. The five levels of invasion of malignant melanoma according to Clark. (From Clark WH Jr, Fran L, Bernardino FA et al: The histogenesis and biologic behavior of primary human malignant melanoma of the skin. Cancer Res 29:705, 1969.)

than a 0.76 mm thickness of epithelium. In a 5-year period, there has been no mortality and all the patients have remained disease-free. Unfortunately, no data were presented on lymph node metastasis or local recurrence other than the statement that these situations rarely, if ever, occur with these so-called "thin tumors." An earlier report by the principal author[30] described a series of 98 melanoma patients of whom 45 had lesions that were less than 0.76 mm deep, no wider than 5 mm, and less than 6.01 mm in cross-sectional area on the fixed specimen. Except in one of these patients, there was no local recurrence of tumor or development of metastasis. Unfortunately, these data were collected on cases involving the extremities, and their relevance to the head and neck can only be inferential.

In an analysis of 510 melanomas by Smith,[23] a correlation between lesion thickness in millimeters and Clark level of penetration was made (Fig. 10–2). Table 10–1 correlates Clark level of Stage I melanoma with 5- and 10-year survival (Bergsen-Gage), and Table 10–2 correlates depth of penetration with survival. Stage I was defined as a primary melanoma that is not a recurrent primary and that has no metastasis. Within these limitations, it is apparent that tumors fulfilling the criteria for Clark Levels I, II, and III and with penetration depths of less than 0.99 mm have an excellent prognosis.

Mucosal melanomas of the head and neck form a special group. They have a much poorer prognosis than cutaneous lesions of the same region, but are fortunately rare, with those involving the oral mucosa making up 0.4 to 14 per cent of all melanomas. Much less common sites of involvement include the nose, tonsils, paranasal sinuses, and larynx. Hormia and Vuori[31] reviewed 7253 cases of malignancy of the upper aerodigestive tract and found only 11 malignant melanomas. In a review of four large series of head and neck melanomas, Batsakis[22] compiled 930 cases of which only 71 involved the mucous membranes.

Melanotic pigmentation of the mucosa is characteristic of the Negro race but is less common in Caucasians, except for those of Latin descent. Mucosal melanoma is exceedingly rare in Negroes, has a predilection for males, and has its highest incidence in the age group of 20 to 70 years. Although primary rather than secondary lesions are reported to be by far the most common in the head and neck region, this has not been the

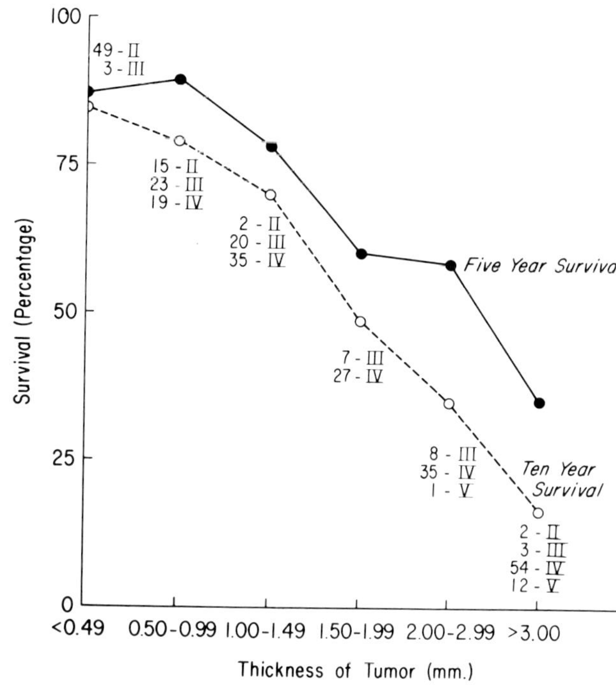

Figure 10–2. Graph relating the survival of patients with malignant melanoma to lesion thickness and to Clark level. (From Smith JL: Neoplasms of skin and malignant melanoma. *In* Histopathology and Biologic Behavior of Malignant Melanoma. Chicago, Year Book Medical Publications, 1976, p 321.)

Table 10–1. SURVIVAL OF STAGE I PATIENTS ACCORDING TO CLARK LEVEL OF INVASION*

Total No. of Patients	Males/Females	Stage	Level	5-Year Survival	10-Year Survival
68	26/42	1	II	87.8	83.7
66	27/39	1	III	86.0	74.6
170	80/90	1	IV	56.2	40.7

*From Smith JL: Neoplasms of skin and malignant melanoma. *In* Histopathology and Biologic Behavior of Malignant Melanoma. Chicago, Year Book Medical Publications, 1976, p 320.

Table 10–2. SURVIVAL OF STAGE I PATIENTS ACCORDING TO THICKNESS OF TUMOR*

Total No. of Patients	Males/Females	Stage	Thickness of Tumor (mm)	5-Year Survival	10-Year Survival
55	19/36	1	<0.5	87.2	84.8
58	21/37	1	0.5–0.99	89.5	79.0
57	25/32	1	1.0–1.49	78.4	70.0
36	15/21	1	1.5–1.99	60.4	48.8
49	27/22	1	2.0–2.99	58.5	35.2
82	43/29	1	>3.0	35.3	18.4

*From Smith JL: Neoplasms of skin and malignant melanoma. *In* Histopathology and Biologic Behavior of Malignant Melanoma. Chicago, Year Book Medical Publications, 1976, p 321.

case in the author's experience. I have found the oral and nasal septal mucosa to be a much more common site of secondary melanoma than primary.

The prognosis for mucosal melanoma is poor because of the frequency of metastases, delay in recognition and diagnosis, the richness of lymphatic drainage, and the often inadequate resection of the lesion.

DIAGNOSIS

The diagnosis of head and neck melanoma is suggested by any color change in a pigmented lesion. A thickening or nodularity in a Hutchinson's freckle or junctional nevus usually denotes malignant degeneration. Ulceration and bleeding, a halo of inflammation, and satellitosis are even stronger indications of malignant change. In Conley's series of head and neck melanomas, 8 per cent were amelanotic. The absence of pigment is more common in the mucosal form of the disease than in the cutaneous. The frequency of occurrence of cutaneous melanomas of the head and neck in the series reviewed by Batsakis[22] is illustrated in Figure 10–3.

The lesions occur most frequently in the neck, scalp, and cheek,[22, 32] where the skin has the highest melanocyte density. However, lesions in these sites have the best prognosis, whereas affliction of the skin of the external ear carries the worst prognosis. In a series of 42 cases occurring in this site, Pack and Conley[33] describe the lesion's most frequent occurrence in the helix and anthelix.

The rate of metastasis to regional lymph nodes is difficult to determine. Most series summarize the experience of a large referral center where many patients are sent who either have failed primary treatment and have a local recurrence or are already metastatic and therefore difficult to manage. Thus these lesions are automatically more aggressive and more advanced. Conley,[34] for example, observed a 48 per cent rate of metastasis to cervical lymphatics when the patient was first seen, but in only 10 per cent of the cases was he the first physician to excise the primary. In fact, in 25 per cent of his 175 cases, two or more excisions had already been done before the patient's first visit to see him. In contrast, the series of Storm et al[35] contained 69 patients of whom only 17 represented cases of local recurrence following therapy done elsewhere. Only 15 patients in this series (21.7 per cent) had manifest cervical metastasis when first seen by the authors. Southwick et al[36] had 17 of 38 patients (44.7 per cent) who presented with regional metastases, and Simons[37] had 78 of 265 (29.4 per cent) with cervical node involvement. Both of these authors saw a large number of patients with previously treated disease.

The site of the lesion and the depth of penetration strongly influence the metastatic rate. As already mentioned, metastases are rarely seen in cases of lentigo maligna melanoma, and Clark Level I melanoma metastases are similarly unusual. The regional metastatic rate for Clark Level II is from 2 to 5 per cent; for Level III, approximately 20 per cent; for Level IV, 40 per cent; and for Level V, 70 per cent.[21] Lesions of the skin of the cheek and neck infrequently metastasize and have a good prognosis, whereas melanomas of the external ear and scalp have a higher metastatic rate and a poorer prognosis. Conley[32] quotes a 50 per cent rate of cervical

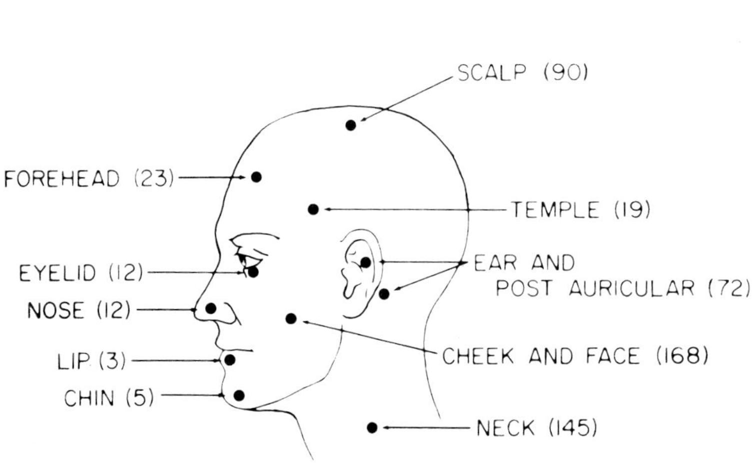

Figure 10–3. Topographic distribution of 179 cutaneous malignant melanomas of the head and neck. (From Batsakis JG: Tumors of the Head and Neck: Clinical and Pathological Considerations. Baltimore, Williams & Wilkins, 1974, p 335.)

secondaries for primary tumors of the scalp, with frequent bilateral neck involvement. His pessimism regarding scalp lesions is shared by Southwick et al,[36] who had only 2 of 9 patients survive 5 years.

Mucosal melanomas can present as flat lesions but are usually nodular. They are almost exclusively confined to the maxillary portion of the head, with the palate the most common site of origin. Lesions of the tongue and mandibular gingiva are uncommon. In the nasal cavities, the tumor may present on either the septum or turbinates and rarely may primarily involve the maxillary or ethmoid sinuses.

The oral lesions may ulcerate and bleed and may involve bone and become painful. Gingival involvement eventually results in loosening of the teeth. Nasal cavity melanomas cause symptoms of nasal obstruction, epistaxis, and foul nasal discharge.

Mucosal melanoma has a high incidence of regional and distant metastases with an attendant poor prognosis. The same relationships of Clark staging and Breslow penetration depth to metastatic rate and survival pertain. Unfortunately, most of these lesions are quite extensive before they are diagnosed, resulting in tragic consequences. This is borne out by the series of both Chaudry et al[38] and Allen,[39] who cite a 4 to 6 per cent 5-year survival rate for patients with oral melanoma.

The diagnosis of malignant melanoma is established primarily by the biopsy of a suspicious lesion. Electrodesiccation of moles and other pigmented lesions or their relegation to the trash can after excision is to be decried. Only biopsies that skirt the lesions by at least a narrow margin of healthy tissue and extend into the subcutaneous layer are sufficient. All specimens must be submitted for histologic examination. In the case of a large lesion it is often not reasonable to do a total excision because of the resultant large defect and the potential for having to do a major revisional operation if the lesion is malignant. There is no evidence available to indicate that incisional biopsy followed by definitive resection increases the local recurrence rate, increases the frequency of local and distant metastases, or diminishes survival.[22]

Because of the common development of distant metastases in the absence of cervical adenopathy, scans of potential distant metastatic sites are advisable in all Level IV and V and most Level III melanomas. Disseminated disease will produce a generalized change in cutaneous pigmentation and even melanouria.

TREATMENT

The precise histologic classifications of Clark and Breslow have revolutionized the surgical management of malignant melanoma. Heretofore the dictum was that all melanomas had to be resected with a 4- to 6-cm margin of surrounding healthy tissue in order to ensure complete excision. It has become increasingly apparent that adequate removal of lentigo maligna and Clark I melanomas can be achieved with a 1-cm resection margin. Breslow and Macht[29] found in their experience that the "thin" melanoma—one measuring less than 0.76 mm in depth—could be safely excised with a narrow resection margin. They followed 62 patients who had excision of a thin lesion in which the resection margin varied from 0.1 to 5.5 cm. A remarkable 32 per cent of the margins were 1 cm or less. All patients were free of disease at the end of the 5-year observation period.

When the lesion penetrates the epithelial surface to the deep III, IV, or V levels, or measures greater than 0.76 mm in thickness, satellitosis, local recurrences, and regional metastases are common. These lesions require a wide margin of excision. A margin of healthy tissue at least 4 to 6 cm wide will adequately encompass the disease in most instances. Care must be taken not only to adequately skirt the lesion but to excise sufficient depth as well. The pernicious nature of melanoma dictates the most radical of excisions.

In thin melanomas of small diameter, it is often possible to close the defect by primary approximation of the wound edges. This is relatively safe because of the low incidence of local recurrence of these lesions. In wider excisions, the defect may be covered with a split-thickness skin graft, a full-thickness skin graft, or a flap. The problem with using a flap is the potential for obscuring local recurrences. To a degree, the same problem pertains to the full-thickness graft. Although the split-thickness graft is the safest method of wound coverage, it is also the most esthetically disagreeable. The surgeon is often faced with the dilemma of choosing between patient safety and cosmetic appearance.

Table 10–3. FIVE-YEAR FOLLOW-UP STUDY OF 224 PATIENTS WITH MALIGNANT MELANOMA OF THE HEAD AND NECK*

		Died				**Alive**			
		Uncontrolled Disease		*Other Cause*		*With Disease*		*Well, without Disease*	
Procedure	**All Patients**	*No.*	*Per Cent*	*No.*	*Per Cent*	*No.*	*Per Cent*	*No.*	*Per Cent*
Excision without nodal dissection	133	53	40	13	10	6	5	61	45
Excision with nodal dissection for positive nodes	37	25	68	1	3	0	0	11	29
Regional nodal dissection; no treatment to primary lesion	29	23	79	0	0	2	7	4	14
Excision with prophylactic nodal dissection	25	7	28	2	8	0	0	16	64
Total	224	108	48	16	8	8	4	92	41
Excision with late dissection for positive nodes†	28	23	82	0	0	0	0	5	18

*From Simons JN: Malignant melanomas of the skin of the head and neck. Am J Surg 124:487, 1972.
†Patients were in group that had undergone excision without nodal dissection.

Radical Neck Dissection

Indications

The presence of palpable cervical lymphadenopathy is a definitive indication for a radical neck dissection, provided there is no evidence of distant metastases. However, the role of elective neck dissection remains highly controversial.

The low incidence of regional metastases in thin melanomas rules out the serious consideration of elective neck dissection for these lesions. A review of the literature by Bernstein et al[40] showed that in a number of large series there was good evidence of the efficacy of elective neck dissection in cases of thick melanomas. One of the major problems in analyzing the statistics on this issue is the lack of conforming data among series. Sisson and McMahan[41] have neatly summarized the major areas of discrepancy. The major problem is the small number of cases available for study, with variations in statistical method, the use of different classification systems, and the fact that patients are not always randomized to treatment groups all adding to the difficulty of drawing solid conclusions.

An analysis of the data of Simons[37] on 224 patients with head and neck melanoma shows that those who had a prophylactic neck dissection did statistically significantly better than those who had excision and a delayed therapeutic dissection once regional secondaries became manifest (Table 10–3). Tables 10–4, 10–5, and 10–6 illustrate the efficacy of

Table 10–4. END RESULTS OF TREATMENT IN 116 DETERMINATE CASES*

		Five-Year Definitive Cures	
Therapy	**Total**	*No.*	*Per Cent*
Local excision only	42	26	62.0
Local excision and elective neck dissection			
Negative nodes	17	13	76.5
Positive nodes	8	2	25.0
Local excision and radical neck dissection with proven secondary	56	6	10.4

*From Conley JJ, Pack GT: Melanoma of the head and neck. Surg Gynecol Obstet 116:26, 1963. By permission of Surgery, Gynecology & Obstetrics.

Table 10–5. RESULTS OF REGIONAL NODE DISSECTIONS (Five-Year Postoperative Follow-up of 185 Cases)*

Histology	Living and Well	Recurrence	Lost to Follow-up	Dead†	Total
Nodes Microscopically Negative					
Clinically negative	69 (56%)	6 (5%)	12 (10%)	37 (30%)	124
Clinically "positive"	3 (27%)	0	2 (18%)	6 (55%)	11
Nodes Microscopically Positive					
Clinically negative	6 (30%)	2 (10%)	1 (5%)	11 (55%)	20
Clinically "positive"	3 (10%)	0	3 (10%)	24 (80%)	30
Total					185

*From Gumport SL, Harris MN: Results of regional lymph node dissection for melanoma. Ann Surg 179:107, 1974, Table 2.

†Death from all causes.

elective neck dissection in three other series of patients with head and neck melanoma. On the other hand, Sisson and McMahan[41] point to a report by Veronesi et al,[42] who analyzed a prospective randomized study of 557 patients of whom 267 had immediate resection and regional node dissection and 286 had local excision and adenectomy only when metastases became manifest. When the patients were controlled as to sex, age, and lesion extent and site of origin there was no significant difference in survival. One of the major drawbacks for our purposes to this study is that it unfortunately was done only on melanoma confined to the extremities.

Technique

The neck dissection for malignant melanoma differs somewhat from that for squamous cell carcinoma. Because of the distribution of cutaneous lymphatics, the platysma[43] must be included in the resection. An extensive lymphatic network in the subpapillary dermis leads to a dense lymphatic plexus in the dermal-hypodermal junction, providing ample opportunity for tumor spread.[44]

In addition, for tumors involving the temporal scalp, ear, and cheek, a total parotidectomy should be done. The wealth of superficial and deep parotid lymph nodes draining these areas mandates this additional step. The posterior belly of the digastric and stylohyoid muscles should also be included in these resections.

Although the conservation neck dissection has gained some popularity in the clinically negative neck in selected cases of squamous cell tumor, it is contraindicated in cases of melanoma. The propensity of the disease for extension beyond the areas of gross clinical involvement militates against doing a less than radical operation, because of the risk of leaving behind occult residual disease. Thus sacrifice of the internal jugular vein, spinal excessory nerve, and sternocleidomastoid muscle is essential to an adequate resection.

The unknown primary is less common in melanoma than in other head and neck cancers, occurring in only approximately 2.5 per cent of cases.[45] Survival following radical neck dissection in these patients is about the same as for those in whom the primary was found.

Table 10–6. ELECTIVE NODE DISSECTION 1954–1964, 259 PATIENTS

Histology	No. of Patients	Cure 5-Year	Cure 10-Year
Negative nodes	219	83%	79%
Positive nodes	40 (15%)	42%	42%
Microscopic focus	9	67%	67%
One node	18	50%	50%
Multiple nodes	13	15%	15%
Total	259	76%	73%

*From Fortner JG, Woodruff J, Schottenfield D, MacLean B: Biostatistical basis of elective node dissection for malignant melanoma. Ann Surg 186:102, 1977, Table 1.

Management of Specific Sites

Scalp

The scalp is a source of a particularly aggressive form of melanoma. Most lesions in this area are nodular in type and tend to develop both satellitosis and bilateral cervical metastases. Wide-field local excision with a

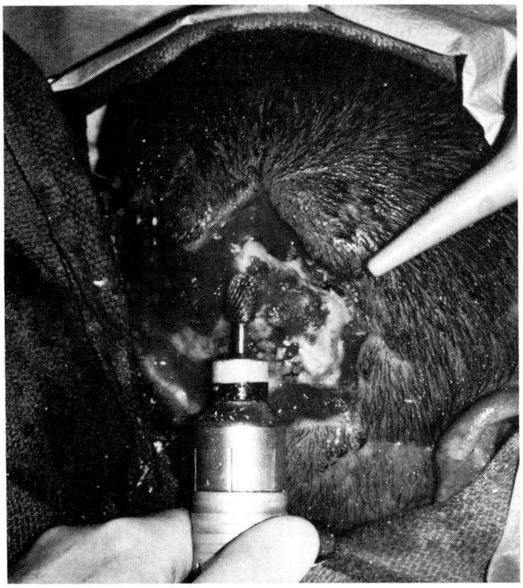

Figure 10–4. Calvarium being prepared with multiple bur holes for a split-thickness skin graft.

4- to 6-cm margin is advisable. If the tumor is predominantly on one side, an ipsilateral neck dissection is done. However, if bilateral metastases are present, a bilateral neck dissection is required. A somewhat pessimistic view is unavoidable in cases in which there is bilateral disease. Scalp melanoma has the poorest prognosis of all cutaneous melanomas and always requires a bilateral radical neck dissection.

A split-thickness skin graft is used to cover the wound. If the Clark level is IV or V, excision of the underlying periosteum and outer table of skull will be necessary to achieve an adequate margin. The bone excision is also necessary to supply a sufficient vascular bed for graft take. If some periosteum is removed and portions of the graft slough, the areas of denuded bone may be revascularized. All dead bone is removed, and multiple small penetrations through the outer table into the diploë are made with a bur (Fig. 10–4). A subsequent growth of granulation tissue will serve as a bed for reapplication of the skin graft.

Cheek

The commonest site for the most benign forms of melanoma is the mid-face. The lentigo maligna variety is most frequently seen on the cheek of elderly females. Radical neck dissection is not necessary in these cases, and a narrow margin of about 5 mm is usually sufficient to ensure adequate excision. During the resection of the primary lesion, care must be taken to avoid damage to the branches of the facial nerve. This can be achieved by keeping the dissection plane at the level of the subcutaneous fat, similar to the plane of a face lift.

Closure can be done with the Kuhnt-Szymanowski rotation flap (Fig. 10–5) or, for smaller defects, the bilobed flap (Fig. 10–6). The unsightly scar of a split-thickness skin graft is not only ugly but unnecessary in the thin melanoma. Great care must be taken in designing the flap when the lesion approximates the lower eyelid. If the Kuhnt-Szymanowski flap is used, the incision lateral to the lateral canthus of the eye must be swept superiorly enough to prevent the development of ectropion once the flap is rotated.

Nodular melanoma may also occur at this site. A wide excision must be planned along with a parotidectomy and radical neck dissection (Fig. 10–7). The optimal closure in terms of facilitation of follow-up is a skin graft. In a lesion such as the one in Figure 10–7, the residual esthetic deformity resulting from such a maneuver would be devastating. Wound coverage in this particular case was done using a large rotation flap. A permanent tarsorrhaphy was necessary to prevent ectropion.

The temporal region is somewhat intermediate between the cheek and the scalp proper in terms of lesion severity. Figure 10–8 is the postoperative photograph of a patient with a Clark Level II superficial spreading melanoma. He was managed by resection with a 1-cm margin and application of a split-thickness skin graft. Because thin melanomas rarely produce occult metastasis to regional nodes, radical neck dissection was not done.

A lesion greater than 0.76 mm in depth or deeper than Clark Level II would require wide-field resection, parotidectomy, radical neck dissection, and a split-thickness skin graft for coverage.

Ear

The external ear is an uncommon site for melanoma, comprising, according to Pack and Conley,[33] only 14.5 per cent of melanotic lesions of the head and neck region. Figure 10–9 illustrates the distribution of sites of origin in their series of 42 patients. The helix, being the most sun exposed area, was the

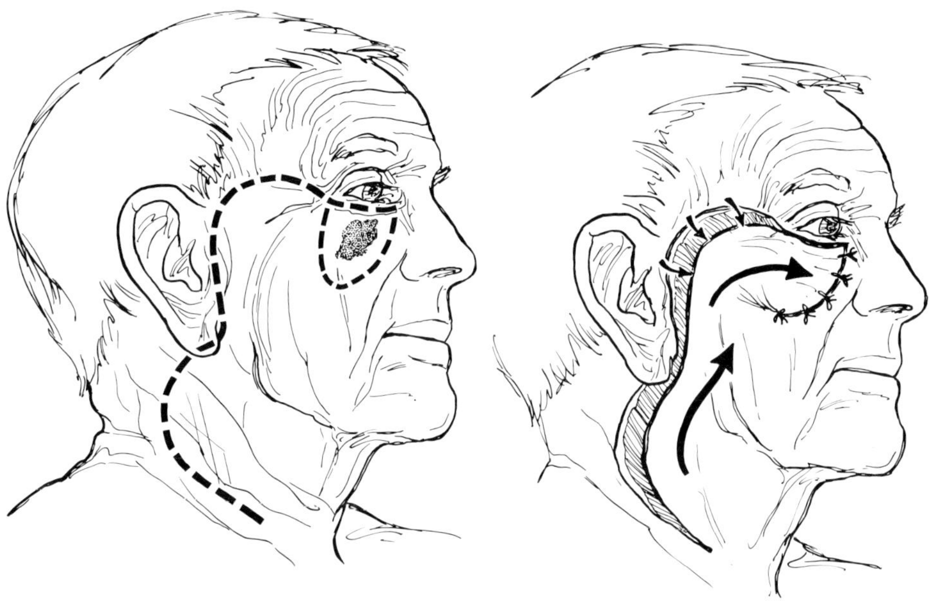

Figure 10–5. Kuhnt-Szymanowski rotation cheek flap.

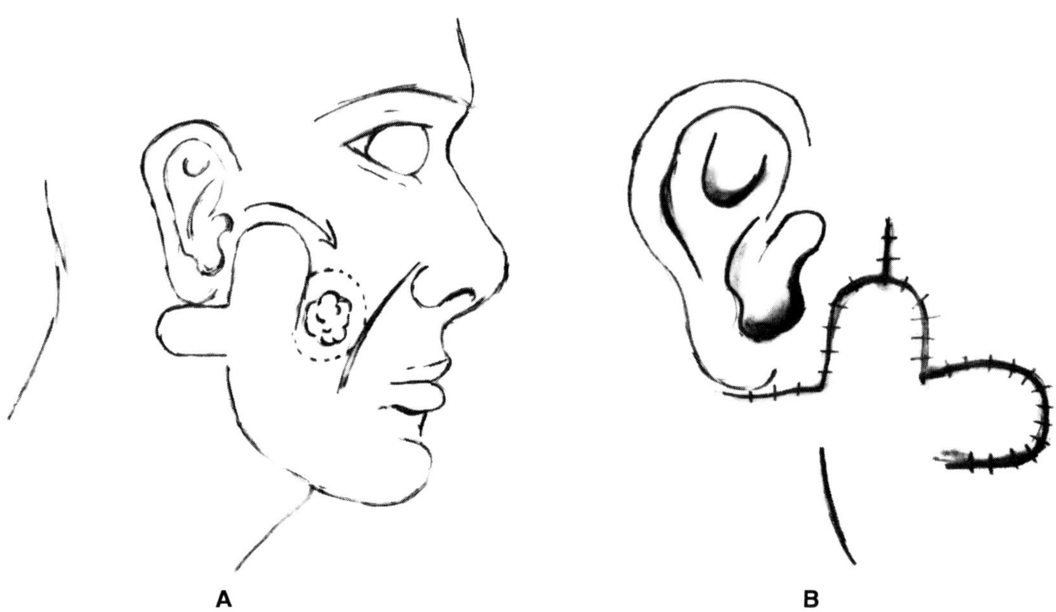

Figure 10–6. Bilobed flap. *A,* Lesion to be excised and bilobed flap outlined. *B,* Larger flap rotated into defect. Smaller flap used to close defect left by the first flap. Defect from smaller flap closed in a straight line.

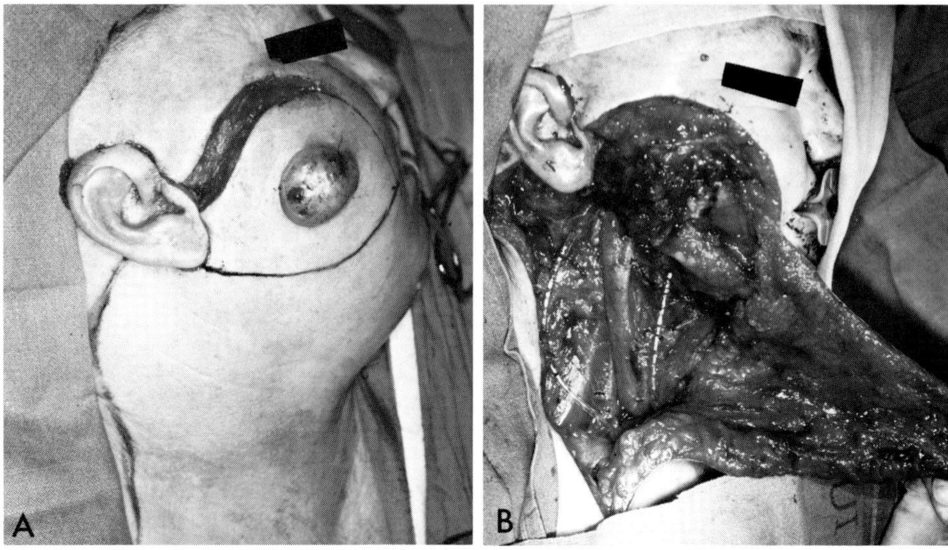

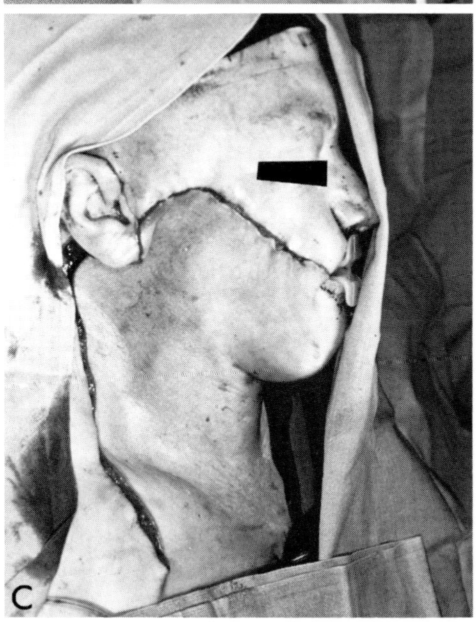

Figure 10–7. *A,* Nodular melanoma of the face. *B,* Wide-field resection, parotidectomy, and radical neck dissection. *C,* Large rotation flap used to close defect. Incision extends beneath the auricle down the posterior neck and curves onto the chest.

site with the highest incidence. One third of the patients presented with cervical lymphadenopathy, representing the highest incidence of lymph node involvement among all head and neck melanomas, which illustrates the aggressiveness of these lesions. Because of the proximity of the external auditory canal to the parotid gland and the free access of lymphatics via the fissures of Santorini, there are excellent routes for the spread of auricular melanoma to the parotid salivary gland. Lymphatics of the auricle also drain to the lymph nodes in the occipital triangle.

The superficial lesions can be managed by wedge resection and primary approximation of the auricle. Resection of more extensive melanomas must include total auriculectomy (Fig. 10–10), total parotidectomy, radical neck dissection, and dissection of the occipital triangle. The incision for this resection is similar to that for temporal bone excision (see Chapter 7, Fig. 7–16). Enough exposure can be achieved with a back cut through the parietal scalp to clearly visualize and dissect the occipital nodes. Smoothly curving incisions that interconnect at right angles permit

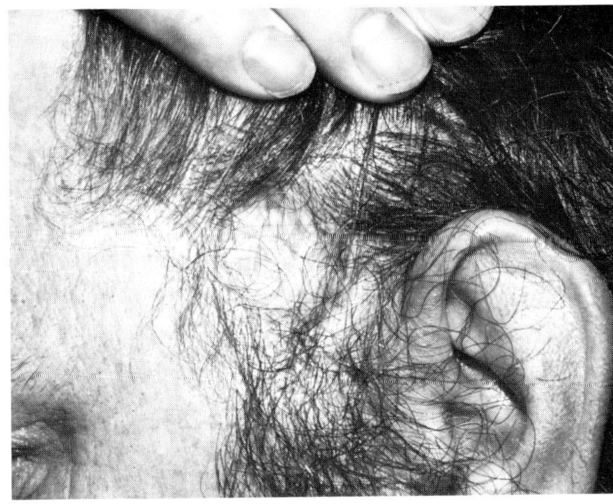

Figure 10–8. Local excision for Clark level II melanoma of the temporal scalp utilizing a 1-cm margin. Defect covered with a split-thickness skin graft. Narrow margins are safe in "thin" melanomas.

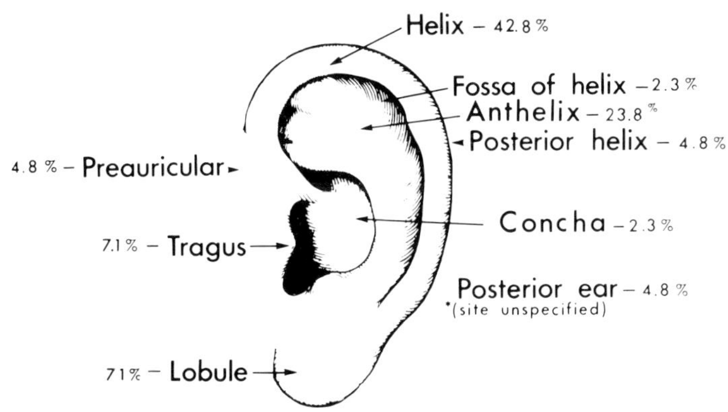

Figure 10–9. Frequency distribution of malignant melanoma of the ear. (From Pack GT, Conley J, Orepeza R: Melanoma of the external ear. Arch Otolaryngol 92:106, 1970.)

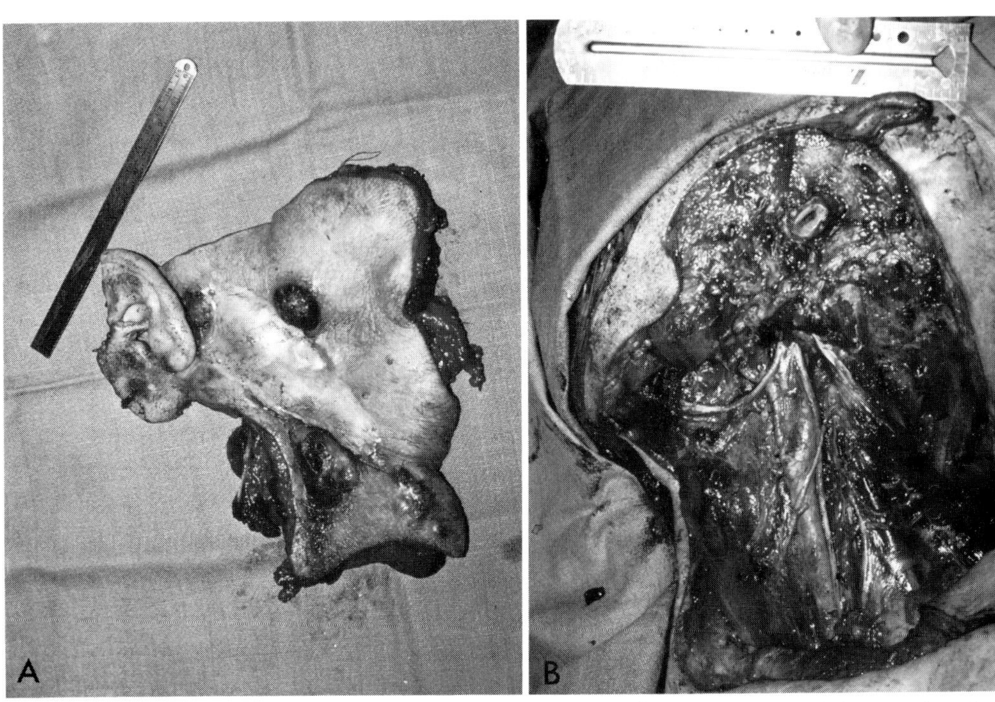

Figure 10–10. Total auriculectomy for malignant melanoma. *A,* Specimen following widefield resection of nodular melanoma. *B,* Defect following widefield local resection and radical neck dissection.

adequate exposure and promote optimal hearing. If the lesion is stuck to the mastoid tip, a lateral temporal bone resection is advisable (see Chapter 7).

One must be on guard against being lulled into a state of complacency by the seemingly innocuous appearance of a small auricular melanoma. Most of these lesions are deeply invasive and characteristically metastatic early. The literature is replete with examples of inadequate, piecemeal, "whittling" operations in which the surgeon was always one step behind the progress of the disease. Faintheartedness in the management of this insidious lesion has devastating consequences to the patient.

Giant Hairy Nevus

Management of the giant hairy nevus is very problematic. The lesion usually presents at birth (Fig. 10–11). Even when the lesion is in as esthetically unobtrusive an area as the one depicted in Figure 10–11, excision will demand a reconstructive effort of considerable magnitude. Subsequent deformity of some degree is inevitable. The incidence of malignant melanoma developing in a congenital giant hairy nevus is between 15 and 42 per cent.[46] Great care must be exercised in making a diagnosis of malignancy when biopsies are taken in the first year of life, since at this stage there is a marked tendency for much cellular atypia to appear in these lesions despite an entirely benign clinical course.[46]

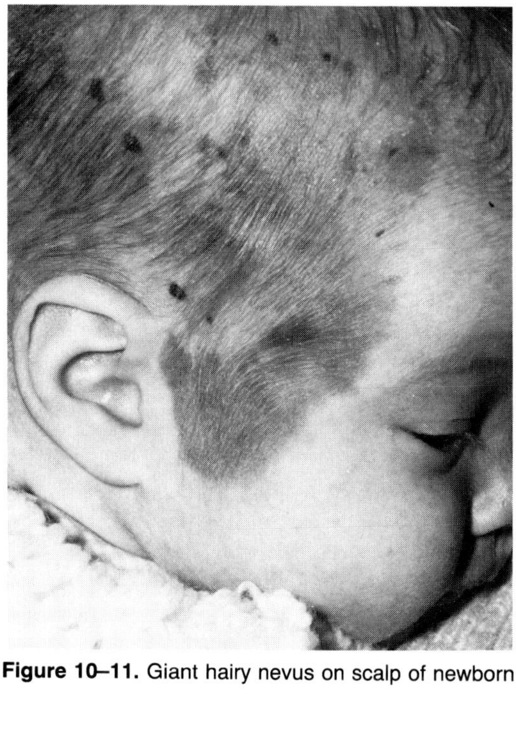

Figure 10–11. Giant hairy nevus on scalp of newborn.

Excision is usually done in stages, beginning in the prepubertal years. An attempt is made to resect individual anatomic esthetic facial units. The areas are usually resurfaced with split-thickness skin. A gap of 6 to 9 months is usual between stages. The region of the forehead together with the periorbital and cheek areas is one of the most challenging. For the lips, local flaps should be used if possible.

The concern regarding the danger of incising into the substance of the lesion during the serial resection, with its possible potential for inducing malignancy, has been somewhat dispelled by the experience of Ariel.[46] He reports having had not one instance of melanoma appearing at the incision line when doing staged excisions.

There are some reports that if deep dermabrasion is done during the first year of life, most or all of the pigment can be eliminated.[47, 48] Muti[49] describes a cryotherapeutic technique that unfortunately produces the same unesthetic result as skin grafting. The problem of not being able to detect recurrent malignancies in their early stages when either dermabrasion or cryotherapy is used has yet to be resolved.

Mucosal Melanoma

Mucosal melanoma is extremely difficult to manage because of its silent nature until substantial size has been achieved and because of the relative obscurity of the sites in which it originates. A high index of suspicion must be maintained whenever a pigmented lesion in the mucosa of a Caucasian is apparent. Melanotic pigmentation in the nasal chambers is especially rare and is highly suspect (Fig. 10–12). The possibility of the upper aerodigestive mucosa as the site of deposition of secondary melanoma must always be entertained.

The treatment of choice is wide-field resection with, whenever possible, en bloc radical neck resection. In the region of the nasal cavities and the paranasal sinuses, en bloc dissection is impossible. However, Shah and Goldsmith[50] demonstrated no significant difference in survival between those patients in whom a neck dissection was done in continuity and those in whom it was discontinuous.

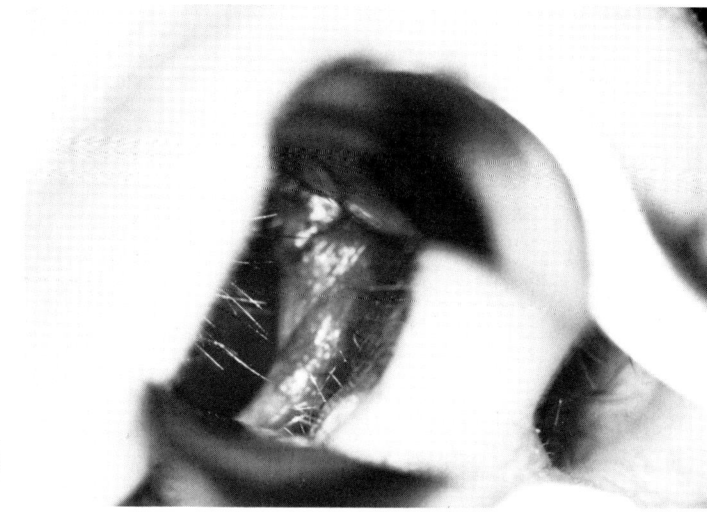

Figure 10–12. Melanotic pigmentation in nasal cavity with malignant melanoma of nasal mucosa.

The frequency of occult metastases (25 per cent and higher) leaves little argument against prophylactic neck dissection in the clinically negative neck.

The resection must widely skirt the primary lesion. A margin double or triple that conventional for squamous cell tumor resection is required. Split-grafts or mucosal-to-skin closures are mainly impractical for the oral cavity lesions. Reconstruction with flaps is the only method whereby adequate function and acceptable cosmesis can be attained. (See Chapters 1 and 5.)

The most unfortunate aspect of mucosal melanoma is the frequency of blood-borne metastases even in the absence of lymphatic secondaries. Mucosal melanoma has the poorest prognosis of all melanomas of the head and neck. Oddly enough, although melanomas are generally relatively radioinsensitive, those involving mucosa are more responsive to gamma irradiation. However, the best opportunity for cure is early diagnosis and radical resection, including neck dissection.

The lesion of the patient in Figure 10–13 demonstrates the protean behavior of malignant melanoma even in a mucosal site. This melanoma had a desultory course for 40 years until it reached an accelerated growth phase and, despite two radical resections that spared only the eyes, continued to grow (Fig.

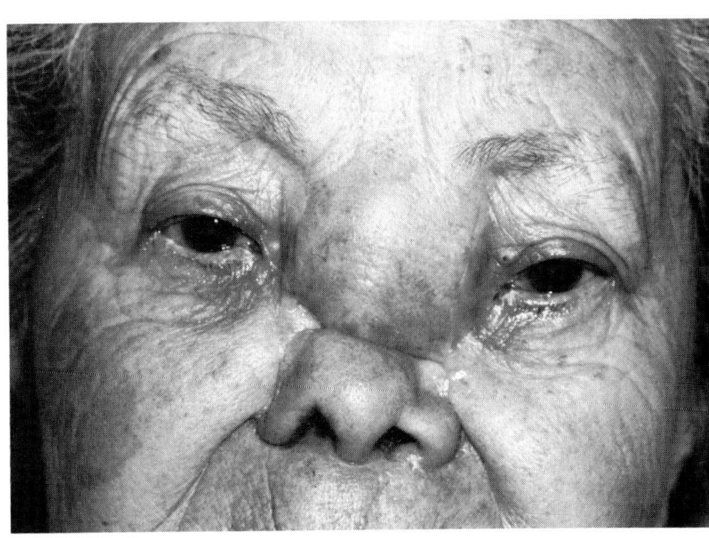

Figure 10–13. Intranasal melanoma that was controlled with intermittent local resections for 40 years, until it reached an accelerated growth phase.

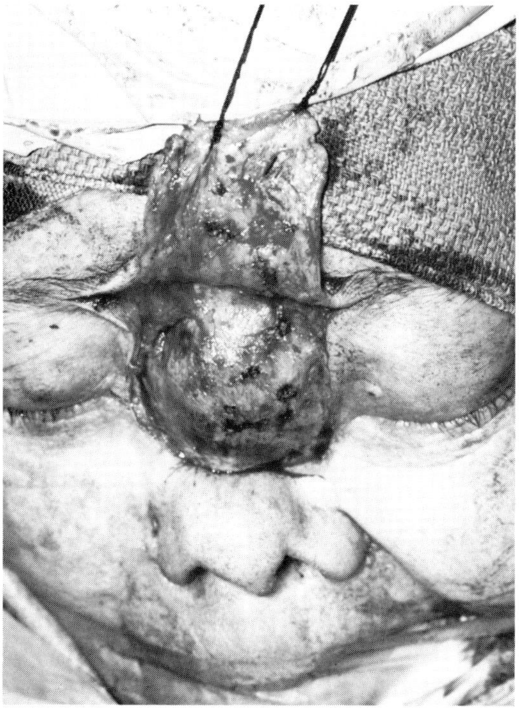

Figure 10–14. Intraoperative view of extensive nasal mucosal melanoma that invaded both maxillary antra and ethmoid blocs.

10–14) and finally extended intracranially (Fig. 10–15).

PROGNOSIS

Head and neck melanoma offers the best chance of survival of all the sites of melanoma. The one notable exception to this is when the lesion involves mucosa; for these cases, the 5-year survival rates are only 6 to 16 per cent,[22] ranking second only to anorectal melanoma in bleakness.

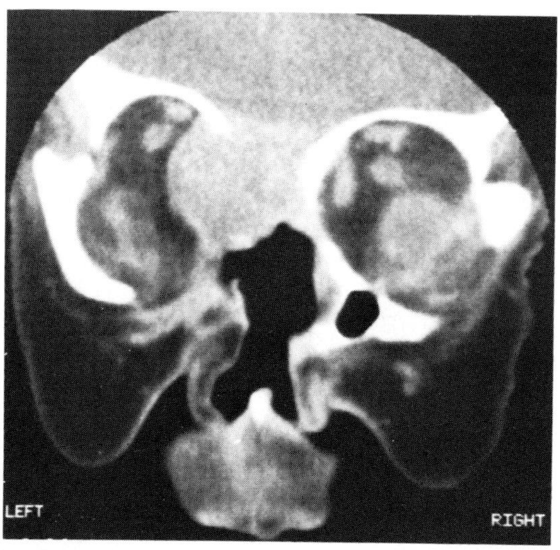

Figure 10–15. CAT scan showing both intranasal and intracranial extent of lesion in patient from Figures 10–13 and 10–14.

In melanoma, 5-year survival rates are not as meaningful as 10-year rates. In fact, it is not uncommon to read reports of individuals surviving 20 to 25 years before succumbing to their disease. The overall survival rate in Conley's series of 200 patients was 35 per cent.[32] However, it should also be noted that when local excision alone was required, the figure leapt to 62 per cent. Local excision combined with elective neck dissection when the nodes were histologically negative yielded a 76.5 per cent survival rate.

Catlin[51] reports a 5-year survival rate of 40.7 per cent in his series of 179 patients, while Ballantyne[52] reports a 65.7 per cent 5-year survival in a series of 405 patients. The presence of metastasis correspondingly diminishes the survival, as can be seen by referring to Tables 10–4, 10–5, and 10–6.

The superficiality of the tumor in terms of penetration is, as has been mentioned, of the utmost influence with regard to a favorable prognosis. Finally, those melanomas that have originated on sun-damaged skin also have a more favorable prognosis.

The heretofore unponderable nature of the degree of host immunity plays a vital role. The dramatic effect of BCG administration[53] on the arrest and involution of often widespread melanoma has provided an exciting glimpse into what appears to be the hope of the future in the management of this devastating malignancy.

References

1. Ronsdahl MM, Cox IS: Biological aspects of pigment cells and malignant melanoma. *In* Neoplasms of the Skin and Malignant Melanoma (Proceedings of the M.D. Anderson Hospital and Tumor Institute Symposium). Chicago, Year Book Medical Publications, 1976, p 251.
2. Pack GT, Davis J: The pigmented mole. Postgrad Med 27:370, 1960.
3. McNeer G, Das Gupta TK: Prognosis in malignant melanoma. Surgery 56:512, 1964.
4. Hugo ME: Malignant melanoma: brief review of current therapy. Milit Med 134:52, 1969.
5. Silverberg E: Cancer statistics. Cancer 29:15, 1979.
6. MacDonald EJ: Malignant melanoma in Connecticut. *In* The Biology of Melanomas. New York Academy of Science (special publication) 4:71, 1948.
7. MacDonald EJ: Incidence and epidemiology of melanoma in Texas. *In* Neoplasms of the Skin and Malignant Melanoma (Proceedings of the M.D. Anderson Hospital and Tumor Institute Symposium).

Chicago, Year Book Medical Publications, 1976, p 279.
8. Davis NC, Herron JJ, McLeod GR: Malignant melanoma in Queensland: analysis of 400 skin lesions. Lancet 2:407, 1966.
9. Pack GR, Gerber DM, Scharnagle IM: End results of the treatment of malignant melanoma: a report of 1140 cases. Ann Surg 136:905, 1952.
10. White LP, Linden G, Breslow L, et al: Studies in melanoma. The effect of pregnancy on survival in human melanoma. JAMA 177:235, 1961.
11. George PA, Fortner JG, Pack GT: Melanoma with pregnancy. Cancer 13:854, 1960.
12. Miller TR, Pack GR: The familial aspect of malignant melanoma. Arch Dermatol 86:35, 1962.
13. Anderson DE: Clinical characteristics of the genetic variety of cutaneous melanoma in man. Cancer 28:721, 1971.
14. Bahn AK, Rosenwaike I, Hemann J, et al: Melanoma after exposure to PCB's (letter). N Engl J Med 296:108, 1977.
15. Bahn AK, Grover P, Rosenwaike I, et al: PCB and melanoma (reply to previous letter). N Engl Med 296:108, 1977.
16. Albert DM, Puliafito CA: Choroidal melanoma—possible exposure to industrial toxin (letter). N Engl J Med 296:634, 1977.
17. Houten L: Increased risk of cancer among workers in metal-related occupations (abstract). Public Health Rep 91:569, 1976.
18. Morton WE, Starr GF: Epidemiologic clues of the cause of melanoma. West J Med 131:263, 1979.
19. Currie GA: Cancer and the immune response. Chicago, Year Book Medical Publications, 1974, p 25.
20. Clark WH Jr, Fran L, Bernardino FA, et al: The histogenesis and biologic behavior of primary human malignant melanoma of the skin. Cancer Res 29:705, 1969.
21. Goldsmith H: Melanoma. *In* Practice of Surgery. Hagerstown, MD, Harper & Row, 1978, pp 1–26.
22. Batsakis JG: Tumors of the Head and Neck. Baltimore, Williams and Wilkins, 1974, p 332.
23. Smith JL: Neoplasms of skin and malignant melanoma. *In* Histopathology and Biologic Behavior of Malignant Melanoma (Proceedings of the M.D. Anderson Hospital and Tumor Institute Symposium). Chicago, Year Book Medical Publications, 1976, p 293.
24. Fortner JG, Woodruff J, Schottenfield D, et al: Biostatistical basis of elective node dissection for melanoma. Ann Surg 186:101, 1977.
25. Das Gupta TK: Results of treatment of 269 patients with primary cutaneous melanoma: a five-year prospective study. Ann Surg 186:201, 1977.
26. Wanebo HJ, Woodruff J, Fortner JG: Malignant melanoma of the extremities. A clinicopathologic study using levels of invasion (microstage). Cancer 35:666, 1975.
27. Gumport SL, Harris MN: Melanoma of the skin. *In* Andrade R, Gumport SL, Popkin GL, et al (eds): Cancer of the Skin, Vol II. Philadelphia, WB Saunders, 1976, p 950.
28. Conley JJ, Pack GT: Melanoma of the head and neck. Surg Gynecol Obstet 116:15, 1963.
29. Breslow A, Macht SD: Evaluation of prognosis in Stage I cutaneous melanoma. Plast Reconstr Surg 61:342, 1978.
30. Breslow A: Thickness, cross-sectional area and depth of invasion in the prognosis of cutaneous melanoma. Ann Surg 172:902, 1970.
31. Hormia M, Vuori EEJ: Mucosal melanoma of the head and neck. J Laryngol Otol 83:349, 1969.
32. Conley J: Concepts in Head and Neck Surgery. New York, Grune & Stratton, 1970, p 277.
33. Pack GT, Conley J, Oropeza R: Melanoma of the external ear. Arch Otolaryngol 92:106, 1970.
34. Davis NC, McLeod GR, Beardmore GL, et al: Primary cutaneous melanoma: a report from the Queensland melanoma project. CA—A Cancer Journal for Clinicians 26:80, 1976.
35. Storm KF, Eilber FR, Morton DL, et al: Malignant melanoma of the head and neck. Head Neck Surg 1:123, 1978.
36. Southwick HW, Slaughter DP, Hinkamp JF, et al: The role of radical neck dissection in malignant melanoma. Arch Surg 85:63, 1962.
37. Simons NJ: Malignant melanoma of the head and neck. Am J Surg 124:485, 1972.
38. Chaudry AP, Hampel A, Garlin RJ: Primary malignant melanoma of oral cavity: review of 105 cases. Cancer 11:923, 1958.
39. Allen AC: The Skin, 2nd ed. St Louis, CV Mosby, 1967, p 967.
40. Bernstein L, Donald PJ, Chole RA: Prophylactic radical neck dissection in melanoma of the face and scalp. *In* Snow JB (ed): Controversies in Otolaryngology. Philadelphia, WB Saunders, 1980, p 239.
41. Sisson GA, McMahan JT: Prophylactic radical neck dissection for melanoma may not be indicated. *In* Snow JB (ed): Controversies in Otolaryngology. Philadelphia, WB Saunders, 1980, p 245.
42. Veronesi V, Adomus DC, Bandiers DC, et al: Inefficacy of immediate node dissection in Stage I melanoma of the limbs. N Engl J Med 297:627, 1977.
43. Oropeza R: Melanoma of special sites. *In* Andrade R, Gumport SL, Poplin GL, et al (eds): Cancer of the Skin, Vol II. Philadelphia, WB Saunders, 1976, p 974.
44. Bloom W, Fawcett DW (eds): Textbook of Histology, 10th ed. Philadelphia, WB Saunders, 1975, p 593.
45. Ballantyne AJ: Malignant melanoma of the head and neck region. *In* Neoplasms of the Skin and Malignant Melanoma (Proceedings of the M.D. Anderson Hospital and Tumor Institute Symposium). Chicago, Year Book Medical Publications, 1976, p 345.
46. Ariel IM: Moles and malignant melanoma of the preadolescent child. *In* Malignant Melanoma. New York, Appleton-Century-Crofts, 1981, p 87.
47. Johnson HA: Permanent removal of pigmentation from giant hairy nevi by dermabrasion in early life. Br J Plast Surg 30:321, 1977.
48. Johnson HA: A registry of results obtained by the abrasion of giant nevi in early infancy. Plast Reconstr Surg 67:258, 1981.
49. Muti E: Cryotherapy in the treatment of some facial nevi. Ann Plast Surg 9:167, 1982.
50. Shah JP, Goldsmith HS: Dissection for malignant melanoma. Cancer 26:610, 1970.
51. Catlin D: Cutaneous melanoma of the head and neck. Am J Surg 112:512, 1966.
52. Ballantyne AJ: Malignant melanoma of the skin of the head and neck. An analysis of 405 cases. Am J Surg 120:425, 1970.
53. Eilber FR, Townsend CM Jr, Martin DL: Results of BCG adjuvant immunotherapy for melanoma of the head and neck. Am J Surg 132:476, 1976.

11

PEDIATRIC MALIGNANCIES

Paul J. Donald, M.D.

Malignancies in the pediatric age group are, fortunately, quite rare. Approximately 5 per cent of all malignant tumors in childhood arise in the head and neck. The psychological impact of a child with cancer is devastating on parents and physician alike. One of the major difficulties in formulating a plan of attack on these tumors is the general lack of experience in the management of pediatric cancers by any one surgeon or group. In addition, unlike cancers seen in adults, which are nearly always of epithelial origin, the vast majority of pediatric neoplasms are of mesodermal derivation, with those of epithelial origin being distinctly rare.

Malignant neoplasms are second only to accidents as a cause of mortality in children, accounting for the deaths of 7 to 8 per 100,000 of children between the ages of 1 and 14.[1] Head and neck malignancies make up approximately 27 per cent of this group.[1, 2] By far the largest group is represented by the lymphomas, especially Hodgkin's disease and lymphosarcoma.[3] Rhabdomyosarcoma is the next most common, being the most common soft tissue sarcoma and occurring with the highest frequency in the head and neck.[4, 5] Fibrosarcoma, neurosarcoma, thyroid malignancy, and salivary gland cancer in that order are the next most frequent.

LYMPHOMA

Lymphomas of the entire body present most commonly with a lump in the neck. In the M.D. Anderson series, 84 per cent of children with Hodgkin's disease had their primary presentation in the cervical nodes.[2] This is in general agreement with other series.[6, 7, 8] Males outnumber females by 7 to 3. The children afflicted are almost always over the age of 10 and are usually over the age of 15. Most often the regional adenopathy is the only locus of the disease.

The current system of histologic classification of the lymphomas is outlined in Table 11–1. Lymphocytic lymphosarcoma is the most common,[3] with the neck being the primary presenting site in 45 per cent of cases. Approximately 5 per cent of all lymphosarcomas are found in the pediatric age group.[2]

Lymphosarcoma and reticulum cell sarcoma when presenting with cervical adenopathy have unilateral nodes most of the time (75 per cent for lymphocytic and 90 per cent when the disease is of the reticulum cell type). Most lymphocytic lymphomas develop in the upper chain, whereas reticulum cell sarcomas are found only half the time in the upper chain, with the other half being supraclavicular in location.[3] The nodes are rubbery, firm, nontender, and eventually coalesce into large masses.

These tumors may occur outside the neck. The tonsil is the commonest site, with the disease presenting as a nontender, nonulcerating enlargement. The nasopharynx, salivary glands, lingual tonsils of the tongue, maxilla, and mandible are less commonly involved. The maxilla and maxillary sinuses are more commonly involved than the mandible.[9] Lym-

Table 11–1. HISTOLOGIC CLASSIFICATION OF MALIGNANT LYMPHOMAS†

Predominating Component Cell(s)	*Rappaport Classification*	*"Old Classification"*
Primitive reticular cell	Malignant lymphoma, reticulum cell type, undifferentiated*	
Histiocyte	Malignant lymphoma, reticulum cell type, histiocytic*	Large cell lymphosarcoma; reticulum cell sarcoma
	(Malignant lymphoma Hodgkin's type)*	
Histiocyte and lymphocyte	Malignant lymphoma, mixed cell type (histiocytic-lymphocytic)	Large cell lymphosarcoma; lymphoblastic lymphosarcoma
Lymphocytic cells Poorly differentiated lymphocyte	Malignant lymphoma, lymphocytic type, poorly differentiated*	
Differentiated lymphocyte	Malignant lymphoma, lymphocytic type, well-differentiated*	Small cell lymphosarcoma; lymphocytic lymphosarcoma
*Malignant lymphomas with follicular pattern have been integrated into this classification and are designated by adding follicular to the cytologically appropriate term		(Giant) follicular lymphoma

†From Ferguson CF, Kendig EL: Pediatric Otolaryngology, Vol II, 2nd ed. Philadelphia, WB Saunders, 1972, p 1136.

phosarcoma can also arise in the skin of the face and scalp.[3]

One of the tragedies of these two tumors is the risk of leukemic transformation, which may occur in as many as 50 per cent of those with head and neck involvement.

Ten to 15 per cent of all cases of Hodgkin's disease occur in the pediatric age group. Cervical adenopathy is the primary presenting symptom 80 per cent of the time. Unilateral disease was present in 82 per cent of the children in Rosenberg's large series.[9] Supraclavicular nodes were involved only 25 per cent of the time, and upper cervical and occasionally preauricular nodes were affected in the majority of cases. When the supraclavicular nodes have disease, mediastinal extension is common. The nodes are commonly multiple and matted together. Extranodal disease is uncommon.

Burkitt's lymphoma, an undifferentiated lymphoma, was initially thought to be an endemic disease exclusively afflicting African children.[10] Since it was first identified, however, its worldwide distribution has become apparent.[11] The tumor characteristically afflicts the mandible and maxilla, and when untreated rapidly progresses to a generalized, fatal disease. It is curious that, while cervical adenopathy is uncommon, abdominal nodes are present in 80 per cent of cases.[12] Furthermore, the jaws are usually the only bones affected. The tumor occurs exclusively between the ages of 2 and 14, with the peak age being 5 and 6 years. In Uganda, Burkitt's tumor accounts for 50 per cent of all childhood malignancies and in Kenya 40 per cent.[13] In children outside Africa the jaws are much less affected and the disease itself is rare.

The lesion begins in the medullary cavity of the jaw and progresses to the alveolar bone, where the deciduous teeth become loosened and extrude. Maxillary alveolar involvement rapidly spreads into the adjacent antrum and then into the ethmoid and sphenoid sinuses and the orbit, producing proptosis.[14] Involvement of the abdominal viscera, retroperitoneal soft tissues, central nervous system, and salivary and thyroid glands rapidly follows, producing a fatal course in untreated cases.[15]

The treatment of pediatric head and neck lymphomas varies somewhat with both cell type and extent of disease. Lymphosarcoma and reticulum cell sarcoma, when limited to extranodal sites in the head and neck, may be cured by simple excision. For example, Rosenberg[9] reported a 50 per cent cure rate with tonsillectomy when the lymphoma involved only the tonsil and had not extended to the cervical nodes. Similarly, parotid gland lesions were cured by parotidectomy when no nodes were involved. Irradiation is more applicable to nasopharyngeal, maxillary sinus, lingual, and cervical nodal disease, as the majority of these tumors are highly radiosensitive. The overall prognosis in the management of lymphosarcoma and reticular cell sarcoma is much better in head and neck lesions (52 per cent)[16] than when other parts of the body are involved (28 per cent).[3] The addition of multiple drug chemotherapy has vastly improved the survival rates. Specifically, use of vincristine, prednisone, cyclophosphamide and methotrexate in combination with wide-field radiotherapy has improved 2-year, disease-free survival rates to 80 per cent in Stage I and Stage II disease.[17] Hodgkin's disease is also highly radiosensitive; thus radiotherapy is the mainstay of therapy. Often only 3000 to 4000 rads is all that is needed to ablate this disease.

The addition of cyclophosphamide, procarbazine, vincristine, and prednisone to the therapeutic armamentarium has vastly improved the survival rates in patients with Stage III and IV disease.[18]

Burkitt's tumor is highly sensitive to chemotherapy, albeit briefly. Cytoxan causes brief remissions, and a combination of surgery and chemotherapy produces an occasional cure.

RHABDOMYOSARCOMA

This tumor is the most common nonlymphomatous malignancy of the head and neck in children. It is primarily a disease of the first decade of life.[19, 20] In 166 patients with rhabdomyosarcoma of the head and neck studied by Dito and Batsakis,[21] 129 (77.7 per cent) were between the ages of 1 and 12. Five of these patients had their tumors at birth. As Batsakis[20] eloquently points out, rhabdomyosarcomas are malignant neoplasms that recapitulate the embryologic development of the myocyte. The progression of the primitive anlage, a small round cell, through the stages of a spindle cell and finally the characteristic multinucleated, straplike myocyte, complete with its typical cross-striations, is seen in the various forms of the tumor. Neoplasms whose cell of predominance is of the more primitive variety lack the cross-striations and in the past were often designated as other than rhabdomyosarcoma. Presently the cellular types are classified as pleomorphic, embryonal, or alveolar, with occasionally the designation of a subclass—botryoid.

The pleomorphic variety demonstrates some relatively normal appearing myocytes, others that appear undifferentiated although retaining their cross-striations, and a further type of a somewhat more undifferentiated variety but still with striations. The embryonal type possesses cells that are more characteristic of those of the developing muscle cell in the early embryonic period. At the 7- to 10-week stage, round and spindle-shaped cells of varying size predominate. Their dearth of cytoplasm has often led to their being confused with lymphomas. The alveolar type may be simply a variant of the embryonic tumor. It is characterized by round cells aligned in an acinar fashion, resembling a glandular structure. Although spaces between the cells occur near the lumen of the pseudogland, cytoplasmic continuity is maintained at the periphery. The botryoid subclassification is used mainly to describe the grapelike exuberant quality characteristic of some of these tumors. Botryoid tumors always originate on a mucosal surface but have no pathognomonic histologic pattern. Since the appellation serves only to describe gross appearance, the utility of the term is questionable. Most botryoid rhabdomyosarcomas are of the embryonal type histologically. The commonest form in children is the embryonal type.

Next to the orbit and eyelid, the commonest site of occurrence of rhabdomyosarcoma in the pediatric age group is the facial soft tissues. The next most frequent site is the nasopharynx (Table 11–2). Rhabdomyosarcoma can occur anywhere in the head and neck as a painless mass until bone erosion or neural invasion ensues. This is especially true of primaries in facial soft tissue (Fig. 11–1). Sarcomas in the ear often present as a polyp that causes bloody otorrhea. Those in the orbit cause proptosis or appear as fungating masses. Laryngeal and hypopharyngeal lesions present with dysphagia and hoarseness or airway compromise. Some tumors arising in the nasopharynx or nose and paranasal sinuses are so large that their site of origin is indeterminate. One such patient in our own experience presented with a massive neoplasm that filled the nasal cavities, nasopharynx, and maxillary and ethmoid sinuses, and encroached on the middle cranial fossa. The tumors are rapid-growing, and medical attention is nearly always sought within 6 months and usually before 2 months.[15]

Metastasis to regional lymph nodes is variably reported. Lawrence et al[23] reported

Table 11–2. INCIDENCE OF RHABDOMYOSARCOMA

	Author(s)						
Site	*Jaffe*[3]	*Batsakis*[15]	*Healy*[19]	*Schuller*[22]	*Sutow & Montague*[4]	*Heyn*[27]	***Total***
Orbit and Eyelid	2	54	2	8	9	10	85
Ear and Temporal Bone	4	19	3	2	8	7	43
Cervical Facial Soft Tissue	3	44	5	7	8	4	71
Oral Cavity	2	27	—	3	1	8	41
Oropharynx	1	3	—	5	—	—	9
Nasopharynx	6	16	1	3	8	3	37
Hypopharynx	—	3	—	3	1	2	9
Nose and Sinuses	1	3	1	2	3	—	10
Total							305

lymph node involvement in only 3 out of 96 head and neck sarcomas. Donaldson et al,[24] on the other hand report an incidence of 26 per cent in a group of 19 patients. In Schuller's series only 3 of 35 cases had nodal disease.[22] All reports agree in one respect, and that is that lymphatic metastasis from orbital rhabdomyosarcomas are extremely rare.[22-25] This illustrates the ability of the orbit to contain the tumor within its bony confines, which is likely responsible for its good prognosis relative to other sites.

Unfortunately, the favorable prognosis of orbital rhabdomyosarcoma is not reflected by these tumors in the rest of the head and neck. The head and neck area in general has the worst prognosis of all the regions in the body.[25] The prognosis of the disease seems to be related to the stage of the disease. Unlike the TNM system of tumor staging that

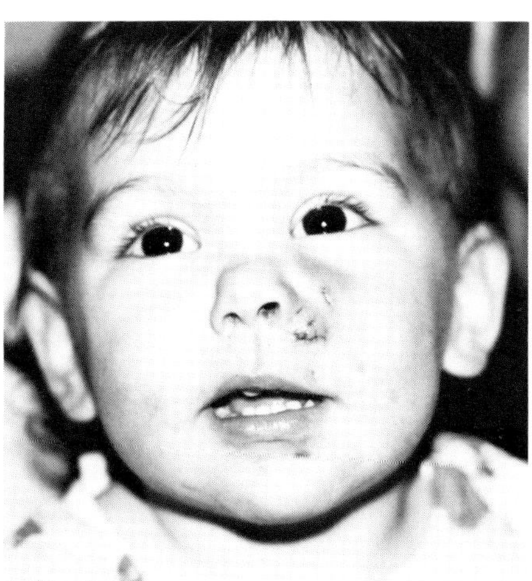

Figure 11–1. Patient with rhabdomyosarcoma of soft tissue area adjacent to nose.

Table 11–3. CLINICAL STAGING SYSTEM FOR RHABDOMYOSARCOMA*

Group I—Localized disease, completely resected
Group II—Localized disease, microscopic residual
- (A) Grossly resected tumor with microscopic residual; no evidence of regional node involvement
- (B) Regional disease, completely resected; no known microscopic residual
- (C) Regional disease with involved nodes, grossly resected, but with evidence of microscopic residual.

Group III—Incomplete resection or biopsy with gross residual disease
Group IV—Distant metastatic disease present at onset

*Intergroup Rhabdomyosarcoma Study.

we all have become accustomed to, the system used to classify rhabdomyosarcomas, devised by the Intergroup Rhabdomyosarcoma Study,[26] is based on a consideration of past surgical therapy as well as extent of disease (Table 11–3). The final designation is often based on the pathologist's findings following histologic examination of the specimen.

Treatment

Treatment for rhabdomyosarcoma in children has undergone considerable evolution in the past decade. Formerly these lesions were managed with either surgery or radiation therapy. Johnson[28] provides a concise historical review of this method of management. He quotes a study done in 1965 which reviewed the preceding 5 years' experience with surgical management of 64 cases of rhabdomyosarcoma of all sites. There were 24 cases in which complete tumor extirpation had been performed, with only 5 of the patients surviving 5 years. These were the only survivors in the entire group of 64; thus there was only a 7.8 per cent overall survival rate. Johnson further reviewed a number of series of cases in which either irradiation or surgery alone was the method of treatment. The overall survival rate in this group was approximately 12 per cent.

Complete excision of the neoplasms is often exceptionally difficult not only because of the invasive nature of the cancer but also because of the inherent reluctance on the part of the patient's parents, the pediatrician, and the surgeon to perform multilating surgery on a child. The difficulty in completely encompassing these tumors surgically is reflected in Donaldson's experience, in which only 3 of 19 resections resulted in a total excision with tumor-free margins.[24]

The evolution of triple therapy, combining surgery with irradiation and chemotherapy, has produced a heartening improvement in prolonged survival rates in these children.[27] In Donaldson's series of 16 incomplete excisions out of 19 resections, 74 per cent of the children were alive without evidence of disease at 2 years.[24] With aggressive triple therapy Ghavimi et al[29] reported a 67 per cent actuarial 3-year survival rate in 6 patients with head and neck lesions. For all sites throughout the body they had a 100 per cent 3-year survival rate for the 200 patients who had Group I and Group II disease. Wilbur et al[30] reported a series of 11 selected cases of inoperable nasopharyngeal and oropharyngeal tumors that were treated with radiation therapy and chemotherapy alone. At the time of treatment none had proved distant metastatic disease. Cervical nodes were involved in 4 patients. A regimen of 5000 to 6500 rads of Co^{60} irradiation was given to most patients. A combination of vincristine, actinomycin D, and cyclophosphamide was given during the radiotherapy in a maintenance schedule as outlined in Table 11–4. After 2 years the chemotherapy was discontinued. Of the 11 children, 9 were alive and free of disease at 28 to 62 months from the onset of therapy, with a median disease-free survival time of 41 months.

The present method of management of these lesions involves resection of all disease, if possible, without creating a huge defect that severely compromises the patient. The recent advances in head and neck reconstructive surgery, especially the use of musculocutaneous and free flaps, have permitted wider field resections that will enable the surgeon to do more adequate cancer surgery without crippling the patient. If there is node involvement, a radical neck dissection is done. Prophylactic neck dissections are not done. It is apparent, however, that chemotherapy and irradiation are vital elements of the treatment plan. For large tumors with widespread local infiltration, a debulking procedure reduces the total tumor load for ablation by chemotherapy and irradiation. A carefully coordinated, well-planned, multidisciplinary approach has resulted in vastly improved survivorship. Although the delayed effects of the toxic medications and the high dose of irradiation are as yet undetermined and can only be speculated upon, the 2- and 3-year disease-free survival rates of 50 to 75 per cent certainly seem to justify such treatment.[22, 27, 29-31]

FIBROSARCOMA

Fibrosarcoma is the third most common head and neck malignancy in children, with 25 per cent of all pediatric fibrosarcomas occurring in this region.[19] Histologically there are two basic types, differentiated and undifferentiated. The well-differentiated tumors have a tendency to local recurrence but rarely metastasize. The poorly differentiated metastasize early and widely and have an expect-

Table 11–4. VAC COMBINATION CHEMOTHERAPY FOR RHABDOMYOSARCOMA*

Drug	*Dosage*
Vincristine	2 mg/m² IV weekly × 12 weeks (max. 2 mg)
Actinomycin D	0.075 mg/kg/course IV over 5–8 days (max. 0.5 mg/kg/day) every 3 months × 5 courses
Cyclophosphamide	2.5 mg/kg/day PO for 2 years

*From Wilbur JR, Sutow WW, Sullivan MP: The changing treatment of rhabdomyosarcoma in children, particularly in treatment for inoperable rhabdomyosarcoma of the nasopharynx and oropharynx. *In* MD Anderson Hospital: Neoplasia of the Head and Neck. Chicago, Year Book Medical Publications, 1974, p 281.

edly poor prognosis. The degree of differentiation, and even the distinction between fibrosarcoma and benign fibromatoses such as desmoid tumor, dermatofibrosarcoma, and nodular fasciitis, are difficult problems. Moreover, the metastatic potential of a given lesion is not always possible to predict from histologic examination. In addition, the histologic appearance of a variety of other soft tissue sarcomas mimics fibrosarcoma.

In both adults and children fibrosarcomas have a predilection for males.[32] They can occur at any age and may even be present at birth.[33, 34] Fortunately the prognosis in children is better than in adults. This is exemplified by the 23 patients reviewed by Stout,[35] of whom 9 had recurrences, 2 developed metastases, but only 3 died of the disease. In Jaffe's series,[3] the 5-year disease-free survival rate was 79 per cent for patients with well-differentiated lesions and 33 per cent for those with the undifferentiated type. Fortunately, the cases of well-differentiated tumors outnumber those of poorly differentiated by a ratio of 3 or 4 to 1. The biologic behavior of fibrosarcoma is unlike that of any other malignancy of the head and neck in that late recurrences up to 15 years following resection have been reported.[36]

The most effective treatment is resection.[3] In Conley's series of 22 fibrosarcomas in children, only 2 were undifferentiated, and both patients died despite treatment.[1] The remainder of the tumors were well-differentiated and were resected; 5 years after surgery, 16 of the patients were alive and free of disease and 4 were alive with disease. Lymph node metastases are rare, so routine neck dissection is unwarranted. Because of the tendency for local recurrence, wide resection is the rule. Radiotherapy and chemotherapy do not result in cure.

NEUROBLASTOMA

Neuroblastoma, although the commonest solid tumor in the pediatric age group, is rare in the extracranial portion of the head and neck.[42] In the M. D. Anderson series,[2] the head and neck region was the site of 7 per cent of all neuroblastomas seen, while Bodian[37] reported 5 per cent of 129 cases and Gross et al[38] 2 per cent of 217 cases to be located in the head and neck. Although the tumor can arise de novo in cervical sympathetic ganglia, neuroblastomas in the head and neck often represent metastatic disease from distant sites.

This tumor demonstrates a rather curious biologic behavior. Neuroblastomas are discovered in 0.5 per cent of all autopsies done on infants under the age of 3 months.[39] Since the overall incidence of the tumor is 1/10,000, an active immune defense mechanism must exist for these neoplasms. Indeed, Hellström[40] has demonstrated antineuroblastoma activity in the lymphocytes and plasma of affected patients. Furthermore, Lauder and Aherne[41] have established that the duration of survival is positively related to the amount of round cell infiltration seen in reaction to the tumor. Ten per cent of neuroblastomas are congenital, and half of all congenital tumors are neuroblastomas.[3]

The presence of a neuroblastoma causes the production of urinary catecholamines; specifically VMA (3 methoxy-4-hydroxymandelic acid) and cystathionine. Elevated levels of these metabolites not only indicate the presence of disease but are a reliable indicator of residual or recurrent disease as well.

The prognosis of the disease hinges on a number of factors. Patients under the age of 1 have a 60 per cent chance of survival, but those over the age of 1 have only a 16 per cent chance. The more differentiated the cells composing the tumor, the better the prognosis. Neuroblastomas of the head and neck have an overall better prognosis than those in any other site. In view of the aforementioned comments concerning the immunologic reaction to these tumors, it is not surprising that they have a relatively high incidence of spontaneous regression. Another strange behavioral characteristic of these tumors is their tendency to differentiate into a mature ganglioneuroma.

When presenting in the head and neck, neuroblastomas usually appear as a rapidly growing cervical mass. Rarely the primary tumor may originate in the nasopharynx, maxillary sinus, orbit, nose, scalp, or lip. The nasopharynx is the most common of these latter sites. The mass is initially painless and displaces or invades the surrounding structures. The supraclavicular fossa is a common cervical site, and invasion of the brachial plexus and even cervical vertebrae can occur, especially in the more undifferentiated varieties. Primaries occurring higher in the cervical sympathetic chain may invade the cranial nerves so that impairment of nerves X, XI, and XII may become apparent. Before

Table 11–5. SURVIVAL RATES FOR EXTRA-ADRENAL NEUROBLASTOMAS*

Author(s)	No. of Patients	Survival No.	Survival Per Cent	Duration (years)
Bodian	51	19	37	1
Fortner et al	48	8	17	5
King et al	13	13	100	2
Koop	68	26	38	4
Phillips	20	7	35	3
Young et al	17	9	53	5

*From Batsakis J: Neoplastic and non-neoplastic tumors of skeletal muscle. *In* Tumors of the Head and Neck. Baltimore, Williams & Wilkins, 1974, p 206.

initiating therapy, one must make a thorough search for metastatic disease, keeping in mind that the cervical disease may very likely represent a metastasis from a distant site.

Localized disease is best managed by surgical resection. Severe compromise of function or drastic alterations in esthetic appearance may be avoided by leaving some residual tumor and "mopping up" with postoperative irradiation of the bed. Although generally this principle is to be decried in the management of head and neck malignancy, it appears to be effective in curing neuroblastoma. Widespread metastatic disease can be successfully treated with chemotherapy, and even hepatic metastases can be eliminated, especially if the patient is less than 1 year of age.[3] The wide discrepancy of reported survival rates is indicated in Table 11–5.

OSTEOSARCOMA

Osteogenic sarcomas, chondrosarcomas, and Ewing's sarcoma are fortunately rare in children. The most usual site is the mandible or the skull. The zygoma and maxilla, especially the alveolar processes of the latter, are also involved. The body of the mandible is most commonly affected.

Most of the information on these tumors is derived from single case reports. Ewing's sarcoma is especially rare in the head and neck. In a review of the Massachusetts General Hospital experience over a 22-year period, 50 cases throughout the body were discovered.[46] Only 2 were located in the head and neck; one in the mandible of a 14-year-old child who died 30 months after resection, and another in the same site of a 29-year-old who was alive 2 years following irradiation therapy. A review of the literature by Roca et al[47] that covered the period from 1949 to 1967 revealed 37 Ewing's sarcomas of the jaw, with special note made of the frequency of mandibular involvement. Approximately 50 to 65 per cent of these tumors occur in the first two decades of life, most commonly between the ages of 10 and 20.[43, 44] Males are affected more than females by a ratio of 2 to 1. The tumor appears to originate in the mesenchymal cells of bone marrow and causes local swelling, pain, tenderness, and fever. A radiograph of a lytic lesion in the affected bone, showing increased density, expansion of the cortex, and increased periosteal thickening, coupled with the clinical picture, often creates confusion with an inflammatory lesion. Blood-borne and lymphatic metastases are common, with up to 25 per cent of patients demonstrating metastases at the time of diagnosis.[48]

The most effective treatment is the judicious combination of surgery, radiation, and chemotherapy. Goepfert et al[44] demonstrated a 20 per cent 5-year survival rate using this approach. Jaffe et al,[49] using mainly a combination of vincristine, actinomycin D and cyclophosphamide coupled with irradiation therapy, treated 14 patients with Ewing's sarcoma outside of the head and neck. Of the 9 who had no metastases at the time of diagnosis, 2 died of pulmonary metastases and the remaining 7 are alive without disease at 4 months' to 4 years' follow-up. Those who had metastases at the time of diagnosis experienced decreased survival times.

Chondrosarcomas are exceptionally rare in the head and neck. Considerable difficulty is experienced in the histologic differentiation between chondroma and chondrosarcoma. Moreover, the biologic behavior is not always commensurate with the histologic picture. To add further confusion, chondrosarcomatous foci may appear in an osteogenic sarcoma.[50] This latter fact prompted Conley[1] to group these lesions together as osteochondrosarcomas. Head and neck osteogenic sarcoma and chondrosarcoma are most commonly seen in the mandible and maxilla. The mandible[51] is the more frequent site for osteogenic sarcoma (a ratio of 2 to 1 over the maxilla), while the maxilla is a more common site of chondrosarcoma, accounting for about 60 per cent of all cases involving bony structures of the head and neck.[45] Chondrosarcomas may arise in a pre-existing benign chondroma. Individuals with Ollier's disease (familial multiple exostoses and enchondromatosis) are highly predisposed to developing chondrosarcoma, with malignant degeneration tending to develop around the time of puberty.[51]

Bone that has been irradiated is predisposed to the development of osteogenic sarcoma. Kragh[52] reports 4 cases of mandibular osteosarcoma that occurred following irradiation. Mandibular lesions tend to remain localized; they have a marked propensity for local recurrence, but rarely cause regional or distant metastasis. Fibrous dysplasia is an additional predisposing factor, being a precursor in 12 cases of osteogenic sarcoma recorded by Yannopoulos.[53]

Both chondrosarcoma and osteogenic sarcoma are radioresistant, so that successful therapy depends upon the ability to adequately resect the lesion. The mandibular tumors have a fairly good prognosis. Kragh et al[52] reported a 33 per cent 5-year survival rate in a study of 35 patients with osteosarcoma. Tumors of the maxillary alveolar ridge have a more favorable prognosis than those of the antrum in that the former can be adequately encompassed by a radical resection. Radical neck dissection is reserved for those individuals with manifest cervical metastases.

Mandibular reconstruction with bone grafting using either rib grafts or a metal tray containing cancellous bone chips will successfully rehabilitate the child. Adjustment will have to be made and revisions will be required as growth proceeds.

MALIGNANT HEMANGIOPERICYTOMA

This neoplasm arises from the pericytes of Zimmerman. Since its discovery in 1942 by Stout and Murray, 300 cases have been reported, of which approximately a third originated in the head and neck.[54] Kauffman and Stout[55] reported 9 of 31 cases in children having developed in the head and neck. The sites of origin are the nose and paranasal sinuses, neck, oral cavity, scalp, skull, orbit, larynx, and nasopharynx.[3, 54, 55] Histologic differentiation between benign and malignant forms is extremely difficult.

Management is by wide local excision, as the tumor, despite its vascularity, is radioresistant. Regional metastases are far less common with head and neck lesions than with those located elsewhere. Because the major problem in management is the frequency of local recurrence, radical excision is essential. Radical neck dissection is reserved for lesions with manifest regional nodes. Malignant hemangiopericytomas have a marked tendency for late recurrence, with tumor reappearing 10 years and even longer after apparently successful excision.

RARE LESIONS

Angiosarcoma, liposarcoma, leiomyosarcoma, malignant schwannoma, and neuroepithelioma are very rarely seen in children. Guidance in therapy is usually based on individual case reports rather than series of cases containing significant numbers.

Angiosarcomas appear as purplish masses, usually in skin or mucous membrane, and are most commonly found in the scalp. As they spread in the dermal layer they impart a violaceous hue to the skin adjacent to the lesion. Conley[1] had only 2 angiosarcomas in his series of 88 pediatric tumors. Only 1 patient who was treated by a radical maxillectomy survived 5 years. Jaffe[3] also had 2 cases in his large series. Wide excision is the treatment of choice, with radiotherapy reserved for unresectable cases and chemotherapy for distant metastatic disease. These tumors are among the few types of sarcoma that metastasize to lymph nodes, with this occurring in 30 to 50 per cent of cases.

Leiomyosarcoma is very rare but has a good prognosis. Treatment is wide excision. Liposarcoma is a curiosity in the head and neck, although a very common sarcoma elsewhere in the body. It usually occurs in persons over age 30. In our experience, a 10-year-old boy with this tumor in the buccal fat pad was treated by incomplete excision followed by radiation and chemotherapy. The patient succumbed to extensive local disease and widespread metastases 2 years later.

Malignant schwannoma usually occurs in patients suffering from von Recklinghausen's disease. Multiple sites of origin may be found. Wide-field excision is essential because of the tumor's tendency to spread along the sheath of the involved nerve. Blood-borne metastases are common, and the prognosis is generally poor.[56]

Neuroepithelioma is also very rare in the pediatric age group and is amenable to radiotherapy.

References

1. Conley J: Concepts in Head and Neck Surgery. New York, Grune & Stratton, 1970, pp 181–192.
2. Sutow WW, Montague ED: Pediatric tumors. *In* McComb, WS, Fletcher GH (eds): Cancer of the Head and Neck. Baltimore, Williams & Wilkins, 1967, pp 428–446.
3. Jaffe BF: Neck masses and malignant tumors of the head and neck. *In* Ferguson CF, Kendig EL Jr (eds): Disorders of the Respiratory Tract in Children, Vol 2: Pediatric Otolaryngology. Philadelphia, WB Saunders, 1972, p 1135.
4. Sutow WW, Sullivan MR, Ried HL, et al: Prognosis in childhood rhabdomyosarcoma. Cancer 25:1384, 1970.
5. Kilman JW, Clatworthy HW, Newton WA, et al: Reasonable surgery for rhabdomyosarcoma: a study of 67 cases. Ann Surg 78:346, 1973.
6. Bailey RJ, Burgert EO, Dahlin DC: Malignant lymphomas in children. Pediatrics 28:985, 1961.
7. Pierce MI: Lymphosarcoma and Hodgkin's disease in children. Fourth National Cancer Conference Proceedings, 1960. Philadelphia, JB Lippincott, 1961, p 559.
8. Rosenberg SA, Diamond HD, Dargeon HW, et al: Lymphosarcoma in childhood. N Engl J Med 259:505, 1958.
9. Rosenberg SA, Diamond BD, Jaslowitz B, et al: Lymphosarcoma: a review of 1269 cases. Medicine 40:31, 1961.
10. Burkitt D: A sarcoma involving the jaws in African children. Br J Surg 46:218, 1958.
11. Burkitt D: Burkitt's lymphoma outside the known endemic area of Africa and New Guinea. Int J Cancer 2:562, 1967.
12. Wright, DH: Burkitt's tumor: a postmortem study of 50 cases. Br J Surg 51:245, 1964.
13. Cliff RA, Wright DH, Clifford P: Leukemia in Burkitt's lymphoma. Blood 22:243, 1963.
14. Williamson JJ: Blood dyscrasias. *In* Gorlin RJ, Goldman HM (eds): Thoma's Oral Pathology, Vol II. St. Louis, CV Mosby, 1970, pp 948–951.
15. Schnitzer B, Weaver DK: Lymphoreticular disorders. *In* Batsakis, JG (ed): Tumors of the Head and Neck. Baltimore, Williams & Wilkins, 1974, pp 359–362.
16. Catlin D: Lymphosarcoma of the head and neck. Am J Roentgenol 59:354, 1948.
17. Murphy SB: Childhood non-Hodgkin's lymphoma. N Engl J Med 299:1446, 1978.
18. DeVita VT Jr, Lewis BJ, Rosencweig M, et al: The chemotherapy of Hodgkin's disease: past experiences and future directions. Cancer 42:979, 1978.
19. Healy GB: Malignant tumors of the head and neck in children: diagnosis and treatment. Otolaryngol Clin North Am 13:483, 1980.
20. Batsakis, JG (ed): Neoplastic and non-neoplastic tumors of skeletal muscle. *In* Tumors of the Head and Neck. Baltimore, Williams & Wilkins, 1974, pp 206–210.
21. Dito WR, Batsakis JG: Rhabdomyosarcoma of the head and neck: an appraisal of the biological behavior in 170 cases. Arch Surg 84:582, 1962.
22. Schuller DE, Lawrence TL, Newton WA: Childhood rhabdomyosarcomas of the head and neck. Arch Otolaryngol 105:689, 1979.
23. Lawrence W Jr, Hays DM, Moon TE: Lymphatic metastasis with childhood rhabdomyosarcoma. Cancer 39:556, 1977.
24. Donaldson SS, Castro JR, Wilbur JR, et al: Rhabdomyosarcoma of the head and neck in children. Cancer 31:26, 1973.
25. Sutow WW, Sullivan MR, Ried HL, et al: Prognosis in childhood rhabdomyosarcoma. Cancer 25:1384, 1970.
26. Maurer HM, Moon T, Donaldsen M, et al: The Intergroup Rhabdomyosarcoma Study: a preliminary report. Cancer 40:2015, 1977.
27. Heyn RM, Holland R, Newton WA Jr, et al: The role of combined chemotherapy in the treatment of children with rhabdomyosarcoma. Cancer 34:2128, 1974.
28. Johnson DG: Trends in surgery for childhood rhabdomyosarcoma. Cancer 35 (Suppl): 916, 1975.
29. Ghavimi F, Exelby PR, D'Angio GJ, et al: Multidisciplinary treatment of embryonal rhabdomyosarcoma in children. Cancer 35:677, 1975.
30. Wilbur JR, Sutow WW, Sullivan MP: The changing treatment of rhabdomyosarcoma in children, particularly in treatment for inoperable rhabdomyosarcoma of the nasopharynx and oropharynx. *In* MD Anderson Hospital: Neoplasia of the Head and Neck. Chicago, Year Book Medical Publications, 1974, pp 281–288.
31. Healy GB, Jaffe N, Cassady JR: Rhabdomyosarcoma of the head and neck: diagnosis and management. Head Neck Surg 1:334, 1979.
32. Stout AP, Lattes R (eds): Tumors of the Soft Tissues. Washington DC, Armed Forces Institute of Pathology, 1966, pp 101–106.
33. Gross RE, Faber S, Martin LW: Neuroblastoma sympatheticum. Pediatrics 23:1179, 1959.
34. Weingrad DN, Rosenberg SA: Early lymphatic spread of osteogenic and soft tissue sarcomas. Surgery 84:231, 1978.
35. Stout AP: Fibrosarcoma in infants and children. Cancer 15:1028, 1962.
36. Horne CHW, Slavin G, McDonald AM: Late recurrence of juvenile fibrosarcoma. Br J Surg 55:102, 1968.
37. Bodian M: Neuroblastoma. Pediatr Clin North Am 6:449, 1959.
38. Gross RE, Farber S, Martin LW: Neuroblastoma sympatheticum: a study and report of 217 cases. Pediatrics 23:1179, 1959.
39. Beckwith JR, Perrin EV: *In situ* neuroblastomas: a contribution to the natural history of neural crest tumors. Am J Pathol 43:1089, 1963.
40. Hellström I, Hellström KE, Sjögren NO, et al: Demonstration of cell-mediated immunity to human neoplasms of various types. Int J Cancer 7:1, 1971.
41. Lauder I, Aherne W: The significance of lymphatic infiltration in neuroblastoma. Br J Cancer 26:321, 1972.
42. de Lorimier AA, Bragg KU, Linden G: Neuroblastoma in childhood. Am J Dis Child 118:441, 1969.

43. McCormack LJ, Dockerty MB, Ghormley RK: Ewing's sarcoma. Cancer 5:85, 1952.
44. Goepfert H, Rochlin DB, Smart CR: Palliative treatment of Ewing's sarcoma. Am J Surg 113:246, 1967.
45. Kragh LV: Bone tumors of the jaws. *In* Gorlin RJ, Goldman HM (eds): Thoma's Oral Pathology, Vol I, 6th ed. St. Louis, CV Mosby, 1970, pp 560–576.
46. Wang CC, Schultz MD: Ewing's sarcoma—a study of 50 cases treated at the Massachusetts General Hospital, 1930–1952 inclusive. N Engl J Med 248:571, 1953.
47. Roca AN, Smith JL, MacComb WS, et al: Ewing's sarcoma of maxilla and mandible. Oral Surg 25:194, 1968.
48. Falk S, Alpert M: Clinical and roentgen aspects of Ewing's sarcoma. Am J Med Sci 250:492, 1965.
49. Jaffe N, Traggis I, Salian S, et al: Improved outlook for Ewing's sarcoma with combination therapy (vincristine, actinomycin D, cyclophosphamide) and radiation therapy. Cancer 38:1925, 1976.
50. Spjut HJ, Darfman HD, Fechner RE, et al: Tumors of bone and cartilage. *In* Atlas of Tumor Pathology, Fascicle 5, 2nd ed. Washington DC, Armed Forces Institute of Pathology, 1971, pp 104–110.
51. Garrington GE, Scofield HH, Cornyn J, et al: Osteosarcoma of the jaws: analysis of 56 cases. Cancer, 20:377, 1967.
52. Kragh LV, Dahlin DC, Erich JG: Osteogenic sarcoma of the jaws and facial bones. Am J Surg 96:496, 1958.
53. Yannopoulos K, Bom AF, Griffiths CO, et al: Osteosarcoma arising in fibrous dysplasia of the facial bones: case report and review of the literature. Am J Surg 107:556, 1964.
54. Walike JW, Bailey BJ: Head and neck pericytoma. Arch Otolaryngol 93:345, 1971.
55. Kauff, SL, Stout AP: Hemangiopericytoma in children. Cancer 13:695, 1960.
56. D'Agostino AN, Soule EN, Miller RH: Sarcomas of the peripheral nerves and somatic soft tissues associated with multiple neurofibromatosis (von Recklinghausen's disease). Cancer 16:1015, 1963.

12

THE ROLE OF RADIOTHERAPY IN COMBINED TREATMENT OF MALIGNANT NEOPLASMS OF THE HEAD AND NECK

David A. Deer, M.D.

In recent years there have been concerted efforts to improve results in head and neck cancer by combining surgery and radiotherapy. The "either/or" approach, practiced in the past by many radiotherapists and surgeons, has been abandoned in selected clinical presentations in favor of a cooperative effort with the purpose of improving local regional control and survival, while decreasing morbidity. The inclusion of the prosthodontist, speech pathologist, rehabilitative nurse, social worker, and dietitian has enhanced this team effort. Recently, with the availability of effective chemotherapeutic agents, the role of the medical oncologist has become more important.

The choice of any specific treatment modality or combination is dependent on a number of factors, including the possibility of local and regional tumor control, potential salvage with secondary therapy, social and nutritional factors, morbidity (including early and late complications), functional and cosmetic rehabilitation, and patient acceptance. For many oncologists, the predominating factor in the decision regarding choice of treatment modality is local tumor control. Unfortunately, very few prospective randomized studies have been performed that indicate the optimal therapy for local control. In general, retrospective studies, fraught with bias and errors, have been used in selecting a particular treatment modality. Furthermore, the decision-making process is confused by the differing results reported in the scientific literature. This is not surprising, since many variables exist among institutions with regard to patient selection, staging schemes, surgical techniques, and radiation techniques and doses. Therefore, it is often difficult to select the optimal treatment program for the patient with advanced cancer.

This chapter will discuss the general principles of radiotherapy, the general indications for using combined radiotherapy and surgery, and the multidisciplinary interactions involved in the combined approach. The primary emphasis will be on the patient with advanced cancer rather than the patient with early disease, for whom only one treatment modality may be indicated.

PRINCIPLES OF RADIOTHERAPY

Radiation Cell Kill—An Exponential Function

It has been an empirical observation for many decades that radiotherapy is more effective in controlling small localized cancers than large advanced malignancies. The reason for this was first demonstrated in the laboratory in the 1950's with the use of mammalian tissue culture techniques. Figure 12–1 depicts a cell survival curve typical of both in vivo–in vitro mammalian cells.[1-3] The fraction of surviving cells is plotted on a logarithmic scale against a known dose of radiation on a linear scale. The resulting curve is characterized by a shoulder followed by a straight-line, exponential function. In simplistic terms, the shoulder represents the ability of the cell to repair sublethal damage whereas the straight-line slope represents the radiosensitivity of the cell. Once the exponential function of the curve is reached, the same dose of radiation will kill a constant fraction of cells. The clinical implications of these data are obvious. Cure is achieved only when the last clonogenic cell is destroyed. A larger number of cancer cells requires a corresponding increase in radiation dose for control. When the radiation dose is limited by normal tissue tolerances, the probability of local tumor control decreases as tumor size increases.

Further laboratory experience, using both in vivo and in vitro tissue culture techniques, has demonstrated that mammalian cells, whether benign or malignant, have approximately the same cell survival curve—that is, one characterized by an initial shoulder followed by an exponential, straight-line function. Despite this fact, it has been demonstrated clinically that radiation can selectively destroy malignant neoplasms while preserving normal tissues. The reason seems to be that normal tissues have a greater capacity to repair sublethal damage. Thus, a course of radiotherapy that delivers a number of treatments over a prolonged time will preferentially spare normal tissue. This is demonstrated in Figure 12–2, in which it is seen that normal tissues, represented by the solid line, have a greater ability to repair radiation injuries than do malignant tissues.[3] After a given number of treatments (fractions), the normal tsisues have survived most of the radiation damage while the malignant tumor has not been able to repair and survive. Furthermore, the normal tissue repair is enhanced by migration of peripheral stem cells into the area from adjacent unirradiated tissue.

The Oxygen Effect

The oxygen effect refers to the fact that oxygenated cells are 2.5 to 3.0 times as sensitive to conventional radiation than hypoxic cells (data generated by in vitro tissue culture

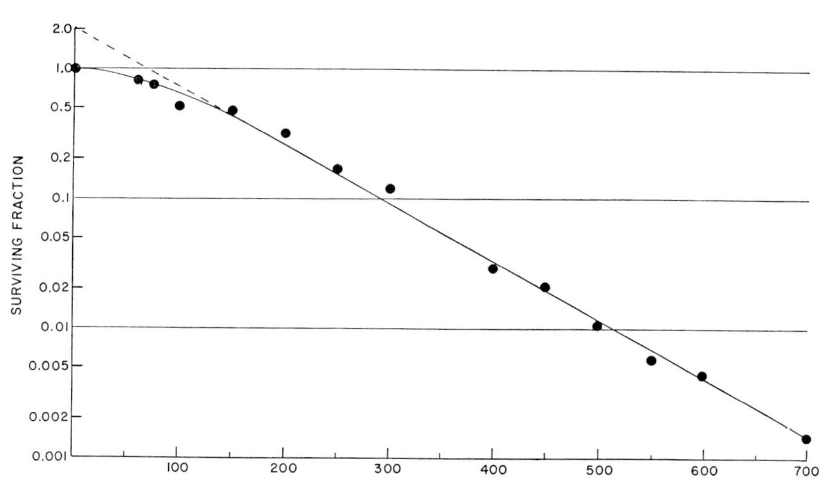

Figure 12–1. Cell survival curve illustrating the initial shoulder at doses of less than 150 rads and exponential cell kill at higher doses. (From Puck TT, Marcus PI: Action of x-rays on mammalian cells. J Exp Med 103:653, 1956.)

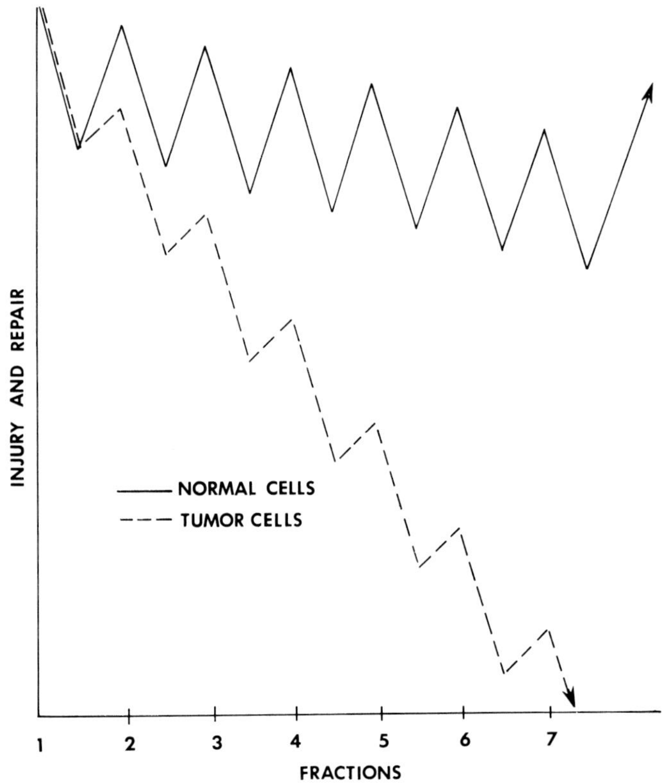

Figure 12–2. Neoplastic and normal tissue sustain the same amount of cell kill, but normal tissues have a greater capacity to repair radiation injury; after several fractions, the differential effect is apparent. (From Kligerman MM: Principles of radiation therapy. *In* Holland JF, Frei E (eds): Cancer Medicine. Philadelphia, Lea & Febiger, 1973.)

techniques).[4] In vivo experiments on mammalian tumor systems have demonstrated that hypoxic cells play an important role in radiation cell survival.[5]

In 1955, Thomlinson and Gray presented convincing evidence that human bronchogenic carcinomas contain significant numbers of hypoxic cells.[6] First, they demonstrated that these tumors grow in solid cores, with areas of necrosis developing in the center after tumor diameters of 160 to 200 microns have been reached. Next, using basic calculations involving oxygen diffusion coefficients and the respiratory rate of tissues, they showed that the tissue oxygen tension dropped off rapidly as the distance from the vascular supply increased. At a distance of 150 to 200 microns from the capillary, the tissue oxygen tension was calculated to be essentially zero. Between the central necrotic component and the peripheral oxygenated tumor component, it was assumed that there are hypoxic cells that remain clonogenic and relatively radioresistant.

From the above data we know that hypoxic cells play an important role in the radiotherapy of malignant neoplasms. Large tumors may contain a significant hypoxic cell fraction, which may be partially responsible for the difficulty in controlling advanced tumors with radiotherapy. If, indeed, human tumors contain a hypoxic cell component that is more radioresistant, then nearby oxygenated normal tissue may suffer more damage given the same dose of radiation. However, we know that the clinical situation does not confirm this rationale in all cases. The reason for this discrepancy is thought to be that a fractionated course of radiotherapy, long known to be more effective than single doses of radiation in achieving local tumor control and minimizing normal tissue damage, allows for reoxygenation between repeated doses of radiation.

However, many large tumors probably contain a significant number of hypoxic cells that never reoxygenate during a course of fractionated radiotherapy. In an attempt to overcome this potential cause of radiation failure in local control, many centers have irradiated malignant neoplasms under hyperbaric, oxygenated conditions. Some studies have shown this method to have potential benefit in local tumor control, but the overall results have not been significantly better to justify routine use of hyperbaric chambers.[7, 8] Many radiation oncologists, believing that hyperbaric chambers are unable to completely reoxygenate hypoxic cells, look to radiosensitizers of hypoxic cells to improve local tumor control. These drugs mimic oxygen in their radiation-sensitizing effect, yet are not metabolized. Therefore, they slowly diffuse into the hypoxic areas and deprive the cells of their hypoxic radiation protection. Clinical trials using these drugs are being conducted throughout the United States.

Radiosensitivity and Cell Age

In the cell cycle, cells in mitosis are more sensitive to ionizing radiation than cells in the DNA synthesis phase. In an asynchronous population of tumor cells, cells in the "S" phase would sustain less cell kill than cells in mitosis when exposed to a single large dose of radiation. A multifraction course of radiotherapy, allowing cells to proceed through the cycle between doses, would irradiate cells throughout the cycle and therefore be more effective.

CLINICAL APPLICATIONS

On the basis of empirical observation substantiated by laboratory data, it is widely accepted that a multifraction course of radiotherapy is more effective than a single large dose in destroying tumors while minimizing normal tissue damage. Multifractionation of radiation doses allows for reoxygenation of tumor cells, redistribution of radioresistant "S" phase cells in the cell cycle, repair of sublethal damage of normal cells, and repopulation of the irradiated area by normal cells from adjacent unirradiated areas. Again, the ultimate goal of radiotherapy is to kill all clonogenic tumor cells while avoiding irreparable damage to normal tissue.

Subclinical Disease

The term subclinical disease refers to the presence of microscopic disease (1 cubic mm contains 10^6 cells) that is not clinically detectable. As outlined in the preceding paragraphs, the quantity of radiation dose required to kill epithelial tumors of the head and neck is dependent on tumor volume and oxygenation. Clinical studies have shown that 5000 rads given over a 5-week period is adequate to eliminate well-oxygenated subclinical or microscopic disease.[9]

Gross Disease

Once a cancer has reached 1 cubic cm, it may contain 10^9 cells, some of which may be hypoxic. Surgery may increase the hypoxic cell component by disrupting the blood supply. As the tumor volume and the number of hypoxic cells increase, the increased radiation dose required, together with the greater amount of tissue that needs to be irradiated, raises the risk for complications. The upper limits of radiation dose (6500 to 8000 rads) are determined by normal tissue tolerance. The damage to normal tissues can be minimized in various ways, such as by reducing the field size after 5000 rads, employing electron beams to spare underlying normal tissues, and using interstitial therapy.

Dose-Effect Curve

In many anatomic sites, it is thought that the dose-effect for tumor response or normal tissue complication is best described by a sigmoid curve, plotting effect on the vertical axis and dose on the horizontal axis.[3, 10] As depicted in Figure 12–3, the optimal dose for a given tumor maximizes local control and minimizes complications. Usually the curves overlap to some extent, so that 100 per cent local control cannot be achieved without a significant complication rate. Depending on the spatial relationship of the curves to one another, a small increase in dose may cause a large increase in tumor control with only a small increase in complications. It should also be pointed out that there is a threshold dose below which no effect will be seen. As the tumor size increases, the sigmoid curve for the tumor response shifts to the right and decreases the changes for local control if the same radiation dose is given.

MULTIDISCIPLINARY INTERACTIONS

Nutritional Care

The ability of head and neck cancer patients to successively complete a course of

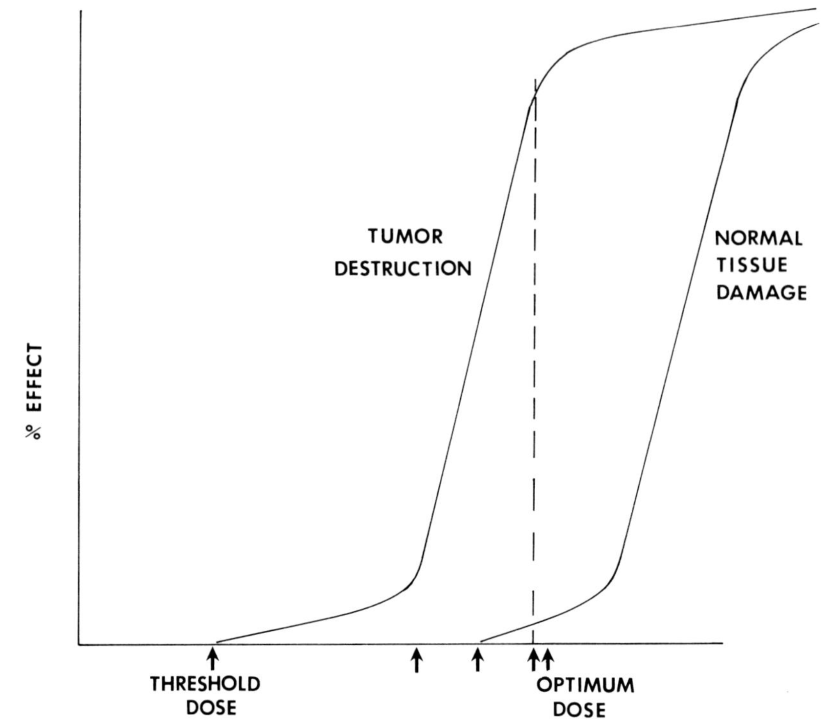

Figure 12–3. Measurement of effect (tumor destruction or normal tissue damage) against radiation dose. Relationship of curves is dependent on many factors, including tumor volume, amount of hypoxic cells, and type of normal tissue. (From Kligerman MM: Principles of radiation therapy. *In* Holland JF, Frei E (eds): Cancer Medicine. Philadelphia, Lea & Febiger, 1973.)

combined therapy is dependent on their nutritional status. The malignant process interferes with normal alimentation and may lead to negative nitrogen balance. Unless positive measures are taken to reverse this problem, extensive surgical procedures may be complicated by wound breakdown and/or delayed healing, which may interfere with the initiation of postoperative radiotherapy. The problem is further magnified by side effects from radiotherapy, which often lead to continued weight loss and necessitate an unwelcome break in the radiotherapy program. Also, many of these patients continue to use tobacco and alcohol, further compounding the problem. Needless to say, the nutritional care of these patients is extremely important.

Dental Care

Radiation portals often include major portions of salivary gland tissue and mandible, which can lead to radiation caries and osteoradionecrosis of the mandible. All dentulous patients in whom radiation therapy is contemplated should be seen by a dentist before any therapy is started. In order to minimize the morbidity from therapy, a major dental care program should be available.

SURGICAL-RADIOTHERAPEUTIC CONSIDERATIONS

Many factors enter into the decision-making process that lead to using combined therapy for head and neck patients. The success of either modality alone in controlling local and regional disease, the ability of one modality to salvage failures from the primary modality, and increased morbidity from the combined approach are but three factors that are relevant. Furthermore, surgery and radiotherapy may be used to treat different areas. For example, surgery can be used to remove a large primary tumor while radiotherapy is being employed to treat the N_0 neck that is at significant risk for microscopic disease.

The rationale for combining irradiation and surgery has been well described in the literature. Radiotherapy can destroy microscopic disease that has been inadvertently left behind at the time of surgery. On the other hand, surgery can remove large tumors that are poorly controlled with radiotherapy because of high tumor burden and cellular hypoxia. Thus, these two modalities can be expected to be complementary in many anatomic sites.

In general, the combined use of surgery and radiotherapy is recommended when the control of local and regional disease is significantly better than with either modality alone and the potential salvage of failure with the other modality is dismal. However, the improvement in local and regional control may not translate into improved survival, because of deaths due to intercurrent disease, second primaries, metastatic disease, or treatment complications.

Sequence of Combined Therapy

The above rationale can be applied to either preoperative or postoperative radiotherapy. The choice of time sequence is somewhat controversial and each approach has ardent proponents, usually based on results from retrospective clinical studies. The theoretical advantages for preoperative radiotherapy include the possible conversion of inoperable lesions into operable lesions and a decrease in distant metastases as a result of the radiation's interfering with the viability of tumor cells that may spread via the vascular system at the time of surgical resection. Also, the unoperated primary site and regional lymphatics, with an intact blood supply, may contain less hypoxic cells. The disadvantages of preoperative therapy include the risk of increased morbidity and mortality due to poor wound healing, the inability of the surgeon to recognize original tumor margins when significant regression of disease has taken place, and the delay in surgery which may allow a radioresistant tumor to grow and possibly metastasize.

The potential advantages of postoperative radiotherapy include facilitation in radiation treatment planning by knowing the extent of the tumor, the ability to give higher radiation doses, and the lack of interference with surgical healing. Disadvantages include possible postponement of initiating therapy in the event of delays in surgical healing, which could lead to repopulation of tumor before radiation can begin; the possibility of increased distant metastases via intravascular spread at the time of surgery; compromise in blood supply in the operative site, leading to tumor hypoxia and radioresistance; and increase in the treatment volume necessary to cover the operative site.

Preoperative Radiotherapy

Preoperative irradiation is occasionally used for patients who are surgically inoperable because of fixed nodes in the neck. The primary site and entire neck are treated with 5000 rads in 5 to 6 weeks. Based on the clinical response at the primary and nodal site, the decision is then made either to attack the primary and/or neck residual by surgery or to carry the radiation dose to tumoricidal levels. In one series, the combined approach controlled 8 of 9 necks with fixed nodes, while surgery controlled 5 of 11, and irradiation 7 of 15 necks.[11]

The potential advantage of decreasing the incidence of distant metastases with preoperative irradiation is theoretical, but has experimental support.[12, 13] The clinical data to substantiate a decrease in distant metastases is inconclusive. Merino et al, in a retrospective review in which the incidence of distant metastases was evaluated with either preoperative or postoperative therapy, found an advantage in the preoperative irradiation group.[14] However, other prospective studies using low-dose preoperative irradiation failed to confirm this benefit.[13, 15] The Radiation Therapy Oncology Group, comparing high-dose preoperative irradiation with postoperative irradiation in a randomized study of head and neck cancer patients, failed to demonstrate a decreased incidence in distant metastases with preoperative therapy.[16]

The choice of preoperative or postoperative radiotherapy has been compared in two recent prospective randomized studies. Vandenbrouck et al[17] reported on a prospective randomized series in hypopharyngeal carcinoma, comparing preoperative and postoperative radiotherapy with a dose of 5500 rads. Survival rate was significantly better in the postoperative group, although this may have been due to uncontrolled case selection as explained in the article. Recently, the Radiation Therapy Oncology Group reported their data from a prospective randomized trial comparing preoperative radiotherapy (5000 rads) and postoperative radiotherapy (6000 rads) in tumors involving the oral cavity, oropharynx, supraglottic larynx, and hypopharynx.[16] In addition, a third treatment plan—irradiation only, followed by surgical salvage for failures—was used for lesions of the oral cavity or oropharynx. To date there have been no differences in survival between the preoperative and postoperative groups. The group that had radiation alone followed by surgical salvage had slightly less satisfactory survival rates and a higher complication rate. The local and regional control is significantly better for the postoperative group in the hypopharynx and supraglottic larynx.

Many surgeons are concerned with an increased complication rate following high-dose preoperative radiotherapy.[18, 19] The report by Vandenbrouck and coworkers,[17] in which 5500 rads was used preoperatively in hypopharyngeal carcinomas, confirms this potential problem. In their study, the interval between radiotherapy and surgery was 2 weeks, and this may explain the increased complication rate. The RTOG study, using 5000 rads preoperatively, found no difference in severe complications compared with postoperative radiotherapy.[16] It is quite likely that the difference in complication rates in these two studies reflects the widely held belief that a small increase in radiation dose inordinately increases the complication rate, as explained earlier in this chapter under "Clinical Applications."

Thawley,[20] in an excellent review of the literature and analysis of data from his institution, looked at complications from combined therapy for cancers involving the larynx and inferior hypopharynx. From a review of the literature, he concluded that there was no significant difference in complication rates between preoperative (3000 to 5000 rads) and postoperative (5000 to 6000 rads) radiation therapy. Analysis of his own data revealed no significant difference in complication rate between pre- and postoperative therapy for laryngectomy patients. With supraglottic laryngectomy, the total complication rate as well as the incidence of involved margins was higher for the postoperative group. When all surgical groups were considered, there was no significant difference in the rate of severe complications (i.e., wound slough, fistula, carotid blowout, chronditis, and death) between preoperative and postoperative therapy. The lack of difference in complication rates is attributed to improved surgical techniques with regard to protection of the carotid artery, optimal placement of incisions, use of flaps, and control of orocutaneous fistulas.

Preoperative radiotherapy has been advocated in two other situations. Moderately advanced lesions are given a trial of irradiation. After 5000 rads, tumors that have responded poorly are selected for curative resection while patients with good tumor responses are treated with definitive high-dose radiotherapy. Although this practice is common in many centers, there are no data to support its usefulness. Preoperative irradiation has been used when reconstructive surgery will delay postoperative radiotherapy by more than 6 weeks.

Postoperative Radiotherapy

Postoperative therapy should be a planned event rather than an afterthought. Often, the choice of the surgical procedure will depend on the use of irradiation in the control of subclinical disease in the neck. The postoperative radiation may permit selection of an operation that will yield less morbidity and improved function.

By carefully planning the surgical incisions, the surgeon can often influence the morbidity from the postoperative therapy. For example, needless extensions of the operative field into the submental, infraclavicular, and other areas force the radiotherapist to enlarge his treatment volume, thereby increasing the patient's morbidity. Effective interaction between the physicians utilizing the two modalities is necessary to eliminate these problems, Also, the surgical oncologist must keep in mind the importance of the time interval between the surgical procedure and the initiation of irradiation. Progressive growth of microscopic tumor can be expected to occur during the immediate postoperative period. Therefore, radiotherapy should not be delayed any longer than necessary for wound healing to take place. Vikram,[21] in a small series of patients, showed a marked improvement of survival in patients whose postoperative treatment was started within 7 weeks after surgery when compared with patients who had prolonged delays.

The amount of radiation required to eliminate subclinical disease in the postoperative patient is not well defined. As stated earlier, 5000 rads in 5 weeks has been shown to sterilize subclinical disease in surgically unviolated tissues over 90 per cent of the time. After radical surgery, there is extensive scarring in the operative bed, resulting in interruption of normal vasculature and decreased oxygenation of the cells in that region. Therefore, it can be expected that doses greater

Table 12–1. NUMBER OF PATIENTS WITH FAILURE WITHIN THE PRIMARY TREATMENT FIELD ACCORDING TO DOSE AND REASON FOR ADDING POSTOPERATIVE IRRADIATION*

	Primary Reason for Adding Postoperative Irradiation (Failures within Field/Total Patients)								*Total*	
Dose (rad)	*Positive Margins*	*Questionable Margins*	*Perinodal Extension*	*Perineural Involvement*	*Thyroid Cartilage Invasion*	*Mandible Involvement*	*Multiple Nodes*	*Misc.*†	*No.*	*(%)*
<5000	0	1/2	0	0	0/1	0	1/1	0	2/4	(50)
5000–5499	1/2	1/1	0/1	0	2/4	0	0	0/1	4/9	(44)
5500–5999	2/3	1/3	1/3	1/2	0/2	0	2/7	0/5	7/25	(28)
6000–6499	2/4	0/1	0/1	0	0/2	2/2	0/1	0/3	4/14	(28)
≥6500	0/7	0/1	0/1	0/1	0/2	0/1	0	0	0/13	(0)
Total	5/16 (31%)	3/8 (38%)	1/6 (17%)	1/3 (33%)	2/11 (18%)	2/3 (67%)	3/9 (33%)	0/9 (0%)	17/65 (26%)	

*From Marcus RB, Million RR, Cassisi NJ: Postoperative irradiation for squamous cell carcinoma of the head and neck: analysis of time-dose factors related to control above the clavicles. Int J Radiat Oncol Biol Phys 5:1943, 1979.

†Treated for reasons not clear in chart.

than 5000 rads will be necessary to control microscopic tumor. Marcus reviewed the indications for postoperative irradiation in 71 patients and correlated failure with radiation dose (Table 12–1).[22] With increasing dose, there was a corresponding decrease in local and regional failure. It was also demonstrated that split-course treatments, popular because of decreased acute morbidity, had a higher failure rate. These data suggest that a dose of 6500 to 7000 rads may be required for control of clinically involved, operated sites, whereas only 5000 rads may be sufficient for uninvolved, nonoperated areas.

Often, the radiotherapist may not see the patient until the postoperative period. A diligent review of the clinical, surgical, and pathologic findings is necessary before the recommendation for postoperative irradiation is made. When the risk for local-regional failure is greater than 20 to 30 per cent, adjuvant therapy should be considered. The presence of positive margins[23] or extracapsular nodal extension[24] carry a high risk for local-regional failure and require high doses of postoperative irradiation.[22] Other indications for adjuvant irradiation may include multiple involved neck nodes, perineural invasion, high-grade histology, and bone or cartilage invasion.

Carcinogenesis from Combined Treatment

Many studies have demonstrated that low-dose radiation in childhood for benign conditions carried definite risk for radiation-induced neoplasms in adulthood. The extrapolation of these data as a relative contraindication to radiotherapy for treatment of head and neck cancer patients is not warranted. At the Curie Institute, only 4 out of 1000 irradiated patients (minimum follow-up 5 years) developed a malignant neoplasm in the treatment field of different histology from the original tumor.[25] The M.D. Anderson Hospital reviewed 1163 patients surviving greater than 5 years after treatment for head and neck cancer and found that irradiation does not increase the risk for squamous cell carcinoma in the radiation field.[26]

SELECTED TUMOR SITES

The overall management of any given individual patient is dependent on many factors. These include site and stage of disease, medical operability of the patient, social and nutritional status, possibility of local-regional control with a single modality vs. combined treatment, potential salvage with secondary therapy, morbidity, and patient acceptance. Because of these variable factors, the purpose of the following discussion will be to point out relevant data that may serve as general guidelines for the management of head and neck cancer patients. Most of the data is retrospective and subject to many variables, including different staging schemes. The American Joint Committee staging system[27] will be used in this chapter unless otherwise specified.

Oral Cavity

The lip, floor of mouth, oral tongue, buccal mucosa, upper and lower gingiva, hard palate, and retromolar trigone make up the oral cavity. Because of the tremendous variation in anatomy, patterns of spread, and treatment, each site must be discussed separately.

Lip. Small carcinomas at this site are easily cured with radiotherapy or surgical excision. Lesions of moderate size, which may require extensive plastic repair or compromise the oral stoma, may be treated with radiotherapy alone with excellent results.[28–31] Advanced lesions with bone, nodal, or nerve involvement may require combined therapy for optimal results.

Floor of Mouth. The primary lymphatic drainage is to the submaxillary or subdigastric nodal chain. In most series, at least 30 per cent of patients will have clinical involvement of lymph nodes (N^+) at presentation.[32, 33] With elective neck dissection, Southwick et al[34] reported 39.9 per cent of clinically negative necks (N_0) to contain microscopic metastases. This high risk for occult tumor infestation of lymph nodes is verified by other data that show that 20 to 35 per cent of N_0 necks will develop nodal metastases without neck treatment.[35–37] For T_1, T_2, T_3, and T_4 lesions, the incidence of nodal metastases on presentation is reported to be 9 to 11 per cent, 29 per cent, 44 to 68 per cent, and 54 per cent respectively.[32–38]

The early lesions (T_1 and early T_2) can be managed equally well with either surgery or radiotherapy.[38] Local control for T_1N_0 and T_2N_0 tumors treated with radiotherapy alone varies from 68 to 98 per cent and 65 to 94 per cent respectively.[38–40] Surgical salvage is possible in a large percentage of patients.

Moderately advanced lesions (late T_2 and T_3) are difficult to manage because of potential cosmetic and functional disability. These patients often present with regional node metastases. Guillamondegui and Jesse report survival rates approaching 60 per cent with surgery or x-ray therapy, but do not mention the number of irradiated patients salvaged with surgery.[41] By contrast, Fu et al report local control in 100 per cent (6 out of 6 patients) and 25 per cent (4 out of 32 patients) of T_3 lesions treated with combined therapy or radiotherapy alone, respectively.[38] If mandibular continuity can be preserved with rim or coronal resection, combined therapy may give superior results in the T_3 lesions while maintaining function and cosmesis. The M.D. Anderson Hospital reported 20 T_3–T_4 patients with periosteal or bone invasion who were treated with surgical procedures that maintained mandibular continuity, followed by postoperative radiotherapy.[41] At 1 year, there was only 1 local failure, while 4 failed in the neck and 2 died of distant metastases.

T_4 lesions are seldom controlled with radiotherapy alone.[41] If the patient has fixed nodal disease, preoperative radiotherapy is recommended. Otherwise, I advise surgical resection of the primary followed by radiotherapy. In patients with massive disease from tumor extension to skin, neck, or base of tongue, curative therapy may not be feasible.

Oral Tongue. The primary lymphatic drainage is to the subdigastric and submaxillary lymph nodes. At presentation, 35 to 45 per cent of patients will be clinically N^+.[32, 33, 42] Decroix and Ghossein[42] reported that 34 per cent of 244 patients with N_0 necks had occult metastases on elective neck dissection. For T_1 to T_4 lesions, the nodes are clinically involved in 14, 30, 47.5, and 76.5 per cent respectively.[32]

The local control and survival for T_1, T_2, and early T_3 lesions treated with surgery or radiotherapy are similar in retrospective series from the Curie Institute and Memorial Hospital.[43, 44] Favorable results with primary radiotherapy are reported by others.[40, 45, 46] However, superior results with surgery for treatment of T_2–T_3 lesions are reported by White and Byers of the M.D. Anderson Hospital and Tumor Institute.[47] In their experience local control with surgical treatment was achieved in 96 per cent of T_2 and 76 per cent of T_3 and T_4 lesions. By contrast, local control with radiotherapy in T_2 and T_3–T_4 lesions was 79 per cent and 29 per cent respectively.

Combined treatment is probably more effective for local-regional control of advanced lesions (late T_3–T_4). This is suggested by retrospective studies[47, 48] as well as a prospective, randomized study currently being conducted by the Radiation Therapy Oncology Group.[16] In patients with cancer of the oral cavity and oropharynx randomized to treatment groups of preoperative, postoperative, or radiotherapy alone, the local-regional control at 2 years is reported to be 56, 53, and 39 per cent while 2-year survival for cancer of the oral cavity is 53, 59 and 42 per cent respectively.[16] Although the differences are not statistically significant, a trend in favor of combined treatment is suggested.

Buccal Mucosa. The lymphatic drainage is to the submaxillary and subdigastric nodes. Lymph node metastases are present in 31 to 42 per cent of patients.[49, 50] In one series, 30 per cent of patients with clinically negative necks were found to have occult infestation of nodes at the time of elective neck dissection.[50]

Local excision alone for lesions smaller than 1 cm is adequate. Lindberg and Fletcher[51] report local control rates of 90 per cent for T_2–T_4 lesions treated with radiotherapy, although Vegers et al report superior results with surgery.[50] Based on the Memorial Hospital experience, in which 5-year determinate survival rates of 27 per cent for Stage III and 18 per cent for Stage IV lesions were reported, combined therapy should be considered for advanced lesions.[52]

Hard Palate and Gingiva. The lymphatic drainage is to the submaxillary and subdigastric nodal stations. Clinical regional nodal spread is seen in approximately 40 per cent of patients with squamous cell carcinoma of the lower gingiva and 25 per cent of patients with hard palate lesions.[49, 53]

Surgery has been the treatment of choice in most institutions. With T_1 and T_2 lesions, surgery is curative in approximately 80 per cent of cases.[54, 55] The experience with radiotherapy at this site is limited, but Chung et al[53] reported 8 of 12 irradiated patients to be free of recurrence at 24 months, as compared with 6 of 12 patients treated with surgery. Postoperative radiotherapy is recommended for cancers showing positive surgical margins, perineural invasion, and extensive nodal metastases, although re-excision is usually necessary for positive surgical margins.

Oropharynx

The soft palate, tonsil, and base of tongue account for the majority of cancers in the oropharynx. The posterior pharyngeal wall will be discussed under "Hypopharynx" (p. 353).

Lymphatics. The subdigastric node is the primary lymphatic drainage for this region. The incidence of clinically positive nodes is 70 to 83 per cent for lesions of the base of the tongue, 44 to 47 per cent for lesions of the soft palate, and 66 to 76 per cent for tonsillar fossa tumors.[32, 33, 56] The risk for lymph node involvement is directly related to increasing T stage at all sites.[32, 56]

Base of Tongue. The optimal treatment for this site is unknown. Because of the functional and cosmetic deformity with surgical resection, many favor primary radiotherapy.

Favorable results, in terms of local-regional control, have been reported by three different institutions utilizing radiotherapy alone (Table 12–2).[56–58] Parsons et al report absolute and determinate 5-year survival rates for Stages I and II, Stage III, and Stage IV to be 100, 50, and 22 per cent, and 100, 86, and 24 per cent respectively.[56] In this series of 110 patients, 15 were excluded from curative therapy because of distant metastases (3 patients) or advanced local-regional disease and poor medical condition (12 patients). Unfavorable results with radiotherapy alone are reported by Rollo and coworkers.[59] In their series, 18 patients received doses of from 1800 to 7000 rads; of these patients 35 per cent had less than 6000 rads to the primary. Five of 15 patients who died within 5 years had local-regional failure, while the majority died of intercurrent disease, second primaries, or distant metastases.

Others have advocated surgical resection as the primary modality. Whicker et al,[60] in a retrospective review of the Mayo Clinic experience, reported a 42 per cent survival rate in 102 selected patients of whom 46 had surgery only.[60] Thirty-seven patients (33 per cent) had some degree of local or regional failure. Spiro and Strong, in a retrospective review of the M.D. Anderson Hospital experience in the treatment of 34 advanced

Table 12–2. LOCAL CONTROL RATES AT 2 YEARS IN CARCINOMA OF THE BASE OF THE TONGUE

	Institution			
Stage	*University of Florida*[56]	*M.D. Anderson*[58]	*Michigan*[57]	***Total (%)***
T_1	6/8	23/32	13/14	42/54 (78)
T_2	10/15	23/49	15/19	48/83 (58)
T_3	14/22	33/64	19/33	66/119 (55)
T_4	3/24	6/29	9/26	18/79 (23)

cancer patients with surgery alone, reported determinate survival at 5 years to be 20 per cent, with local-regional control achieved in 27 per cent of the patients at 2 years, and a 17.6 per cent operative mortality rate.[62]

Combined therapy has been reported to be superior to single modality therapy. Rollo et al[59] reported 50 per cent of 63 patients treated with preoperative radiotherapy alive at 5 years, as compared with 3 of 18 patients treated with radiotherapy alone. However, the radiotherapy (< 6000 rads) was not curative in 35 per cent of patients, although only 5 patients died from local-regional failure. Rabuzzi et al[63] had favorable results in 58 selected patients with oropharyngeal carcinoma treated with 5000 rads preoperatively. They report absolute 3-year survival rates in Stages I and II, III, and IV to be 67 per cent (8/12), 65 per cent (11/17), and 28 per cent (8/29), and determinant 3-year survival rates to be 67 per cent (8/12), 79 per cent (11/14), and 38 per cent (8/21) respectively. The overall survival rate was 47 per cent.

It is hoped that preoperative randomized studies will provide answers to the question of what is the optimal treatment at this site. An interim report from the RTOG study on combined treatment shows no statistical improvement in local control and survival at 2 years in oropharyngeal carcinoma.[16]

Tonsil. Radiotherapy alone achieves local control in 80 per cent of early lesions.[64, 65] Surgery is usually effective in controlling radiation failures. For advanced lesions, the optimal treatment is not known. While Perez et al[65] report a 32 per cent local-regional failure rate with radiotherapy alone in T_3 lesions, Kaplan et al[64] report 71 per cent. Both Perez and Kaplan report poor local-regional control in T_4 lesions (30 and 40 per cent respectively) treated with radiotherapy.[64, 65] Because of these poor results, many institutions use combined therapy. Perez et al, in a retrospective review of patients treated with preoperative low-dose radiation or radiotherapy alone, found no difference in tumor recurrence.[65] Weichert et al,[66] utilizing 4500 rads preoperatively, report improved results in Stage III disease, with a 63 per cent actuarial 3-year survival rate for a group of 8 patients. Favorable results with high-dose preoperative radiation are also reported by Rabuzzi et al,[63] in the treatment of oropharyngeal carcinomas. These favorable results are also confirmed by Shrewsbury et al,[67] who report a 76 per cent 2-year survival rate in 21 patients with T_3 lesions treated with 4500 to 5000 rads preoperatively.[67] However, the interim report from the RTOG study shows no difference in 2-year survival rates between combined therapy and radiotherapy alone in oropharyngeal carcinoma.[16]

Soft Palate. As with other sites, early lesions (T_1–T_2) can be controlled equally well with radiotherapy or surgery.[51, 68–70] Because of functional morbidity with resection of the soft palate, many prefer radiotherapy. Local control rates with T_3–T_4 lesions treated with radiotherapy are reported to be from 64 to 83 per cent.[51, 69, 70] For lesions of a diffuse nature, Ratzer and colleagues from New York's Memorial Hospital recommend radiotherapy alone, while combined therapy is preferred for "extensive local involvement plus regional lymph node metastases."[71]

Nasopharynx

Malignant tumors of the nasopharynx are characterized by a number of features that separate them from other sites. The central location at the base of the skull makes resection untenable, and radiotherapy has been the major therapeutic modality. Epidemiologic studies have suggested the role of three causative factors: genetic predisposition, environmental influence, and the Epstein-Barr virus.[72]

Lymphatics. The submucosal lymphatics are extensive, accounting for the high incidence of neck metastases. Because of midline crossover of lymphatics, bilateral or contralateral metastases are not uncommon. Lymphatic drainage to the neck may occur via three different lymph node stations: the jugular chain, the spinal accessory chain, and the retropharyngeal nodes. Unilateral neck metastases present in 60 to 90 per cent of cases, and bilateral neck involvement in approximately 50 per cent.

Pathology. Carcinomas account for approximately 85 per cent and lymphomas for 10 per cent of the malignant lesions. So called lymphoepitheliomas and transitional cell carcinomas are thought to be histologic variants of the undifferentiated carcinoma. Other rare histologic types include adenocarcinoma, melanoma, plasmacytoma, sarcoma, and juvenile angiofibroma.

Spread Patterns. Because of the inaccessibility of these lesions to thorough clinical examination, the extent of disease is often underestimated. Cranial nerve involvement and bone involvement, as diagnosed by routine radiographs, are late manifestations of advanced disease. The use of computerized tomography should increase our ability to define disease extensions so that appropriate treatment techniques can be employed.

Clinical Evolution. A painless upper neck mass secondary to lymphatic dissemination is the most common presenting complaint. Nasal obstruction, epistaxis, and hypoacusis are often present. Cranial nerve involvement represents superior or lateral extension, and trismus indicates involvement of the pterygoid region. Sore throat is a symptom of inferior extension into the oropharynx.

Staging. Although not uniformly accepted, the American Joint Committee staging system is the most widely used.[27] For the primary site, the staging system is as follows:

- T_{IS} Carcinoma in situ
- T_1 Tumor confined to one site of nasopharynx, or no tumor visible
- T_2 Tumor involving two sites
- T_3 Extension of tumor into nasal cavity or oropharynx
- T_4 Tumor invasion of skull, cranial nerve involvement, or both; nodal invasion of skull, cranial nerve involvement, or both

Treatment. In most situations, radiotherapy is the primary modality. Exceptions include juvenile angiofibroma, for which I favor surgical management because of the young age of the patient and recent improvements in surgical technique.

Malignant lymphomas confined to the nasopharynx are usually managed with radiotherapy alone. With regional involvement (Stage II) the risk for systemic disease increases substantially, and combined radiotherapy and systemic chemotherapy may be indicated. Stage III and Stage IV lymphomas are managed primarily by chemotherapy.

Carcinomas are managed with radiotherapy. Primary neck dissection is used infrequently, both because of the relative effectiveness of radiotherapy in controlling neck disease and because of the potential involvement of the retropharyngeal nodes, an area that is not resected in the classic neck dissection. If the primary lesion is controlled but residual neck disease is still present at the completion of radiotherapy, a neck dissection should be considered.

Technique of Treatment. A thorough knowledge of the anatomy and routes of spread is fundamental to treatment planning. Differences in histology or grade of tumor do not alter the techniques, which are outlined in detail in standard radiotherapy texts.[73] Three general principles that need to be followed in all cases are the application of large-volume irradiation to the primary tumor, entire bilateral neck irradiation, and shrinking the field when possible. The required radiation dose is dependent on stage and histology. Lymphomas are controlled with doses of 4000 to 4500 rads, whereas squamous cell carcinomas require 6500 to 7000 rads.[73]

Acute Sequelae. Owing to the large volume of irradiated tissue, which includes the nasopharynx, oropharynx, supraglottic larynx, posterior nasal cavity, and entire neck, morbidity is high, often requiring multidisciplinary care. Because most, if not all, salivary gland tissue is included in the treatment volume, xerostomia is the rule, and with the higher doses used to treat the carcinomas, permanent dryness in the mouth will result. Sore throat and loss of taste can be expected to resolve in most patients after therapy has finished. Serous otitis with hypoacusis, caused by obstruction of the eustachian tube, may require tympanostomy tubes.

Chronic Sequelae. Some degree of xerostomia occurs in all patients. Trismus may result from fibrosis of the pterygoid musculature or fibrosis around the temporal mandibular joint. The inclusion of the hypothalamus, temporal lobes, and pituitary in the large volume carries the risk of brain necrosis, but this is seldom seen. However, pituitary dysfunction secondary to radiotherapy has been reported.[74] Radiation myelitis of the brain stem or cervical cord is a risk but can be minimized by shrinking the fields and using proper technique. Other unusual complications include impaired vision or loss of vision resulting from retrobulbar optic neuritis or retinopathy, and cranial nerve paralysis caused by nerve entrapment from fibrosis.

Results of Treatment. The 5-year survival rates for carcinomas vary from 37 to 59 per cent, the best results probably reflecting the least number of advanced cases.[75, 78] Tables 12–3 and 12–4 show local and regional control rates from three different institutions.[76–78] Treatment failure due to distant metastases is a significant problem and awaits the development of effective systemic treatment. Lymphoepitheliomas are reported to have a better prognosis than the other epithelial neoplasms.[76, 79]

Table 12–3. LOCAL CONTROL RATES IN CARCINOMA OF NASOPHARYNX

	Institution			
Stage	*M.D. Anderson*[76]	*Stanford*[77]	*University of Florida*[76]	***Total (%)***
T_1	23/36	33/38	4/4	60/78 (77)
T_2	55/65	15/16	4/5	74/86 (88)
T_3	32/42	13/19	9/10	54/71 (76)
T_4	29/48	04/09	10/20	43/77 (56)

Larynx

The primary therapeutic goals at this site are to maximize local-regional control and to preserve voice function when feasible. In early lesions, these objectives can usually be accomplished by radiotherapy or conservation surgery. In advanced lesions, the strategy becomes more complex, and one of the above objectives must be compromised depending on treatment selection.

Lymphatics. The major lymphatic drainage for the supraglottic lesion is in the upper and mid-jugular region. Clinical involvement of nodes is present in 23 to 55 per cent of cases, increasing directly with the extent of T stage.[32, 80, 81] For T_1 to T_4 lesions, the risk for clinical involvement varies from 15 to 39 per cent, 33 to 42 per cent, 23 to 65 per cent, and 52 to 75 per cent respectively.[32, 80–83] Contralateral involvement is present in 23 per cent of all cases.[32] Because of sparse lymphatics, early glottic cancers rarely present with clinically involved nodes, whereas advanced lesions have nodal involvement in 15 to 31 per cent of cases.[83]

Supraglottic Larynx. Early lesions with minimal nodal involvement can be managed with primary radiotherapy or supraglottic laryngectomy.[81, 82, 84] With a bulky T_2 or exophytic T_3 lesions, some institutions advocate a trial of radiotherapy. If a favorable tumor response is seen after 4500 to 5000 rads, curative doses of irradiation are administered; otherwise a laryngectomy is indicated.

Patients who present with early primary lesions in conjunction with unresectable neck disease are treated with definitive radiotherapy. If the neck disease becomes resectable after 5000 rads, then therapeutic neck dissection follows in 4 to 6 weeks. However, such salvage surgery is frequently not possible, and persistent unresectable neck disease is treated with further irradiation at higher doses, as control with irradiation alone is possible.[11] The primary lesion is treated to curative doses if a favorable response is observed; otherwise surgical resection must be considered.

Postoperative radiotherapy is indicated with most T_4 lesions and advanced resectable neck disease. This combined approach not only improves local regional control[86] but also results in significant improvement in survival as compared with surgery alone.[51]

In the RTOG study comparing preoperative and postoperative irradiation, the local regional control is significantly better at 2 years in the postoperative group.[16] However, there is no significant difference in survival between these two groups.

Stage IV unresectable disease can occasionally be controlled with high-dose radiotherapy. Fletcher, in a review of 23 surgically unresectable patients, reported local-regional control in 14 patients. Intercurrent disease and distant metastases accounted for 13 deaths, leaving only one 5-year survival.[87]

Glottis. Early lesions can be managed by definitive radiotherapy, with surgery reserved

Table 12–4. REGIONAL CONTROL RATES IN CARCINOMA OF THE NASOPHARYNX

	Institution		
Nodal Involvement	*M.D. Anderson*[76]	*Stanford*[77]	***Total (%)***
N_0	24/24	23/24	47/48 (98)
N_1	15/17	23/25	38/42 (90)
N_2	39/46	13/15	52/61 (85)
N_{3A}	69/94	16/18	85/112 (76)
N_{3B}			

for radiation failure, or with conservation surgery. Voice quality is usually superior with radiotherapy.

Advanced lesions (T_3–T_4) are managed in most institutions by surgery. The major exception is the Princess Margaret Hospital in Toronto, where it is felt that radical irradiation with surgery for salvage has the advantage of voice preservation and is equal in overall survival to combined treatment.[88] However, their survival results seem to be inferior to other centers where surgery is the primary treatment.[89, 90]

Indications for postoperative radiotherapy include (1) prior tracheostomy as the risk for subsequent stomal recurrence is increased;[91] (2) cartilage invasion or extension into surrounding tissues; (3) extensive subglottic growth because of the increased risk for stomal recurrence;[92] (4) multiple positive nodes or when the risk for occult nodal involvement is significant. This is present in lesions greater than 2 cm and in those with poor differentiation, infiltrating margins, or nerve sheath invasion.

Hypopharynx

The hypopharynx usually includes the pyriform sinus, postcricoid area, and posterior hypopharyngeal walls. Because the routes of spread are similar, the pharyngeal walls of the oropharynx will also be included in this section.

Because of the rich supply of lymphatics in this region, the silent nature of the early lesion, and patient delay in presentation, these cancers are often advanced at diagnosis. In one series of 418 pyriform sinus lesions, 83 per cent were T_3–T_4 and 74 per cent were N+ at presentation.[93] Pharyngeal wall lesions are reported to have positive lymph nodes in 59 to 73 per cent of cases.[32, 90, 93] Advanced cancers in this region are known not only for the difficulty in obtaining local regional control but also for a high incidence of patients dying with distant metastases.

Lymphatics. The jugular chain forms the primary lymphatic drainage site, but the spinal accessory chain is also at risk. Any treatment plan should also consider the retropharyngeal nodes, which were positive in 42 per cent of pharyngeal wall lesions in one surgical series.[94]

Pharyngeal Walls. For T_1N_0–T_2N_0 lesions, 3- to 5-year survival with radiotherapy alone is reported to be approximately 50 per cent, while advanced lesions are seldom cured.[95, 96] Using combined surgery and radiotherapy for advanced lesions, Meoz-Mendez of M.D. Anderson Hospital reported local regional control in 15 to 20 patients (75 per cent), as compared with 55 of 108 patients (51 per cent) treated with irradiation alone.[97] Because of the potential increased morbidity with high-dose preoperative irradiation, postoperative radiotherapy is usually preferred for advanced lesions.[97, 98] Radiation doses of 5000 rads to the unoperated, clinically negative neck and doses of 6000 to 7000 rads to the operative bed should be considered. Special techniques to avoid underdosage or overdosage at the junction between the upper and lower neck fields are needed.

Pyriform Sinus. Acceptable results for local control of early lesions (T_1–T_2) are achieved with either radiotherapy or surgery. Million and Cassisi[99] report 17 of 24 patients with T_1–T_2 lesions controlled at 2 years with radiotherapy alone, and ultimate control with surgical salvage was achieved in 20 of the 24 patients. In the selected T_3 patients (exophytic tumors), local control was obtained in only 50 per cent (3 out of 6).

Although results are not unanimous, most series report improved local-regional control and survival rates in advanced carcinoma of this site treated with the combined approach. The optimal sequence of therapy is controversial. While Goldman and coworkers[100] reported excellent survival and acceptable complication rates in their retrospective, high-dose (5500 rads) preoperative series, Vandenbrouck et al,[17] using the same dose in a prospective randomized group of patients, reported improved survival and decreased morbidity with postoperative irradiation. Possible explanations for these different conclusions include patient selection and timing of surgery. Also, the Goldman series included patients with laryngeal cancer, a more favorable site.

In a retrospective series from the M.D. Anderson Hospital, 5-year survival with combined therapy was 40 per cent, as compared with 25 per cent for the group treated by surgery alone.[93] Although the patients were not randomized, the number of advanced cases in each group was approximately the same, providing more validity to the results and conclusions. On the basis of these results and the potential increase in morbidity with high-dose preoperative radiotherapy, the author favors postoperative radiotherapy.

The radiation technique, as with lesions of the pharyngeal walls, must include all lymph node chains at risk, including the retropharyngeal nodes. Special techniques to ensure dose homogeneity (wedges or tissue compensations) and to prevent overdosage of the spinal cord must be used.

Nasal Vestibule, Nasal Cavity, and Paranasal Sinuses

Lymphatics. Compared with other sites in the head and neck, the incidence of lymphatic metastases is low. In a series of 36 patients with carcinoma of the nasal vestibule, 5 patients (14 per cent) presented with lymph node metastases; of these 5 patients, 1 was graded T_1, 1 was T_2, and 3 were T_3.[101] For the nasal cavity and maxillary sinus, lymph node involvement is also low, ranging from 0 to 15 per cent.[102–105] Once the cancer extends beyond the confines of the involved sinus, the incidence of lymphatic involvement is higher.

Treatment. Squamous cell carcinomas of the nasal vestibule are relatively rare. In a 3-year follow-up of a group of 31 patients who were treated with radiotherapy alone, Wang[101] reported no evidence of disease in 20 of 25 patients with T_1–T_2 lesions and in 3 of 6 patients with T_3 lesions. For the advanced primary tumors, Wang recommends radical surgery with or without preoperative radiotherapy.

The selection of treatment for lesions of the nasal cavity is dependent on size, location, and histology. Midline lethal granulomas are treated by some with radiotherapy alone, whereas inverting papillomas are managed by surgery.

Carcinomas of the nasal cavity are managed with surgery or radiotherapy. Frazell and Lewis[107] report superior results with surgery over radiotherapy, but the radiotherapy techniques and doses were suboptimal and outdated by current standards. Recent reports indicate favorable results with radiotherapy alone.[102, 103, 106] For example, Ellingwood and Million[106] reported 95 per cent local control in 15 patients, with an absolute 5-year survival rate of 54 per cent.

Esthesioneuroblastoma of the nasal cavity is a rare tumor of neural crest origin. Elkon et al,[108] in a review of the world literature since 1966, found no significant survival difference in Stage A and Stage B patients treated with surgery, radiotherapy, or combined treatment. Combined treatment is recommended for advanced (Stage C) disease.

Management of carcinomas of the maxillary sinus is dependent on the extent of disease. Surgery alone may be adequate for early lesions involving the infrastructure. Unfortunately, these lesions usually present at a late stage. When the base of the skull or the nasopharynx is involved, surgery is contraindicated, except in selected cases. Otherwise, combined treatment is recommended by most institutions,[104, 105, 109] although Amendola et al[110] report superior results with radiotherapy alone as compared with surgery. In a review of combined treatment, Jesse found no survival difference between preoperative and postoperative radiotherapy.

Carcinomas of the ethmoid and sphenoid sinuses are rare, which accounts for the paucity of retrospective data. Historically, Frazell and Lewis[107] reported 40 per cent and 20 per cent 5-year cure rates in ethmoid carcinomas treated with radiotherapy and surgery, respectively. Ellingwood and Million[106] recently reported 71 per cent local control in 17 patients who were followed for more than 2 years.

Major Salivary Glands

The therapeutic management of salivary gland malignancies is based on location, histology, and extent of disease. Historically, surgery has been the sole treatment modality, owing to the misconception that the neoplasms are radioresistant. Recent literature suggests that combined therapy improves both local control and survival in many clinical situations.

The failure rate in major salivary gland malignancies is dependent on stage and histology. Spiro et al[111] reported the recurrence rate in Stages I, II, and III to be 7, 21, and 58 per cent respectively, with an overall recurrence rate of 27 per cent in 268 parotid gland tumors. Beahrs et al[112] reported local failure rates of 37.6 and 72.5 per cent respectively in patients with moderately malignant and highly malignant tumors. Tapley et al,[113] from the M.D. Anderson Hospital, reported local failures in 3 of 38 low-grade parotid tumors and in 16 of 44 high-grade tumors. Acinic cells and low-grade mucoepidermoid carcinomas were considered low grade, while the high-grade malignancies included squamous cell carcinomas, adenocarcinomas, undifferentiated carcinomas, high-grade mucoepidermoid carcinomas, malignant mixed tumors, and adenoid cystic carcinomas. Combined therapy for high-grade malignant tumors improves local control and probably survival. Tapley[114] reported local failures in 16 of 54 patients (27.6 per cent) who were treated by surgery alone, as compared with a 9.1 per cent failure rate (3 out of 33 patients) for combined treatment. Fu et al analyzed a group of patients with positive or close surgical margins. Local recurrence occurred in 54 per cent of those who were managed with surgery alone, in contrast to only 14 per cent of those who received postoperative irradiation.[115] Survival in advanced lesions is also increased with combined treatment. Shidnia et al[116] reported 5-year survival rates of 65.4 per cent (17 of 26 patients) and 28.5 per cent (4 of 14 patients) in Stage III and Stage IV disease treated with combined treatment and surgery respectively.

Radiation alone is recommended for patients who refuse surgery, patients with unresectable lesions, and those who are medically inoperable. Shidnia et al reported 100 per cent local control in 6 patients who refused surgery and received high-dose radiotherapy.[116] A similar experience was reported by Rossman in 5 patients.[117]

References

1. Puck TT, Marcus PI: Action of x-rays on mammalian cells. J Exp Med 103:653, 1956.
2. Hewitt HB, Wilson CW: A survival curve for mammalian cells irradiated in vivo. Nature 183:1060, 1959.
3. Kligerman MM: Principles of radiation therapy. *In* Holland JF, Frei E (eds): Philadelphia, Lea & Febiger, 1973, pp 541–546.
4. Read J: The effect of ionizing radiation on the broad bean root. X. The dependents of the x-ray sensitivity on dissolved oxygen. Br J Radiol 25:89, 1952.
5. Powers WE, Tolmach LF: A multicomponent x-ray survival curve for mouse lymphosarcoma cells irradiated in vivo. Nature 197:710, 1963.
6. Thomlinson RH, Gray LH: The histological structure of some human lung cancers and the possible implications for radiotherapy. Br J Cancer 9:539, 1955.
7. Cade IS, McEwen JB: Clinical trials of radiotherapy in hyperbaric oxygen at Portsmouth—1964–1976. Clin Radiol 29:333, 1978.
8. Henk JM, Kunkler PB, Smith CW: Radiotherapy and hyperbaric oxygen in head and neck cancer. Lancet 2:101, 1977.
9. Fletcher GH: Clinical dose response curve of subclinical aggregates of epithelial cells and its practical applications in the management of human cancers. *In* Friedman M (ed): Biological and Clinical Basis of Radiosensitivity. Springfield, IL, Charles C Thomas, 1974, pp 485–501.
10. Mendelsohn ML: The biology of dose-limiting tissues. *In* Bond VP, Suit HD, Marcial V (eds): Time and Dose Relationships in Radiation Biology as Applied to Radiotherapy. Springfield, IL, Clearinghouse for Federal, Scientific, and Technical Information, 1970, pp 154–159.
11. Votava C, Fletcher GH, Jesse RH, et al: Management of cervical nodes, either fixed or bilateral, from squamous cell carcinoma of the oral cavity and faucial arch. Radiology 105:417, 1972.
12. Perez CA: Preoperative irradiation in the treatment of cancer: experimental observation and clinical implications. *In* Front. Radiation Therapy Onc. 5:1–29. Karger. Bard/Muchen/Paris/New York 1970.
13. Ketcham AS, Hoye RC, Chretien PB, et al: Irradiation twenty-four hours preoperatively. Am J Surg 118:691, 1969.
14. Merino OR, Lindberg RD, Fletcher GH: An analysis of distant metastases from squamous cell carcinoma of the upper respiratory and digestive tracts. Cancer 40:145, 1977.
15. Lawrence W Jr, Terz JJ, Rogers C, et al: Preoperative irradiation for head and neck cancer: a prospective study. Cancer 33:318, 1974.
16. Snow JB, Gelber RD, Kramer S, et al: Comparison of preoperative and postoperative radiation therapy for patients with carcinoma of the head and neck. Acta Otolaryngol 91:611, 1981.
17. Vandenbrouck C, Sancho H, Le Fur R, et al: Results of a randomized clinical trial of preoperative irradiation versus postoperative in treatment of tumors of the hypopharynx. Cancer 39:1445, 1977.
18. Joseph DL, Shumrick DA: Risks of head and neck surgery in previously irradiated patients. Arch Otolaryngol 97:381, 1973.
19. Donald PJ: Complications of combined therapy in head and neck carcinomas. Arch Otolaryngol 104:329, 1978.
20. Thawley SE: Complications of combined therapy and surgery for carcinoma of the larynx and inferior hypopharynx. Laryngoscope 91:677, 1981.
21. Vikram B: Importance of the time interval between surgery and postoperative radiation therapy in the combined management of head and neck cancer. Int J Radiat Oncol Biol Phys 5:1837, 1979.
22. Marcus RB, Million RR, Cassisi NJ: Postoperative irradiation for squamous cell carcinomas of the head and neck: analysis of time-dose factors related to control above the clavicles. Int J Radiat Oncol Biol Phys 5:1943, 1979.
23. Looser KG, Shah JP, Strong EW: The significance of positive margins in surgical resected epidermoid carcinomas. Head Neck Surg 1:107, 1978.
24. Johnson JT, Barnes EL, Myers EN, et al: The extracapsular spread of tumor in cervical node metastases. Arch Otolaryngol 107:725, 1981.
25. Steeves RA, Batrini JP: Neoplasms induced by megavoltage radiation in the head and neck region. Cancer 47:1770, 1981.
26. Kogelwik HD, Fletcher GH, Jesse RH: Clinical course of patients with squamous cell carcinoma of the upper respiratory and digestive tracts with no evidence of disease 5 years after initial treatment. Radiology 115:423, 1975.

27. American Joint Committee for Cancer Staging and End Results Reporting (AJC): Manual for Staging of Cancer. Chicago, AJC, 1978, pp 27–52.
28. Baker SR, Krause CJ: Carcinoma of the lip. Laryngoscope 90:19, 1980.
29. MacComb WS, Fletcher GH, Healey JE: Intraoral cavity. *In* MacComb WS, Fletcher GE (eds): Cancer of the Head and Neck. Baltimore, Williams & Wilkins, 1967, pp 89–151.
30. del Regato JA, Sala JM: The treatment of carcinoma of the lower lip. Radiology 73:839, 1959.
31. Petrovich Z, Kuisk H, Tobochnik N, et al: Carcinoma of the lip. Arch Otolaryngol 105:187, 1979.
32. Lindberg RD: Distribution of cervical lymph node metastases from squamous cell carcinoma of the upper respiratory and digestive tracts. Cancer 29:144, 1972.
33. Blady JV: The present status of treatment of cervical metastases from carcinoma arising in the head and neck region. Am J Roentgenol Radium Ther Nucl Med 111:56, 1971.
34. Southwick HW, Slaughter DP, Trevino EJ: Elective neck dissection for intraoral cancer. Arch Surg 80:905, 1960.
35. Ash CL: Oral cancer: a twenty-five year study. Am J Roentgenol Radium Ther Nucl Med 87:417, 1962.
36. Campos JL, Lampe I, Fayos JL: Radiotherapy of carcinoma of the floor of the mouth. Radiology 99:677, 1971.
37. Million RR: Elective neck irradiation for T_XN_0 squamous carcinoma of the oral tongue and floor of mouth. Cancer 34:149, 1974.
38. Fu KK, Lichter A, Galante M: Carcinomas of the floor of mouth: an analysis of treatment results and the sites and causes of failures. Int J Radiat Oncol Biol Phys 1:829, 1976.
39. Chu A, Fletcher GH: Incidence and causes of failure to control by irradiation the primary lesions in squamous cell carcinomas of the anterior two-thirds of tongue and floor of mouth. AJR 177:507, 1973.
40. Mendenhall WM, Van Cise WS, Bova FJ, et al: Analysis of time-dose factors in squamous cell carcinoma of the oral tongue and floor of mouth treated with radiation therapy alone. Int J Radiat Oncol Biol Phys 7:1005, 1981.
41. Guillamondegui OM, Jesse RH: Surgical treatment of advanced carcinoma of the floor of the mouth. Am J Roentgenol Radium Ther Nucl Med 126:1256, 1976.
42. Decroix Y, Ghossein NA: Experience of the Curie Institute in treatment of cancer of the mobile tongue: II. Management of the neck nodes. Cancer 47:503, 1981.
43. Decroix Y, Ghossein NA: Experience of the Curie Institute in treatment of cancer of the mobile tongue: I. Treatment policies and result. Cancer 47:496, 1981.
44. Spiro RH, Strong EW: Discontinuous partial glossectomy and radical neck dissection in selected patients with epidermoid carcinoma of the mobile tongue. Am J Surg 126:544, 1973.
45. Puthawala AA, Syed N, Neblett D: The role of afterloading (Ir^{192}) implant in the management of carcinoma of the tongue. Int J Radiat Oncol Biol Phys 7:407, 1981.
46. Pierquin B, Chassagne D, Baillet F, et al: The place of implantation in tongue and floor of mouth. JAMA 215:961, 1971.
47. White D, Byers RM: What is the preferred method of treatment for squamous cell carcinoma of the tongue? Am J Surg 140:553, 1980.
48. Hamberger AD, Fletcher GH, Guillamondegui OM, et al: Advanced squamous cell carcinoma of the oral cavity and oropharynx treated with irradiation and surgery. Radiology 119:433, 1976.
49. Fletcher GH, MacComb WS, Braun EJ: Analysis of sites and causes of treatment failure in squamous cell carcinomas of the oral cavity. Am J Roentgenol Radium Ther Nucl Med 83:405, 1960.
50. Vegers JW, Snow GB, vander Waal I: Squamous cell carcinomas of the buccal mucosa. Arch Otolaryngol 105:192, 1979.
51. Lindberg RD, Fletcher GH: The role of irradiation in the management of head and neck cancer: analysis of results and causes of failure. Tumori 64:313, 1978.
52. Bloom ND, Spiro RH: Carcinoma of the cheek mucosa: a retrospective analysis. Am J Surg 140:556, 1980.
53. Chung CK, Rahman SM, Lim ML, et al: Squamous cell carcinoma of the hard palate. Int J Radiat Oncol Biol Phys 5:191, 1979.
54. Cady B, Catlin D: Epidermoid carcinoma of the gum: a 20-year survey. Cancer 23:551, 1968.
55. Byers RM, Newman R, Russell N, et al: Results of treatment for squamous cell carcinoma of the lower gum. Cancer 47:2236, 1981.
56. Parsons JT, Million RR, Cassisi NJ: Carcinoma of the base of tongue: results of radical irradiation with surgery reserved for irradiation failures. Laryngoscope 92:689, 1982.
57. Fayos, JV: Carcinoma of the oropharynx. Radiology 138:675, 1981.
58. Spanos WJ, Shukovsky LJ, Fletcher GH: Time, dose, and tumor volume relationships in irradiation of squamous cell carcinomas of the base of tongue. Cancer 37:2591, 1976.
59. Rollo J, Rozenbom CV, Thawley S, et al: Squamous carcinoma of the base of the tongue: a clinicopathologic study of 81 cases. Cancer 47:333, 1981.
60. Whicker JH, DeSanto LW, Devine KD: Surgical treatment of carcinoma of the base of the tongue: Laryngoscope 82:1853, 1972.
61. Spiro RH, Strong EW: Surgical treatment of cancer of the tongue. Surg Clin North Am 54:759, 1974.
62. Dupont JB, Guillamondegui OM, Jesse RH: Surgical treatment of advanced carcinomas of the base of the tongue. Am J Surg 136:501, 1978.
63. Rabuzzi DD, Mickler AS, Clutter DJ, et al: Treatment results of combined high-dose preoperative radiotherapy and surgery for oropharyngeal cancer. Laryngoscope 92:989, 1982.
64. Kaplan R, Million RR, Cassisi NJ: Carcinoma of the tonsil: results of radical irradiation with surgery reserved for radiation failure. Laryngoscope 87:600, 1976.
65. Perez CA, Lee FA, Ackerman LV, et al: Nonrandomized comparison of preoperative irradiation and surgery versus irradiation alone in the management of carcinoma of the tonsil. AJR 126:248, 1976.
66. Weichert KA, Aron BS, Maltz R, et al: Carcinoma of the tonsil: treatment by a planned combination of radiation and surgery. Int J Radiat Oncol Biol Phys 1:505, 1976.
67. Shrewsbury D, Adams GL, Duvall AJ, et al: Car-

cinoma of the tonsillar region: a comparison of radiation therapy with combined preoperative radiation and surgery. Otolaryngol Head Neck Surg 89:979, 1981.

68. Healy GB, Strong MS, Uchmakli A, et al: Carcinoma of the palatine arch. Am J Surg 132:498, 1976.
69. Cheng V, Shetty KS, Deutsch M: Carcinoma of the anterior tonsillar pillar and the soft palate-uvula: treatment by radiation therapy. Radiology 134:497, 1980.
70. Chung CK, Constable WC: Squamous cell carcinoma of the soft palate and uvula. Int J Radiat Oncol Biol Phys 5:845, 1979.
71. Ratzer ER, Schweitzer RJ, Frazell EL: Epidermoid carcinoma of the palate. Am J Surg 119:294, 1970.
72. Ho JHC: An epidemiologic and clinical study of nasopharyngeal carcinomas: Int J Radiat Oncol Biol Phys 4:183, 1978.
73. Fletcher GH, Million RR: Nasopharynx. *In* Fletcher GH (ed): Textbook of Radiotherapy, 3rd ed. Philadelphia, Lea & Febiger, 1980, pp 364–388.
74. Samann NA, Bakdash MM, Caderao JB et al: Hypopituitarism after external irradiation: evidence for both hypothalamic and pituitary origin. Ann Intern Med 83:771, 1975.
75. Moench HC, Phillips TL: Carcinoma of the nasopharynx: review of 146 patients with emphasis on radiation dose and time factors. Am J Surg 124:515, 1972.
76. Chen KY, Fletcher GH: Malignant tumor of the nasopharynx. Radiology 99:165, 1971.
77. Hoppe RJ, Goffinet DR, Bagshaw MA: Carcinoma of the nasopharynx: eighteen years' experience with megavoltage radiation therapy. Cancer 37:2605, 1976.
78. Gefter JW: Carcinoma of the nasopharynx. Tenth Annual Radiation Therapy Clinical Research Seminar, April 24–26, 1980, pp 220–235. Gainesville, Florida, Division of Radiation Therapy, University of Florida, 1981.
79. Hoppe RT, Williams J, Warnke R, et al: Carcinoma of the nasopharynx—the significance of histology. Int J Radiat Oncol Biol Phys 4:199, 1978.
80. Kirchner JA, Owen JR: Five hundred cancers of the larynx and pyriform sinus. Results of treatment by radiation and surgery. Laryngoscope 87:1288, 1977.
81. Ogura JH, Sessions DG, Spector GJ: Conservation surgery for epidermoid carcinoma of the supraglottic larynx. Laryngoscope 85:1808, 1975.
82. Cashin Y: Supraglottic carcinomas: the early cases. Laryngoscope 85:1617, 1975.
83. Biller MF, Davis WH, Ogura JM: Delayed contralateral cervical metastases with laryngeal and laryngopharyngeal cancers. Laryngoscope 81:1449, 1971.
84. Ghossein NA, Bataini JP, Ennuyer A, et al: Local control and site of failure in radically irradiated supraglottic laryngeal cancer. Radiology 112:187, 1974.
85. Fletcher GH, Lindberg RD, Hamberger A, et al: Reasons for irradiation failure in squamous cell carcinoma of the larynx. Laryngoscope 85:987, 1975.
86. Goepfert H, Jesse RH, Fletcher GH, et al: Optimal treatment for the technically resectable squamous cell carcinoma of the supraglottic larynx. Laryngoscope 85:14, 1977.
87. Fletcher GH, Lindberg RD, Hamberger A: Reasons for irradiation failure in squamous cell carcinoma of the larynx. Laryngoscope 85:987, 1975.
88. Harwood AR, Hawkins WV, Beale FA, et al: Management of advanced glottic cancer: a 10-year review of the Toronto experience. Int J Radiat Oncol Biol Phys 5:899, 1979.
89. Ogura JH, Sessions DG, Spector GJ: Analysis of surgical therapy for epidermoid carcinoma of the laryngeal glottis. Laryngoscope 85:1522, 1975.
90. Woodhouse RJ, Quivey JM, Fu KK, et al: Treatment of carcinoma of the vocal cord: a review of 20 years' experience. Laryngoscope 91:1155, 1981.
91. Keim WF, Shapiro MJ, Rosin HD: Study of postlaryngectomy stomal recurrence. Arch Otolaryngol 81:183, 1965.
92. Schneider JJ, Lindberg RD, Jesse RH: Prevention of tracheal stomal recurrence after total laryngectomy by postoperative irradiation. J Surg Oncol 7:187, 1975.
93. El Badaw SA, Goepfert H, Herson J: Squamous cell carcinoma of the pyriform sinus. Laryngoscope 92:357, 1982.
94. Ballantyne AJ: Principles of surgical management of cancer of the pharyngeal walls. Cancer 20:663, 1967.
95. Wang, CC: Radiotherapeutic management of carcinoma of the posterior pharyngeal wall. Cancer 24:894, 1971.
96. Talton BM, Elkon D, Kim J, et al: Cancer of the posterior pharyngeal wall. Int J Radiat Oncol Biol Phys 7:597, 1981.
97. Meoz-Mendez RT, Fletcher GH, Guillamondegui OM, Peters LJ: Analysis of the results of irradiation in the treatment of squamous cell carcinoma of the pharyngeal walls. Int J Radiat Oncol Biol Phys 4:579, 1978.
98. Marks JE, Freeman RB, Lee F, et al: Pharyngeal wall cancer: an analysis of treatment results, complications and patterns of failure. Int J Radiat Oncol Biol Phys 4:587, 1978.
99. Million RR, Cassisi NJ: Radical irradiation for carcinoma of the pyriform sinus. Laryngoscope 91:439, 1981.
100. Goldman JL, Silverstone SM, Roffman JD, et al: High dosage pre-operative radiation and surgery for carcinoma of the larynx and laryngopharynx—a 14-year program. Laryngoscope 82:1869, 1972.
101. Wang, CC: Treatment of carcinoma of the nasal vestibule by irradiation. Cancer 38:100, 1976.
102. Badib AO, Kurohara SS, Webster JH, et al: Treatment of cancer of the nasal cavity. Am J Roentgenol Radium Ther Nucl Med 106:824, 1969.
103. Chung CT, Rabuzzi DD, Sagerman RH, et al: Radiotherapy for carcinoma of the nasal cavity. Arch Otolaryngol 106:763, 1980.
104. Lee F, Ogura JH: Maxillary sinus carcinoma. Laryngoscope 91:133, 1981.
105. Ahmad K, Cordoba RB, Fayos JV: Squamous cell carcinoma of the maxillary sinus. Arch Otolaryngol 107:48, 1981.
106. Ellingwood KE, Million RR: Cancer of the nasal cavity and ethmoid/sphenoid sinuses. Cancer 43:1517, 1979.
107. Frazell EL, Lewis JS: Cancer of the nasal cavity and accessory sinuses. Cancer 16:1293, 1963.
108. Elkon D, Hightower SI, Lim ML, et al: Esthesioneuroblastoma. Cancer 44:1087, 1979.
109. Cheng VS, Wang CC: Carcinomas of the paranasal sinuses. Cancer 40:3038, 1971.

110. Amendola BE, Eisert D, Hazna TA, et al: Carcinoma of the maxillary antrum: surgery or radiation therapy. Int J Radiat Oncol Biol Phys 7:743, 1981.
110a. Jesse RH: Preoperative versus postoperative radiation in the treatment of squamous carcinoma of the paranasal sinuses. Am J Surg 110:552, 1965.
111. Spiro R, Huvos A, Strong E: Cancer of the parotid gland. Am J Surg 130:452, 1975.
112. Beahrs OH, Woolner LB, Carveth SW, et al: Surgical management of parotid lesions. Review of 760 cases. Arch Surg 80:890, 1960.
113. Tapley N, Guillamondegui O, Byers R: The place of irradiation in the treatment of the salivary glands. Curr Probl Cancer, 1:13, 1976.
114. Tapley ND: Irradiation treatment of malignant tumors of the salivary glands. Ear Nose Throat J 56:110, 1977.
115. Fu KK, Leibel SA, Levine ML, et al: Carcinoma of the major and minor salivary glands: analysis of treatment results and sites and causes of failures. Cancer 40:2882, 1977.
116. Shidnia H, Hornbach NB, Hamaker R, et al: Carcinoma of major salivary glands. Cancer 45:693, 1980.
117. Rossman, KJ: The role of radiation therapy in the treatment of parotid carcinomas. Am J Roentgenol Radium Ther Nucl Med 123:492, 1975.

13

CHEMOTHERAPY

Bernard R. Greenberg, M.D.

The treatment of head and neck cancer with chemotherapy, until recently, offered little hope of significantly prolonging the lives of patients, in spite of the fact that carcinoma of the head and neck region is in general more sensitive to the effects of chemotherapy than are solid tumors in the majority of other sites. Usually patients selected for systemic chemotherapy have already failed surgical and radiation therapeutic attempts at controlling their cancer, have far advanced disease, and are poorly nourished. Despite these negative factors, however, a sizable porportion of these patients were observed to have some reduction in the size of their tumor. The use of the intraarterial route, and combined irradiation and chemotherapy have not gained wide acceptance because of the enhanced toxicity that occurred with these methods with only marginal improvements in survival. Furthermore, the early trials of combination chemotherapy did not meet with the same success in head and neck cancer as they did in other varieties such as Hodgkin's disease and testicular carcinoma. In addition, the early clinical studies were plagued by the lack of prospective randomized trials and the failure to analyze several important prognostic features.

During the past several years, however, we have seen a resurgence of interest in the role of chemotherapy in the management of patients with head and neck cancer. This renewed interest is due to several factors, including the introduction of new and effective agents, better methods of administering older agents, and, perhaps most important, acceptance of the need for treating patients early, while they are still well-nourished and before prior therapy has severely limited the access of chemotherapeutic drugs to the site of the tumor. Many important clinical trials of early chemotherapy are now in progress, and the preliminary results of some appear promising.

The treatment of the majority of patients with head and neck cancer requires a truly multidisciplinary approach. The efforts of surgeons, radiation therapists, medical oncologists, prosthodontists, and pathologists are necessary for a successful outcome. All involved in this treatment should understand the principles and current applications of chemotherapy for head and neck cancer patients. In this chapter I will review the factors influencing the response to chemotherapy, the most commonly used agents and their mechanism of action, combination and intraarterial chemotherapy, irradiation plus chemotherapy, and finally, what is probably the most promising area, the preoperative and preirradiation administration of single or multiple agents.

FACTORS AFFECTING RESPONSE

Until recently, the site of origin was disregarded as an important prognostic factor. In fact, in most studies the site is not even mentioned. Bertino was the first to bring the importance of site to our attention by describing the responses he observed with methotrexate therapy according to site of origin.[1] He observed that the highest frequency of responses occurred in lesions of the oral cavity and oropharynx, with intermediate frequency in laryngeal lesions and lowest frequency in lesions of the hypopharynx and nasopharynx.[1] Furthermore, tonsillar and oral tongue lesions had the longest responses, whereas palatal, oropharyngeal, floor of mouth, and hypopharyngeal had the shortest. Thus, some of the sites with high frequency of response (e.g., oropharynx) were associated with a short median duration of response (2 months), while other sites (e.g., hypopharynx) had both a low frequency of response and a short duration.

The stage or extent of disease affects the likelihood of a beneficial effect. The smaller primaries, T_1 and T_2, are much more likely to respond than massive T_4 lesions, which may contain poorly perfused portions that may not receive an adequate concentration of the chemotherapeutic agent.

Prior therapy with surgery or irradiation will significantly affect the chances for response to chemotherapy, particularly as regards the possibility of a complete response. Both surgery and irradiation may severely limit the blood supply to the tumor. In addition, in previously treated lesions more tumor cells may be in a latent or resting stage (G_0) and thus be less responsive to drugs such as methotrexate, which exert their effect on dividing cells.

Equally important is the increased toxicity observed following prior therapy, especially radiation therapy. Mucositis is a common side effect accompanying the administration of two widely used agents, methotrexate and bleomycin. In patients who have received prior radiation therapy, particularly in the previous 6 months, the frequency, severity, and duration of mucositis is markedly increased.

The patient's overall clinical status, usually stated in terms of the Karnofsky performance score, also affects the chances for response and toxicity.[2] In general, debilitated patients with a low performance status are poor candidates for chemotherapy, whether it be single agent or combination therapy

Next to prior therapy, the patient's nutritional status is perhaps the most important factor in determining tolerance to chemotherapy. Many patients are poorly nourished and deficient in folic acid, making them very susceptible to the side effects of methotrexate, particularly mucositis. One of the primary reasons for the poor nutritional status is dysphagia, which may be due to local tumor growth, radiation-induced fibrosis, surgical defects, or pharyngocutaneous fistulas. Before initiating chemotherapy, it is important to restore patients to an adequate nutritional status, a process that may require parenteral alimentation in some patients.

All of the factors discussed above significantly affect the frequency, magnitude, and duration of response and accompanying side effects of chemotherapy. They also contribute to the wide variation in responses and toxicity reported with similar treatment regimens. A comparison between regimens is of little value unless these factors are included in the final analysis.

In discussing response to chemotherapy, the terms "complete response," "partial response," and "stable disease" are usually used. Complete response (CR) is defined as a complete resolution of all measurable disease, without the appearance of new lesions and accompanied by symptomatic improvement. Partial response (PR) is defined as a 50 per cent reduction in the product of the diameters of the lesions followed, without the appearance of new lesions. Stable disease refers to a response that is less in magnitude than a PR.

SYSTEMIC CHEMOTHERAPY WITH SINGLE AGENTS

Before discussing the individual agents employed in the treatment of head and neck cancer, I would like to briefly review the general principles of cancer chemotherapy. The drugs employed can be divided into those that affect the DNA macromolecule directly, such as alkylating agents (e.g., nitrogen mustard, cyclophosphamide) and antitumor antibiotics (e.g., bleomycin, adriamycin), and those that affect the biosynthesis of nucleic acids (e.g., the antimetabolites). The alkylating agents produce cross-linkages between the single strands of DNA so they cannot separate for replication. Bleomycin produces scission of single-stranded DNA. Methotrexate, an antimetabolite, is structurally similar to folic acid and competes for the enzyme dihydrofolate reductase. A block is produced in the conversion of dihydrofolate to tetrahydrofolate, interfering with the synthesis of thymidylate, a nucleic acid, and thus blocking DNA synthesis. The mechanism of action of *cis*-platinum has not been well established, but it is thought to behave like an alkylating agent.

The renewing populations of cells that make up the bone marrow, mucous mem-

Table 13–1. ACTIVITY OF CONVENTIONAL DOSES OF SYSTEMIC METHOTREXATE*

Dose Schedule	No. of Patients	Number of Responses† PR	CR	Investigator(s)
Weekly or Biweekly				
25–50 mg q 4–7 days IV	27	14	4	Lane et al[4]
60 mg/m²/wk IV or 40 mg/m² 2 × wk	35	20	11	Leone et al[5]
40 or 60 mg/m²/wk IV	23	8	—	DePalo et al[6]
15–100 mg/m²/wk IV	40	3	—	Priestman[7]
Monthly				
25 mg/day × 5 IV	23	4	—	Papac et al[8]
15–20 mg/day × 5 PO	23	4	—	Papac et al[8]

*Modified from Carter SK: The chemotherapy of head and neck cancer. Semin Oncol 4:413, 1977.
†PR = partial response; CR = complete response

branes, gametes, and hair follicles are the most susceptible to injury by chemotherapeutic agents. Thus, bone marrow suppression, mucositis, and alopecia are common side effects. With the introduction of new agents such as bleomycin and *cis*-platinum, unusual and severe toxicities such as pulmonary fibrosis and renal failure have been observed.

Methotrexate. No other agent has been as widely used in the treatment of head and neck cancer as methotrexate. However, despite many years of experience, questions still remain regarding the best route and schedule of administration. Methotrexate may be administered intravenously, orally, intramuscularly or intra-arterially. The majority of this compound is excreted unmetabolized in the urine, and thus the dose must be markedly reduced in patients with renal impairment. The principal side effects include leukopenia, mucositis, and reversible abnormalities in liver enzymes, particularly SGOT.

When administered systemically, methotrexate is usually given intravenously, weekly or biweekly. This schedule produces a partial remission in about one third to one half of patients and appears superior to monthly courses, which are usually given for 5 consecutive days. The full dose of methotrexate on a once-weekly schedule is about 60 mg/m², but many investigators start at a lower dose (e.g., 40 mg/m²) and escalate in small increments until moderate toxicity develops. Patients heavily treated with radiation therapy will frequently develop significant and sometimes prolonged mucositis at a weekly dose considerably below 60 mg/m².

Table 13–1 is a summary of studies employing conventional doses of methotrexate on a weekly, biweekly, or monthly schedule. The best results were reported by Leone[5] with a weekly or biweekly schedule. Though the total response rate of 57 per cent and the complete response of 31 per cent are impressive, the duration of complete response of only 17 weeks is disappointing and is responsible for only a minimal prolongation of survival. In Table 13–2 are listed the responses to systemic methotrexate as a function of the site of origin of the tumor.

Methotrexate with Leucovorin. In an attempt to improve the therapeutic index of methotrexate, investigators have employed high doses followed by the administration of citrovorum factor or leucovorin (leucovorin rescue). Methotrexate competitively inhibits the activity of the enzyme dihydrofolate reductase. Citrovorum factor is N_5N_{10} formyl tetrahydrofolate, the usual product of the reaction the agent inhibits, and when administered it prevents most of the toxicity of the high-dose methotrexate—hence the use of

Table 13–2. RESPONSE TO SYSTEMIC METHOTREXATE AS A FUNCTION OF SITE OF ORIGIN*

Site	No. of Patients	Response Rate (%)	Median Duration of Response (Months)
Palate	6	67	2.0
Oropharynx	5	60	2.0
Alveolar ridge	9	56	2.8
Tonsil	10	50	4.5
Tongue			
Oral	10	50	4.2
Posterior	6	50	2.8
Floor of mouth	10	50	2.0
Larynx	9	44	2.5
Nasopharynx	4	25	—
Hypopharynx	17	18	2.3

*Data from Bertino JR, Boston B, Capizzi RL: The role of chemotherapy in the management of cancer of the head and neck: a review. Cancer 36:752, 1975.

Table 13–3. SYSTEMIC MODERATE AND HIGH DOSE METHOTREXATE (MTX) PLUS CITROVORUM RESCUE*

Investigator(s)	*Time of MTX Infusion (hr)*	*Dose (g/m²)*	*No. of Responding Patients (%)*
Levitt et al[9]	36–42	0.24–0.36 (to 1.08 maximum)	11/28 (39)
Mills[10]	4	0.1	11/28 (39)
Capizzi et al[11]	24	0.24	13/21 (62)
Khandekar & Wolff[12]	24	0.50–4.00	24/32 (75)
Buechler et al[13]	24	0.60–2.00	6/28 (21)
Woods et al[14]	Bolus	0.5	7/27 (26)
DeConti & Schoenfeld[15]	Bolus	0.24	19/80 (24)

*Modified from Muggia FM, Rozencweig M, Louie AE: Role of chemotherapy in head and neck cancer: Systemic use of single agents and combinations in advanced disease. Head Neck Surg 2:196, 1980.

the term "rescue." The exact mechanism of the potentially improved therapeutic effectiveness of high-dose methotrexate with rescue is unknown, but it is postulated that normal cells possess a common carrier transport mechanism for citrovorum factor and methotrexate that is lacking in tumor cells. When a very high concentration of methotrexate is reached (10^{-3} to 10^{-4} mole), it enters the tumor cells by diffusion or another mechanism. However, citrovorum factor cannot enter these cells because of the absence of the transport mechanism. Both methotrexate and citrovorum factor enter normal host cells that contain the carrier transport mechanism. Thus, normal cells are "rescued," while tumor cells are not.

One of the first studies employing high-dose methotrexate with leucovorin rescue in head and neck cancer patients was reported by Levitt et al in 1973.[9] In this study, 16 patients received maximally tolerated doses of methotrexate alone in 30-hour infusions, and 44 per cent responded. Singificant leukopenia was noted, and there were four drug-related deaths. Twenty-five patients received higher doses of methotrexate followed by leucovorin rescue, which produced a 60 per cent response rate and fewer instances of severe toxicity. Though the response rate was higher with the combined approach, the median duration of response was only 11 weeks (12 weeks with methotrexate alone). Since this initial study, numerous others have been reported with variable results. In Table 13–3 are listed studies with 20 or more patients.

Woods et al[14] recently reported on the results of a study in which 72 patients were randomized to receive weekly methotrexate at three different dose levels. No significant difference in duration of survival was observed between those patients who received low-dose (50 mg/m²), medium-dose (500 mg/m²), or high-dose (5 g/m²) methotrexate. The higher response rate in the high-dose group was offset by increased toxicity, and these authors could not recommend high-dose methotrexate as initial therapy. This is in agreement with the results of a large prospective randomized trial conducted by the Eastern Cooperative Oncology Group and reported by DeConti and Schoenfeld.[15] In this study, 259 patients with Stage III and Stage IV cancers were randomized to receive either weekly standard doses (40–60 mg/m²), moderately high doses biweekly (240 mg/m²) with leucovorin, or moderately high doses with leucovorin combined with cyclophosphamide and cytosine arabinoside. Little difference was observed in the response rates between the three arms, but the standard methotrexate alone arm had the best duration of response and survival. Thus, this study also failed to confirm an improved therapeutic index for moderately high dose methotrexate with leucovorin rescue and confirmed that the weekly IV schedule with conventional doses is the standard with which other schedules and combinations must be compared. One possible criticism of this latter study is that higher doses of methotrexate (e.g., 1–7 g/m²) were not included in the comparison.

Considering the duration of response, toxicity, cost, and nursing and medical time necessary for administration, moderate- or high-dose methotrexate does not appear superior to a weekly schedule with conventional (low) doses. The higher-dose approach should be reserved for clinical research trials and optimally should include a comparison with different dose levels. Using conventional doses we can expect that approximately 30 to 50 per cent of patients will respond, with the majority of responses being partial in extent and several months in duration. This therapy is usually well tolerated, the principal side effects being mucositis (greater in heavily irradiated patients) and leukopenia.

Bleomycin. Bleomycin is the next most frequently studied chemotherapeutic agent in the treatment of head and neck cancer. It is the generic name for a group of antibiotics isolated from *Streptomyces verticillus*. The optimal route of administration—i.e., either intravenous bolus, intramuscular injection, or continuous intravenous infusion—has not been well established, although the last is theoretically superior. This drug is concentrated in the skin and lungs, and common side effects include dermatitis (particularly involving the hands) and pulmonary toxicity. Though the dermatitis is rarely severe, the pulmonary toxicity may be fatal. This latter complication is more frequent in patients who are elderly and have underlying lung disease. Other side effects include mucositis (most pronounced in previously irradiated areas), fever, and chills. Since bleomycin is not myelosuppressive, it quickly became a popular agent, especially in combination regimens.

The response rates observed with bleomycin as a single agent range between 6 and 45 per cent.[3] The dose and route of administration also vary considerably. A good estimate of the chance for response is in the range of 15 to 25 per cent; however, this figure may be depressed because many patients had been previously treated with methotrexate. The responses to bleomycin are short, averaging 3 months, and are rarely complete. Further studies employing the continuous infusion route and the simultaneous administration with radiation therapy are now under way, but presently this agent must be considered inferior to methotrexate.

***Cis*-platinum.** *Cis*-platinum or *cis*-diamminedichloroplatinum 11 (DDP) is a newly released drug that has already assumed a major role in the chemotherapy of advanced head and neck cancer. Although the overall response rate in previously treated patients is only about 30 per cent (Table 13–4), the responses appear early and the duration is usually longer than that observed with other single agents.[17] Most exciting, however, is the very high response rate—approaching 70 per cent—obtained in previously untreated patients with less advanced disease. This agent is now being used prior to surgery and radiation therapy in patients with advanced operable disease or in combination with radiation therapy in inoperable patients. This will be discussed later.

Cis-platinum must be administered intravenously, but neither the optimal dose (high vs. low) nor the optimal method (bolus vs. continuous infusion) has yet been established. The principal toxicity is renal, causing tubular damage, and this may be irreversible and fatal. Since this is dependent upon drug concentration, it may be significantly reduced or prevented by vigorous diuresis. Many oncologists employ mannitol or furosemide together with generous amounts of intravenous saline, and this has reduced the nephrotoxicity considerably. Nausea with vomiting is another major side effect and is frequently refractory to antiemetics. Other side effects include anorexia, tinnitus, high-frequency hearing loss, and moderate myelosuppression. In spite of its toxicities, this agent is very active, particularly when administered early in the treatment course. It may also be effectively and safely employed in various combination regimens.

Information on the other standard cancer chemotherapeutic agents in head and neck cancer is much less complete, and the response rates may be falsely high because of the lack of uniform response criteria. The only drug for which data on more than 100 patients is available is 5-fluorouracil (5-FU), with an overall response rate of 15 per cent. This drug, however, has undergone more extensive studies when used in combination with radiation therapy. Less experience has been accumulated with the standard alkylating agents, cyclophosphamide and mechlorethamine (nitrogen mustard). In Table 13–5

Table 13–4. *CIS*-PLATINUM AS A SINGLE AGENT IN RECURRENT HEAD AND NECK CANCER*

Year of Study and Reference	*Dose*	*No. of Patients*	*CR† (Duration in Months)*	*PR† (Duration in Months)*	*CR + PR (%)*
1977[18]	3 mg/kg q 3 wk	26	2(2+,6+)	6(1−,8+)	31
1978[19]	40 mg/m²/wk	13	1(2)	3(1+,2,3+)	31
1978[20]	80 mg/m² q 3 wk	18	1(6+)	6(4)	39
1978[21]	50 mg/m²/days 1 & 8 q 4 wk	26	—	8	31
1978[22]	120 mg/m² q 3 wk	15	2(7)	3(4)	33
	20 mg/m² days 1–5 q 3 wk	15	1(8)	3(4)	27

*Modified from Jacobs C: The role of cisplatin in the treatment of recurrent head and neck cancer. *In* Prestayko AW, Crooke ST, Carter SK (eds): Cisplatin: Current Status and New Developments. New York, Academic Press, 1980, Chapter 30.

†CR = complete response; PR = partial response. Plus sign indicates duration was longer than the described number of months; minus sign means duration was less than the described number of months.

Table 13–5. ACTIVITY OF SINGLE AGENTS IN HEAD AND NECK CANCER ADMINISTERED SYSTEMICALLY (EXCLUDING METHOTREXATE AND *CIS*-PLATINUM)*

Drug	No. of Evaluable Patients	No. of Patients with 50% Regression	Overal Response Rate (%)	Range of Response Rates (%)
Bleomycin	298	64 (10 complete)	22	6–45
5-Fluorouracil	118	18	15	0–33
Cyclophosphamide	77	28	36	0–39
Mechlorethamine	66	5	7.5	0–12
6-Mercaptopurine	45	6	12	0–15.6
Vinblastine	35	10	29	—
Chlorambucil	34	5	14.7	—
Doxorubicin	34	8	23	—
Procarbazine	31	3	10	—
Hydroxyurea	18	7	39	—

*Modified from Carter SK: The chemotherapy of head and neck cancer. Semin Oncol 4:413, 1977.

the activity of single agents, excluding methotrexate and *cis*-platinum, is summarized.

COMBINATION CHEMOTHERAPY

Until recently, little experience had been acquired in the use of combination chemotherapy in head and neck cancer. Although numerous studies have been conducted in the past several years and many are still in progress, the superiority of combination chemotherapy over use of a single agent remains to be established. This is unlike the experience in acute leukemia, lymphomas, and certain solid tumors (such as testicular and breast carcinomas), in which combination regimens have been amply demonstrated to be far superior to single agents, not infrequently resulting in cures despite widespread disease.

The principles of combination chemotherapy remain the same for all types of malignancies. Only agents that have been shown to be effective as single agents are combined in a regimen. A desired but not always achieved goal is to combine agents with non-overlapping toxicities, so that full or nearly full doses of each drug can be given. In the formulation of a combination, it may be helpful to select drugs in which there is a biochemical basis for synergism. Ideally, the drugs should have different mechanisms of action at the molecular level and act at different points in the cell cycle. Most combinations are administered in brief courses, to allow for recovery of marrow and immunologic function. The most important thing, however, is to select drugs that have been proved to be effective and that have non-overlapping toxicities.

Combinations of drugs are considered to be more effective than single agents because of the additive effects of full or nearly full doses of two or more potent agents. In addition, synergistic effects may be observed that can be significantly greater than the expected additive effects. Finally, combinations may prevent or delay the appearance of a population of resistant tumor cells.

Certainly there is no lack of drugs with non-overlapping toxicities capable of producing at least a partial shrinkage of head and neck cancers. However, most of the earlier studies with combinations yielded disappointing results accompanied by increased toxicity. The combination of bleomycin and methotrexate has been studied by several investigators without demonstrating an advantage over the use of either agent alone.[23–25] The increased incidence of mucositis was expected; however, the severe bone marrow suppression occasionally encountered was not. Other regimens usually employ three or more drugs, and though there may be a slight increase in response frequency, the median duration of remission is frequently short; thus responders experience only a minimal survival advantage. The "COB-MAM" from M.D. Anderson Hospital utilizes six different agents (cyclophosphamide, vincristine, bleomycin, methotrexate, adriamycin, and methyl CCNU), all with some activity in head and neck cancer, but unfortunately the response frequency of this combination is inferior to what one would have anticipated with such an aggressive regimen.[26] An 18 per cent complete response (CR) rate (5/28) and a 25 per cent partial response (PR) rate (7/28) were reported, yielding a total response rate of only 43 per cent, not dissimilar to the results reported for methotrexate alone, although with COB-MAM more CR's were obtained. The median duration of response to "COB-MAM" is a highly respectable 25 weeks, which appears to be superior to single agent therapy. However, toxicity is much greater.

Before the availability of *cis*-platinum, the majority of regimens contained methotrexate, bleomycin, vincristine, and an alkylating agent, such as cyclophosphamide. In most studies with combinations there is only one treatment arm; i.e., no comparison is made with single-agent therapy. Furthermore, in many studies important prognostic factors have not been carefully analyzed. It is apparent, however, that patients who have been treated with both surgery and radiation therapy and who may be in a precarious nutritional balance can still tolerate rather aggressive chemotherapy.

In Table 13–6 are summarized the results of combinations not containing *cis*-platinum. It is difficult to draw adequate conclusions from these studies, owing to lack of randomization and other factors. In addition, although the number of total and complete responses in some studies is encouraging, the impact on survival frequently is minimal. For example, in the study of Holoye et al[30] the median survival time of the complete responders (42 weeks) was only 7 weeks greater than that for partial responders (35 weeks), and only 13 weeks greater than for nonresponders (29 weeks). The combination reported by Cortes et al[34] is probably the most promising. In this regimen bleomycin was administered by continuous intravenous infusion for 3 days in the majority of patients and was well tolerated. One third of the responses were complete, with a median duration of 11 months. An impact on survival was demonstrated by the 15-month median survival of complete responders versus only 4 months for patients with progressive disease. In this study, 84 per cent of the patients had been previously treated with radiation therapy. It would be unusual to see complete remissions of this duration with single-agent therapy in previously treated patients. This leads one to feel that perhaps the increased toxicities of combination chemotherapy are justified because of the potential for occasionally producing sustained remissions and a favorable impact on survival.

A number of studies on the use of *cis*-platinum in combination with other agents have already been reported. The popularity of this new agent in combinations was to be

Table 13–6. COMBINATION CHEMOTHERAPY NOT INCLUDING *CIS*-PLATINUM ADMINISTERED SYSTEMICALLY (20 OR MORE PATIENTS)

Regimen*	No. of Evaluable Patients	Response Rate (%) Total	Response Rate (%) Complete	Duration of Response (R) or Survival (S) (Months)†	Reference
"COB-MAM" (CTX-VCR-BLM/MTX-ADM-MeCCNU)	28	43	18	6 (R)	26
VCR-BLM-MTX	42	71	10	Not indicated	27, 28
CTX-ADM-MTX-BLM	26	35	0	2.5 (R)	29
BLM-CTX-VCR-MTX-5FU	22	59	18	CR: 42 wk (S) PR: 35 wk (S) NR: 29 wk (S)	30
VCR-BLM-MTX-HCT-5FU + LV	68	63	Not indicated	Not indicated	31
VLB-MTX-BLM	33	27	9	CR: 14 (R) PR: 4 (R)	32
VLB-BLM-MTX (low-dose)	60	62	32	CR: 6.9 (R) PR: 3.9 (R)	33
BLM-CTX-MTX-5FU	39	54	18	CR: 15 (S); 11 (R) PR: 10 (S); 7 (R) NR: 4 (S)	34
CTX-BCNU-ADM	31	35	3	PR: 8.8 (S)	35

*CTX = Cytoxan (cyclophosphamide); VCR = vincristine; BLM = bleomycin; MTX = methotrexate; ADM = Adriamycin (doxorubicin); MeCCNU = methyl CCNU; 5FU = 5-fluorouracil; VLB = Velban (vinblastine); HCT = hydrocortisone; LV = leucovorin

†CR = complete response; PR = partial response; NR = no response

expected, since it produces no mucositis and only mild or moderate myelosuppression. Employing hydration with mannitol and/or furosemide, several investigators have amply demonstrated relative safety from nephrotoxicity in head and neck cancer patients. The emesis and anorexia produced by *cis*-platinum remains formidable, and it is not uncommon for patients to discontinue therapy even though they are responding satisfactorily.

In Table 13–7, the results of several recently reported regimens that include *cis*-platinum are summarized. In most it is apparent that previously untreated patients have a total and complete response rate superior to that of previously treated patients. Since untreated patients usually receive surgery or radiation therapy following chemotherapy, the duration of response cannot be ascertained. Certainly the response rates in excess of 70 per cent with complete responses in the range of 18 to 22 per cent seen when chemotherapy is used as initial therapy are promising enough to consider the greater use of *cis*-platinum–containing regimens prior to surgery or radiation therapy in patients presenting with advanced (T_3 and T_4) tumors. Whether or not this will improve survival is now being evaluated in a randomized study sponsored by the National Cancer Institute. The role of chemotherapy as initial therapy is discussed further later on in this chapter.

Although the majority of investigators hospitalize patients receiving *cis*-platinum, Vogl and Kaplan[40] have satisfactorily demonstrated that with hydration and diuresis a dose of 50 mg/m^2 can be administered in combination on an outpatient basis with only a minor risk of mild nephrotoxicity. Furthermore, their regimen produced a high response rate in previously treated patients, as well as a long duration of complete remission resulting in substantially improved survival.

With careful attention to hydration and diuresis the nephrotoxicity of *cis*-platinum has been minimized, thus making emesis and anorexia the major toxicities. Use of the newer antiemetics, alone or in combinations, has resulted in adequate control of emesis in a substantial proportion of patients. Further studies, particularly randomized trials, will be necessary to document whether regimens containing *cis*-platinum are significantly superior to those not containing this agent to justify utilizing the drug despite these side effects.

INTRAARTERIAL CHEMOTHERAPY

Intraarterial chemotherapy in head and neck cancer was first introduced over 20 years ago; however, considerable controversy still exists as to its efficacy and superiority over systemic chemotherapy. With this route of administration chemotherapeutic agents, singly or in combination, are continually infused into the arterial blood supply of the cancer, usually through the aid of a bedside or portable infusion pump. The drugs are infused over several hours or days, and usually this is followed with a course of radiation therapy or surgery. This form of therapy has been administered to patients with advanced cancers who have a high incidence of local recurrence following standard therapy. By producing significant tumor shrinkage it is expected that some inoperable tumors may become operable or that the chances for complete eradication with radiation therapy will be improved.

With intraarterial administration, higher regional concentrations of cytoxic agents are produced than can be achieved safely with the systemic route. The tumor is thus exposed to high levels of active drug, while other areas—such as the bone marrow and gastrointestinal tract—are exposed to much lower levels, resulting in less toxicity. Furthermore, extraction by the liver of active drug and metabolites may aid in lowering systemic toxicity.

Despite these theoretical advantages, the complications and need for technical expertise and hospitalization have tended to limit the use of intraarterial chemotherapy in the United States, although many European investigators still advocate its application. The complications are frequently local and include thrombosis, skin infection, leakage of drug, and slippage of the catheter. Distal vascular complications (i.e., embolization) and systemic toxicity have also been reported.

An accurate evaluation of this method of administering cytotoxic chemotherapy is extremely difficult owing to the lack of randomized trials involving, for example, intraarterial versus standard systemic chemotherapy in patients of equal stage and performance status. In reviewing the literature on this form of treatment, one is struck by the diversity of chemotherapy regimens and the duration

Table 13–7. SYSTEMIC COMBINATION CHEMOTHERAPY WITH *CIS*-PLATINUM

		Response Rate (%)					
		Previously Untreated Patients		*Previously Treated Patients*			
Regimen*	**Number of Evaluable Patients**	*Total*	*Complete*	*Total*	*Complete*	**Duration of Response (R) or Survival (S) (Months)†**	**Reference**
CP-BLM	21	71	19			Received RT following chemotherapy	36
CP-BLM	39	76	20			Many patients underwent surgery after chemotherapy	37
CP-BLM-HDMTX + LV (single course only)	26	73	18	55	0		38
MTX-BLM-CP (high-dose)	19			58	16	4 (R)	39
MTX-BLM-CP (outpatient schedule)	31			61	22.5	CR: 13 (R) PR: 3 (R)	40
MTX-VLB-BLM-CP	21	48	0			Patients received RT or surgery post chemotherapy	41
CP-MTX-BLM-VCR	29			24	10	CR: 8.7+ (R) PR: 7.7+ (R)	42
CP-VCR-BLM (single course only)	27	40	0	50	0	Not indicated	43
VLB-BLM-CP	45	74	22	45	9	Untreated: 10 (R) Previously treated: 4 (R)	44

*CP = *cis*-platinum; BLM = bleomycin; HDMTX = high-dose methotrexate; LV = leucovorin; VLB = Velban (vinblastine); VCR = vincristine
†RT = radiation therapy; CR = complete response; PR = partial response

of administration of drugs. Furthermore, although this is not usually mentioned in the reports, one tends to believe that patients selected for intraarterial chemotherapy are as a group probably in a higher performance status and have more localized disease than patients receiving systemic chemotherapy.

Carter, in a 1977 review of the literature on continuous intraarterial infusion of methotrexate,[3] found a 53 per cent cumulative response rate in 340 cases. This response rate is similar to the one obtained with systemic methotrexate. Furthermore, in several of the intraarterial studies considerable toxicity was reported which not infrequently led to fatalities. In one series with 25 patients, 4 treatment deaths were reported, and in another larger series with 68 patients, 8 succumbed to hemorrhage and 4 had major embolization.[3]

The choice of methotrexate as the agent for intraarterial administration may be a poor one. This drug is highly diffusible, and with the intraarterial route only slightly higher tissue levels are achieved in the region supplied by the artery as compared with intravenous injection. In addition, this drug is strongly dependent on time of exposure for its cytotoxicity.[45]

With modern radiographic equipment precision positioning of the catheter for selective intraarterial injection is now much less difficult. In more recent studies, the complications reported are usually less serious and less frequent, but they still remain a problem. Investigators now have several active agents to choose from in place of methotrexate as a single agent. Table 13–8 summarizes the results of some of the more recent studies, the majority of which have been conducted outside of the United States. Having been disappointed with the earlier results, investigators in this country apparently are reluctant to use this technique.

It is evident that, as with systemic chemotherapy, intraarterial therapy is most effective in previously untreated patients. The high response rate reported by Donegan and Harris[46] in previously treated patients was associated with only brief remissions, which tend to have little impact on survival. The complication rate remains quite varied, and it appears that combining agents results in greater toxicity. Unfortunately, because of the lack of randomized studies, we cannot properly evaluate the role of intraarterial chemotherapy and determine whether it is superior to systemic chemotherapy or preoperative radiation therapy alone with regard to local control and survival. Further clinical trials should focus on advanced tumors in the oral region with clinically negative nodes. Those patients with positive nodes are probably not suitable for intraarterial therapy. Previously untreated, well-nourished patients with intact vascular access to their tumor appear to respond best to chemotherapy whether it is administered systemically or intraarterially.

RADIATION THERAPY AND CHEMOTHERAPY COMBINED

For over a decade investigators have attempted to improve the survival of patients with advanced head and neck cancer by combining radiation therapy and chemotherapy. The chemotherapy in these trials is usually single agent, but occasionally combination regimens have been employed. The route of chemotherapy administration is most often intravenous, but there are several studies in which the intraarterial route has also been used. To properly evaluate the impact of this combined approach upon survival, carefully conducted, prospective randomized clinical trials are necessary. Unfortunately these are few in number and in general the results obtained to date have been discouraging.

The two principal goals of this combined therapy are to improve the local control rate and to decrease the incidence of distant metastases. Local control should be improved if, by combining chemotherapy and radiation, a greater tumor cell kill occurs, which will result in a greater likelihood of eradication of tumor cells within the irradiated region. The chemotherapeutic agent is thus viewed as a "radiopotentiator" augmenting the local effects of irradiation. The theoretical basis for this concept is that large tumors, by virtue of their size or prior surgery, frequently are poorly vascularized and contain significant numbers of hypoxic cells, usually in the central area. Hypoxic cells are resistant to radiation, and thus inferior results are obtained when larger tumors are irradiated. Should chemotherapy shrink the tumor mass, the ability of radiation to eradicate the tumor is enhanced.

Though the majority of patients dying from head and neck cancer succumb to local tumor effects, a significant number—approaching 30 per cent—develop distant metastases. These

Table 13–8. INTRAARTERIAL CHEMOTHERAPY OF HEAD AND NECK CANCER

Regimen*	Evaluable Patients	Response Rate (%) Previously Untreated Patients: Total	Response Rate (%) Previously Untreated Patients: Complete	Response Rate (%) Previously Treated Patients: Total	Response Rate (%) Previously Treated Patients: Complete	Duration of Response (R) or Survival (S) (Months)†	Comments	Reference
5FU-MTX-BLM	15			87	20	2.5 (R) (32% 12-month survival)	No treatment deaths One patient developed a transient hemiparesis that resolved In general, toxicity was acceptable but remissions were brief	46
Mitomycin C	15	62(5/8)	0	0(0/7)	0	Not indicated (chemotherapy followed by RT)	Superselective angiographic techniques used No serious complications and no systemic toxicity None of the previously treated group responded	47
VCR-MTX-BLM-ADM	47	62.5	19			Resp: 51.6 (S) Nonresp: 5.4 (S)	Chemotherapy followed by RT in all patients Considerable toxicity: 57.5% developed BLM pulmonary toxicity, which was fatal in 18% (5/27); hepatotoxicity frequently observed (44.6%)	48
BLM-MTX + LV	31	64.5 (Combined response rate for untreated and previously treated patients)	Not indicated			9.7 (R) (But chemotherapy was combined with RT in 27/31 patients)	In patients treated with IV chemotherapy, response rate was only 20%; however, this group tended to have more advanced disease No discussion of complications or toxicity	49
ADM-BLM-VCR ADM-BLM-MTX	112	75	Not indicated			CR: 77% 3-yr (S) NR + PR: 18–23% 3-yr (S) (Majority of patients underwent surgery or RT post chemotherapy)	Favorable survival only in group who had planned surgery post chemotherapy (52% 3-yr survival)	50

*5FU = 5-fluorouracil; MTX = methotrexate; BLM = bleomycin; VCR = vincristine; ADM = Adriamycin (doxorubicin); LV = leucovorin
†RT = radiation therapy; CR = complete response; PR = partial response; NR = no response

distant metastases are frequently microscopic in size and not detectable by conventional means such as physical examination, x-rays, or radioisotope scans. Systemic chemotherapy administered with radiation has the potential benefit of eradicating occult microscopic tumor located outside the radiation field.

As would be expected, the agent most often combined with radiation therapy is methotrexate. In Table 13–9 are listed studies with 40 or more patients in which the methotrexate is given intravenously, orally, or intraarterially. The severity of the toxicities observed in these studies was quite variable and depended on the dose, duration, and route of administration of methotrexate. The common side effects, as anticipated, were mucositis and myelosuppression, which occasionally were so severe that the patient could not complete the full course of therapy. In general, mucositis developing with combined therapy was more severe than that associated with radiation therapy alone.

The results of the largest randomized study comparing radiation therapy alone versus radiation therapy plus methotrexate have recently been published by Fazekas et al[55] (see Table 13–9). In this study, conducted by the Radiation Therapy Oncology Group, one group of patients received five doses of intravenous methotrexate immediately preceding full-course irradiation. Only very modest improvements in the 5-year median survival rate (1 to 4 months) were observed with the combined therapy. The authors did not recommend this combination for routine clinical practice but suggested that other adjuvant programs be investigated.

Hydroxyurea is an agent that interferes with the conversion of ribonucleotides and is classified as an antimetabolite. As a single agent it has been reported to have only moderate activity in advanced head and neck cancer. Its most widespread application, however, is in combination with radiation therapy, to take advantage of the potential ability of hydroxyurea to sensitize tumor tissue to the effects of irradiation. This drug has the unique property of synchronizing cellular mitoses in addition to arresting mitoses in the radiosensitive S (DNA synthesis) stage.[56] Experiments in laboratory animals and in cell cultures have demonstrated synergistic tumor-cell killing when hydroxyurea is combined with irradiation.[57]

A large uncontrolled study by Richards and Chambers[58] indicated that patients who received combined therapy (hydroxyurea plus radiation therapy) had a higher likelihood of surviving 5 years than patients treated with irradiation alone. The combined therapy group also had a higher local control rate. Unfortunately, the lack of randomization made an accurate analysis of the true efficacy of this combined therapy extremely difficult. Furthermore, two randomized studies have not supported the beneficial effect of hydroxyurea plus irradiation. Steffani et al[59] in a study of 95 evaluable patients reported no survival benefit or improved local control with combined therapy. Similar results were reported by Hussey and Abrams[60] in their study of 40 evaluable patients. They found no statistically significant difference in the regression, local control, or 24-month no-evidence-of-disease (NED) rates between the group receiving radiotherapy alone and the group treated with combined hydroxyurea and radiotherapy.

5-Fluorouracil (5-FU) is an antimetabolite commonly used in breast and gastrointestinal carcinomas. The University of Wisconsin has accumulated the most experience with this agent in combination with radiation therapy for the treatment of advanced squamous cell carcinomas of the head and neck. In 1961 researchers there began a randomized study comparing 5-FU plus radiation therapy with radiation therapy alone. In their most recent update[61] 136 patients were analyzed, with the combined treatment group showing improved local control and survival rate. Only in the oral cavity patient population, however, was this difference statistically significant. Furthermore, acute and late complications were much more frequent in the combined therapy group, and only in this group were major complications observed. In spite of the toxicity, however, the results of these University of Wisconsin trials appear promising enough to warrant further randomized trials with larger patient groups.

Bleomycin, which is most effective in killing cells in the mitotic and premitotic (G_2) phases, has also been employed as a radiosensitizer. The largest experience with this agent is from India, where squamous cell carcinomas of the oral cavity are the most common cancers and the majority of patients present in advanced stages. In 1971 a study was begun in which patients with T_3 and T_4 oral squamous cell carcinomas were randomized to receive either irradiation alone or bleomycin and irradiation. As of 1977, 136 patients had completed this trial.[62] The com-

Table 13–9. COMBINED METHOTREXATE (MTX) AND RADIATION THERAPY (RT)*

Author	Sites	No. Patients	Route of MTX	Results: *RT Alone*	Results: *Combined Therapy*	Comments
Lustig[51]	All sites advanced disease	48	PO			
		74 randomized	35 IV 39 RT *alone*	*3-yr survival:* 10%	IV—20% PO—33%	PO MTX + RT produced statistically superior survival, but there was much greater oral toxicity in the oral MTX group
Knowlton[52]	All sites Stage III and IV	98	IV—5-day course or high-dose with leucovorin rescue	*3-yr survival:* 16.6% *Local control:* 31.2%	13.6% 22.9%	No significant differences in local control, survival, or incidence of distant metastases
Condit[53]	All sites advanced disease	40	IV	*Remission:* 12/20 *Duration of remission:* 3 to 4 mo	8/10 5.1+ mo	No significant differences in number or duration of remission or local failure rate
Bagshaw & Doggett[54]	All sites T_3 and T_4	41	IA with leucovorin rescue	*Local control:* 6/16 *Distant metastases:* 0/16	7/22 0/22	
Fazekas[55]	All sites T_3 and T_4 and nodal cervical disease	638	IV—5-day course just prior to RT	*Adjusted median survival (mo)* Oral cavity: 11.8 Oropharynx: 13.6 Supraglottic larynx: 17.2 Hypopharynx: 9.7	 12.4 13. 19.2 13.4	Minimal improvement in survival in combined therapy group

*Modified from Borgelt BB, Davis LW: Combination chemotherapy and irradiation for head and neck cancer: a review. Cancer Clinical Trials 1:49, 1978.

bined therapy group (74 patients) demonstrated much higher rates both for complete local control (77.0 versus 20.9 per cent) and crude 3-year survival (50 versus 20 per cent).

Two other randomized studies, however, have demonstrated increased side effects without improved survival for combined bleomycin and irradiation. In the preliminary results of a randomized E.O.R.T.C. Head and Neck Cooperative Group Study,[63] mucositis and epidermitis were far more frequent with combined therapy (72 versus 21 per cent) and necessitated a delay in irradiation in 22 per cent of patients. Furthermore, there was no statistical difference in tumor regression 6 weeks after irradiation, and at 15 months' follow-up the median survival was the same in the irradiation alone and irradiation plus bleomycin groups. Similar results were noted by Shah et al,[64] who reported an 82.6 per cent incidence of side effects in the combined therapy group without an improvement in median survival time. In both the E.O.R.T.C. study and the one by Shah, the dose of bleomycin was 15 mg. The Northern California Oncology Group has shown that a dose of 5 units twice weekly is well tolerated and no compromise has to be made in the administration of irradiation.[65] This group is presently conducting a randomized study comparing low-dose bleomycin plus irradiation to irradiation alone.

Varied combinations of chemotherapeutic agents have been combined with irradiation in hopes of improving both local control and survival, but unfortunately some of these trials have not been randomized (Table 13–10). The chemotherapy has been administered systemically in most cases, and occasionally intraarterially.

Bitter[66] employed irradiation together with a combination of bleomycin and methotrexate administered intraarterially in 20 patients with T_3 lesions and reported a 50 per cent complete response rate. Four additional patients (20 per cent) were rendered free of disease after surgery. Stomatitis, as expected, was severe.

Fu et al[67] treated 15 patients with advanced inoperable squamous cell carcinomas with a combination of cyclophosphamide, vincristine, and bleomycin concurrent with radiation therapy, followed by cyclophosphamide, bleomycin, and methotrexate post radiation. In this pilot study, sponsored by the Radiation Therapy Oncology Group, complete disease control was achieved in 7 patients (47 per cent). The side effects, which included enhanced radiation stomatitis and infection, were severe, and 3 patients developed fatal complications. These authors considered the toxicity of this regimen to be prohibitive and did not proceed with a randomized trial.

Bezwoda et al[68] randomized 58 patients with advanced head and neck cancer to treatment with either radical radiation therapy alone or radiation therapy plus a combination chemotherapy regimen consisting of vincristine, adriamycin, bleomycin, 5-FU, and methotrexate. Though no significant difference was observed in response rates, the patients who received combined therapy had a significantly prolonged survival (36 weeks versus 18 weeks). Stomatitis was greater with combined therapy, and in about one third of the patients it interfered with swallowing. The survival rates in the group receiving radiation therapy alone were relatively short and inferior to the results of most other studies. A statistically superior 4-year disease-free survival rate has been reported for the combination of vincristine, bleomycin, and methotrexate (VBM) plus radiation when compared with radiation alone (56.5 versus 21.8 per cent).[69] However, intense mucositis was observed in the combined therapy group, and approximately one third of these patients required nasogastric tube feeding for an undefined period of time.

In a recent pilot study by Petrovich et al,[70] 23 patients with Stage IV unresectable squamous cell carcinomas were randomized to receive radiation therapy or radiation therapy plus vincristine and high-dose methotrexate with leucovorin rescue. The response rate was higher with combined therapy (67 versus 36 per cent), as was the duration of remission (6 versus 2.3 months), but the median survival was only modestly improved (12 versus 5.6 months). This regimen was well tolerated in the combined treatment group, with all patients experiencing at most only moderate mucosal reaction without an increase in the amount of local or regional reaction.

It appears that further randomized studies will be necessary before the role of combined chemotherapy with radiation therapy is clearly defined. Many of the previous attempts have not produced a significant enough improvement in survival to warrant the added toxicity, cost, and inconvenience. In future studies, in addition to randomization, it will be important to carefully analyze the data by both anatomic site and stage.

Table 13–10. COMBINATION CHEMOTHERAPY AND RADIATION THERAPY (RT)

Author(s)	*Number of Patients*	*Chemotherapy Regimen**	*Response Rate†*	*Survival*	*Comments*
Bitter[66]	20	MTX-BLM (intraarterial)	50% CR	80% at 1 yr	Severe stomatitis, nonrandomized
Fu et al[67]	15	CTX-VCR-BLM	47% CR	40% at 1 yr	Severe toxicity (3 fatalities), nonrandomized
Bezwoda et al[68]	58‡	VCR-ADM-BLM-5FU-MTX	*RT alone:* CR + PR = 50% *Combined:* CR + PR = 60%	RT alone: 18 weeks Combined: 36 weeks	Short survival in RT alone group
O'Connor et al[69]	92‡	VCR-BLM-MTX (VBM)	Not stated	*Disease-free at 4 yr:* RT alone: 21.8% Combined: 56.5%	Severe mucositis in combined group
Petrovich et al[70]	23‡	VCR-HDMTX + LV	*Rt alone:* 9% CR *Combined:* 33% CR	RT alone: 5.6 mo Combined: 12 mo	Significant improvement in response rate with combined therapy, but only marginal improvement in survival

*MTX = methotrexate; BLM = bleomycin; CTX = Cytoxan (cyclophosphamide); VCR = vincristine; ADM = Adriamycin (doxorubicin); 5FU = 5-fluorouracil; HDMTX = high-dose methotrexate; LV = leucovorin

†CR = complete response; PR = partial response

‡Randomized study

PREOPERATIVE AND PREIRRADIATION CHEMOTHERAPY

Even with the most modern surgical and radiotherapeutic techniques, the treatment of patients with Stage III and Stage IV head and neck cancer yields poor results at best. Over 50 per cent of these patients who fail local therapy will develop systemic metastases, and approximately 30 per cent of this group will be noted to have distant metastatic disease as their only site of failure. As mentioned earlier, untreated patients have a far superior response rate to single agent or combination chemotherapy when compared with previously treated patients (50 to 75 per cent versus 30 to 40 per cent). There are several reasons for this finding, but the poor vascular access to the tumor site following surgery and/or radiation therapy is a frequently cited cause. Certainly a precarious nutritional balance will make a previously treated patient far more susceptible to the toxic effects of chemotherapy. In addition, the delay in chemotherapy administration necessitated by prior surgery or radiotherapy allows further time for occult microscopic cancer (micrometastases) to grow in size and in number of sites, making eradication by systemic chemotherapy more difficult. It has been well documented that chemotherapy is more effective when a smaller tumor cell burden is present. This is one of the basic principles of adjuvant chemotherapy as is widely employed in the early treatment of breast cancer and osteogenic sarcoma.

Considering these facts, it seems appropriate and logical to administer chemotherapy prior to surgery or radiation therapy in patients with locally advanced disease. The goal of this early chemotherapy is to increase survival both by improving local control rates and by eliminating possible distant micrometastases. A significant number of studies on this approach have already been published, some reporting promising results. The ultimate impact on survival, however, has not been established.

In the majority of trials employing chemotherapy as initial therapy, combination regimens are usually used, and *cis*-platinum is frequently one of the agents. This is understandable in view of the very high response rate with this drug in untreated patients and the lack of bone marrow and mucous membrane toxicity. Bleomycin is also frequently included in the initial regimen.

One of the first trials of preoperative chemotherapy was performed at the National Cancer Institute, and the results were reported by Tarpley et al.[71] They chose moderate high-dose methotrexate (240 mg/m^2) with leucovorin rescue and, by comparing their 30 study patients to an identical number of randomly selected patients matched for tumor site and stage but treated with surgery alone, were able to show some encouraging results. Methotrexate produced a preoperative decrease in tumor size in 77 per cent of the patients and was not associated with any medical or surgical complications. Though no significant difference in survival was noted between the two patient groups, there was a significantly greater disease-free interval in the methotrexate-treated patients. The authors were encouraged with the antitumor response as well as with the lack of toxicity and recommended that further studies with preoperative chemotherapy be conducted.

In contrast, a Radiation Therapy Oncology Group pilot study employing two cycles of vincristine, bleomycin, and methotrexate (VBM) prior to irradiation produced intolerable morbidity and complications, and could not be recommended for further trials in spite of an initial excellent tumor response.[77] Another preirradiation chemotherapy regimen recently reported also produced similarly disappointing results. Zulke-Temme et al[73] used a triple-therapy protocol consisting of intraarterial chemotherapy with bleomycin and methotrexate followed by radiation therapy, and then, when feasible, surgical resection. With the exception of the treatment of patients with operable Stage III carcinomas of the maxillary antrum, the authors felt that the results of this study did not justify the further use of the preirradiation intraarterial combination.

New regimens employing *cis*-platinum in combination with one or two other agents have produced exciting though preliminary results. Weaver et al[74] administered two courses of *cis*-platinum, oncovin, and bleomycin (COB), followed by surgery if the lesions were judged to be resectable, or radiation therapy if unresectable. The toxicity produced by the combination was considered to be tolerable and did not prevent the use of subsequent surgery or radiation therapy. Of the 75 patients with Stage III and Stage

IV cancer, 80 per cent had a complete or partial response to chemotherapy, and in 35 patients radical surgery became possible. This was not a randomized study, and as expected, patients who attained a complete or partial response to chemotherapy were observed to have a statistically improved survival as compared with patients who had only a minimal or no response.

In another nonrandomized study, 58 patients with Stage III and Stage IV cancers were treated with two courses of high-dose *cis*-platinum and one course of bleomycin by continuous infusion and then evaluated for response.[75] Resectable patients underwent surgery followed by radiation therapy, while unresectable patients were given radiation therapy alone. Twenty per cent of the patients had a complete response to the chemotherapy, and an additional 52.7 per cent a partial response. Twenty-five patients underwent surgical resection. In patients who achieved a complete remission at the end of all therapy, the median survival was in excess of 60 months, compared with only 7.3 months for patients with residual disease post treatment. To better define the usefulness of this induction chemotherapy, these authors are now conducting a controlled randomized study.

In England, the Price-Hill regimen with six different agents (vincristine, bleomycin, hydrocortisone, methotrexate, leucovorin rescue, and 5-FU) is being employed prior to radiation therapy, with promising results.[76] Furthermore, this is an outpatient regimen with minimal side effects. In particular, the prominent nausea and vomiting accompanying *cis*-platinum administrations is not seen.

The National Cancer Institute is presently sponsoring a prospective multi-institutional randomized trial of preoperative *cis*-platinum and bleomycin in patients with advanced head and neck cancer. This study is designed to determine the impact of preoperative chemotherapy on tumor control and survival. The preliminary results indicate a satisfactory resonse rate with minimal toxicity.[77] In particular, there were no delays in surgery due to chemotherapy effects and no significant differences in postoperative complications. Considering the large number of patients in this study, its multi-institutional composition, and its careful design, we should be able to learn a great deal about the value of this preoperative chemotherapy regimen in patients who do poorly with our present standard therapy.

References

1. Bertino JR, Boston B, Capizzi RL: The role of chemotherapy in the management of cancer of the head and neck: a review. Cancer 36:752, 1975.
2. Amer MH, Al-Sarraf M, Vaitkevicius VK: Factors that affect response to chemotherapy and survival of patients with advanced head and neck cancer. Cancer 43:2202, 1979.
3. Carter SK: The chemotherapy of head and neck cancer. Semin Oncol 4:413, 1977.
4. Lane M, Moore JE, Levin H, et al: Methotrexate therapy for squamous cell carcinoma of the head and neck. JAMA 204:561, 1968.
5. Leone LA, Albalba MM, Rege VB: Treatment of carcinoma of the head and neck with intravenous methotrexate. Cancer 21:828, 1968.
6. DePalo GM, DeLena M, Molinari R, et al: Clinical evaluation of high weekly intravenous doses of methotrexate in advanced oropharyngeal carcinoma. Tumori 56:259, 1970.
7. Priestman J: Results in fifty cases of advanced squamous cell carcinoma of the head and neck treated by intravenous chemotherapy. Br J Cancer 27:400, 1973.
8. Papac RJ, Jacobs EM, Foye LV Jr, et al: Systemic therapy with amethopterin in squamous cell carcinoma of the head and neck. Cancer Chemother Rep 32:47, 1963.
9. Levitt M, Mosher MB, DeConti RC, et al: Improved therapeutic index of methotrexate with "leucovorin rescue." Cancer Res 33:1729, 1973.
10. Mills EED: Intermittent intravenous methotrexate in the treatment of advanced epidermoid carcinoma. S Afr Med J 46:398, 1972.
11. Capizzi RL, DeConti RC, Marsh JC, et al: Methotrexate therapy of head and neck cancer: improvement in therapeutic index by the use of leucovorin "rescue." Cancer Res 30:1782, 1970.
12. Khandekar JD, Wolff A: A clinical trial of high dose methotrexate with leucovorin "rescue" (HDMTX) in advanced epidermoid carcinoma of the head and neck. Proc Am Soc Clin Oncol 18:281, 1977 (abstract).
13. Buechler M, Mukherji B, Chasin W, et al: High dose methotrexate (MTX) with and without BCG therapy in advanced head and neck malignancy. Proc Am Soc Clin Oncol 18:329, 1977 (abstract).
14. Woods RL, Fox RM, Tattersall MHN: Methotrexate treatment of squamous-cell head and neck cancers: dose-response evaluation. Br Med J 282:600, 1981.
15. DeConti RC, Schoenfeld D: A randomized prospective comparison of intermittent methotrexate, methotrexate with leucovorin, and a methotrexate combination in head and neck cancer. Cancer 48:1061, 1981.
16. Muggia FM, Rozencweig MR, Louie AE: Role of chemotherapy in head and neck cancer: systemic use of single agents and combinations in advanced disease. Head Neck Surg 2:196, 1980.
17. Jacobs C: The role of cisplatin in the treatment of recurrent head and neck cancer. *In* Prestayko AW, Crooke ST, Carter SK (eds): Cisplatin: Current

Status and New Developments. New York, Academic Press, 1980, Chapter 30.
18. Wittes RE, Cvitkovic E, Shah J, et al: Cis-dichlorodiammineplatinum (II) in the treatment of epidermoid carcinoma of the head and neck. Cancer Treat Rep 61:359, 1977.
19. Randolph VL, Wittes RE: Weekly administration of cis-diamminedichloroplatinum (II) without hydration or osmotic diuresis. Eur J Cancer 14:753, 1978.
20. Jacobs C, Bertino JR, Goffinet DR, et al: 24-hour infusion of cis-platinum in head and neck cancers. Cancer 42:2135, 1978.
21. Panettiere FJ, Lane M, Lehane D: Effectiveness of a new outpatient program utilizing CACP in the chemotherapy of advanced epidermoid head and neck tumors. A Southwest Oncology Group study. Proc Am Soc Clin Oncol 19:410, 1978 (abstract).
22. Sako K, Razack MS, Kalnins I: Chemotherapy for advanced and recurrent squamous cell carcinoma of the head and neck with high and low dose cis-diamminedichloroplatinum. Am J Surg 136:529, 1978.
23. Mosher MB, DeConti RC, Bertino JR: Bleomycin therapy in advanced Hodgkin's disease and epidermoid cancers. Cancer 30:56, 1972.
24. Yagoda A, Lippman AJ, Winn RJ, et al: Combination chemotherapy with bleomycin (BLM) and methotrexate (MTX) in patients with advanced epidermoid carcinomas. Proc Am Soc Clin Oncol 16:247, 1975 (abstract).
25. Bonadonna G, Tancini G, Bajetta E: Controlled studies with bleomycin in solid tumors and lymphomas. Prog Biochem Pharmacol 11:172, 1976.
26. Livingston RB, Einhorn EH, Burgess MA, et al: Sequential combination chemotherapy for advanced, recurrent squamous carcinoma of the head and neck. Cancer Treat Rep 60:103, 1976.
27. Pouillart P, Mathé G: Bleomycin in rational combinations of chemotherapy. Gann 19:279, 1976.
28. Ratkin GA, Brown CA, Ogura JH: Combination chemotherapy in head and neck cancer. Proc Am Soc Clin Oncol 19:330, 1978 (abstract).
29. Wittes RE, Spiro RH, Shah J, et al: Chemotherapy of head and neck cancer: combination treatment with cyclophosphamide, adriamycin, methotrexate and bleomycin. Med Pediatr Oncol 3:301, 1977.
30. Holoye PY, Byers RM, Gard DA, et al: Combination chemotherapy of head and neck cancer. Cancer 42:1661, 1978.
31. Price LA, Bridget T, Hill AH, et al: Improved results in combination chemotherapy of head and neck cancer using a kinetically-based approach: a randomized study with and without adriamycin. Oncology 35:26, 1978.
32. Vanhaelen C, Bertrand M, DeJager R, et al: Vinblastine, methotrexate, and bleomycin in the management of head and neck cancer. Eur J Cancer 15:1315, 1979.
33. Molinari R, Mattavelli F, Cantu G: Results of a low-dose combination chemotherapy with vincristine, bleomycin and methotrexate (V-B-M) based on cell kinetics in the palliative treatment of head and neck squamous cell carcinoma. Eur J Cancer 16:469, 1980.
34. Cortes EP, Kalra J, Amin UC: Chemotherapy for head and neck cancer relapsing after radiotherapy. Cancer 47:1966, 1981.
35. Scarborough JP, Metter GE, Moseley HS: Adriamycin, bleomycin and CCNU as effective induction chemotherapeutic agents in advanced squamous cell carcinoma (COB protocol 7333). J Surg Oncol 10:501, 1978.
36. Randolph VL, Vallejo A, Shiro RH, et al: Combination therapy of advanced head and neck cancer: induction of remissions with diamminedichloroplatinum (II), bleomycin and radiation therapy. Cancer 41:460, 1978.
37. Hong WK, Shapshay SM, Bhutani R, et al: Induction chemotherapy in advanced squamous head and neck carcinoma with high-dose *cis*-platinum and bleomycin infusion. Cancer 44:19, 1979.
38. Elias E, Chretien PE, Monnard E, et al: Chemotherapy prior to local therapy in advanced squamous cell carcinoma of the head and neck: preliminary assessment of an intensive drug regimen. Cancer 43:1025, 1979.
39. Caradonna R, Paladine W, Ruckdeschel JC: Methotrexate, bleomycin, and high-dose cis-dichlorodiammineplatinum (II) in the treatment of advanced epidermoid carcinoma of the head and neck. Cancer Treat Rep 63:489, 1979.
40. Vogl SE, Kaplan BH: Chemotherapy of advanced head and neck cancer with methotrexate, bleomycin, and cis-diamminedichloroplatinum II in an effective outpatient schedule. Cancer 44:26, 1979.
41. Wittes R, Heller K, Randolph V, et al: Cis-dichlorodiammineplatinum (II)–based chemotherapy as initial treatment of advanced head and neck cancer. Cancer Treat Rep 63:1533, 1979.
42. King GW, Halpen JJ, Smith RE: Cis-dichlorodiammineplatinum (II), methotrexate, bleomycin, and vincristine in head and neck cancer: a pilot study. Cancer Treat Rep 63:1735, 1979.
43. Amer MH, Izbicki RM, Vaitkevicius VK, et al: Combination chemotherapy with cis-diamminedichloroplatinum, oncovin, and bleomycin (COB) in advanced head and neck cancer: phase II. Cancer 45:217, 1980.
44. Brown AW, Blom J, Butler WM, et al: Combination chemotherapy with vinblastine, bleomycin, and cis-diamminedichloroplatinum (II) in squamous cell carcinoma of the head and neck. Cancer 45:2830, 1980.
45. Bleyer WA: The clinical pharmacology of methotrexate—a new application of an old drug. Cancer 41:36, 1978.
46. Donegan WK, Harris P: Regional chemotherapy with combined drugs in cancer of the head and neck. Cancer 38:1479, 1976.
47. Brismar J, Björklund A, Elner A, et al: Selective intra-arterial cytostatic injections in malignant head and neck tumors. Neuroradiology 16:434, 1978.
48. Curioni C, Quadu G: Clinical trial of intraarterial polychemotherapy in the treatment of carcinoma of the oral cavity. J Maxillofac Surg 6:207, 1978.
49. Matras H, Bürkle K, Watzek G, et al: Concept of cytostatic therapy in advanced tumors of the head and neck. J Maxillofac Surg 7:150, 1979.
50. Muggia FM, Wolf GT: Intraarterial chemotherapy of head and neck cancer: worth another look? Cancer Clin Trials 3:375, 1980.
51. Lustig RA, DeMare PA, Kramer S: Adjuvant methotrexate in the radiotherapeutic management of advanced tumors of the head and neck. Cancer 37:2703, 1976.
52. Knowlton AH, Bercarpio B, Bobrow S, et al: Methotrexate and radiation therapy in the treatment of advanced head and neck tumors. Radiology 116:709, 1975.

53. Condit PT: Treatment of carcinoma with radiation therapy and methotrexate. Missouri Med 65:832, 1968.
54. Bagshaw MA, Doggett RLS: A clinical study of chemical radiosensitization. Front Radiat Ther Oncol 4:164, 1969.
55. Fazekas JT, Sommer C, Kramer S: Adjuvant intravenous methotrexate or definitive radiotherapy alone for advanced squamous cancers of the oral cavity, oropharynx, supraglottic larynx or hypopharynx. Int J Radiat Oncol Biol Phys 6:533, 1980.
56. Philips FS, Steinberg SS, Schwartz HS, et al: Hydroxyurea. 1. Acute cell death in proliferating tissues in rats. Cancer Res 27:61, 1967.
57. Phillips RA, Tolmach LJ: Repair of potentially lethal damage in x-irradiated HeLa cells. Radiat Res 29:413, 1966.
58. Richards GJ Jr, Chambers RG: Hydroxyurea in the treatment of neoplasms of the head and neck. A resurvey. Am J Surg 126:513, 1973.
59. Stefani S, Eells RW, Abbate J: Hydroxyurea and radiotherapy in head and neck cancer. Results of a prospective controlled study in 126 patients. Radiology 101:391, 1971.
60. Hussey DH, Abrams JP: Combined therapy in advanced head and neck cancer: hydroxyurea and radiotherapy. Prog Clin Cancer 6:79, 1975.
61. Lo TCM, Wiley AL Jr, Ansfield FJ, et al: Combined radiation therapy and 5-fluorouracil for advanced squamous cell carcinoma of the oral cavity and oropharynx: a randomized study. Am J Roentgenol 126:229, 1976.
62. Shanta V, Krishnamurthi S: Combined therapy of oral cancer. Bleomycin and radiation: a clinical trial. Clin Radiol 28:427, 1977.
63. Cachin Y, Jortay A, Sancho H, et al: Preliminary results of a randomized E.O.R.T.C. study comparing radiotherapy and concomitant bleomycin to radiotherapy alone in epidermoid carcinomas of the oropharynx. Eur J Cancer 13:1389, 1977.
64. Shah PJ, Shukla SN, Patel KM, et al: Effect of bleomycin-radiotherapy combination in management of head and neck squamous cell carcinoma. Cancer 48:1106, 1981.
65. Fu KK: Personal communication.
66. Bitter K: Bleomycin-methotrexate-chemotherapy in combination with telecobalt-radiation for patients suffering from advanced oral carcinoma. J Maxillofac Surg 5:75, 1977.
67. Fu KK, Silverberg IJ, Phillips TL, et al: Combined radiotherapy and multidrug chemotherapy for advanced head and neck cancer: results of a Radiation Therapy Oncology Group Pilot Study. Cancer Treat Rep 63:351, 1979.
68. Bezwoda WR, deMoor NG, Derman DP: Treatment of advanced head and neck cancer by means of radiation therapy plus chemotherapy—a randomized trial. Med Pediatr Oncol 6:353, 1979.
69. O'Connor AD, Clifford P, Dalley VM, et al: Advanced head and neck cancer treated by combined radiotherapy and VBM cytoxic regimen—four-year results. Clin Otolaryngol 4:329, 1979.
70. Petrovich Z, Block J, Kuisk H, et al: A randomized comparison of radiotherapy with a radiotherapy-chemotherapy combination in Stage IV carcinoma of the head and neck. Cancer 47:2259, 1981.
71. Tarpley JL, Chretien PB, Alexander JC Jr, et al: High dose methotrexate as a preoperative adjuvant in the treatment of epidermoid carcinoma of the head and neck. A feasibility study and clinical trial. Am J Surg 130:481, 1975.
72. Glick JH, Fazekas JH, Davis LW, et al: Combination chemotherapy-radiotherapy for advanced inoperable head and neck cancer. An RTOG pilot study. Cancer Clin Trials 2:129, 1979.
73. Zulke-Temme BC, Stevens KR, Everts EC, et al: Combined intraarterial chemotherapy, radiation therapy, and surgery for advanced squamous-cell carcinoma of the head and neck. Cancer 45:1527, 1980.
74. Weaver A, Loh JJK, Vandenberg H: Combined modality therapy for advanced head and neck cancer. Am J Surg 140:549, 1980.
75. Hong WK, Bhutani R, Shapshay SM, et al: Induction chemotherapy of advanced previously untreated squamous cell head and neck cancer with cisplatin and bleomycin. *In* Prestayko AW, Crooke ST, Carter SK (eds): Cisplatin: Current Status and New Developments. New York, Academic Press, 1980, Chapter 31.
76. Dalley VM: Radiotherapy and chemotherapy in treatment of head and neck cancer. Int J Radiat Oncol Biol Phys 4:173, 1978.
77. Wolf GT, Makuch RW: Preoperative *cis*-platinum (DDP) and bleomycin (BLM) in patients with head and neck squamous carcinoma (HNSCC):Toxicity and tumor response. Proc Am Soc Clin Oncol 21:400, 1980 (abstract).

14

MAXILLOFACIAL PROSTHETICS

Robert E. Gillis, Jr., D.M.D., M.S.D.

From the beginning of man, it has been generally accepted that bodily deformities compromise an individual's ability to function within a society. Abnormalities that are judged by the individual to compromise socially accepted norms of appearance have long required varying types of intervention. Certainly the ideal type of intervention would restore the patient to normal function utilizing the patient's own tissues and requiring little other than ordinary care and maintenance on the part of the patient. By this definition, maxillofacial rehabilitation, in which artificial materials are used for restoration, must be deemed less than ideal. It should be realized, however, that this type of rehabilitation is often the most satisfactory, especially for patients who have had head and neck cancer. Decisions and judgments regarding the use of prosthetic devices always involve some degree of compromise. Inherent in such decisions is the potential for problems, which will be the main focus of this chapter. For further information on the subject of maxillofacial rehabilitation, the reader is referred to the several excellent texts cited in the References.[1, 2, 3]

GENERAL BACKGROUND

Although relatively little is understood about the psychologic care and evaluation of the head and neck cancer patient, all professionals involved in the patient's care treat the patient's psyche to some extent. An evaluation of the existing literature in this area suggests that our knowledge is rudimentary at best. The area of the face is critically important, with alterations affecting patients in regard to both their self-esteem and their ability to communicate with others.

Gillis[4] describes the current status of our understanding of these factors. The best understanding of the reaction of any individual patient can be acquired from the realization that head and neck cancer constitutes an extreme crisis situation in the life of the patient. The patient will respond, albeit unpredictably, to this stress based on his existing psychologic makeup.

In attempting to understand the response of the head and neck cancer patient to his illness it is helpful to outline the types of crises he is faced with. The first crisis concerns the patient's adaptation to his role of being seriously ill. The second crisis is somewhat disease-specific and relates to the particular fears engendered by cancer as an illness. These include the fear of death and dying, the fear of social stigma or ostracism, and the fear of abandonment by family and friends who may find it uncomfortable to be in the patient's presence. The last crisis centers on the fact that the patient's cancer is located within the facial area. The specific stresses here are fear of facial disfigurement and fear of the loss of self-esteem that accompanies changes in one's total body image. These factors, which are especially significant in the head and neck cancer patient, are discussed at length by Ross.[5] The importance of the face to the total person is discussed by Gillis.[4]

Because of these factors, there is great potential for altered or limited communication between the patient and his physicians, as well as between the patient and his family. Those treating the patient must be aware of the importance of these psychologic responses of the patient, and of the social support system that is necessary for the patient's recovery and rehabilitation.

COMMUNICATION PROBLEMS

It is important to understand also the attitudinal problems that may exist among many members of the rehabilitative team. The underlying difficulty is best described by Conley,[6] who describes the dilemma of the head and neck surgeon:

> He is asked to attack a disease that will kill; his method of attack is . . . mutilative. Imagine the emotional involvement of a sensitive surgeon. Unlike cancer of the stomach or cancer of the lung, his work is constantly on exhibition and he is frustrated. His patients not only die, but they get recurrent cancers. He is failing, the patient is coming apart, the family is after him, the community is after him, and on the whole, he is literally running away from the patient because he cannot absorb the gigantic deluge of emotional feeling which is coming from his lack of success. This is a built-in emotional phenomenon which I think the surgeon should try to analyze. Perhaps we are so mired down, not so much by a lack of technical efficiency as by emotional involvement with failure, mutilation, or potential mutilation.

It is important for the professionals treating these patients to evaluate their own thoughts and feelings regarding such topics as facial disfigurement, disability, and death. Death is the ultimate realization of our limitations and basic human frailty. It is perhaps in this realization that the solution lies. For in accepting our patients as human and dealing with them in a compassionate manner, we can indeed assist them in meeting their most basic human needs:

1. The need to love and be loved.
2. The need for autonomy or being capable of making independent decisions.
3. The need for self-worth.
4. The need to belong, to be a meaningful part of a group.

One of the problems in managing these patients is that of communication between the various professional people involved in their treatment. Each of us has as his goal the restoration of the patient; and each of us approaches this restoration through his own individual discipline. The cure, restoration, and rehabilitation of the cancer patient are complex procedures requiring interdisciplinary care, and cannot at this time be achieved by any one individual. It is extremely important, therefore, that there be good communication among the individuals treating the patient, and that these individuals trust the judgment of their colleagues. There must be a willingness to listen openly, the freedom to question all aspects of the patient's treatment and care, and in the end, a unified definitive plan of treatment for each patient. There are patients whose care is fragmented; who are transferred from one professional to another. After each professional has exhausted the treatment possibilities in his specialty, the patient has received far less than ideal care, and often has an increased number of problems. Examples of this include the surgeon who sends his patients only to the prosthodontist following the completion of the patient's surgery, or the prosthodontist who is unwilling to be involved in any more than the physical restoration of the missing anatomy of his patient. A team approach to the treatment of these patients is essential.

It is as important to treat the emotional problems of the patient as it is to treat the physical aspects of the disease. This is extremely difficult; even psychiatrists do not agree on the proper approach in this area. Certainly, each patient must be dealt with as an individual, even when the patient chooses a course of treatment that the treating physicians may not totally agree with. The role of the treating physician is to advise, inform, and carry out the agreed upon treatment. The patient must be actively involved in the decision-making process. Those treating the patient need to learn to take the time to listen to the patient and to acknowledge the patient's fears. The importance of the role of the patient's family cannot be overemphasized. Patients with strongly supportive families certainly appear to deal with this crisis situation more easily, and are better able to accommodate their lives to their disability than are patients with little or no family support. Furthermore, "family" can include any persons who are significant and have a close relationship with the patient.

PROBLEMS RELATED TO RADIATION THERAPY

A large number of patients who have head and neck cancer receive radiation therapy either as the primary modality or in combination with surgery, chemotherapy, or both. Although radiation therapy is often successful at killing malignant cells, it also has an effect on normal tissues. In general, the effects can be summarized by stating that the surviving tissues have a decreased blood supply, and that the capacity for change in these tissues is severely altered.

In the oral cavity, the side effects of radiation are of prime importance and concern with regard to the salivary glands and bone. There is no cure or solution to these problems. However, a number of measures can and should be taken prior to radiation therapy to prevent possible disastrous sequelae related to these two tissues. All patients who receive head and neck radiation in the megavoltage range should be seen and evaluated by a dentist prior to therapy. The dentist must evaluate not only the present status of the patient's dentition but also its long-term prognosis and the possible prosthetic restoration as well as the ability of the patient to care for and maintain his oral cavity.

Pre-irradiation Evaluation

In dentistry, practitioners are often taught a "wait and see" attitude or a conservative approach to problems. The philosophy here is that the patient can often be motivated to change the habits that are creating problems, and that, given time, the tissues will heal and stabilize. Unlike surgeons dealing with cancer, dentists are not conditioned to seeing patients in a relatively short period of time, obtaining x-rays and records immediately, and deciding on long-term treatment. However, in the case of the head and neck cancer patient, often it is necessary for the dentist to see the patient within a day of being contacted and to make treatment decisions immediately.

It should be remembered that if any oral surgical procedure is required prior to radiation therapy, the patient will have to wait approximately 7 to 10 days to allow for healing before the radiation therapy can begin. There are no data to evaluate what effect this delay has on the outcome of treatment. Many patients, however, do ask this question, and the best response at present is that we don't really know but that we are not aware that the wait changes the ultimate prognosis. It may be of value to know that it is possible to perform necessary extractions during a midtherapy break in treatment. This has been done on a number of patients with satisfactory results. In these cases, it was the judgment of the radiation therapist that the nature of the disease necessitated the immediate start of radiation therapy. In six selected cases, the necessary oral surgery was performed after approximately 2500 to 3000 rads of therapy. No complications were noted.[7] It is critical in the care of the head and neck cancer patient that the patient be seen by the dentist at the same time he is being evaluated for the rest of his treatment. The dentist should be well trained and familiar with the problems involved with all modalities of treatment of the head and neck cancer patient. The dentist also should be capable of making long-term rehabilitation decisions for the patient. Often the dental treatment and sequence will play a critical role in the overall treatment of the head and neck cancer patient. The following case history illustrates this point.

CASE. A man in his middle forties was seen by a head and neck surgeon. The patient was found to have a $T_1N_0M_0$ lesion in the mid-floor of the mouth. There was no involvement of the mandible. The patient was subsequently seen by a second head and neck surgeon and a radiation therapist. The patient had been told that either surgery or irradiation would offer an equal chance of cure for his disease. Over the course of his evaluation, the patient saw a prosthodontist for a pretreatment evaluation of his dentition and oral cavity. He was found to have moderate to severe periodontal disease. If the patient was to receive radiation therapy, it would be necessary to extract all of his remaining maxillary teeth and all but four of his remaining mandibular teeth. It would not be possible to replace the patient's missing dentition for at least several months after the completion of radiation therapy. All of this was explained to the patient prior to treatment. After evaluating all of the problems and all of the modalities of treatment, the patient decided that in this case, surgical excision of the lesion in question would be the best treatment for him. This was based in part on the realization that if he were to have radiation therapy, he would be edentulous for 3 to 4 months (Fig. 14–1).

In the patient who is to receive head and neck irradiation therapy, it is not necessary to extract all of the teeth, nor is it necessary to extract the teeth within the primary beam. A judgment must be made concerning which teeth can be saved. In a patient with good sound dentition, having little or no decay or periodontal disease, there is no question that all of the teeth should be saved.

Many patients with oral cancer have lived 50 or more years with poor oral hygiene habits. It is often difficult to save teeth in a patient with such a history. The patient must be involved in this decision and must be made to understand that all of the teeth will be lost unless he is willing to change his habits drastically. If the patient appears apathetic and has moderate to severe dental disease, extractions should be seriously considered. As a general rule, any teeth with severe carious involvement or severe periodontal involvement should be extracted. In addition, any problems concerning bone contour, malpositioned teeth, impacted teeth, or any other long-term considerations with regard to the restoration of the patient's oral cavity must be resolved prior to radiation therapy.

If the patient has severe end-stage periodontal disease or decay, there is little doubt that the teeth should be extracted. In the remainder of patients, constituting the majority of those with head and neck cancer, the decision to save or extract teeth is often difficult but should be based on the following variables:

1. The patient's age.
2. The prognosis.
3. The importance of each tooth in question to the overall restorative/rehabilitative effort.
4. The presence or absence of caries.
5. The periodontal support remaining.
6. The risk involved in maintaining each tooth in question.
7. The complications involved if the tooth should be lost in the future.
8. The field of irradiation.
9. The mode of therapy.
10. The dosage of irradiation.
11. The primary area of treatment.
12. The location of the tooth (mandible vs. maxilla).

A proper evaluation of these factors and the making of a wise decision requires training and experience in all phases of dentistry, but especially prosthodontics.

Potential Complications of Radiotherapy and Their Prevention

There are several other problems that are related to the side effects of radiation. These are radiation decay, xerostomia, loss of taste, and osteoradionecrosis.

Radiation decay and osteoradionecrosis are best handled by being prevented. The patient should be examined and evaluated prior to radiation therapy, as previously discussed. Custom fluoride carriers should be fabricated for the patient to be used with a 1 per cent fluoride gel[8] (Fig. 14–2). Fluoride rinses generally are not effective in prevent-

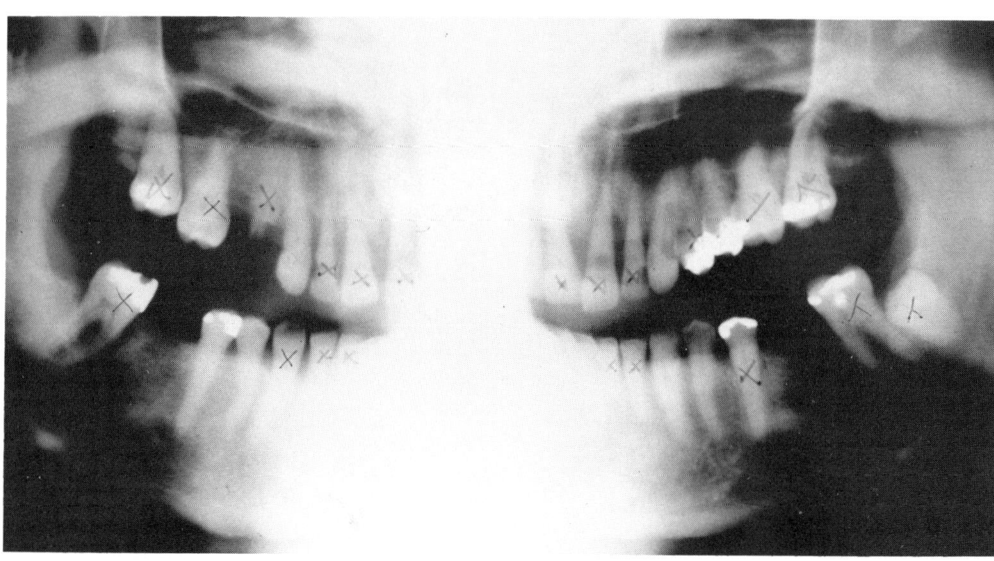

Figure 14–1. Radiographs of a patient seen for evaluation prior to irradiation therapy. There is severe periodontal breakdown requiring extraction of all of the remaining maxillary teeth and all but four of the mandibular teeth.

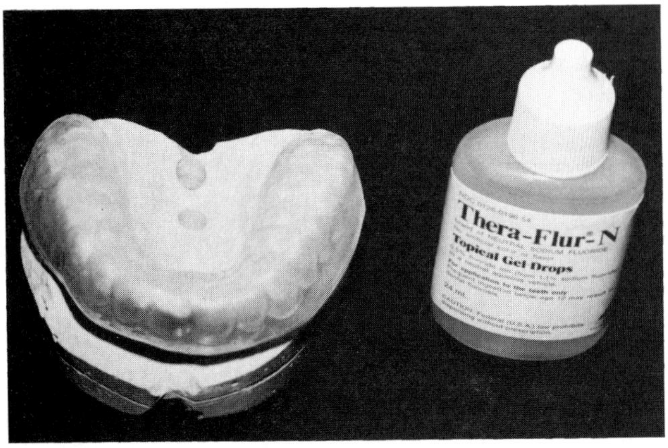

Figure 14–2. Fluoride tray and 1% sodium fluoride gel. A small amount of gel is placed in the tray, and the tray is placed over the teeth for 5 minutes following brushing and flossing.

ing decay and should not be used as a standard treatment for this problem. All patients who receive more than 2000 rads to the salivary gland tissues should receive fluoride therapy. This includes patients with Hodgkin's disease. In patients who have received high-dose radiotherapy, the fluoride should be continued for life. In the case of low-dose therapy, the patient can be taken off the fluoride after 6 to 12 months, and then evaluated at 3-month intervals. If, after a year, there is no appreciable increase in the rate of decay, the fluoride can be totally discontinued and a normal recall schedule instituted. The restoration of decayed teeth after irradiation can be difficult; often the entire circumference of the tooth is involved in the cervical area. It is usually best to restore one half of the tooth at a time, allowing the material to set or cure completely before restoring the second half. The light-cured resin systems have proved invaluable in helping to solve this restorative problem.

Osteoradionecrosis, a serious postradiation complication, is a bony infection that continues because of the compromised postradiation circulation. It is best prevented by a thorough evaluation prior to irradiation therapy. When osteoradionecrosis occurs, it should initially be treated conservatively. The area of exposed bone should be irrigated with a solution composed of one-half 3 per cent peroxide and one-half normal saline. This should be followed by rinses of normal saline, and can be done 4 to 5 times daily. The patient should be followed at 2- to 4-week intervals, and any loose exposed bone should be removed. Bone removal should not involve mucoperiosteal flaps unless an extensive surgical approach is planned. Small localized surgeries often result in greater areas of exposed bone. It is not necessary to place the patient on long-term antibiotics, as the osteoradionecrosis can persist for months to years. However, acute episodes with edema, erythema, fever, lymphadenopathy, and lymphadenitis should most definitely be treated with antibiotics. In the case of infection of areas that communicate with the oral cavity, penicillin is the drug of choice. Cephalosporins or erythromycin also can be used appropriately.

Extractions

When extractions are done prior to radiation therapy, a radical or modified radical alveolectomy should be performed and primary tissue closure achieved. Ordinarily little bone is trimmed following tooth extraction. It should be remembered that bony healing and recontouring will be greatly altered and reduced by the radiation therapy. Therefore idealized bony contours and soft tissues should be attained at the time of surgery.

In the case of carious teeth with periapical infection following radiation therapy, conservative measures such as endodontically treating the teeth should be attempted first. When it becomes essential to extract teeth following irradiation therapy, the patient should be placed on antibiotics prior to the extractions. The antibiotic of choice is penicillin. Radical alveolectomy should be performed, and primary closure attained. Adequate bone removal and tissue undermining should be done to attain tension-free closure with slight eversion of the tissue as illustrated in Figure 14–3. Antibiotic therapy should be continued for 5 to 7 days after extraction.

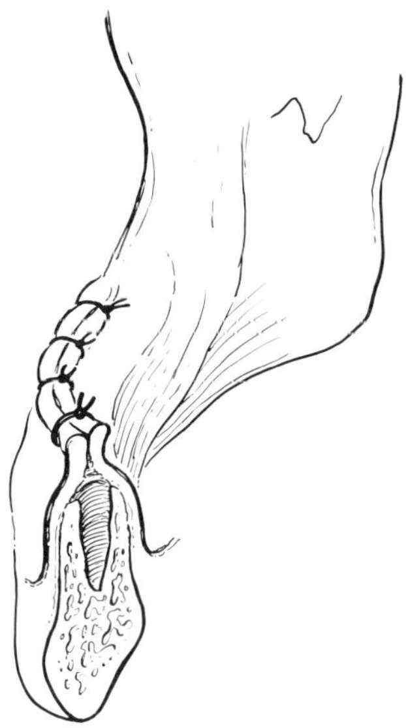

Figure 14–3. Tissue closure at the site of an extracted tooth in an irradiated patient. Note slight eversion of tissue to ensure maintenance of primary closure.

In the postirradiated patient with periodontal involvement, it is best to try to allow chronic periodontal disease to progress to the point where the teeth are surrounded by granulation tissue and can simply be lifted out of the socket. No curettage should take place. Acute episodes in chronically periodontally involved teeth should be treated with antibiotics. Surgery should be avoided if possible (Fig. 14–4).

Hyperbaric Oxygen

Hyperbaric oxygen therapy has been used with some reported success in treating postirradiation complications such as osteoradionecrosis. The reports of this type of therapy state that it greatly enhances healing. Hyperbaric oxygen therapy increases the oxygen tension in the bloodstream and theoretically makes available increased oxygen at the site of the wound. It is known to have specific cellular and biochemical actions, and it facilitates increased vascularity. Hyperbaric oxygen is most valuable as adjunctive therapy. Marx and Ames[9] report on bony reconstruction of irradiated patients using a specific hyperbaric oxygen protocol and rigid evaluation criteria. They note a 94 per cent success rate with use of this treatment. This is especially impressive because of the dismal failures with hyperbaric oxygen in the past.

SURGICAL PROBLEMS

General Considerations

It is extremely important that all of the patient's dental and prosthetic considerations be thoroughly assessed presurgically. It is desirable to obtain past dental records at this stage. If prosthetic rehabilitation of the patient is to be effective, the entire oral situation must be completely evaluated prior to any treatment. There is no doubt that this evaluation places a moderate amount of pressure on both the surgeon and the dentist, because it must be done in a timely fashion so as not to retard the treatment of the patient. A number of general considerations that should always be included in the presurgical assessment are: the remaining dentition of the patient, the bony and soft tissue contours of the oral cavity, the possible placement of flaps or grafts into the defect area, and the function of the remaining tissue following surgery. Surgeons should avoid painting an unrealistically optimistic outlook for the patient with regard to the amount of improvement that can be expected with prosthetic rehabilitation.

A complete and thorough evaluation of the teeth should always be done prior to surgery. This should include an assessment of existing

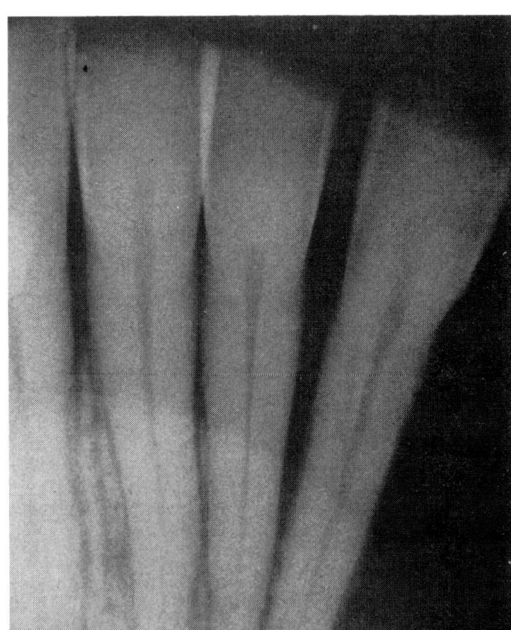

Figure 14–4. Radiograph showing continued chronic bone loss on a tooth in an irradiated patient. This tooth was finally "lifted out" of the alveolus, with the granulation tissue left untouched.

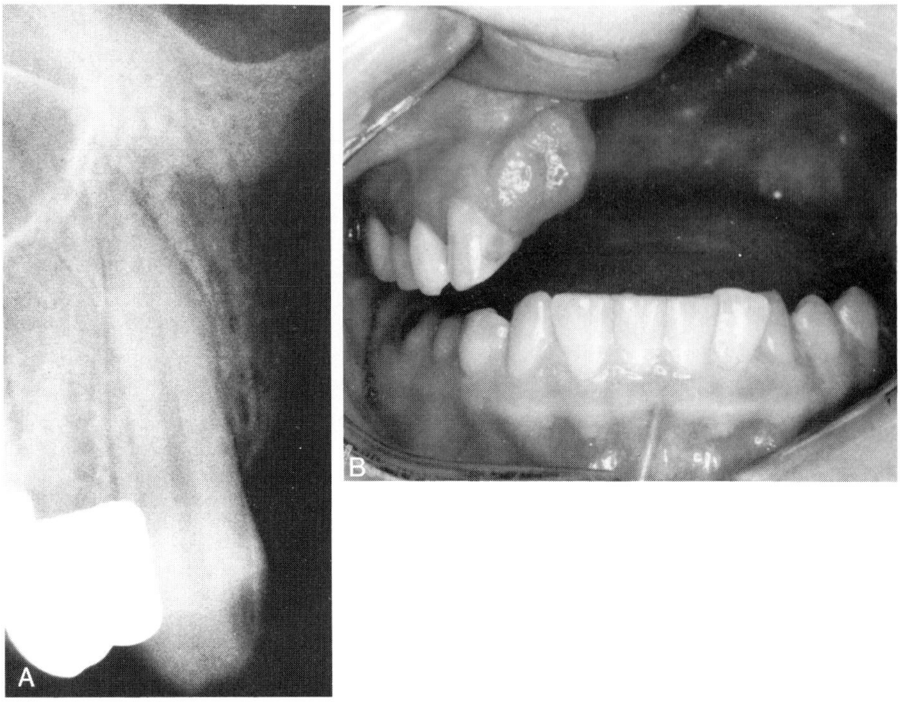

Figure 14–5. Lateral incisor tooth extracted at the time of surgery. Note buttress of bone still remaining medial to cuspid tooth despite the wearing of an obturator prosthesis for 5 years. *A,* Radiograph 5 years post surgery. *B,* Photograph 5 years post surgery.

restorations, periodontal status, occlusal relationships, and the position of teeth in the arch as well as surrounding hard and soft tissue contours. Because the surgeon does not have the training and background in dentistry, he may not realize that some teeth may be more satisfactorily used as abutment teeth than others. It is imperative that the dentist evaluate the patient and consider *all* the facets of his treatment, including the effects of radiation and chemotherapy, when planning for prosthetic rehabilitation. In light of this, there are a number of general principles regarding the dentition and the bony and soft tissue contours of the oral cavity that should be used as guidelines, but not as rigid rules.

Dentition. Since most of these patients will be partially edentulous following surgery, the patient's situation should be evaluated for the placement of some type of cast framework. It should be remembered that the prosthetic devices used for head and neck cancer patients often place increased amounts of stress on the remaining dentition. The design of the prosthesis should allow for movement of the prosthesis in function while placing a minimum amount of stress on the remaining teeth. The surgeon should be advised of key abutment teeth. However, no attempt should be made to compromise the surgical margins and thereby hinder the cure of the patient's primary disease. If the surgeon is aware that a tooth such as a cuspid could be of great assistance in the placement of an obturator prosthesis, there are times when these critical teeth can be saved. The surgeon should also be advised, where it is possible, to make incisions through the middle of an extracted tooth socket and not in an interproximal area between teeth. By doing this, a buttress of bone will more often be provided along the proximal surface of the tooth that will help to prevent gingival stripping by the prosthetic device (Fig. 14–5). Lastly, exostoses and tori should certainly be removed prior to any radiation therapy. This is often best accomplished at the time of the patient's primary surgery.

Bony and Soft Tissue Contours. In evaluating the bony and soft tissue contours, attention should be paid not only to the existing contours but also to those surrounding the potential defect that will exist. Consideration and discussion should be given to the placement of skin grafts when possible. There is little doubt among prosthodontists that skin grafts greatly improve prosthesis placement in these patients. Skin is a better stress-bearing tissue than the attached mucosa that normally makes up the tissues of the hard palate and those directly around the teeth. Unattached mucosa is a poor substitute; often the pseudostratified columnar epithelium found in the sinus cavities will not support a prosthetic device if any pressure is placed on the soft tissue. Radiation therapy simply compounds this problem. During the initial evaluation and planning, it is critical to anticipate the projected potential functioning of the tissues involved following surgery. When possible, reconstructive surgical treatment and a program of rehabilitation should be determined. Ideally this should include a written plan outlining the steps to be followed in prosthetic rehabilitation, speech therapy, physical therapy, nursing care, follow-up, and psychologic support and assistance, the last of which should include an evaluation of the patient's family and support structure.

Trismus

Trismus can be a severe problem in both maxillectomy and mandibulectomy patients. In the maxillectomy patient, control of scar tissue is important. If the area of the coronoid process is exposed surgically, consideration should be given to removing it. This excision will not adversely affect mandibular movement to any great extent, and it may prevent the trismus that might otherwise occur as a result of the formation of scar tissue between the coronoid and surrounding structures.

Control of scar tissue is also critical in mandibulectomy patients. Placing the patient in intermaxillary fixation immediately postoperatively will prevent both mandibular deviation and sometimes trismus. Once trismus occurs, it should be treated immediately with mobilization and physical therapy. Mobilization can be provided by threaded screw devices or guide prostheses, or simply with the use of tongue blades prying the jaws apart within the limitation of pain. In the recalcitrant patient a forceful opening under general anesthesia may be necessary.

Maxillectomy

In the patient who is to have a maxillectomy, there are many factors to be considered. If at all possible, teeth should be saved, because they will certainly assist in the placement, stability, and retention of a prosthetic device. The prosthodontist is certainly aware of the many factors that aid in obturator retention, since many of these are similar to those involved in the placement of partial dentures. Several authors have discussed these factors extensively,[10, 11] and the surgeon should be familiar with the problems involved. Several factors are critical to the surgical treatment of the patient's disease: the contour and alignment of the defect; the timing of the placement of the obturator; the placement of scar bands in both the vertical and horizontal planes; the predictability of the margins; and the removal of the obturator for the first revision. These will all be discussed briefly.

Contour and Alignment of Defect. It is important that the alignment of the defect be coordinated with the alignment of the remaining supporting structures, whether these be the residual alveolar ridge and teeth or the ridge alone. The key here is that the long axis of the bulk of the defect should be parallel to the majority of the supporting structures. Certainly undercut areas that exist both along the hard palate and at the juncture of the defect area laterally at the buccal mucosa will allow for compound paths of insertion and increased retention of the prosthetic device (Fig. 14–6). In addition, extensions can often be obtained superior to the remaining soft palate tissue. This will also allow for increased retention of the prosthesis.

Hard and Soft Palate Defects. When the soft palate is involved, a number of considerations must be taken into account. If the tumor involves the soft palate and the sur-

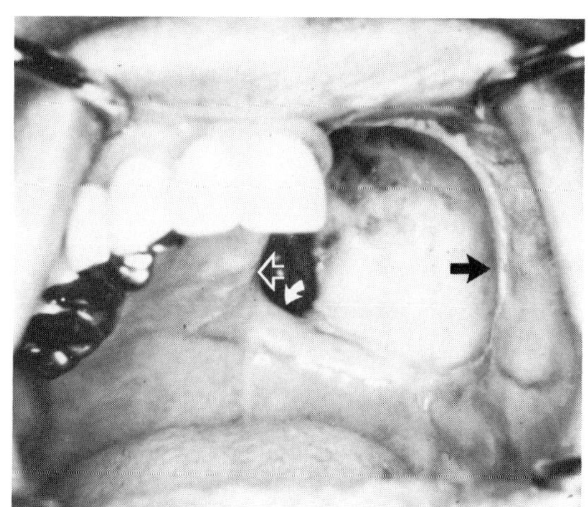

Figure 14–6. Arrows indicate areas of the hand and soft palate available for retention. Note also lateral area with skin graft, which greatly facilitates retention.

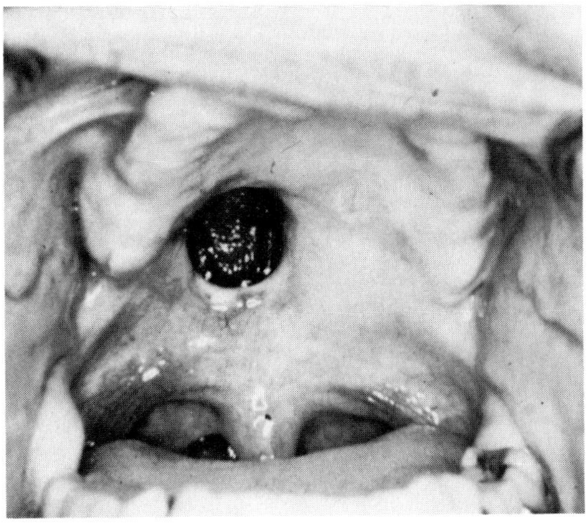

Figure 14–7. Defect at the juncture of the hard and soft portions of the palate.

geon is considering saving some portion of it, at least 1 cm of tissue should be preserved in an anterior posterior direction if the soft palate is to be functional. Usually the extent of the tumor is such that an insufficient portion of the soft palate can be maintained in an anterior posterior direction. However, it may still be helpful if at least half of the width of the soft palate can be salvaged. It is important in such cases, however, not to attempt to use this tissue to obtain partial closure of the defect. This allows for greater movement of the remaining soft palate tissue, which will assist in velopharyngeal closure.

The location of the potential defect in relationship to the juncture of the hard and soft palate may also be critical. Small defects in the region of the junction of the hard and soft palate can be extremely difficult to obturate, because of the amount of movement in this area (Fig. 14–7). Patients often have problems with some leakage because of the lack of a seal. If no planning is done presurgically and the bony defect area is simply allowed to heal, this tissue becomes covered with a modified pseudostratified columnar epithelium. This type of epithelial tissue does not tolerate pressure. In order to adequately obturate the defect, the tissue of the area must be capable of withstanding the pressure of the prosthesis. Several options exist. The first consideration of the surgeon should always be to obtain adequate surgical margins for tumor excision. Within this framework it is suggested that the bony excision in any area of the hard palate be approximately 0.5 cm wider than the soft tissue excision. This will create a 0.5-cm flap of attached mucosa that can be placed into the defect. This will provide increased tissue support in an area of stress. When possible, skin grafts should also be used (Fig. 14–8).

Placement of Scar Tissue. The placement of the scar tissue that will result from normal healing may be critical to good function and peripheral sealing of the obturator prosthesis. In the horizontal axis, it is important that the scar band be placed above Stensen's duct. Care must be taken not to occlude this structure or interfere with its function. If the scar band is located too high in the defect, it will be difficult to obtain an adequate seal with

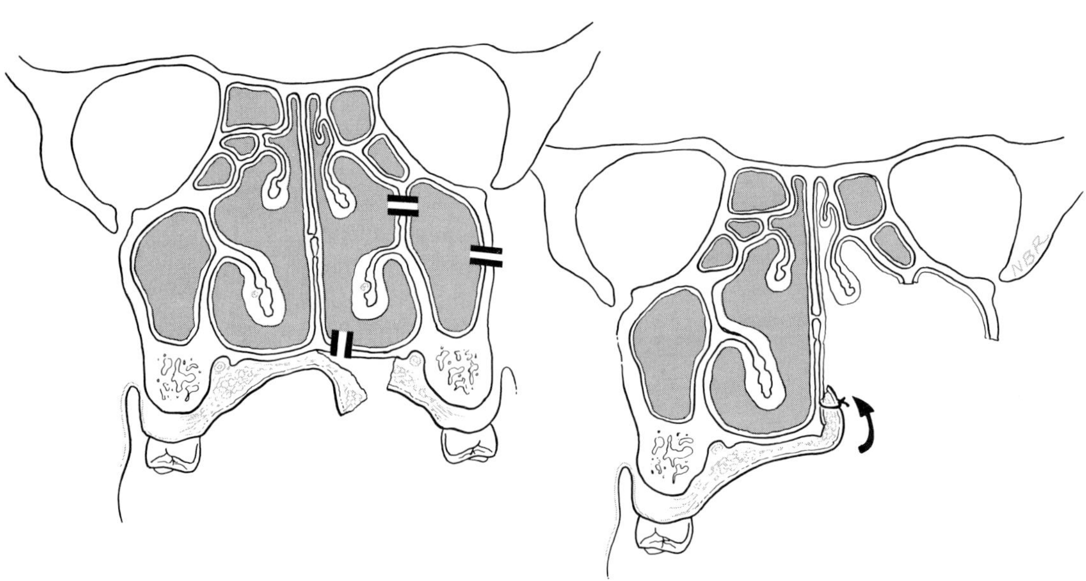

Figure 14–8. Design of surgical incision to allow placement of palatal mucosa into wall of bony defect.

the obturator. If the scar band is located too low on the remaining buccal mucosa, the normal function of the buccinator will be interfered with and the obturator will tend to be displaced. In addition, the scar bands in this area tend to lead to puckering and retraction of the cheek and buccal mucosa. Vertical disposition of scar tissue can also be important, especially in the area of the upper lip. Excessive scar contraction here can cause retraction of the upper lip, producing an appearance similar to that of a badly scarred cleft lip defect. This too interferes with the placement of an obturator, from both a functional and an esthetic point of view. Reconstruction of a defect area with the patient's own tissues is always preferred over the placement of a prosthesis when the functional and esthetic results are equivalent. If the patient will need to wear a prosthetic device, it would be wise to consult a prosthodontist prior to performing reconstructive surgery if there is any chance that the procedure will interfere with the total rehabilitation of the patient.

Timing of Obturation. The timing of the obturator prosthesis is important. Most authors indicate that some type of immediate obturation of the defect is desirable. The definition of "immediate obturation," however, differs from author to author. In the strictest sense, an immediate obturator is one that is placed at the time of surgery. However, at times this definition is also used to describe an obturator that is placed several days after surgery. There is disagreement even among prosthodontists regarding the optimum timing for the placement and the extent of the obturator prosthesis. Certainly if a skin graft is in place, some type of pressure needs to be maintained on the grafted tissue immediately. This can be accomplished either by adequate packing or with the obturator. The obturator can simply be made to conform to the periphery of the defect area. The dressing placed in the defect can seal those margins of the defect that are not contacted by the prosthesis but still maintain pressure on any skin graft which has been placed.

It is always difficult to predict the exact margins of the defect prior to surgery, and it is virtually impossible to fabricate an obturator that will conform to all of the defect areas prior to the surgery itself. At times, it may be possible to add some type of material, such as tissue conditioning material, to the obturator to adapt it to the defect. This will allow extremely accurate adaptation of the surgical prosthesis to the defect area. This requires, however, either that the prosthodontist be present at the time of surgery or that the surgeon be skilled in the use of these materials. Depending on the setting, this may or may not be possible. Probably the most critical time in the postsurgical phase is the time at which the dressing in the surgical defect is removed. It is essential at this point that the obturator prosthesis conform accurately, especially against the lateral walls of the defect. This can be accomplished in several ways. One is to make an impression of the entire defect area and surrounding oral structures; then an interim obturator prosthesis can be fabricated from acrylic resin and placed into the defect. This has some definite advantages in that the interim obturator prosthesis can be more easily kept clean and is easily maintained both in the remaining healing phase following surgery and if the patient is to undergo further treatment such as radiation therapy. An alternative method that can prove satisfactory, especially if prosthodontic or laboratory support is somewhat limited or if prosthodontic care is not available, is to add tissue conditioning material to the surgical obturator prosthesis so that it will conform to the defect area. It is critical that this phase of care be well coordinated. Lack of attention to detail during this phase of care can lead to uncontrolled placement of scar tissue, facial disfigurement, and extreme difficulty in definitive obturation of the surgical defect.

Maxillectomies can also cause lack of orbital support and other eye problems (Fig. 14–9). Once the scarring has occurred, little can be done to correct the problem prosthetically. The surgeon must be involved in preventing this problem by means of good surgical technique and timely prosthetic intervention.

There are a number of controversies that presently exist in prosthodontics with regard to the obturator prosthesis; among the questions yet to be resolved are:

1. Should the obturator be hollow or solid?
2. Should the superior surface of the obturator be convex or concave?
3. Should the obturator be fabricated from processed acrylic resin or should some type of semipermanent soft material such as silicone be used?

The advantages and disadvantages to each of these approaches are covered in several texts,[12, 13] to which the reader is referred for

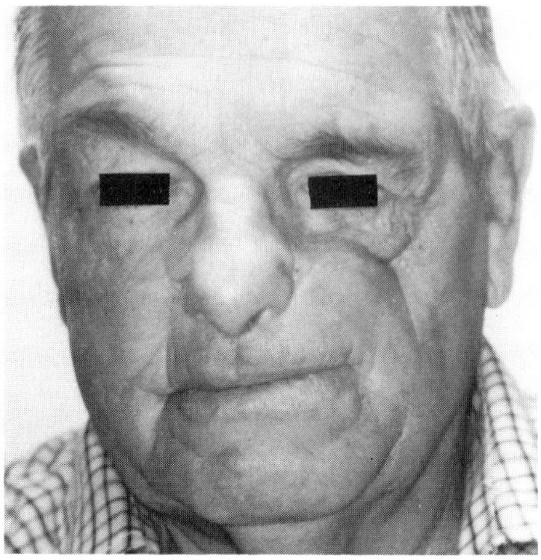

Figure 14–9. Loss of support for left eye, creating facial defect and causing double vision.

further discussion. It should be noted here, however, that variations in the contour and construction of the obturator should be individualized for each patient. If a maxillary obturator prosthesis is to function maximally, its placement and maintenance must be well integrated with the remainder of the treatment of the patient.

Mandibulectomy

General Background

Patients with mandibulectomies have varying types of defects depending on the physical extent of surgery, the involvement of other surrounding structures (such as the tongue), the amount of neural involvement, the amount of scarring at the surgical site, and the amount of deviation during mandibular movement. Curtis has classified patients who undergo mandibulectomies into 3 categories based on the amount of bony involvement.[14] The three basic categories are radical alveolectomy, anterior resection, and hemimandibulectomy (Fig. 14–10).

Radical Alveolectomy

In the patient with a radical alveolectomy, all of the usual prosthetic considerations come into play, as discussed by Sharry.[15] One of the most important of these is the management of the surrounding soft tissues. Two factors are important here: (a) wound closure with coverage of the mandible and (b) mobility of the tongue.

Wound Closure. When the soft tissues from the floor of the mouth or tongue are approximated to those of the buccal mucosa, thus effecting primary closure of the defect, it is often difficult to place a prosthesis in this area. There are two reasons for this. The first is that the mandible is not covered with firm supporting tissues, while the unattached mucosa that is normally present in the buccal mucosa is not well suited to provide prosthetic support. The second reason is that this type of closure often introduces tissues that are highly movable and thus will cause a great deal of movement in any prosthesis that is placed over them.

Mobility of the Tongue. Several authors have discussed the importance of the tongue in the management of any prosthetic device—

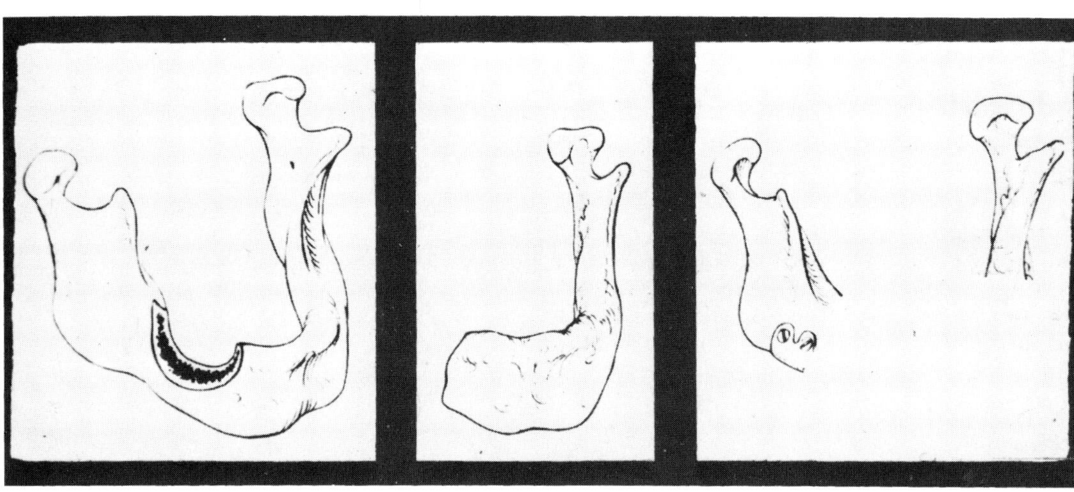

Figure 14–10. Basic mandibulectomy categories.

especially a removable one—that is placed in the mandible.[16–18] This is important not only with regard to the need for mobility of the tongue, which enables it to physically manage various aspects of mastication, deglutition, and speech, but also with respect to its kinesthetics, in light of the fact that decreased sensations of proprioception seem to markedly decrease the ability of the patient to speak and eat normally.

The principal problem that arises from radical alveolectomy is the loss of a ridge that will fix and support a denture. If the adjacent ridges are insufficient, an alveoloplasty may be necessary (see Chapter 1).

Anterior Resection

To date, patients who have undergone anterior resections of the mandible have not been well rehabilitated prosthetically. The problems of lack of control of saliva, lack of normal proprioceptive function of the skin of the lips and face, lack of stability of the mandible, altered maxillomandibular relationships, and loss of teeth all markedly interfere with prosthetic rehabilitation. The solution to these problems in the future will lie in combined surgical and prosthetic rehabilitation of the patient. An example of this type of treatment is shown in Fig. 14–11. (See also Chapter 1.)

Hemimandibulectomy

Patients who have had a classic hemimandibulectomy are perhaps the most challenging, both surgically and prosthetically. These patients hardly constitute a unified group, and for this reason the discussion here will be further subdivided in order to fully cover each of the factors involved in the rehabilitation of the hemimandibulectomy patient. These factors are: the degree of temporomandibular joint function, the amount of remaining bone structure, the loss of the muscles of mastication and the supra- and infrahyoid musculature, the degree of function of the muscles of the tongue, neuromuscular integration, the movement of the mandible, the teeth remaining, and lastly, the types of adjuvant therapy employed. Obviously these factors, although discussed separately in the following paragraphs, must be considered in an integrated fashion as they apply in each individual case. There is great variety in the types of rehabilitation possible for the hemimandibulectomy patient, and reconstructive surgery may make a significant contribution to prosthetic rehabilitation.

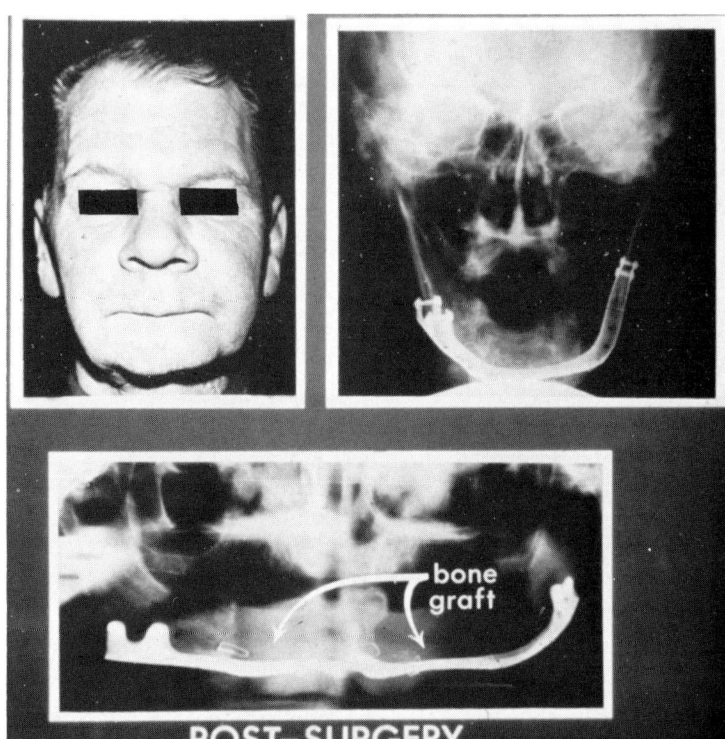

Figure 14–11. A patient with an anterior resection of the mandible, rehabilitated with a combination of surgical and prosthetic reconstruction.

The Temporomandibular Joint. The loss of the temporomandibular joint creates problems in mandibular motion that are most critical in mastication, the patient otherwise being capable of both speech and deglutition. It is rare to have a patient with head and neck cancer who loses only temporomandibular joint function, or whose only structural loss involves the condylar head and surrounding structures. The patient who has lost the temporomandibular joint on just one side suffers two problems: instability and lack of lateral movement from centric relation to the side *opposite* the defect.

The loss of the condyle involves the loss of the external pterygoid muscle on the side of the defect. This muscle is primarily responsible for lateral movement from centric relation to the opposite side of the defect. This movement becomes important during the chewing cycle; most individuals do not chew in a straight vertical plane but in a somewhat teardrop-shaped fashion as described by Posselt.[19] The external pterygoids act as a muscle pair with slight antagonism. Considering these muscles in light of the force vectors they can create, the vectors possible are bilateral and at an angle of approximately 45° to the frontal plane. Obviously, acting unilaterally and unopposed, these force vectors will create a deviation to the side of the defect. This is in part responsible for the deviation of the mandible to the side of the defect in the patient with a hemimandibulectomy. The relative importance of this factor is not entirely known.

Remaining Bone Structure. The next factor is the amount of mandibular bone structure remaining. Essentially, this can be divided into three categories according to bony loss: the ascending ramus, the mandibular body from cuspid to angle, and the body from the symphysis posteriorly. All hemimandibulectomies result in mandibular discontinuity. With an increasing deficit of bone structure, there is a progressive loss of stability in any prosthetic device that is fabricated, and other factors involved become more and more critical, especially the presence or absence of teeth and the amount of residual functioning tongue. It is not absolutely clear how important the amount of residual mandible is. However, in a small study that evaluated mandibular movement in mandibulectomy patients, the patient who had been surgically reconstructed so that only the ascending ramus of the mandible was missing exhibited mandibular movements somewhat analogous to the norm.[20] The loss of bony structure often precludes the extension of any prosthetic device into the area of the defect, especially in the edentulous patient. This creates a serious problem, because any forces that are generated on the remaining mandible are not counteracted and there is not enough lateral stability to stop the generated rotational forces.

Muscles of Mastication and Supra- and Infrahyoid Musculature. The loss of the muscles of mastication and of the supra- and infrahyoid musculature on the side of the defect also creates some instability. This is discussed at some length by Beumer et al.[21] The forces generated in this situation tend to be of the type that will dislodge the prosthesis rather than stabilize it. In addition, the muscles of mastication, which are responsible for the closing movements of the mandible, and the supra- and infrahyoid muscles, which are responsible for the opening movements of the mandible, are paired, bilateral structures. When these structures are required to function unilaterally, it is necessary for the patient to learn to control the mandible in an entirely new way, which is extremely difficult because the mandibular movements involved in chewing and speaking are essentially instinctive movements. Little is known about the best manner in which to approach this problem. Certainly, further research is needed.

Muscles of the Tongue. The role of the tongue in maintaining a prosthetic device in the mandible is well known. Both Wright[16] and Desjardins[17] have described how the tongue, especially its position and movement during function, can act either to maintain or displace the prosthesis. Patients who have lost portions of their tongue obviously will have altered function. In addition, adjacent scarring often restricts the movements of the tongue remmnant or even an intact tongue, and may be a cause for prosthetic instability.

Neuromuscular Integration. Neuromuscular integration involves sensory feedback, proprioception, and neural integration of the oral tissues. Normal sensory feedback allows for a subconscious perception of the position of the hard and soft tissues in space and in relationship to each other, as well as the presence, absence, or position of any other material in the oral cavity, such as a prosthesis or a bolus of food. Without adequate neural integration and sensory feedback, complicated movements such as placing food in the mouth and properly masticating it becomes extremely difficult, if not impossible. Patients often complain of large amounts of food becoming lodged in the area of the defect or of losing food through the lips because they are not aware of its presence. In addition, the coordination of movements required during chewing, such as moving a bolus of food back onto the chewing table or swallowing, requires proprioception and neural integration.

Mandibular Movement. It is important, too, in understanding potential prosthesis design, to understand the movements of the mandible of a patient with a hemimandibulectomy. The normal movements of the mandible are described in many texts, and the literature on the subject is well summarized by Sharry.[15] The normal movements of the mandible must be analyzed first before the altered mandibular movements in the mandibulectomy patient can be fully understood. The patient with a mandibulectomy opens and closes his mouth in a somewhat diagonal fashion. In addition, the dentition tends to make contact on the defect side first. Following contact of the teeth on the defect side, there is a net rotational movement that occurs with a continued lateral slide. Following contact of the dentition (natural or artificial) on the non-defect side, there actually is disarticulation of the teeth on the defect side.

Remaining Dentition. It becomes critical in patients with a mandibulectomy to maintain the remaining dentition if at all possible. There are two reasons for this. First, if it is necessary to restore missing dentition, it becomes very difficult for the patient to adequately masticate food. This difficulty seems to be proportional to the number of teeth lost. Second, as with fabrication of any prosthetic device, the absence of teeth creates a problem because of the loss of stability of the prosthetic device. Even patients with their own remaining natural dentition will still have a number of the problems outlined above and may have seriously compromised function. Restoration of missing teeth, when some of the dentition remains, is still a major problem.

Adjuvant Therapy. Lastly, adjuvant therapy often can further complicate the situation of the hemimandibulectomy patient. This is especially true of radiation therapy, which often creates further scarring at the site of the defect with resultant distraction, partial fixation, and loss of mobility of the mandibular fragment. In addition, there is a reduction in saliva, which tends to decrease prosthesis retention and create additional, frictional resistance between the remaining oral tissues and the prosthesis. In short, radiation therapy tends to magnify the problems that already exist because of the surgical excision.

FACIAL PROSTHESES

It is especially true in the case of facial reconstruction that adequate restoration of the missing anatomy with the patient's own tissue is always preferable. Often, however, such surgical restoration requires multiple procedures, and the end result is not as satisfactory as that achieved with a facial prosthesis. The innate disadvantages and advantages of facial prostheses must also be taken into account.

Disadvantages. A facial prosthesis must be removed to be cleaned, and the surrounding tissues must also be carefully cleansed and maintained. Facial prostheses deteriorate over a period of time, requiring alteration and, at times, refabrication. With extremely large facial defects, fixation of the prosthesis is still an extremely difficult and serious problem; many times external means such as straps need to be employed. Implants may in the future help to resolve this problem. Small facial prostheses, such as those for the ear, nose, and orbital area, can often be maintained by the use of facial adhesives alone (Fig. 14–12). There are a number of adhesives available, all of which are gum-based materials that adequately hold the prosthesis in place. Intermediate-sized prostheses often can be maintained with a combination of adhesives and some type of retentive device attached to an additional intraoral prosthesis. Examples of these types of retentive devices are magnets, hooks, buttons, or grooves (Fig. 14–13).

Advantages. There are a number of advantages to a facial prosthesis. The surgical site can be continuously cleaned and inspected. This is especially important during the first few years after treatment, when recurrence of disease is most likely. Facial contours can often be very accurately reproduced or even altered to suit patient preferences. For instance, a nose that the patient had considered too large prior to surgery can be replaced with a nasal prosthesis that is small or more pleasing. Large defects that are unamenable to surgical restoration can be totally reconstructed, enabling the patient to more comfortably integrate back into society. Numer-

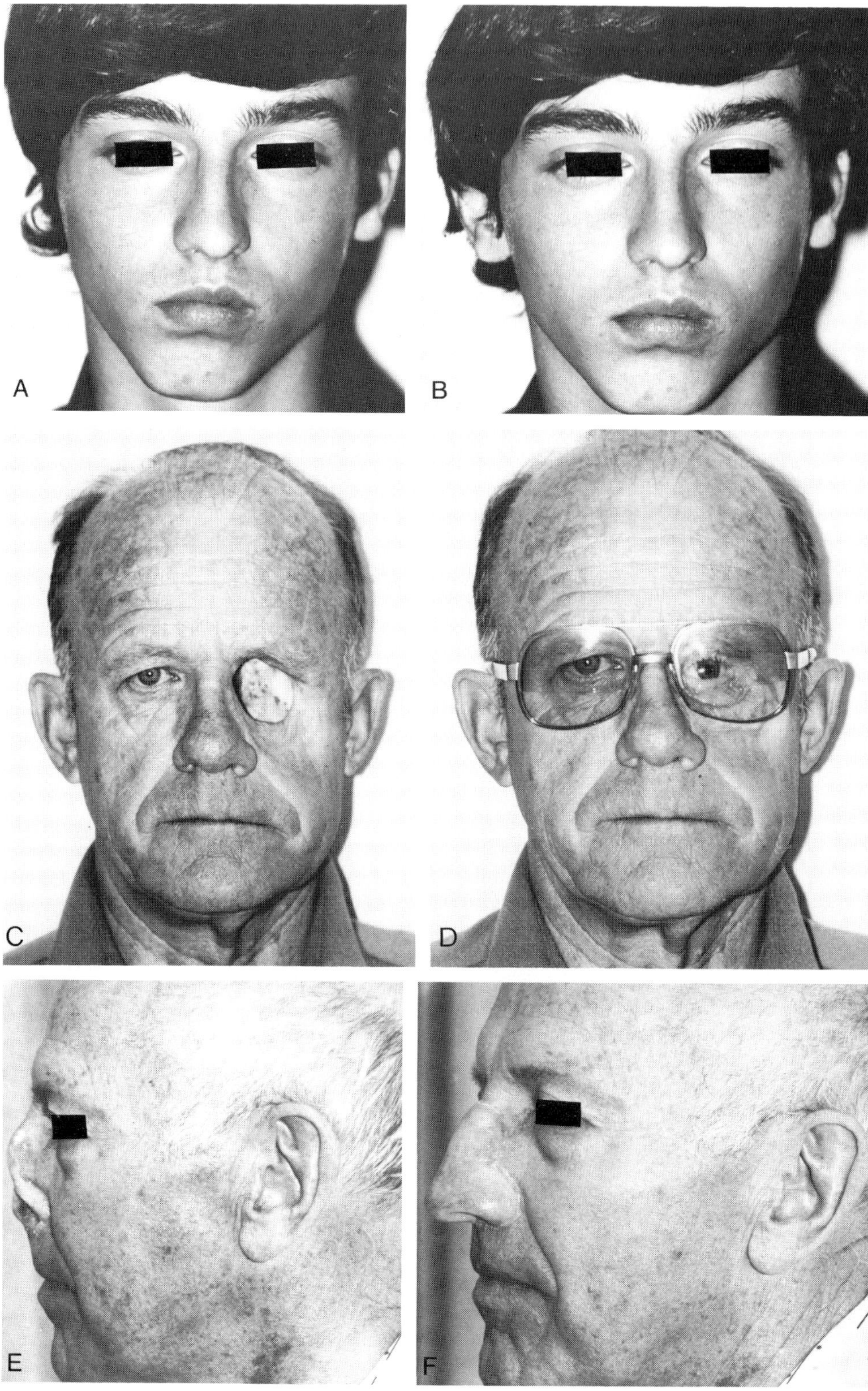

Figure 14–12. Several patients with and without prosthesis. *A* and *B*, Ear. *C* and *D*, Eye. *E* and *F*, Nose.

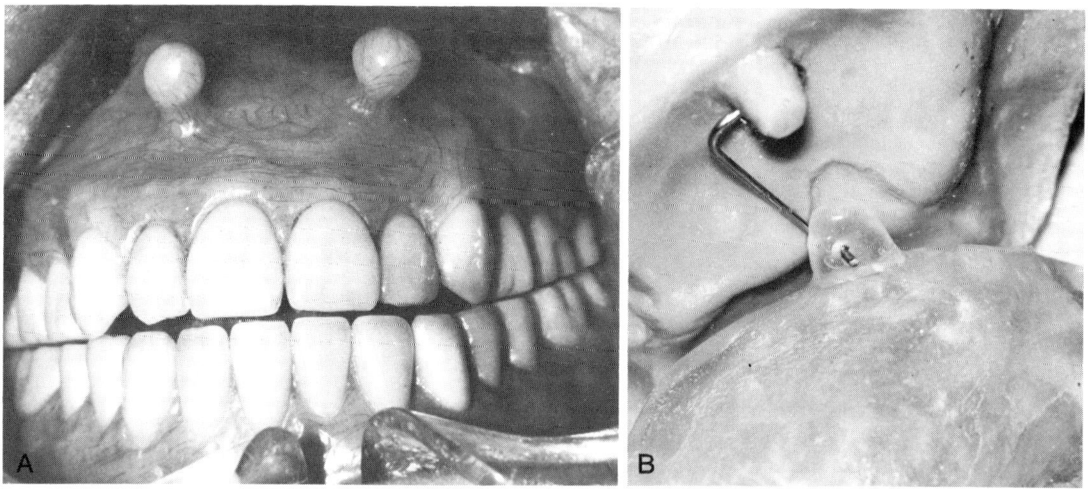

Figure 14–13. Examples of prosthesis retention. *A,* Buttress used to retain facial prosthesis. *B,* Wire hook on inner aspect of facial prosthesis, which attaches to groove in obturator as shown in Figure 14–14.

ous examples of such types of rehabilitation exist (Fig. 14–14).

As with other prosthetic devices, it is important when designing a facial prosthesis that adequate discussion take place between the surgeon and the prosthodontist so that reasonable rehabilitative goals can be set and the most satisfactory result obtained. When possible, skin is the most satisfactory surface for retaining a facial prosthesis. This will at times necessitate lining areas such as the nasal cavity with a skin graft following surgical excision. The tissue surfaces and tissue contours must be carefully prepared to enhance the fit and retention of a prosthesis. An especially difficult problem is to construct a prosthesis that will allow for adequate movement in the lip and cheek areas. Although it is quite possible for some movement with a facial prosthesis, especially when a flexible material such as silicone is used, movements that are essential to form certain common facial expressions are often not possible. In addition, satisfactory control of saliva can be difficult, if not impossible. If a patient should have a recurrence of tumor in the facial area, consultation should again take place between the surgeon and the prosthodontist before surgery is undertaken. If these areas are reexcised without adequate consultation, it may be extremely difficult or impossible to fabricate a new facial prosthesis.

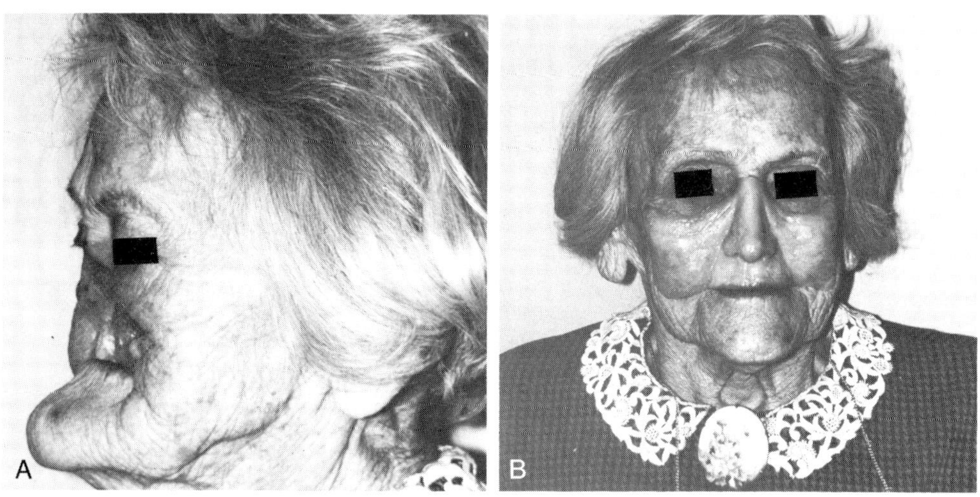

Figure 14–14. *A,* Large facial defect. *B,* After restoration with intraoral and facial prosthesis.

CONCLUSION

A prosthetic device can be a critical part of the total treatment of the head and neck cancer patient. There are inherent limitations to, as well as advantages of, this type of rehabilitation, as has been discussed. The ideal care of the patient requires thorough integration of prosthetic treatment with all other phases of treatment.

References

1. Chalian V, Drane J, Standish M (eds): Maxillofacial Prosthetics. Baltimore, William & Wilkins, 1971.
2. Laney WR (ed): Maxillofacial Prosthetics. Post Graduate Dental Handbook Series. Littleton, MA, PSG Publishing Co, 1979.
3. Beumer J, Curtis TA, Firtell DN: Maxillofacial Rehabilitation. St Louis, CV Mosby, 1979.
4. Gillis RE: Psychological implications of patient care. *In* Laney WR (ed): Post Graduate Dental Handbook Series. Littleton, MA, PSG Publishing Co, 1979, p 21.
5. Ross BR: The clinician and the head and neck cancer patient. *In* Beumer J, Curtis TA, Firtell DN: Maxillofacial Rehabilitation. St Louis, CV Mosby, 1979, p 1.
6. Conley J. *In* Healy JEJ (ed): Ecology of the Cancer Patient. Washington DC, Interdisciplinary Communications Association, 1970.
7. Gillis RE: Unpublished data.
8. Driezen S, Daly T, Drane JB: Prevention of xerostomia related dental caries in irradiated cancer patients. J Dent Res 56:99, 1977.
9. Marx RE, Ames JR: The use of hyperbaric oxygen therapy in bony reconstruction of the irradiated and tissue deficient patient. J Oral Maxillofac Surg 40:412, 1982.
10. Henderson D, Steffel VL: McCrackens' Removable Partial Prosthodontics. St Louis, CV Mosby, 1981.
11. Terkla L, Laney WR: Partial Dentures. St Louis, CV Mosby, 1963.
12. Laney WR (ed): Maxillofacial Prosthetics. Post Graduate Dental Handbook Series. Littleton, MA, PSG Publishing Co, 1979, p 115.
13. Beumer J, Curtis TA, Firtell DN: Maxillofacial Rehabilitation. St Louis, CV Mosby, 1979, p 205.
14. Curtis TA, Cantor R: Prosthetic management of edentulous mandibulectomy patients. Part I. Anatomic, physiologic and psychologic considerations. J Prosthet Dent 25:446, 1971.
15. Sharry J: Complete Denture Prosthodontics. New York, McGraw-Hill, 1974.
16. Wright CR: Evaluation of the factors necessary to develop stability in mandibular dentures. J Prosthet Dent 16:414, 1966.
17. Desjardins RP: The tongue as it relates to complete dentures. JADA 88:814, 1974.
18. King GE, Martin JW, Munson TJ: Functional mandibular surgical stents: use in primary reconstruction of the cancer patient. J Prosthet Dent 49:217, 1983.
19. Posselt U: Studies in the mobility of the human mandible. Acta Odont Scand 10 (Suppl):90, 105, 114, 1952.
20. Gillis RE, Curtis TA: A pantographic study of hemimandibulectomy patients. Unpublished.
21. Beumer J, Curtis TA, Firtell DN: Maxillofacial Rehabilitation. St Louis, CV Mosby, 1979, p 106.

15

NURSING ASPECTS

Ann E. Furiel Sievers, R.N., M.A.

This chapter covers the problems that nurses face in dealing with the complicated care of patients with head and neck cancer. The function of the nurse is to be a highly trained coordinator and patient advocate.

MULTIDISCIPLINARY APPROACH

Allied health personnel can and should be a powerful influence in the care of patients with head and neck tumors. Representation of individuals from varied disciplines—such as nurses, psychologists, social workers, dieticians, speech pathologists, and volunteers—is essential to a comprehensive plan of care.

It is important to understand that nowhere else in the body are scars, defects, and asymmetry as evident to others as in the head and neck area. The face as a focal point for communication and identity is very important in our society. Trauma and wounds of the head and neck area not only cause disfigurement but also involve organs that function to meet the basic human needs of air, fluid, and food intake. These organs also serve to assess the environment via the special senses of sight, hearing, taste, and smell. Radical surgery for the treatment of cancer may involve these same special tissues or may require the removal of, or changes in, the organs used for speech. Any interference with facial appearance, the ability to obtain basic human needs, or the ability to communicate can be a devastating experience for the patient and family. Being sensitive to those reactions and providing meaningful support are only part of the challenge in caring for these patients.[1]

The most challenging aspect of care is to provide the emotional, psychological, and physical support needed to help these patients return to as normal a life as possible. Because of their numerous problems with eating, breathing, and communication, our purpose is to help them attain an optimal level of function. The families must be involved and must understand that this is a cooperative planning and decision-making effort. *The secret of the care of the patient is in caring for the patient.*

Much has been written about the multidisciplinary approach to treating patients with extensive life-threatening illnesses, especially cancer. This method of intervention brings the best minds together to care for the patient. However, a leader of the team must be clearly identified, and this is usually the attending physician. In our experience the team should consist of surgeons, chemotherapists, radiation oncologists, dentists, clinical nursing specialists, social workers, psychiatrists, visiting nurses, speech pathologists, and nutritionists. Each should establish a rapport with the patient and family to ensure successful hospitalization and rehabilitation. Clear lines of communication must be kept open for the team to function. The key to success of such a team is open, close, and honest communication.

COUNSELING OF PATIENTS AND FAMILIES

In the past decade, numerous advances have taken place in the surgical treatment and nursing management of the patient with head and neck cancer. In addition to innovative techniques, appliances and speech aids have been developed, and large numbers of speech pathologists have been trained to teach laryngectomees alaryngeal speech. In general, our overall knowledge of the rehabilitation needs of laryngectomees has increased dramatically, and we have recognized that this includes their need for information, instruction, and psychological support. Unfortunately, despite this knowledge, countless patients with laryngeal cancer still show evidence of inadequate counseling, particularly during the preoperative period. They have misconceptions about their disease and its treatment, the physical sequelae of laryngectomy, self-care, and the various steps involved in total rehabilitation. When the patient and close relatives are not informed about these matters, postoperative adjustment tends to become increasingly difficult and prolonged. The impact of this lack of presurgical counseling has been documented by a number of investigators.[3]

Studies have revealed many misconceptions regarding surgery and its sequelae. Lack of knowledge of the disease and normal functioning, as well as ignorance of general health care measures required after surgery, has been well documented. It is therefore very important that patients and families receive intensive counseling throughout the treatment process, especially during the preoperative period. The nursing staff must be made aware of the specific types of surgical intervention and their implications for rehabilitation, e.g., the difference between a total and supraglottic laryngectomy.

One of the most interesting and rewarding ways to counsel patients is in a patient support group. Explained in detail later in this chapter (see Psychologic Rehabilitation, p. 409), the group meetings provide a comfortable environment for the exchange of ideas and information. Patients are the real experts, and in such a group they can freely exchange their knowledge. In addition, a good deal of emotional support is demonstrated. Patients address such issues as "Should I get a second opinion?" and "How can I get mad at my doctor without fearing retribution?" They also discuss how to cope with the death of fellow group members.

With such a group base, information regarding hospitalization can easily be addressed. Patients can give information that only someone who has gone through the experience is able to give. Such a basis is invaluable for the medical staff to build upon.

Concrete information must be delivered. All patients undergoing laryngectomy at our institution are given *Looking Forward—A Guide Book for the Laryngectomee,* by Robert Keith. This book offers a wealth of information presented in a simple and concise manner. Patients are also given *Self Help for the Laryngectomee,* by Edmund Lauder. Both books answer questions like "How do I take a shower?" and "Can I speak again?"

Extensive support from the speech pathologist is critical for all patients who have head and neck cancer. The ability to communicate is extremely important in our society, and maintenance of a functioning language system can make a great deal of difference during the hospitalization and rehabilitation.

Materials from the American Cancer Society, Health and Human Services Department, and National Cancer Institute are used extensively in teaching and counseling. Patient education should be an ongoing process beginning before admission to the hospital. In most cases, the more information patients receive, the better prepared they are for their surgery. It is important to start with very basic information and then gradually expand their knowledge.

During the process of diagnosis, treatment, and follow-up, the patient often may feel a loss of control as well as a loss of privacy. The constraints, especially time limitations, that are often imposed upon patients can be overwhelming. Sensitivity to the patient's emotional need for control and self-determination often is lost by hospital staff members, who are mainly involved in the physical aspects of patient care. In defense of the staff, patients who have extensive surgery or complications may indeed require a high degree of time intervention. However, it is important to remember that allowing the patient and family time to themselves to think, talk, and conduct their own "business" often provides a welcome respite from medically related activities. It is often reciprocated by a patient who becomes more willing to endure the frequent dressing changes and numerous tests that are required. The process of building a nursing care plan together with the patient allows him to participate in his own care. When the plan is developed and followed by both staff and patient, it is usually more successful in directing energies toward getting the patient well.

Family and friends should not be forgotten.

They should be informed about where to wait during the surgery, how long the visiting hours are in the Intensive Care Unit, and how long the patient will stay in Intensive Care before being moved to the regular hospital floor. Factual information can make the difference between an extremely anxious family and one that feels they can participate in the care of the patient.

Preparation for discharge also can be a very trying time for family and patient. Providing consistent patient education and concrete information is paramount to making a smooth transition from hospital to home. Requiring patients and family to assume their own care for at least 48 hours in the hospital under direct supervision allows them to practice their responsibilities while retaining the opportunity to ask questions of physicians and staff.

Discharge from the hospital is often a very frightening time for both patients and their families. Even the best prepared patients have related that the reality of being responsible for their own care at home was very frightening for the first few days. Here the services of a visiting nurse can be invaluable. The nurse who will be coordinating care at home should first visit the patient in the hospital. This allows both parties to meet each other in a non-stressful situation. Upon leaving the hospital, patients should be given written information about their surgery, instructions for follow-up care, and emergency phone numbers.

SPECIFIC ASPECTS OF CARE

Artificial Airways

There are many controversial theories about the care of artificial airways. This is because the field is changing so quickly. It is important to understand the basic concepts relevant to the clinical situation. A staff skilled in the care of patients with artificial airways can prevent many complications. *Prevention is the rule.*

Routine care procedures may often be neglected. Because the principal functions of the upper airway are bypassed as a result of a tracheostomy means that such factors as humidification, filtration, and warmth are often forgotten. However, if routine procedures are meticulously attended to, major problems can usually be avoided. Supplying mist to the airway, ensuring adequate hydration, and instilling normal saline, as well as filtration and suctioning and periodic bagging are all important measures in airway care. Mist can be supplied as a warm or cool mist or by intermittent ultrasonic nebulization. Normal saline can be instilled in amounts of 2 to 4 cc every 2 to 3 hours as needed to assist in the moisturizing and mobilization of secretions. Patients at home can be taught how to make their own saline solution and instill it with an eyedropper. Saline instillation is not, however, a replacement for adequate systemic hydration either by oral liquids or by nasogastric or intravenous replacement. The equivalent of 8 to 10 glasses of water per day is adequate to promote pulmonary clearance and assist the function of the normal pulmonary escalator.

Suctioning and bagging are very important in the immediate postoperative period. Maintenance of adequate tidal volume (V_T) and vital capacity (VC) will prevent postoperative pulmonary complications. Aggressive pulmonary toilet may appear to be more critical with patients who have undergone thoracic and abdominal surgeries. However, a high percentage of patients with head and neck cancer have extensive smoking histories and often have some chronic obstructive pulmonary disease, requiring good pulmonary toilet to prevent atelectasis and pneumonia after lengthy anesthesia. Sterile suction catheters and gloves should be used to prevent inoculation of microorganisms into the pulmonary system. These and the irrigation fluid for the catheter should be changed after each use.

Filtration of the airway is not as critical in the hospital as it is in the home or the outside environment. Dusting bath powders, paint fumes, and even vinyl curtains can be irritating to the airway. A stoma shield of cotton or foam can be used to provide some protection (Fig. 15–1). Coverings of matching cloth or jewlery, available from the local Lost Cord Club or the American Cancer Society, are both attractive and functional. The airway does become "acclimatized" after a period of time varying from 4 to 6 months.

Tracheostomy and Stoma Care

Care of a tracheostomy or stomal wound is simply a matter of keeping the wound clean. This is true of all wounds no matter how complex. Application of a solution of hydrogen peroxide and normal saline should maintain a clean wound site. The use of

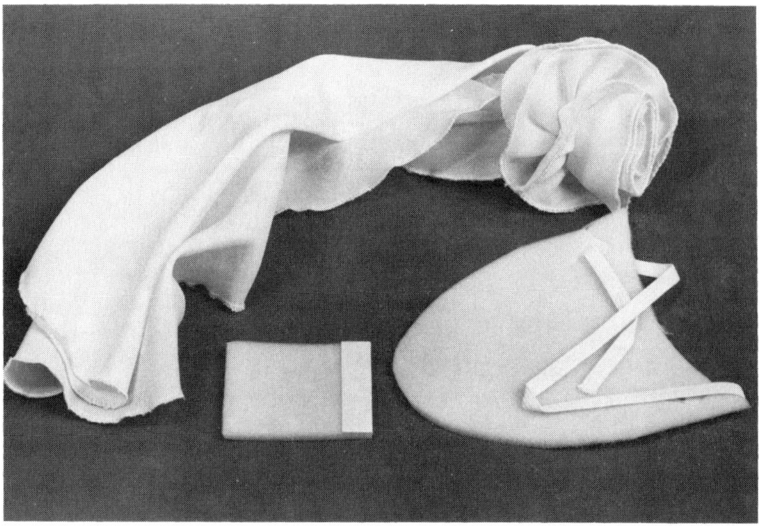

Figure 15–1. Stoma shield.

dressings, sterile Q-tips, and clean technique is acceptable. It is critical to use sterile supplies when doing wound care, but the procedure itself is considered clean. There is some evidence that in a hospital setting, in terms of preventing infection and avoiding contamination, clean technique is equivalent to sterile technique.

An antibiotic ointment may be used around the wound site after cleansing. This helps to avoid crusting at the incision sites on permanent stomas. Patients are taught clean technique for home use, including strict handwashing and frequent cleaning of equipment.

For patients who have severely excoriated skin around the stoma or tracheostomy wound site, the skin is thoroughly cleansed and dried, and Stomahesive is applied to the affected area. This protects the skin and allows it to heal, yet is comfortable to the patient. The tracheostomy dressing is applied over the Stomahesive and acts as an absorbant for secretions. Cotton dressings should *never* be cut and placed directly over the wound, because the threads separate and become embedded in the healing wound. Precut and stitched dressings, such as the Soft-Wik Drain Sponges manufactured by Johnson and Johnson, are excellent. Patients prefer the drain sponges because of their high absorbancy and soft texture.

In clinical medicine, tracheostomy has four basic indications: (1) to bypass an upper airway obstruction; (2) to assist or control respirations over prolonged periods; (3) to facilitate the chronic care of respiratory tract secretions; and (4) to prevent aspiration of oral and gastric secretions.[5]

Care of the patient with a tracheostomy is not difficult if the needs of each particular patient are clearly defined. An awareness of the goals of care, daily maintenance requirements, and possible complications is necessary.[6] Complications of tracheostomies can be classified into immediate, delayed, and late (after extubation). Table 15–1 lists some

Table 15–1. COMPLICATIONS OF TRACHEOSTOMIES

I. Immediate
1. Aspiration
2. Hemorrhage
3. Difficulty in immediate placement
4. Pneumothorax
5. Air embolism
6. Subcutaneous emphysema
7. Injury to recurrent laryngeal nerve
8. Penetration of posterior wall
9. Airway obstruction
10. Accidental extubation
11. Vagal stimulation
12. Bronchial obstruction
13. Atelectasis

II. Delayed
1. Airway obstruction
2. Infection
3. Hemorrhage
4. Dysphagia
5. Tracheoesophageal fistula
6. Tracheomalacia
7. Tracheopleural fistula
8. Granulation tissue in airway
9. Atelectasis
10. Cuff malfunction
11. Accidental extubation and mediastinal intubation

III. Late (Following Extubation)
1. Granulation tissue
2. Scar
3. Tracheostenosis
4. Tracheocutaneous fistula

Table 15–2. TRACHEOSTOMY TUBES

1.	***Acute Care***
	Lanz Critikon Inc. (Fig. 15–2)*
	Argyle
	Harris-Lake
	National Catheter
	Ohio
	Portex
	Shiley (Fig. 15–3)*
	Surgitek
	Bivona
2.	***Airway Maintenance***
	Shiley (Fig. 15–4)
	Pilling (Fig. 15–5)
	Portex
3.	***Vocalization***
	Pitt Talking Tracheostomy Tube (Fig. 15–6)
	Tucker Valve (Fig. 15–8)
	Fenestrated Pilling and Shiley (Fig. 15–7)
4.	***Laryngectomy***
	Pilling
	Shiley
5.	***Specialized***
	Pitt Talking Tracheostomy Tube
	Cane-shaped Pilling
	Extra-long Pilling
6.	***Buttons***
	Olympic
	Kistner
	Hyer-Schulte

*Has a pressure relief valve.

of the more frequent problems. The complications are significant, requiring careful observation and aggressive nursing care, but fortunately most can be treated with good results. Unusual or severe complications in tracheostomy often can be avoided by careful attention to meticulous technique and highly disciplined postoperative care.[7]

There are many types of tracheostomy tubes available to practitioners. The list given

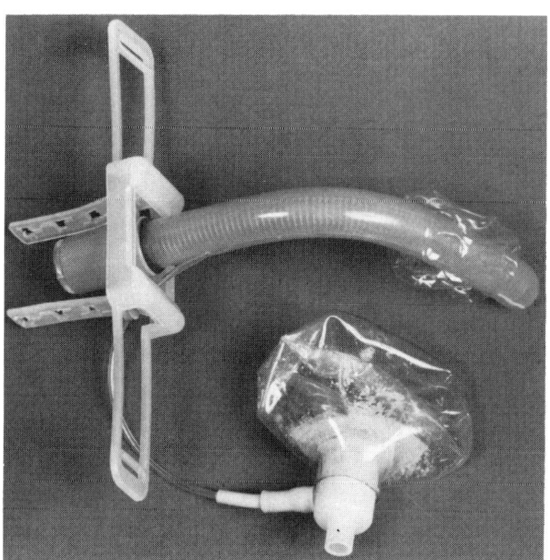

Figure 15–2. Lanz tracheostomy tube.

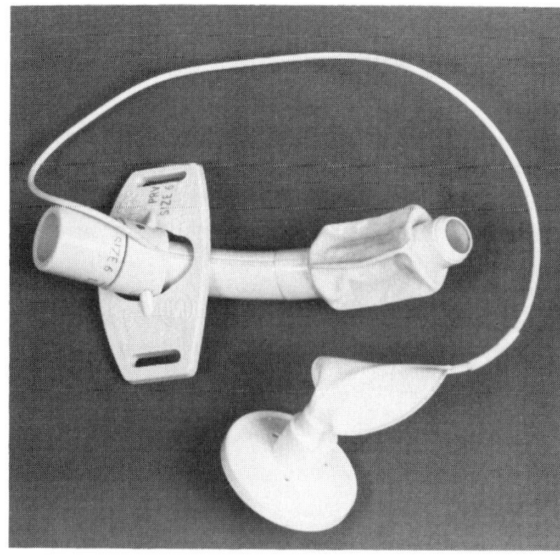

Figure 15–3. Shiley tracheostomy tube with pressure relief valve.

in Table 15–2, which categorizes the tubes according to six general uses, is not complete but will serve as a guide.

Explanation of Selected Types of Tracheostomy Tubes

The Pitt Tracheostomy Tube seals the airway, allowing for mechanical ventilation, yet provides air flow through the vocal folds for vocalization independent of respiration (Fig. 15–6). An alternate use for the Pitt tube—in the evaluation and treatment of aspiration—is well described by Shavari.[8]

Fenestrated tubes made by Pilling and Shiley, Inc., are often used during the process of decannulation or for vocalization. The fenestration provides a route for air flow through the upper airway (Fig. 15–7).

Tucker valved tubes made by Pilling are used for vocalization and do not require plugging the tube or placing a finger over the tube opening. Designed with a gravity-dependent flutter valve that opens on inhalation and closes on exhalation, the tube is used for those people who require long-term use of a tracheostomy tube yet still maintain use of their vocal cords. This tube is used for patients who have little or no pulmonary disease, as it often requires an increased effort in breathing in order to ventilate past the obstruction of the tube (Fig. 15–8).

Cuffs

The purpose of the cuff on a tracheostomy or endotracheal tube is to seal the airway. It

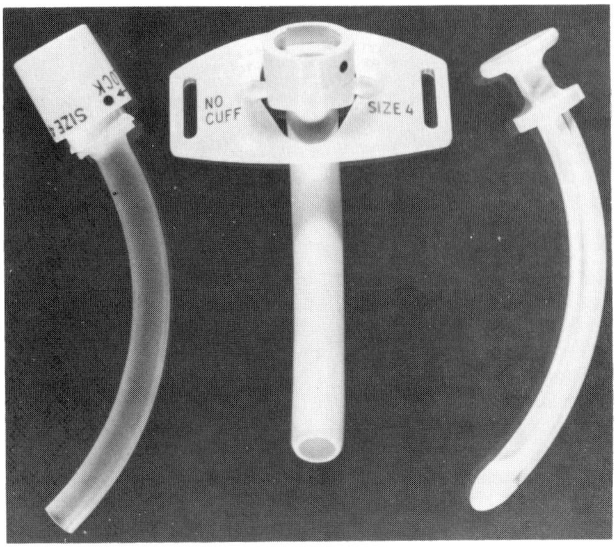

Figure 15–4. Shiley tracheostomy tube.

allows for use of positive-pressure mechanical ventilation and protects the airway. Contrary to what many believe, it does not hold a tube in place, although it does center the tube in the airway. If a cuff pressure greater than 30 mm Hg is maintained for a prolonged period, progressive tracheal wall necrosis results, with erosion into adjacent structures.[9]

The cuff used today is a large-volume, floppy, thin-walled balloon that on inflation conforms to the shape of the trachea and seals with a low pressure. This is an improvement over the small, relatively stiff balloons used in the past, which created high pressures. The low-pressure cuff, probably more than anything else, minimizes the risk of tracheostenosis, which often results from cuffed tracheostomy tubes. The best protection from stenosis lies in using the minimal amount of pressure sufficient to seal the trachea with a large thin-walled cuff that does not distort the shape of the trachea when inflated. The cuff of the tracheostomy tube should be inflated only when ventilatory assistance is needed or if aspiration during swallowing is a problem.[10]

Tracheostenosis cannot be prevented by intermittent deflation or by using alternating cuffs at different levels. In general, cuffs should be deflated approximately every 8 hours, or each nursing shift. The purpose of deflation is to (1) re-establish the seal of the cuff, and (2) remove the secretions above the cuff site.

The procedure for cuff deflation is as follows:

1. Suction posterior pharynx.
2. Suction airway, using sterile technique.
3. Upon exhalation, either voluntary or by means of an anesthesia bag, Ambu bag, or ventilator, deflate the cuff.
4. Suction airway.
5. Remove oral secretions.
6. Suction airway if needed.
7. Reinflate the cuff.

The primary principle in cuff inflation is to inflate the cuff with just enough air to seal the airway. The Lanz and Shiley systems each have pressure relief valves to maintain cuff pressure at no greater than 25 mm Hg. The McGuinness Valve of the Lanz system consists of a very compliant pressure-limiting external balloon that distends at pressures over 25 torr. It must be used with a large residual volume cuff. Overinflation by 25 ml of air beyond that needed to seal results in a slight decrease of tracheal mucus pressure to

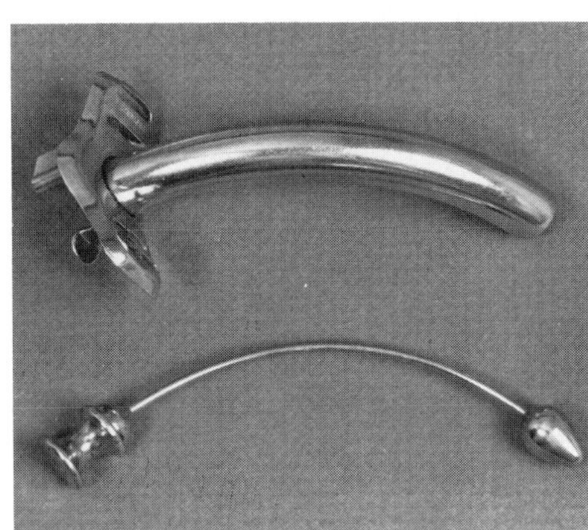

Figure 15–5. Pilling tracheostomy tube, noncuffed.

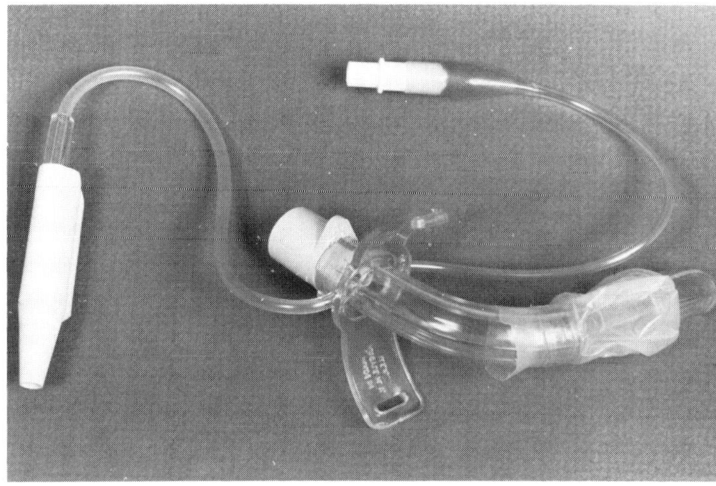

Figure 15–6. Pitt talking tracheostomy tube.

22 torr. The McGuinness Valve prevents rapid loss of cuff volume during continuous positive-pressure ventilation, thus avoiding leakage when peak pressures exceed 25 torr.[12]

When using cuffs without overinflation devices, the tracheal cuff pressures must be measured by a manometer. The correct procedure for cuff measurement is well described by Cox and Shatz.[13] By using an aneroid manometer, a four-way stopcock, and a simple Y connector, accurate measurements can be made.

Decannulation

Decannulation of the patient with a tracheostomy tube often involves a confusing series of decisions. For decannulation to be feasible, the following three criteria must be fulfilled: (1) the patient must not require mechanical ventilation; (2) VC (vital capacity) must be greater than 14 ml/kg body weight, and IF (inspiratory force) must be greater than 25 cm H_2O negative pressure; and (3) the patient must be able to manage his own oral secretions, perform a good swallow, and produce an effective cough.[14] Although the first two criteria are objective and fairly easy to evaluate, the third often requires keen judgment.

Swallowing can be tested by having the patient drink methylene blue dye, then watching for traces of blue in the sputum when the patient coughs. A more accurate method is to have the patient swallow a thin barium solution under observation by fluoroscopy. Every patient with an artificial airway in place has some swallowing dysfunction. This is caused by the relative inability to properly elevate the larynx due to the tethering caused by the stoma. There is also some current discussion that lack of use of the laryngeal musculature leads to a "lazy swallow." This has not yet been proved but is often observed. Clinical observation shows that patients must practice in order to develop an adequate swallow with a tube in place.

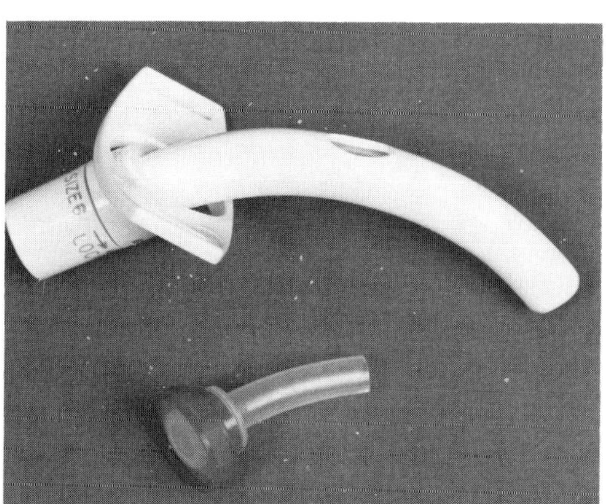

Figure 15–7. Shiley fenestrated tracheostomy tube.

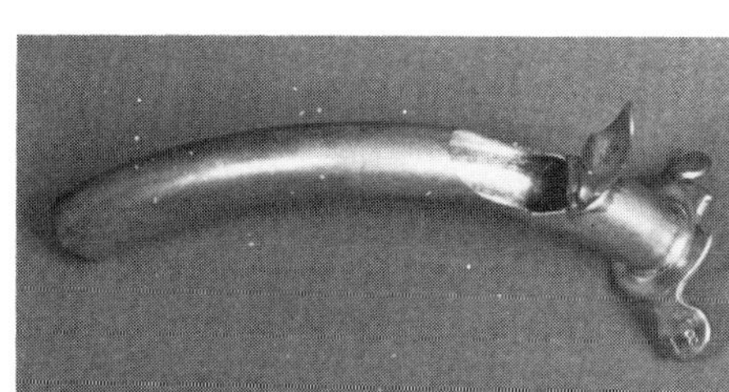

Figure 15–8. Tucker valve.

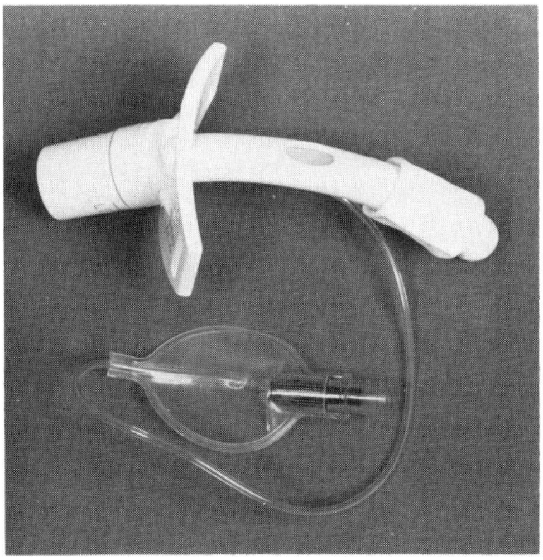

Figure 15–9. Fenestrated cuffed tube.

If the swallowing study demonstrates aspiration, the clinician may (1) elect to leave the tracheostomy tube in place with the cuff inflated, although this may make swallowing more difficult; (2) have the patient practice swallowing with a staff member present for suctioning (the patient should use the "supraglottic" method of swallowing described later in this chapter); or (3) remove the tube, place an occlusive dressing over the stoma, and observe swallowing carefully. There is reason to believe that when the cuff is inflated, pressure is directed posteriorly through the common wall into the esophagus. This pressure decreases the esophageal lumen size and impedes the smooth passage of the bolus.

If the patient is able to swallow, the usual procedure for decannulation is as follows (based on the patient's passing each step successfully):

1. Leave the cuff deflated for 24 hours. Observe the patient for ability to handle both oral and pulmonary secretions.
2. Place a noncuffed tube, preferably fenestrated, for 24 hours, or use a smaller noncuffed tube.
3. Cap the fenestrated tube for 24 hours.
4. Remove the tube. Instruct the patient to place his hand over the stomal bandage to prevent air leaks. Have a spare tube at the bedside, one size smaller than the one removed.
5. Observe for wound closure.

Precautions

1. It is very dangerous to cap or plug a cuffed tube even with the cuff deflated. Cuffs used today are generally high-volume redundant cuffs, and even when deflated occupy a considerable volume of the trachea. Therefore, if the tube is plugged the resultant obstruction may exceed 50 per cent of the airway lumen, a stiff test for even the healthiest patient.
2. The practice of using a fenestrated cuffed tube (Fig. 15–9) as an intermediate tube or to shorten the decannulation process may be fraught with problems. If the cuff is not deflated and the tube is plugged to utilize the fenestration, a significant airway obstruction will exist.

These two situations emphasize the danger of attempting the weaning process and proceeding with decannulation without first switching from a cuffed to a noncuffed tube.

Wound Care

Wound care is probably the most critical aspect of the postoperative management of head and neck cancer patients with which nurses will be involved. As in the care of artificial airways, *prevention is the rule.* The nursing staff must be acutely aware of the process of wound healing. Many factors are associated with wound healing, but the two most critical are blood supply and nutrition.

The maintenance of blood supply to flaps and grafts ensures their viability. Blood supply can be optimized postoperatively by reducing tissue swelling and ensuring adequate drainage with Hemovacs. Swelling can be minimized by following the principles of gravity drainage and avoiding dependent positioning. Elevating the head of the bed 30 to 40 degrees is routine to (1) decrease tension on sutured flaps, (2) alleviate swelling, and (3) enhance pulmonary gas exchange. Tension on suture lines, constricting dressings, and use of tape, oxygen masks, and tracheostomy tapes over flaps, especially flap pedicles, must be avoided at all cost. Tracheostomy tubes or laryngectomy tubes may be sutured to the skin, or secured to Stomahesive with tracheostomy ties.

Note: Pain cannot usually be relied on to indicate flap viability, since most patients with extensive head and neck surgery have very little pain (as compared with someone, for instance, who has undergone gallbladder surgery).[15]

Care of the patient's flaps and grafts is a high priority nursing staff function. Hourly checks of color, temperature, and capillary filling are critical in the first 48 hours after surgery. Maintenance of adequate Hemovac drainage is the key to flap and graft survival. The Hemovac drains prevent accumulation of blood under the neck flaps. They are generally placed to 20 mm Hg wall suction. Any air found leaking into the tubes is suggestive of air leaking from a suture line into the wound. This can occur from separation of the cutaneous suture line, a dehiscence into the upper aerodigestive tract, or an extrusion of part of the drainage tubing that causes the drain to be sucking room air. Air leakage should receive immediate attention. Any leakage of air through the skin incision is stemmed by placing more sutures at suspicious sites and then covering the area with copious amounts of antibiotic ointment. If the tubing has partially slipped out, it and the surrounding skin are carefully prepped with an antiseptic solution, and then the drain is carefully advanced until all the holes are well under the neck flaps and the tube is secured with a heavy silk purse-string suture.

If these methods are ineffective, the leak is presumably from a dehiscence in the internal mucosal suture line. Occasionally a minor manipulation of the tube will re-establish a vacuum seal, but usually this maneuver is unsuccessful. Such a leakage must not be allowed to continue, since persistent suction of pharyngeal or oral contents through the wound will almost assuredly result in an enterocutaneous fistula. A decision must be made to disconnect the Hemovac from suction and convert the tubes to a simple form of gravity drainage system. A large pressure dressing is applied to the wounds, and the tubes are cut and covered with a heavy absorbent pad.

Dressings over flaps should be changed as needed. Rolled up composite dressings, such as ABD pads, can be used to milk the flap. Gently rolling the pad from the distal to the proximal entry of the Hemovac tube will encourage any fluid to escape via the tube. This should be done a few times every hour in the immediate postoperative period to ensure proper drainage and solid seating of the neck flap.

Occasionally the Hemovac tubing will plug. This becomes apparent when drainage ceases and the neck flaps begin to swell as fluid collects beneath them. This is a critical situation. Reinstitution of drainage is essential for the viability of the neck flaps; failure to re-establish function mandates immediate reoperation and tube replacement. A simple maneuver judiciously applied may reinstitute tube function. Approximately 10 cc of sterile normal saline can be injected through each carefully prepped tube. This flushing may dislodge enough clots to restore function. Flushing of the tubes is not a routine procedure but should be used only in cases of obstruction that do not respond to other methods of intervention.

Another cause of tube obstruction is too high a suction level in the drain. A careful check of the suction gauge will prevent subcutaneous fat "corks" from being sucked into the drain.

All wounds should periodically be cleaned with hydrogen peroxide, washed with normal saline, and have antibiotic ointment applied. Full-strength hydrogen peroxide should not be allowed to stay on the wound, as it may cauterize the wound edges. *Meticulous wound care is the rule.* The importance of cleanliness and the prevention of crusting and residual secretions cannot be overemphasized. Patients should be taught to maintain this cleanliness when they begin to do their own care, and the need for strict handwashing must be stressed.

The nutritional aspect of wound healing has been outlined earlier. Adequate tissue nutrition is critical for all head and neck cancer patients. Nursing staff must be aware of proper methods of nasogastric feeding and the use of both total parenteral and partial parenteral nutrition.

Fistula Care

Fistulae may form because of infection, poor nutrition, inadequate wound care, radiation therapy, recurrent cancer, or any combination of these factors. Whenever wounds break down and fistulae form, aggressive wound care is indicated. It is at this time that the nursing staff must be innovative and ingenious in devising dressings that are both functional and comfortable.

Fistulae may be detected by a methylene blue test, which, although not 100 per cent reilable, will give a general idea as to the integrity of tissues. Use 1 cc of dye in 1 cup of water and have the patient drink the solution. If dye is detected in the dressing over the area of suspicion, it confirms the presence of a fistula. Small amounts of dye are often coughed out via the tracheostomy tube, as most patients with artificial airways aspirate. Large amounts of dye produced in this way indicate significant aspiration.

When fistulae are discovered, the wounds are cleaned and packed frequently to prevent stasis of secretions. When there is excessive salivary drainage, as with orocutaneous fistulae, multi-eyed suction catheters may be used in the pharynx to remove secretions. These catheters may be placed in the fistula itself but are usually inserted via the nares. Low constant suction or intermittent suction is used. Diversion of the salivary stream away from the airway and the healing wound is imperative.

The wound is cleaned with hydrogen peroxide and normal saline or povidone-iodine and packed with 0.25 per cent acetic acid–soaked dressings or iodoform gauze. Dressings should be changed every 4 hours, or more frequently if necessary, with allowances made for adequate rest periods for the patient between dressing changes. In most cases, fistulae will heal spontaneously with meticulous aggressive wound care, and surgical closure is only occasionally necessary.

Carotid Blowout

If the wound breaks down over the carotid artery, the consequences are ominous. All nursing staff must be aware of the possibility of carotid "blowout" or rupture. The patient and family must be apprised of the situation and taught what to do if the bleeding occurs at home or when a nurse is not present. However, rarely will a patient be discharged if the risk of a carotid blowout is present.

If imminent carotid rupture is suspected, the patient should be placed on "carotid precautions," which indicates to everyone that this patient is at high risk and must be watched diligently. This is accomplished by moving the patient to a room near the nurses' station or to an ICU. Carotid blowout precautions include (1) measures for airway control; (2) suction equipment; (3) an intravenous line large enough for blood products; (4) the availability of blood products; and (5) dressing supplies to control bleeding. A "carotid blowout tray" with all the necessary equipment can be placed at the patient's bedside.

With the patient on precautions, the nursing staff must be diligent in their wound care and observation. The carotid artery must be kept moist, as drying of the artery is often an immediate precursor to blowout. An aneurysm is also an important premonitory event to rupture. The wound must be kept clean to prevent infection, and nutrition should be optimized to promote wound healing.

Usually, but not always, a herald bleed will occur before the carotid ruptures. This is a small amount of bright red blood and usually appears 6 to 8 hours before the carotid ruptures. If, despite all precautions, the artery ruptures, immediate pressure is placed over the bleeding site. This measure is rapidly followed by transporting the patient to the operating room for carotid ligation. Carotid blowout is a life-threatening situation, and immediate response is essential for patient survival.

Postoperative Facial Edema

Postoperative facial edema can be a very distressing consequence of radical neck dissection, especially when a bilateral operation is performed. Patients and family must be warned preoperatively about this situation and have the cause explained. In a unilateral neck dissection, because the jugular vein is sacrificed and the lymph and venous return are significantly altered only on one side, facial swelling, if it occurs at all, is usually gone in 2 to 4 weeks, although in rare instances it may last as long as 2 to 6 months.

When a bilateral neck dissection is required, the operations are usually staged to allow for compensation of venous blood flow. A modified neck dissection on the side of least involvement, preserving the jugular vein, significantly reduces the amount of swelling and the length of time required for resolution. The swelling may be very severe and may never completely resolve. When neck dissections are done and flaps are used for reconstruction there is always the danger that swelling may compromise the blood supply of the flap, causing necrosis.

Nursing care aimed at reducing postoperative swelling should include the following: (1) adequate nutrition; (2) appropriate fluid therapy administration, with care to avoid overhydration; (3) avoidance of pressure dressings or tight bandages or tracheostomy ties; (4) early ambulation; (5) elevation of the head of the bed 30 to 40 degrees at all times; and (6) the occasional use of carefully administered ice packs. Occasionally isoxsuprine or even low-dose anticoagulants may be used in an attempt to save a flap with a marginal blood supply.

Preoperative and Postoperative Pulmonary Care

Following lengthy anesthesia and surgical intervention, postoperative pulmonary complications are the most frequent cause of morbidity and death. Schlenker and Hubay[16] reported a 50 per cent incidence of severe atelectasis when the duration of anesthesia exceeded 4 hours. The incidence decreased to 19 per cent when the procedure was 2 hours or less. Schwartz et al[17] found that respiratory failure is either a major cause of or a contributing factor to 50 per cent of postoperative deaths.

The goal of preoperative pulmonary evaluation is to identify risk factors and to institute preventive measures that will possibly minimize their adverse physiologic consequences. Of the many risk factors present, respiratory problems and the location of the operative site are the most important.[18]

A high percentage of patients who have cancer of the head and neck are heavy smokers and alcohol abusers. They often present in a nutritionally depleted state and frequently have some degree of aspiration owing to a compromised larynx. Because of a long history of smoking, most patients suffer to some degree from bronchitis, emphysema, and increased sputum production and thus experience significant problems with lengthy anesthesia and long periods of immobility.

Preoperative assessment should include pulmonary function tests, arterial blood gases, routine physical examinations, chest x-ray, and, if metastasis is suspected, computerized axial tomography of the thorax. These studies also act as a baseline for intraoperative and postoperative care.

Nursing staff should instruct patients preoperatively in turning, coughing, deep breathing, and ambulation. For patients who will require an artificial airway after surgery, a thorough explanation of its purpose is necessary. Suctioning should be explained as clearly as possible so that the patient understands its purpose. Patients must be instructed in early ambulation and the hazards of staying in bed. If possible, a physical therapist specializing in chest diseases should be involved in the preoperative teaching plan.

For patients who are admitted with a severely compromised pulmonary system, preoperative chest physical therapy, coughing, deep breathing, suctioning if indicated, and the use of an incentive breathing device is instituted as early as possible.

Postoperative pulmonary care should include turning, coughing, deep breathing, suctioning, airway care, saline instillation, humidification, ambulation, and hydration. Other measures are chest physical therapy, including the manual techniques of percussion, vibration, and shaking; breathing exercises; positioning and bronchial drainage; TENS (Transcutaneous Electrical Nerve Stimulation); and upper extremity mobility exercises. Treatment to modify or prevent respiratory complications is a major focus of care in the postoperative patient.[19] These treatments should continue until the chest x-ray is clear, arterial blood gases return to normal or baseline, and the patient is able to clear his own secretions.

Swallowing

Swallowing is a very complex act that includes both a voluntary and an involuntary phase. Only the oral stage is voluntary; the pharyngeal and esophageal stages are involuntary.

Many muscles in the tongue, palate, and pharynx, as well as those associated with the larynx and hyoid bone, are involved in the swallowing act. They do not act independently or in a random manner but are coordinated sequentially into a patterned performance. The oral stage may be initiated voluntarily but is mainly reflexic. Once the food bolus has triggered receptors distributed around the entrance to the oral pharynx, the entirely reflexive portion of deglutition proceeds inexorably to completion.[20]

The neural control of this highly coordinated muscular activity appears to be centered beneath the temporal lobe near the amygdaloid nucleus, since the stimulation here has elicited the linked performances of chewing and swallowing. Even though swallowing may be initiated voluntarily at higher levels, most normal unsolicited swallowing is believed to be controlled by the brain stem and to occur below the level of consciousness. The coordination with respiration is critical, and normally there is a cessation of respiration during swallowing to allow for the uninterrupted flow of the food bolus into the esophagus, precluding aspiration.[20]

This complex function does not lend itself well to retraining, and much time needs to be spent with the patient, both in evaluation and explanation of the purposes of the learned techniques.

About 10 days after surgery, oral feeding is instituted. The 10-day lapse is to allow for internal sutures to heal, swelling to abate, and normal functions to improve. The nasogastric and tracheostomy tubes are usually removed before swallowing is attempted, since both tubes inhibit the normal swallowing mechanism by securing the larynx in place and keeping the esophageal sphincter open. Bosma describes the tongue, hyoid bone, and larynx as making up an intrinsically mobile column.[21] The nasogastric tube itself may act as a wick for aspiration. When feeding is first attempted clear liquids are used initially because, for most patients, they are easiest to handle. In patients who are suspected of having fistulae or problems with aspiration, a methylene blue test is usually done first, before the institution of a clear liquid diet. Those patients who by the nature of their surgery will have difficulty in swallowing (e.g., supraglottic laryngectomy or glossectomy patients) are *never* initially given clear liquids. Liquids have no substance or texture and are very difficult to handle for someone who has impaired sensation and impaired facilities for swallowing.

Teaching patients to swallow can be time-consuming and very frustrating for both instructor and patient. In addition to the difficulties of learning the technique involved, there is concern for the risks of aspiration and wound breakdown, and for the problem of maintaining adequate nutrition during this relearning process.

Total Laryngectomy

The teaching of patients with total laryngectomy is a simple process, as no respiratory cessation needs to be taught. The total separation of the aerodigestive tract dictates that the patient cannot aspirate. If the surgical wounds maintain integrity, the patient can progress quickly from liquid to solid foods. Staff must be aware of the signs and symptoms of infection heralding fistula formation, which include (1) increase in temperature, (2) general malaise, (3) erythema round the wound area, and (4) pain. Often the only sign of impending fistula is a persistently elevated temperature. When such signs appear, oral feedings must be discontinued and hyperalimentation or nasogastric feedings should be reinstituted until the fistula is healed. The total process of oral alimentation is then begun again.

Supraglottic Laryngectomy and Hemilaryngectomy

Patients who are to undergo supraglottic laryngectomy or hemilaryngectomy must be fully informed of the possible compromises of swallowing and breathing. It has been generally noted that preoperative instruction makes the postoperative period much easier. Swallowing is usually much more difficult for the supraglottic laryngectomy patient than for the patient with a hemilaryngectomy. The most difficulty of all is experienced in the patient who has had an extended partial laryngectomy.

Individualization is the key for the care of such patients. It is generally accepted that liquids are the most difficult to swallow and thick gelled or semisolid foods are the easiest. Applesauce and thick purees of fruits and vegetables may be tried. An extra-thick gelatin can be made by adding an extra packet of gelatin to the recipe. There may be individuals for whom the "rules" do not apply, and generally such patients will quickly be able to define their own eating patterns. When liquids are instituted, begin with carbonated beverages, as these provide a "texture" during the oral and pharyngeal phases of swallowing.

Foods must be pleasing in appearance and taste. Trays should be attractive. Food should be warm or cold, not just room temperature. The addition of extra flavoring may stimulate the "cerebral" phase of eating. The initial attempt at swallowing should be done when the patient is hungry and at regular mealtimes. All attempts at normalcy should be encouraged. Allowing some of the patient's favorite foods to be brought from home often is an impetus to an improved appetite. A suction machine must be present in the event of aspiration that cannot be controlled by a normal cough.

The following instructions are given to the patient for reference and should be kept within plain view during the learning phase. The steps and the reasons for each step are included in the nursing care plan so that each nurse is aware of the importance of following the plan.

Steps	**Reasons**
1. Wash or rinse mouth, brush teeth.	1. To stimulate oral cavity and increase salivation.
2. Sit up in a 90-degree position with head forward.	2. Normal position for eating to prevent aspiration. Head forward to close airway and open esophagus.
3. Cough twice.	3. To clear the airway.
4. Hold your breath.	4. To prevent aspiration and simulate normal respiratory cessation.
5. Take a small bit of food; solids with a spoon and liquids with a short straw.	5. Controlled portions; a straw may help institute the sucking.
6. Double swallow.	6. To clear foods from the oropharynx.
7. Cough twice.	7. To clear the airway.
8. Swallow again.	8. Swallow the final residuum.
9. Repeat the procedure.	

Oral Cavity

Patients who undergo surgery to the oral cavity present a different set of problems. These patients, especially those with oral incompetence, are often the most difficult to nutritionally support by the oral route.

Because the initial phase of swallowing is voluntary, the mixed messages of this phase, because of the oral surgery, are insufficient to adequately initiate the second and third phases of swallowing. The mechanical alterations in the oral cavity are often so great that until reconstruction has been completed oral nutrition is impossible. The use of syringes with catheter tips attached often aids in bypassing the crippled oral cavity (Fig. 15–10).

Motivation is a key factor in the relearning process, and highly motivated patients often do much better than those who are not so motivated. Thick gelled and semisolid foods are the basis for nutrition. Very careful monitoring of weight and nutritional components will quickly identify the patients who are succeeding and those who will require tube feeding.

When oral nutrition is insufficient to support a patient, nasogastric feedings are often instituted. The placement of a small-caliber tube does not preclude oral feeding but can be used for supplementation during the learning period. Furthermore, patients who have been properly instructed and who have received much psychologic support can be taught to place their own tubes for intermittent feeding. Very often patients see the use of tubes as failure on their part to do the correct procedure. It is very important that before any measures are begun, the patient clearly understand the expectations, goals, and alternative procedures.

DISCHARGE PLANNING AND HOME CARE

Planning for discharge should begin even before the patient's hospital admission. During preoperative counseling it must be made clear to the family that resources are available to assist them after discharge. The need for clinic follow-up and the availability of medical and emergency resources are explained.

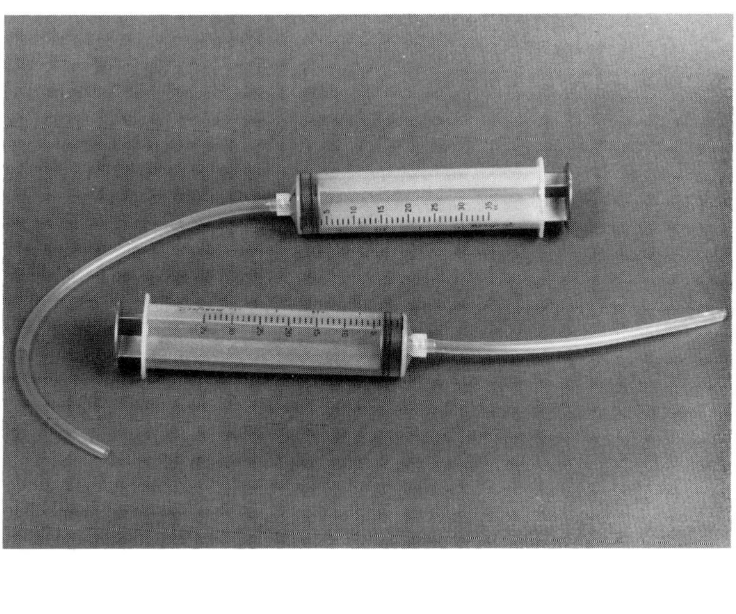

Figure 15–10. Syringe with catheter tip for oral feeding.

During hospitalization, repetition of information and emphasis on available services is important. Because a considerable amount of the patient's care centers on teaching, it is necessary to have a detailed care plan to be certain all aspects of patient education are covered. In most institutions it is not possible for the same nurses to conduct all the teaching sessions required for each patient. A care plan makes it possible for several nurses to participate in the teaching process without duplicating their efforts and without overlooking areas that should be covered.[22]

Coordination with all services involved allows for improved preparation for discharge. Families and patients are provided with the following list of books and pamphlets and are advised as to which will be most helpful according to their particular needs.

1. *Looking Forward—A Guide Book for the Laryngectomee,* by Keith Robert et al. Cancer Rehabilitation Program, Mayo Comprehensive Cancer Center, 1977.
2. *Self-Help for the Laryngectomee,* 1980–1981 edition, by Edmund Lauder.
3. *Eating Hints—Recipes and Tips for Better Nutrition During Cancer Treatment.* US Department of Health and Human Services, National Institutes of Health, August 1980.
4. *Your New Voice,* by William Waldrop and Marie Gould. American Cancer Society, Illinois Division, Chicago, Illinois, 1969.
5. *First Aid for Laryngectomees.* International Association of Laryngectomees, American Cancer Society, 1971.
6. *This Could Save Your Life.* Medic-Alert Foundation, Turlock, California.
7. *Cancer Word Book.* American Cancer Society, 1976.
8. Assorted pamphlets related to the specific site of the cancer (e.g., mouth, larynx), available from the American Cancer Society.
9. *Chemotherapy and You—A Guide to Self-Help During Treatment;* and *Radiation Therapy and You—A Guide to Self-Help During Treatment.* US Department of Health and Human Services, Public Health Service, National Institutes of Health, Bethesda, Maryland.

In addition to these information books, patients are given the supplies listed in Table 15–3, depending on their needs.

Table 15–3. DISCHARGE SUPPLIES

Laryngectomy	
Suction machine	1
Suction catheters, #14 Fr. disposable	20
Sterile Q-tips	100
Bacitracin ointment	2 tubes
Dispos-a-Vial sterile normal saline	1 box
Suture removal sets	2
Hydrogen peroxide	2 bottles
Dressing supplies	
Food supplements	
Medications	
Tracheostomy (Permanent or Temporary)	
Suction machine	1
Suction catheters, #14 Fr. disposable	20
Sterile Q-tips	110
Trach ties	40 ft
Bacitracin ointment	1 tube
Dispos-a-Vial sterile normal saline	1 box
Suture removal sets	2
Trach brushes: small, medium, or large	5
Hydrogen peroxide	2 bottles
Trach dressings: Soft Wik, Johnson & Johnson	30
Stomahesive 4 × 4	2
Food supplements	
Medications	
Dressing supplies	

Patients who are unable to communicate verbally receive the Laryngectomee Emergency Tapes (LET). Through the American Cancer Society and the Easter Seal Society, a set of four tapes is provided with a tape recorder (on loan). The tapes are for (1) police, (2) fire, (3) medical emergency, and (4) conversation. Each tape gives the patient's name, diagnosis, address, and phone. The patients are instructed to answer questions by tapping once for yes, twice for no. Police, fire stations, and emergency vehicles are notified of all persons receiving the tapes, so that accurate identification can be made not only by name and address but also by a preassigned code number. This prevents unlawful use of the tapes.

A simple checklist should be attached to the nursing care plan to alert each nurse to the time teaching was begun and whether it has been completed. Discharge criteria are filed with the head nurse to standardize nursing care and patient education.

All patients who are discharged from the hospital after head and neck surgery should be referred to a home visiting nurse agency. Even if patients are fully independent and in charge of their own care, the transition from hospital to home can be difficult. Being home alone is very different from being in the hospital under supervision, and professional help in the home during the transition time adds essential support. The home health agency also provides feedback to the staff regarding the patient's progress.

The Visiting Nurse Association sends a representative to the weekly tumor clinic and pretreatment conference. This provides continuity of care. Members of the staff are able to follow up on problems, adjust medical care as needed, and meet new patients who will need services after discharge.

Other community resources such as Meals-on-Wheels, the American Cancer Society, the American Lung Association, and the Vocational Rehabilitation and Welfare Department are consulted as necessary for support. A rapport between the Home Health Agency and the medical team is vital in providing continuity of care.

PSYCHOLOGIC REHABILITATION

Patients who have had surgery for head and neck cancer, together with their families, often find it helpful to share their illness-related experiences. This sharing frequently occurs in an informal fashion in the clinic or family waiting rooms. Many patients and families find it helpful to further these casual relationships by establishing formal group meetings designed to promote the exchange of experiences and concerns of illness, surgery, and rehabilitation. The group is not identified as a "therapy group," although it is in fact therapeutic. Group leaders define their role as supportive, encouraging, and intended to help the patients to talk about their feelings and problems. Factual information is provided by the leader as necessary, but it is the patients, by virtue of their experience, who are the real experts on the social and emotional consequences of cancer. The patients are encouraged to care for each other by giving emotional support and advice, and by validating each other's experiences.

In assisting patients and their families, group leaders identify and comment on themes such as anger, fear, death, dying, pain, loss of the ability to communicate, dependency, and family relationships. Reducing the sense of "differentness," yet helping each patient to maintain a sense of identity, is important.

The group is composed of patients, family members, friends, and occasionally children. It is often led by clinical nursing specialists in head and neck surgery and psychiatry. Input from the staff nurses and from speech, nutrition, social service, and operating room personnel lends a base of support to the group structure. Groups can meet weekly or monthly depending on the needs of the patients and families. There is no charge, and a physician's appointment is not necessary to attend the group.

Certain patients may play special roles within the group. Some are defined as "culture carriers"—those who know the group and its purpose and are personally acquainted with the majority of patients. Some extend beyond this into an outreach role, by assisting the staff and making home visits to other patients, and meeting needs other than those addressed within the group itself.

Frequent topics of discussion are the value of a second opinion before surgery, pain control, and such questions as "How can I get mad at my doctor without fearing retribution?" and "Will my sexual function be altered?" Each question is addressed by the group during the session, and only rarely is something tabled because of time restraints until the next week. A diary of each session is kept and reviewed monthly by the staff for their own peer review. Generally, it is the patients with complications who attend these groups. They appear to need outlets not only for their questions and expression of their fears but for their anger as well. The group is an ideal medium for such discussions.

THE PROCESS OF DYING

Dying is a process that keeps the body near the forefront of the mind. Specific symptoms are likely to produce fear, but fear is often present long before symptoms appear. Dying persons, even before physical signs of disintegration begin, fear many things.[23] Patients who have undergone extensive head and neck surgery and then face an unresectable recurrence often display significant depression. They focus on disfigurement, pain, becoming a burden, being left alone, and the problems of supporting the family.

Hospital staff members should become familiar with Elizabeth Kubler-Ross's framework of the five stages of dying: (1) shock and denial; (2) anger; (3) bargaining; (4) depression; and (5) acceptance.[24] It is through these stages that patients deal with death. Staff often accompany these patients through this process—an involvement that is unavoidable and appropriate. Both the health professionals and the patient share with past generations the superstitions and myths about the "unnaturalness" of dying that are rooted in childhood memories and are retained, in many cases, throughout life. One of the hardest misconceptions to correct is the subconscious belief that the patient's terminal illness is an enemy that must be overcome or the inevitable retribution for some wrong he or she has committed. If it is impossible to stave off death, both health professionals and patients may give up in despair, and physicians, nurses, and other health professionals often flee (at least emotionally) because they simply cannot face the fact that they were unable to rescue the patient from death.[25] The surgeon especially feels a sense of failure, often tinged with guilt, at the triumph of the cancerous process over his best efforts. Therapeutic groups for the staff aid greatly in maintaining objectivity. Staff meetings with a psychiatric liaison consultation have become routine in the nursing care of cancer patients.

Comfort, pain relief, and family support make death "more appropriate." Staff should become aware of their limitations to alter the ultimate course, while at the same time understanding the profound supportive effect they may have on both the patient and the family. Weisman and Hackett[26] have coined the term "appropriate death." To achieve this, medical professionals should aid patients to (1) be relatively free of pain; (2) operate on as effective a level as possible within the limits of their disabilities; (3) recognize and resolve residual conflicts; (4) satisfy those remaining wishes that are consistent with existing conditions and ego ideals; and (5) be able to yield control to others in whom they have confidence.

One of the most important criteria by which dying patients judge staff members is that of competence. Patients and families respect those who are able to do the job well, whether it be giving a bath without making the patient cold, or rapidly changing a tracheostomy tube without pain or distress.

It is our philosophy that patients should remain at home or in familiar surroundings until the time they cannot be cared for or are not safe. Hospice care, a philosophical approach to the dying process, is valuable and should be instituted early. This approach to providing care for terminally ill patients and their families provides a way of dealing with dying rather than just being a place to die.[27]

Skilled nurses and volunteers often enable people to remain at home in a safe environment much longer and with a quality of life not afforded in the hospital. However, when it is no longer possible to keep the patient at home, the very difficult decision of placement in a care facility, either a hospital or nursing home, must be made. It is wise to broach this subject early, so that all persons involved can participate in the decision-making process. Demonstrating caring and compassion to the family and patient about such decisions often reinforces the bond that is developed between them and the staff. On the other hand, avoiding the issues seriously weakens this bond.

Communication should be direct and honest. In cases in which the patient and family say they are "not ready to hear the diagnosis," or when family members say "don't tell him he has cancer," bringing them to the point where they are ready is a challenging aspect of care.

The profound effect of a caring staff upon the dying patient and family is evident after the patient's death. Bereavement counseling is often necessary to reaffirm the family's self-image and to reassure family members that everything possible was done for the patient. Staff meetings with the psychiatric liaison team help the staff to better understand their involvement and allow closure to occur.

Acceptance of the death of a loved one takes time to evolve. Time and caring help this resolution and provide emotional support for those who continue to live.

CONCLUSION

The care of patients with head and neck cancer is a tremendous challenge to providers of health care. Because of the many disciplines involved, coordination and communication of the health care team is vitally important to its success. The technical aspects of patient care are rapidly advancing, and the staff must continually strive to incorporate these innovations. Regardless of the techniques in use at any given time, however, there are two principles that must always be fulfilled: the need for meticulous care and the prevention of complications.

There needs to be open honest communication with the patient regarding his illness. An ongoing dialogue should be an integral part of treatment, rehabilitation, and perhaps the process of dying as well.

All of the above culminates in one primary goal: caring for the patient.

References

1. Keith CF: Wound management following head and neck surgery: the challenge of complex nursing intervention. Nurs Clin North Am 14:761, 1979.
2. Dunphy JE: On Caring for the Patient with Cancer. ACS, Professional Education Publication, 1976.
3. Keith R, Lingebaugh D, Cox B: Presurgical counseling needs of laryngectomees: a survey of 78 patients. Laryngoscope 88:1660, 1978.
4. Harris R: Presentation at Society of Otorhinolaryngology and Head and Neck Nurses National Convention, Los Angeles, 1980.
5. Selecky PA: Tracheostomy: a review of present day indications, complications and care. Heart Lung 3(2):272, March–April 1974.
6. Furiel AE, Putnam JS: Patients with tracheostomies: goals of management. Primary Care 5:557, 1978.
7. Kenan PD: Complications associated with tracheostomy: prevention and treatment. Otolaryngol Clin North Am 12(4):807, 1979.
8. Shahvari M, Kigin CM, Zimmerman J: Speaking tracheostomy tubes modified for swallowing dysfunction and chronic aspiration. Anesthesiology 46:290, 1977.
9. Lewis FR Jr, Shiobohm RM, Thomas AN: Prevention of complications from prolonged tracheal intubation. Am J Surg 35:452, 1978.
10. Kenan PD: Complications associated with tracheostomy: prevention and treatment. Otolaryngol Clin North Am 12(4):807, 1979.
11. Powasser MM, Brown MC, Chezam J, et al: The effectiveness of hourly cuff deflation in minimizing tracheal damage. Heart Lung 5:734, 1976.
12. Carroll RG: Evaluation of tracheal tube cuff design. Crit Care Med 1:45, 1973.
13. Cox P, Schatz E: Pressure measurements in endotracheal cuffs: a common error. Chest 65:84, 1974.
14. Greenbaum D: Decannulation of the tracheostomized patient. Heart Lung 5:119, 1976.
15. Jones D, Sigler B: Medical Surgical Nursing: A Conceptual Approach. New York, McGraw-Hill, 1978.
16. Schlenker JD, Hubay CA: The pathogenesis of postoperative atelectasis: a clinical study. Arch Surg 107:313, 1973.
17. Schwartz SI, Shires GT, Spencer FC, et al: Principles of Surgery. New York, McGraw-Hill, 1979, p 495.
18. Riser N: Preoperative and postoperative care to prevent pulmonary complications. Heart Lung 9:57, 1980.
19. Kigin CM: Chest physical therapy for the postoperative or traumatic injury patient. Phys Ther 61:1724, 1981.
20. Hoffman JA, Hoffman RL: Tongue thrust and deglutition. J Speech Hear Dis 30:114, 1965.
21. Bosma JF: Deglutition: pharyngeal stage. Physiol Rev 37:275, 1957.
22. Luckmann J, Sorensen K: Medical-Surgical Nursing: A Psychophysiologic Approach. Philadelphia, WB Saunders, 1980, p 2105.
23. Cassem NH: The dying patient. *In* Hackett TP, Cassem NH (eds): The Massachusetts General Hospital Handbook of General Hospital Psychiatry. St. Louis, CV Mosby, 1978.
24. Kubler-Ross E: On Death and Dying. New York, Macmillan, 1969.
25. Purtilo R: Health Professional Patient Interaction. Philadelphia, WB Saunders, 1978, p 237.
26. Weisman AD, Hackett TP: Predilection to death: death and dying as a psychiatric problem. Psychol Med 23:232, 1961.
27. Coping with Cancer: A Resource for the Health Professional. US Department of Health and Human Services, Public Health Service, National Institutes of Health, Bethesda, MD, September 1980, p 108.

16

NUTRITION

Ann E. Furiel Sievers, R.N., M.A.

NUTRITIONAL SUPPORT FOR THE CANCER PATIENT

Patients with head and neck cancer often initially present with malnutrition.[1] This malnutrition may be caused by a number of factors, including (1) the cancer process itself; (2) pain and discomfort upon chewing or swallowing; (3) side effects of chemotherapy, radiation, or surgical intervention; (4) chronic alcohol consumption; and (5) physical obstruction of the aerodigestive tract by the tumor. Nutritional support is aimed at preventing further nutritional depletion and improving the nutritional status of the severely malnourished patient, thereby enhancing wound healing.[2]

The nutritional status is defined as the degree to which an individual's physiologic needs for nutrients are being met by the intake of food. It is a state of balance between nutrient intake and expenditure of calories.[3] The average daily requirements for weight maintenance, weight gain, or weight loss can be calculated from the following chart, with the values adjusted to suit the patient's current evaluated nutritional status and projected needs.

AVERAGE DAILY CALORIC REQUIREMENTS FOR HEALTHY INDIVIDUALS

Weight Maintenance	25–30 cal/kg
Weight Gain	35–40 cal/kg
Weight Loss	20 cal/kg

Joliffe[4] states that nutritional inadequacy may result from either primary or secondary causes. A primary nutritional inadequacy results from an inadequate intake or imbalance of nutrients either in amount or kind. Secondary (or conditional) nutritional inadequacy is that due to factors other than inadequate food intake, such as a disease process interfering with the ingestion, absorption, or utilization of nutrients. The following checklist developed by Gitlin[5] will objectively help the clinician to determine if a patient is suffering from malnutrition:

1. Recent weight loss exceeding 10% of body weight.
2. Restricted oral intake of >10 days.
3. Basic IV solution >10 days with minimal or no oral intake.
4. History of alcoholism.
5. History of diet faddism.
6. Protracted nutrient loss.
7. Increased metabolic rate.
8. Medications.
9. Major organ disease.

Further nutritional evaluation should include:

1. Anthropometric data (see Table 16–1).
2. Laboratory data (see Table 16–1).
3. Skin testing to define anergy.
4. Testing for nitrogen imbalance.
5. Diet history.
6. Social history.
7. Psychologic history.

The calculation of weight loss based on recalled weight has been shown to be more accurate than that based on ideal weight derived from standard tables.[6] Recalled weight can be defined as the "usual" weight as stated by the patient. Weight loss can be calculated by the following formula:[2]

$$100 \times \frac{\text{Recalled Weight} - \text{Observed Weight}}{\text{Recalled Weight}}$$

During the course of therapy a good protocol for the evaluation of the efficacy of nutritional therapy includes the following:[7]

1. Daily body weight.
2. Twice-weekly nitrogen balance.
3. Weekly total lymphocyte count and serum albumin.
4. Every 3 weeks: anthropometrics, serum transferrin, skin tests.

It is important to consider more than laboratory data and weights in completing a metabolic assessment. A detailed diet history, including social and psychologic implications, will give information on which to base intervention. Food allergies, likes and dislikes, and the person's own description of the problem are very important in making an accurate assessment. It is most important to *listen to the patient.* This may provide more information than all the combined laboratory data.

EFFECTS OF CANCER AND ITS TREATMENT ON NUTRITION

Anorexia, nausea, and vomiting constitute a spectrum of symptoms and signs that result in a reduction of food intake.[8] There are a number of causes of anorexia in advanced cancer. These include abnormalities of taste and smell, disorders of the hunger-satiety mechanism, and, possibly, production by the tumor of intermediate metabolites that can affect central and peripheral mediators of hunger and satiety (the so-called anorexiogenic metabolite hypothesis).[9]

Appetite may also be affected by metabolic changes that occur with tumor growth. Taste distortions are frequently encountered that are as yet not well understood. Some postulate that taste bud cells decrease in size with the presence of tumor, thus decreasing taste. Others feel that the metabolic abnormalities that occur affect threshold of taste, with the altered thresholds then affecting perceptions of taste.

The most striking effect of cancer in many patients is malignant cachexia, clinically manifested by anorexia, marked asthenia, significant loss of body fat and protein, anemia, water and electrolyte abnormalities, and increased basal metabolic rate. The clinical spectrum of cachexia ranges from the patient in the early stages with an undiagnosed neoplasm and minimal weight loss to someone with end-stage disease who has marked weakness and muscle wasting. Wasting of the temporalis major, masseter, and hypothenar muscles are good indicators of this process.[10]

Table 16–1. ANTHROPOMETRIC AND LABORATORY DATA TO ASSESS NUTRITION*

Parameters	*Calculations*	*Values*
1. Weight	$100\,\dfrac{\text{Recalled Weight} - \text{Observed Weight}}{\text{Recalled Weight}}$	kg
2. Height		cm
3. Triceps Skin Fold (TSF)		mm
4. Mid-Arm Circumference (MAC)		cm
5. Mid-Arm Muscle Circumference (MAMC)		cm
	MAMC cm = MAC cm − (3.14 × TSF cm)	
6. Lab Data Serum		
Hemoglobin		
Hematocrit		mm^3
Lymphocytes (total count)		g/100 ml
Serum Albumin		mcg/100 ml
Total Iron Binding Capacity (TIBC)		
Transferrin		
	Serum Transferrin = (0.8 × TIBC) − 43	mg/100 ml
7. Urinary Creatinine (24° sample)		mg
8. Creatinine Height Index (CHI)		
	$\text{CHI} = \dfrac{\text{Actual Urinary Creatinine}}{\text{Ideal Urinary Creatinine}} \times 100$	%
9. Nitrogen Balance Study		
	$\text{N Balance} = \dfrac{\text{Protein (g)}}{6.25} - \left(\begin{array}{c}\text{Urine}\\ \text{Nitrogen} + 2\\ \text{in grams}\end{array}\right)$	

*Adapted from Nutritional Assessment Summary, Ross Laboratories, Columbus, Ohio 43216. Division of Abbott Laboratories.

Secondary Factors

Factors besides the disease process itself, or secondary factors, may also cause malnutrition. Decreases in oral intake are seen in anyone who is in pain, and this problem occurs to an even greater degree when the pain is in the oral cavity or neck area. The character and type of food ingested may drastically change from solid to soft foods or to only liquids, and usually the protein and caloric content of the food decreases along with the amount. Appropriate attention to pain relief before meals may be enough to alter the downward spiral.

Chemotherapy may cause very distressing side effects of nausea and vomiting. Chemoreceptor trigger zones (CTZ) near the floor of the fourth ventricle can be stimulated to produce vomiting, but it is unclear why toxic substances also elicit this stimulation. There are many theories on why chemotherapeutic drugs cause emesis, but none that explain the full story. Whether the reaction results from direct stimulation of the CTZ, from the drug crossing the blood-brain barrier, or from peripheral action, the mechanism is clearly complex.[11] Recent studies using metoclopramide showed this procainamide derivative to be more effective than chlorpromazine, nabilone, or haloperidol in controlling emesis induced by *cis*-platinum chemotherapy.[12] Further investigation in the development and use of antiemetic drugs may significantly reduce the side effects of chemotherapy and radiation.

Radiation causes similar distressing side effects, and the reason is equally unclear. The mechanisms must be more clearly defined before treatment to counteract these side effects can be successful. Research efforts aimed at evaluating the role of central nervous system neurotransmitters, prostaglandins, and gastrointestinal hormones may be fruitful. Treatment of signs and symptoms, attempts at controlling a stable environment, and judicious use of medications before meals and treatment may be helpful.

Oral complications from radiotherapy originate from radiation injury to the salivary glands, oral mucosa, oral musculature, and alveolar bone. Clinical sequelae of such injury (depending on the intensity, duration, and port of therapy) include dryness of the mouth, "mouth blindness" (loss of taste discretion), dental caries, mucositis, osteoradionecrosis, oral infections, and trismus.[13]

Postsurgical scarring, tethering of the tongue, orocutaneous fistulae, or surgical removal of some of the muscles of mastication intervene in the process of deglutition. Patients must be instructed in alternative methods of providing nutrition. Because patients quickly lose energy and weight on basic intravenous solutions,[14] supplementary methods of enteral or parenteral alimentation must be invoked to prevent the insidious onset of the catabolic process.

It is well documented that chronic alcohol abusers are frequently malnourished. These people spend money, time, and energy procuring and ingesting alcohol rather than food. Alcohol decreases the sense of taste and smell, and when combined with smoking results in further depression of these senses. Alcoholism also increases the need for B vitamins.

When normal food intake is insufficient to meet daily requirements, nutritional intervention is indicated. In uncomplicated cases this may be achieved by simply adding calories, protein, fats, and whole milk products to the diet from regular food sources and increasing the amount of food ingested. In some cases, more complex methods, such as total or peripheral parenteral nutrition (TPN, PPN) may be required (see later, under Feeding Administration).

It is important to closely assess the needs of the patient before suggesting a change in diet or other intervention. If a mild nutritional imbalance is present, education and an increase in awareness of basic requirements are often all that is indicated to reverse the process. If special needs are defined, the book "Eating Hints," published by the National Cancer Institute, is especially helpful in outlining simple methods for improving nutrition during cancer treatment. If patients are unable to alter their cooking or food preparation patterns, a nutritionally complete supplement such as Ensure Plus, 1 can/3 or 4 times per day, may be indicated. Similar high-calorie highly refined products are: Sustacal-HC, Magnacal, Forta and Sustacal puddings, Polycose and Citrotine high-protein powders, Carnation Instant Breakfast, and non-fat dry milk solids.

At the University of California at Davis we have found that Carnation Instant Breakfast type supplements are well tolerated and palatable, and provide nutrients and calories in a simple, easy-to-prepare form at a low cost. However, people with milk intolerance will not be able to use this, and soy-based formulas must be used instead. Table 16–2

Table 16–2. COMPARISON OF FORMULAS AND CARNATION INSTANT BREAKFAST*

	Carnation Instant Breakfast/Milk		***Ensure Plus***		***Isocal***		***Vital***	
	9.5 oz	***1000 cc***	***8 oz***	***1000 cc***	***8 oz***	***1000 cc***	***300 cc***	***1000 cc***
Calories	330	1244	355	1500	250	1066	300	1000
Calories per cc	1.24		1.5		1.06		1.0	
Total calories:N	137.5		171		192		150	
Non pro:N	112.5		146		167		125	
Protein (gm)	15	565	16.5	55	10.2	34.2	12.5	41.7
Percentage of calories from protein	18%		14.7%		13.0%		16.7%	
Fat grams	14.5	54.5	15.9	53.3	13.2	44	3.2	10.8
Percentage of calories from fat	39.5%		32%		37%		9.3%	
CHO	35	130.6	60	200	2916	132	56.4	188
Percentage of calories from CHO	42%		53.3%		50.0%		74.0%	
Approximate cost/unit	$.50/265 cc		$1.16/240 cc		$1.22/240 cc		$2.21/300 cc	

*Adapted from calculations by Dietary Department, University of California, Davis Medical Center, 1983.

gives examples of comparison costs of Carnation Instant Breakfast and other frequently used products. Table 16–3 defines the basic formula combination.

If nutritional compliance is a problem, and moderate to severe malnutrition is diagnosed, medical intervention is necessary. Shils et al have compiled an excellent review of liquid formulas that can be used for both oral and tube feeding.[15] The choice of an appropriate formula is as important as the decision to utilize nutritional support at all. Tables 16–4 to 16–8 illustrate the many types of commercially prepared formulas.[16]

If patients are unable to orally ingest adequate nutrients to meet their metabolic needs, tube feeding is indicated. Patients must have functioning gastrointestinal tracts, as is usually the case with head and neck cancer patients. There are six basic types of tube feeding routes: nasogastric, nasoduodenal, nasojejunal, esophagostomy, gastrostomy, and jejunostomy.

The placement of a nasogastric tube is usually a simple procedure that causes minimal discomfort if done correctly. However, in some patients with cancer of the head and neck, this can be a very distressing procedure because of anatomic changes due to surgery or tumor mass, and the use of topical anesthesia, or in rare instances IV sedation, is indicated to make this task more tolerable. Patients can participate by learning to insert their own tubes for intermittent feedings. This gives them a modicum of control over their own nourishment.

Feedings that are delivered directly into the small intestine or by jejunostomy depend on both the upper and lower esophageal sphincters for prevention of regurgitation. Adequate digestion and absorption occur in the small intestine when appropriate formulas are selected. However, when feedings are improperly selected or administered, diarrhea, cramping, dumping syndrome, and hyperglycemia may result. The bactericidal effect of stomach HCl is bypassed, necessitating special attention to formula and equipment sanitation.

There are many types of nasogastric feeding tubes on the market today. The choice of the appropriate tube should be determined by the patient's needs and take into account the following factors: (1) the ability to deliver

Table 16–3. BASIC FORMULA FOR USE OF CARNATION INSTANT BREAKFAST*

Calories (kcal)	***Protein (gm)***	***Instant Breakfast (# pkgs)***	***Whole Milk (oz)***	***Half & Half (oz)***	***Total Volume (oz)***	***Total Volume (cc)***
330	15	1	6	2	9.5	265
990	45	3	18	6	28.5	795
1980	90	6	36	12	56.5	1590
2970	135	9	54	18	85	2385

*Addition of 2 tbsp non-fat milk powder will increase protein and calories (2 tbsp = 2.7 g protein, 27 calories).

Table 16–4. STANDARD FORMULA DIETS: ORAL FEEDING*

Product Name and Manufacturer	*Carnation Instant Breakfast (Carnation)*	*Meritene Liquid (Doyle)*	*Sustacal (Mead Johnson)*
Available Flavors	Vanilla, Chocolate Malt, Eggnog, Strawberry, Chocolate	Vanilla, Chocolate, Eggnog	Vanilla, Chocolate, Eggnog
Form	Powder; add milk	Ready to use	Ready to use
Kcal/ml	1.06	1	1
Carbohydrate Source	Lactose, sucrose, corn syrump	Corn syrup solids, sucrose	Sucrose, corn syrup
Protein Source	Non-fat milk, Na and Ca caseinates, whey, soy protein isolate (chocolates only)	Concentrated skim milk, NA caseinate	Ca and Na caseinates, soy protein isolate
Fat source	Milk fat, cocoa (chocolates only)	Corn oil, mono- and diglycerides	Soy oil
Protein (g/1000 cc)	58	57.6	60
Fat (g/1000 cc)	32	32	23
Carbohydrate (g/1000 cc)	132	110.4	138
mOsm/kg†	677–715	550–610	625
Volume Needed to Meet RDA for Vitamins and Minerals (cc)	1060	1250	1080
Notes	Readily available; requires digestion; high protein; contains lactose	Requires digestion, high protein; contains lactose	Requires digestion; high protein

*From Arnold C: Why that liquid diet may not work (and what to do about it). RN 35:39, 1981.
†Values represent unflavored product. Flavors may increase osmolality.

adequate amounts of feedings; (2) patient comfort; (3) longevity of the tube; (4) the function of the gastrointestinal tract; and (5) ease of placement and maintenance for the patient and staff.

There is currently a preference toward the use of small diameter flexible polyurethane tubes (Fig. 16–1). These tubes often have weighted tips that allow flotation into the jejunum and facilitate jejunal feedings.[17]

Formula Selection

The selection of an appropriate formula should be carefully calculated by a dietician who is familiar with the patient's current and projected needs. The patient's specific requirements for fats, carbohydrates, and protein must be taken into consideration when a formula is chosen. Some patients do not tolerate milk, fats, or formulas with high osmolarity but require high caloric support. Patient tolerance is a crucial factor that must be taken into account in the selection and observation process.

Formula selection should also be based upon the dietician's familiarity with the product and should take into account the availability and cost to the patient. Commercially available formulas are convenience foods. If the patient and family wish, a program of fresh foods can be calculated. Strict attention should be given to a balanced diet and sanitation during preparation and storage.

Before extensive head and neck surgery, patients are often given different types of formulas to taste. This serves three purposes: (1) to introduce the patient to the type of formula that will be used; (2) to allow time for the patient to stabilize on the formula; and (3) to allow the patient to experience "the feeling" of formula nutrition. Clinical observation has shown that those patients who have had time to familiarize themselves with this type of feeding prior to surgery often are better able to tolerate it following surgery.

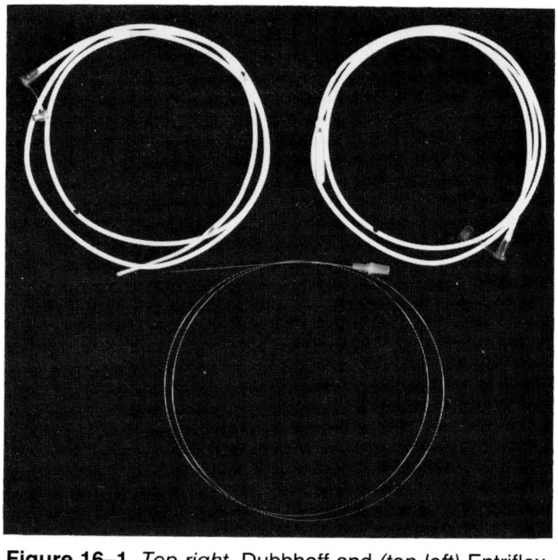

Figure 16–1. *Top right,* Dubbhoff and *(top left)* Entriflex feeding tubes with stylet.

Table 16–5. STANDARD FORMULA DIETS: ORAL OR TUBE FEEDING*

Product Name & Manufacturer	***Ensure (Ross)***	***Ensure Plus (Ross)***	***Precision LR Diet (Doyle)***	***Precision High Nitrogen Diet (Doyle)***
Available Flavors	Vanilla, Chocolate, Black Walnut, Egg Nog, Strawberry, Coffee, plus flavor packets for cherry, pecan, orange, lemon, strawberry	Vanilla, Chocolate, Black Walnut, Egg Nog, Strawberry, Coffee, plus flavor packets for cherry, pecan, orange, lemon, strawberry	Cherry, Lime, Lemon, Orange, Vanilla	Citrus Fruit, Vanilla
Form	Ready to use	Ready to use	Powder	Powder
Kcal/ml	1.06	1.5	1.1	1.05
Carbohydrate Source	Corn syrup solids, sucrose	Corn syrup solids, sucrose	Maltodextrins, sucrose	Maltodextrins, sucrose
Protein Source	Na and Ca caseinates, soy protein isolate	Na + Ca caseinates, soy protein isolate	Egg albumin	Egg albumin
Fat Source	Corn oil	Corn oil	Soy oil	Soy oil
Protein (g/1000 cc)	37	55	26	44
Fat (g/1000 cc)	37	53	1.6	1.3
Carbohydrate (g/1000 cc)	145	197	248	216
mOsm/kg†	450	600	505–549	500–557
Volume Needed to Meet RDA for Vitamins and Minerals (cc)	2000	1500	1710	2850
Notes	Requires digestion	Requires digestion; high caloric density for increased energy needs	Low fecal residue, good bowel prep, requires digestion and fat source for long-term use	Low fecal residue, good bowel prep, requires digestion and fat source for long-term use

*From Arnold C: Why that liquid diet may not work (and what to do about it). RN 35:39, 1981.
†Values represent unflavored product; flavors may increase osmolality.

Table 16–6. STANDARD FORMULA DIETS: TUBE FEEDING*

Product Name & Manufacturer	*Compleat B (Doyle)*	*Isocal (Mead Johnson)*
Form	Ready to use	Ready to use
Kcal/ml	1	1
Carbohydrate Source	Hydrolyzed cereal solids, maltodextrin, vegetables, fruit	Corn syrup, glucose, oligosaccharides
Protein Source	Beef, non-fat milk	Ca and Na caseinates, soy protein isolate
Fat source	Corn oil	Soy oil, MCT oil
Protein (g/1000 cc)	40, 43	34
Fat (g/1000 cc)	40, 43	44
Carbohydrate (g/1000 cc)	120, 128	130
mOsm/kg†	390, 405†	300
Volume Needed to Meet RDA for Vitamins and Minerals (cc)	1600, 1500†	1920
Notes	Requires digestion; commercial blenderized diet; comes in a can or bottle; contains lactose	Isotonic; low Na; requires digestion

*From Arnold C: Why that liquid diet may not work (and what to do about it). RN 35:39, 1981.
†Bottled product.

Feeding Administration

When tube feedings are instituted, patients should be advanced gradually until target goals are reached. Target goals must be clearly defined and intake and output accurately recorded.

Postoperatively, feedings may be started with D_5W solutions or water. Bowel sounds should be present, but some studies show that elemental feedings can be instituted into the jejunum without such gastrointestinal activity. Formula feddings should be advanced from quarter to half to full strength as dictated by patient tolerance. The amount ingested at each feeding should generally stay constant once maximum concentration is achieved. Only one parameter—either strength or amount—should be changed at any one time. This allows for better control over the feeding process.

When problems of patient intolerance occur, it is wise to cut back on both strength and volume and reinstitute the weaning process, advancing one parameter at a time. Intolerance can be manifested by nausea, vomiting, diarrhea, cramping, delayed gastric emptying, and epigastric pain. If the delivery of feedings is slow, especially with bolus feedings, patients are usually able to tolerate most formulas.

There is much controversy over whether feedings should be administered by intermittent bolus or by continuous drip. The general rule of thumb is to allow the patient to make that decision, based on his or her own tolerance. There are obvious advantages and disadvantages to both bolus and continuous feedings. The restriction of mobility during continuous feeding and the drastic change from a normal eating habit are two factors that may negate the success of this administration. On the other hand, bolus feedings in amounts that provide adequate nutrition are frequently not well tolerated. Often an effective compromise is reached by using continuous feedings during the night and bolus feedings during waking hours. This allows patients more freedom during waking hours, yet ensures adequate caloric and nutritional intake.

Another method of feeding is by delivery of an elemental diet directly into the small intestine or by jejunal feedings. Vivonex H-N, Criticare H-N, and Vital are three types of elemental feedings that are used today. Several investigators have studied this type of administration during the immediate postoperative period and have shown that these type of feedings can be instituted before bowel sounds are clinically present, thus preventing the delay of feeding.[18–20]

If enteral feedings are not possible, total parenteral nutrition (TPN) and peripheral parenteral nutrition (PPN) are expensive but appropriate alternatives. There is much controversy about the efficacy of such expensive feeding programs. It is generally recognized that all enteral feeding possibilities should be investigated before TPN is instituted. Dudrick and Ruberg[21] state that parenteral nutrition should be used only for patients who cannot eat, should not eat, will not eat, or cannot eat enough.

Table 16–7. DEFINED FORMULA DIETS: ORAL OR TUBE FEEDING*

Product Name & Manufacturer	*Flexical (Mead-Johnson)*	*Vital (Ross)*	*Standard Vivonex (Eaton)*	*High Nitrogen Vivonex (Eaton)*
Available Flavors	Unflavored	Vanilla, and flavor packets for cherry, lemon, pecan, strawberry	Flavor packets for vanilla, orange-pineapple, strawberry, lemon-lime	Flavor packets for vanilla, orange-pineapple, strawberry, lemon-lime
Form	Powder	Powder	Powder	Powder
Kcal/ml	1	1	1	1
Carbohydrate Source	Corn syrup solids	Sucrose, corn starch, glucose, oligo- and polysaccharides	Glucose, oligosaccharides	Glucose, oligosaccharides
Protein Source	Casein hydrolysate, crystalline amino acids	Soy protein, hydrolyzed whey, meat amino acids	L-Amino acids	L-Amino acids
Fat Source	Soy oil, MCT	Sunflower oil, MCT	Safflower oil	Safflower oil
Protein (g/1000 cc)	22	42	21	42
Fat (g/1000 cc)	34	10.8	1	1
Carbohydrate (g/1000 cc)	152	185	226	210
mOsm/kg†	550	460†	550†	810†
Volume Needed to Meet RDA for Vitamins and Minerals (cc)	2000	1500	1800	3000
Notes	Contains medium-chained triglycerides, an absorbed fat	Low osmolality; separates into layers upon standing; contains medium-chained triglycerides, an easily absorbed fat	Negligible fat, low pancreatic stimulus, absorbed in upper gut; protein in most elemental form; contains chromium, molybdenum, and selenium	Negligible fat, no pancreatic stimulus, absorbed in upper gut; protein in most elemental form; high protein; may need vitamin supplement if given in volumes lower than 3000 cc/day; contains chromium, molybdenum, selenium

*From Arnold C: Why that liquid diet may not work (and what to do about it). RN 35:39, 1981.
†Values represent unflavored product; flavors may increase osmolality.

Table 16–8. SPECIALTY DIETS: ORAL OR TUBE FEEDING*

Product Name & Manufacturer	***Amin-Aid (American McGaw)***	***Hepatic Aid (American McGaw)***
Available Flavors	Orange, Lemon-lime, Strawberry, Berry (instant drinks); Chocolate, Butterscotch (instant puddings)	Chocolate, Custard, Eggnog, Chocolate Mint, Pistachio (instant drinks); Chocolate, Vanilla, Butterscotch (instant puddings)
Form	Powder	Powder
Kcal/ml	2 (instant drink); 4.26 kcal/g (average for instant pudding)	1.63 (instant drink); 3.9 kcal/g (average for instant pudding)
Carbohydrate Source	Maltodextrins, sucrose	Maltodextrins, sucrose
Protein Source	Crystalline essential amino acids, histidine	Crystalline essential amino acids; high in branched chained amino acids, low in aromatic amino acids
Fat Source	Partially dehydrogenated soy oil, lecithin, mono- and diglycerides	Partially dehydrogenated soy oil, lecithin, mono- and diglycerides
Protein (g/1000 cc)	19.6 (instant drink)	42.6 (instant drink)
Fat (g/1000 cc)	46	36.2
Carbohydrate (g/1000 cc)	365	290
mOsm/kg†	1000	950
Notes	For renal disease; requires additional electrolytes, vitamins, and minerals; less than 5 mEq Na^+ per packet	For hepatic disease; requires additional electrolytes, vitamins, and minerals; less than 5 mEq Na^+ per packet

*From Arnold C: Why that liquid diet may not work (and what to do about it). RN 35:39, 1981.
†Values represent unflavored product; flavors may increase osmolality.

TPN, primarily a glucose solution, can be used for primary or supportive nutritional therapy. Any patient who is currently unable to maintain his own nutrition or who will be unable to maintain his nutrition because of proposed intervention is a candidate for TPN. Everyone requires nutrition, and those who are ill usually require augmented nutrition. Nutrition thus is as important to survival and health as surgery is for a ruptured viscus.

Steiger and Grundfest[22] state that the indications for TPN generally fall into five broad categories:

1. Preoperative preparation of malnourished patients, particularly those who have lost more than 10 to 15 per cent of their body weight.
2. Postoperative maintenance of malnourished patients, particularly those who have lost more than 10 to 15 per cent of their body weight.
3. Inflammatory intestinal disease.
4. Patients who are unable to meet their energy needs by oral or nasogastric intake.
5. Patients who are candidates for chemotherapy or radiotherapy, with depressed immune responses as a result of cancer-associated malnutrition.

They also describe four basic principles for the use of TPN:

1. Safe, aseptic catheter placement.
2. Regular catheter care.
3. Proper preparation and delivery of the nutrient solutions and their additives.
4. Careful daily patient monitoring.

The use of subclavian catheter placement, although not without complications, has heralded a safe route for TPN administration. The actual placement of subclavian catheters has been well described by Ryan.[23]

Complications of the placement of these lines and their subsequent use for TPN have greatly diminished as physicians have become more skilled in their use. Complications of central venous catheterization, such as arterial or venous injury, pneumothorax, hydrothorax, or nerve injury, are documented, but their incidence is decreasing. Late complications of catheterization (e.g., thrombophlebitis, superior vena cava thrombosis, sepsis) are also decreasing because of meticulous care and observation by specially trained nursing and surgical staff.

Septic complications are usually due to contamination by draining wounds or accidental disruption of the TPN system. Meticulous catheter care by a trained staff will decrease the incidence of sepsis. Employment of nurses specifically trained in TPN greatly enhances the nutritional program. Their duties include making dressing changes and line changes; inspecting the wound site, keeping track of fever charts, culture reports, and laboratory data; instructing the physician and nursing staff in aspects of TPN with which they may not be familiar; assisting in line placement; and instructing the patient and family on maintenance of home TPN.

If catheter-induced sepsis occurs, blood cultures must be taken, the catheter removed, and appropriate antibiotic therapy instituted. Nutritional support must be continued during this process.

There are also metabolic complications associated with TPN, hyperglycemia, glucose intolerance, hyperosmolar hyperglycemic nonketotic coma, and electrolyte and essential fatty acid deficiencies being only a few. Careful monitoring of the patient and incremental adjustments of solution delivery will help to avoid any potential complications.

Nurses should be instructed to check the patient's urine for acetone and sugar every 6 hours. Solution flow rates are carefully monitored. Catching up is discouraged and may be prevented by the use of sophisticated pump systems. Daily weights and accurate intake and output measurements must be recorded.

While patients are on TPN, lipids are used to prevent essential fatty acid deficiencies and as a source of calories to promote nitrogen sparing. Lipids are the body's main endogenous fuel source. Energy-rich carbon-containing compounds are available for intravenous use. When given with amino acids, as in TPN, they promote protein anabolism. Lipids can be given 3 to 4 times per week.

In peripheral parenteral nutrition, the nutrients used are similar in composition to those for TPN but in slightly different solutions, with peripheral veins being used rather than central veins. The disadvantages of PPN are the limited venous access and limited energy source. Generally PPN is used only for short periods of time to supplement enteral nutrition. The cost is significantly more than that of TPN.

PPN is usually composed of 3 per cent amino acid solution. Delivery depends upon the fluid and electrolyte needs of the patient. Additional electrolytes, vitamins, and minerals may be added as needed during the course of therapy. The use of isotonic amino acids should be discontinued only if the rise in BUN exceeds 5 to 10 mg per 100 ml per day for 3 consecutive days.[24]

The use of intravascular nutrition has greatly enhanced surgeons' ability to care for malnourished patients.

CONCLUSION

Weight loss in cancer patients is due to anorexia and the increased metabolic demands of the tumor. It is often difficult to determine whether one is feeding the host or feeding the tumor when aggressive nutritional intervention is instituted.

It is important to attempt to define the objectives of aggressive therapy at high dollar costs. Institutions must now look at efficacy of treatment for specific patients. The utilization of a nutritional supportive service can only help clinicians provide better care for head and neck cancer patients.

References

1. Putam MR, Jones E, Palmer BU: Postoperative enteral tube feeding in patients with squamous carcinoma of the head and neck. Nutritional Support Services, Vol 2, No 9, p 6.
2. Copeland EM, Daly JM, Dudrick SJ: Nutritional concepts in the treatment of head and neck malignancies. Head Neck Surg 1:350, 1979.
3. Krause M, Mahan K: Food, Nutrition and Diet Therapy, 6th ed. Philadelphia, WB Saunders, 1979, p 220.
4. Joliffe N (ed): Clinical Nutrition, 2nd ed. New York, Harper & Brothers, 1962.
5. Gitlin, N: Malnutrition in the hospitalized patient: etiology, confirmation and significance. Thesis, University of California, San Francisco, April 1952.
6. Morgan DB, Hill GL, Burkinshaw L: The assessment of weight loss from a single measurement of body weight: the problems and limitations. Am J Clin Nutr 33:2101, 1980.
7. Blackburn GL, Bistrian BR, Maini BS, et al: Nutritional and metabolic assessment of the hospitalized patient. JPEN 1:11, 1977.
8. Harris JB: Nausea, vomiting and cancer treatment. CA Cancer J Clinic 28:194, 1978.
9. Theologides A: Anorexia producing intermediary metabolites. Am J Clin Nutr 29:552, 1976.
10. Krause M, Mahan K: Food, Nutrition and Diet Therapy, 6th ed. Philadelphia, WB Saunders, 1979, p 728.
11. Harris JB: Nausea, vomiting and cancer treatment. CA Cancer J Clinic 28:195, 1978.
12. Grallia R, Itri LM, Pisko SE, et al: Antiemetic efficacy of high dose metoclopramide:randomized trials with placebo and prochlorperazine in patients with chemotherapy induced nausea and vomiting. N Engl J Med 305:905, 1981.
13. Eizen G, Daly TE, Drane JB, et al: Oral complications of cancer radiotherapy. Postgrad Med 61:85, 1977.
14. Durdrick SJ: A patient on I.V. therapy need not starve! Consultant, J Med Consult., Cliggott Publishing Co, 1978, p 1.
15. Shils ME, Bloc HAS, Chernoff R: Liquid Formulas for Oral and Tube Feeding, 2nd ed. New York, Memorial Sloan-Kettering Cancer Center, 1979, p 1.

16. Arnold C: Why that liquid diet may not work (and what to do about it). RN 35:39, 1981.
17. Vazquez RM, Craig RM, Slas TJ: Performance and acceptability of Entriflex enteric feeding tube with hydromer lubricated lumen and mercury weight and with placement stylet. Nutritional Support Services 1:9, 1981.
18. Page CP, Carlton PK, Anorassy RJ, et al: Safe cost-effective postoperative nutrition: defined formula diet via needle catheter jejunostomy. Am J Surg 138:939, 1979.
19. Hoover HC, Ryan JA, Anderson EJ, et al: Nutritional benefits of immediate postoperative jejunal feeding of an elemental diet. Am J Surg 139:153, 1980.
20. Moore EE, Junn EL, Jones TN: Immediate jejunostomy feeding. Arch Surg 116:681, 1981.
21. Dudrick SJ, Ruberg RL: Principles and practice of parenteral nutrition. Gastroenterology 61:901, 1971.
22. Steiger E, Grundfest S: Intravenous hyperalimentation: vascular access and administration. *In* Dietel M (ed): Nutrition in Clinical Surgery. Baltimore, Williams & Wilkins, 1980, p 53.
23. Ryan J Jr: Complications of total parenteral nutrition. *In* Fischer JE (ed): Total Parenteral Nutrition. Boston, Little, Brown & Co, 1976.
24. Blackburn G, Flatt JP, Hensle TW: Peripheral amino acid infusions. *In* Fischer JE (ed): Total Parenteral Nutrition. Boston, Little, Brown & Co, 1976, p 379.

17

SPEECH REHABILITATION

Rebecca J. Leonard, Ph.D.

One of the unique, agonizing problems of head and neck cancer is that, at a time of tremendous emotional and physical upheaval, wrought both by the illness and its surgical treatment, there may be severe constraints on a patient's ability to express himself. That is, at a time when the emotional need to communicate is especially keen, the mechanical ability to do so may be seriously impaired. Affording the patient both the opportunity and the means to convey his thoughts is perhaps especially critical during the "perisurgical" period, when coping with the fact of cancer and the experience of a major, even radical surgical procedure may seriously tax personal reserves.

Once the ordeal of surgery is over, and concerns with breathing, swallowing, and eating have been resolved, the patient may begin to focus his efforts on resuming his premorbid lifestyle. At this point, restoration of communication skills to maximal efficiency often becomes a serious priority of the head and neck cancer patient. This chapter will consider the major difficulties encountered in providing such patients with effective communication skills. Special emphasis will be placed on medical-surgical factors that influence the development of alaryngeal speech and compensated speech resulting from orofacial alterations.

SOURCE-FILTER THEORY: A WAY TO VIEW SPEECH PROBLEMS IN HEAD/NECK CANCER PATIENTS

Most of us recognize that to surgically remove or alter some portion of the speech production apparatus may present difficulties for a speaker. However, to understand these surgical effects more fully, it may be of benefit to briefly consider some aspects of normal speech production. A useful model described by Fant[1] divides the peripheral processes of speech into *source, transfer function,* and *output* characteristics.

Source in this model refers to a sound source. In the case of vowel sounds and all consonant sounds that are produced with vibrating vocal folds (i.e., "voiced" speech sounds), the voicing source is the larynx, powered by pulmonary air. Thus, the vocal folds, which can vibrate within audible frequency and intensity levels, and the lungs, the power source that drives the vocal folds, are essential features of human voicing.

The larynx not only permits the *complex, quasiperiodic** voicing source for speech sounds but also allows us to vary the frequency of our voices, which is perceived as a pitch change. In conjunction with the respiratory system, the larynx regulates the intensity, or perceived loudness, of our voices. Thus, a speaker who has the larynx, or some portion of the larynx, removed exhibits a voicing *source deficit* that may alter or prevent voicing altogether, or interfere with pitch and loudness changes.

Removal of the larynx does not mean, however, that a speaker can produce no speech sounds. Many of the speech sounds we make are referred to as "voiceless." These sounds, including /*p, t, k, f, s, sh, ch,* and *th*/, are produced by occluding or constricting

**Complex*—consisting of more than one frequency; *quasiperiodic*—repeating itself at regular intervals.

the vocal tract at a point other than the larynx, and then driving air through or across the point of occlusion. Patients with laryngeal deficits, but with orofacial structures intact, can typically learn to produce these voiceless (*complex* and *aperiodic*) sounds using residual air that remains in the oropharyngeal cavities. For the voiced equivalents of the above consonants, /*b, d, g, v, z, zh, j* and voiced *th*/, two sources are required: a voicing source at the larynx, and an aperiodic noise source generated by the articulators. Obviously, only the noise sources will remain intact in laryngectomy patients.

Sound produced at the larynx, as well as at upper airway sources, does not remain unchanged as it passes through the vocal tract but is modified by the cavities and structures it encounters. This process of modification is referred to in Fant's model as *transfer function.* In essence, the upper airway acts as a filter to sound produced within it. Each time a speaker changes the three-dimensional shape of the tract, its filter function is changed, the most critical aspect of these changes being the locations of the tract's natural resonance frequencies. As is the case with other air-filled containers, the vocal tract has natural resonance frequencies that are modified according to changes in vocal tract size and shape.

The phenomenon of resonance is easily illustrated with the spectrograms of vowel sounds presented in Figure 17–1. In these spectrograms, or "voiceprints," time is represented on the horizontal axis, and frequency on the vertical axis. Intensity is accounted for in a relative way by the degree of blackness, or burn, so that the darker areas in the figure indicate the presence of greater sound energy at particular time and frequency locations. Of interest in the spectrograms are the dark horizontal bands associated with the speaker's productions of "ēē," "ah" and "ōō," respectively. These are called formants and correspond to the natural resonance frequencies of the vocal tract. It can be noted in the figure that the horizontal bands, and thus, implicitly, the vocal tract's resonance locations, are different for each vowel. The ear and brain respond to the uniqueness of these resonance locations in differentiating vowel sounds. In fact, *all* speech sounds have unique resonance characteristics that are important to their accurate perception. And, while resonance characteristics of speech sounds are not the only cues important to speech perception, they are especially vulnerable to the effects of head and neck surgery.

The capacity to quickly effect resonance changes during speech, thereby "articulating" the sounds of speech, is critically dependent on a speaker's ability to constrict and/or occlude the vocal tract in complex ways. Patients with upper airway deficits resulting from maxillectomy, mandibulectomy, pharyngectomy, or glossectomy may have difficulty making such cavity changes, so that the normal articulation of speech is impaired. In addition, size and shape characteristics of the vocal tract determine information present in the speech signal about the speaker, such as identity, age, and sex. How such cues may be affected in certain types of *transfer function deficits* is not well understood.

Output characteristics at the mouth, the final stage of Fant's model, represent the speech signal presented to the listener. This final output is the product of the *source's* having been modified by *transfer function* characteristics, and is increased in amplitude by about 6 decibels as it leaves the oral cavity, owing to the radiation properties of, primarily, the lips. Obviously, surgical factors that influence either source or transfer function characteristics may affect the final speech output. From a general rehabilitative perspective, strategies for restoring effective oral communication skills to patients with either laryngeal or orofacial deficits may be quite good. However, when both the larynx and the upper airway are involved, problems in establishing viable oral communication can be enormous.

REHABILITATIVE PROBLEMS IN PATIENTS WITH LARYNGECTOMY

Finding the optimum alternative voicing source for an individual laryngectomy patient is not an easy task. The problem has become particularly acute in recent years with the influx of new alternatives for the alaryngeal speaker which are often highly touted in both professional and popular media. Every surgeon and speech pathologist in an ENT practice in the last few years has undoubtedly encountered the patient who arrives in the clinic with newspaper clippings, or reports of news items from TV, regarding some new instrument or procedure designed to "restore voice to the voiceless." The patient's question, of course, is "Could this work for me?" It is pleasing to know that the special problems of alaryngeal speakers are better publicized—and, it is hoped, better understood—than at any previous time. But the selection of an alternative voicing source involves more than the simple expression of a preference. In fact, determining the method of choice for each patient is often a complicated process, influenced by many variables. Not every alternative is appropriate for every patient.

Excellent discussions of the many patient variables that influence the communicative potential of the alaryngeal speaker have been detailed elsewhere and will be briefly reviewed here. Initially, it may be worthwhile to consider what investment the use of an alternative voicing source requires from a laryngectomy patient. First, the alaryngeal speaker must be willing to expend time and energy learning how to use the selected alternative. In some instances, this objective may require only a few hours of instruction and practice. In other cases, acquiring the alternative may necessitate additional surgical procedures, with their own attendant risks and problems. Second, essentially all available alternatives require some degree of maintenance and some adaptation of the patient's lifestyle in order to be viable. These activities may range from keeping batteries and special supplies on hand to cleaning a tracheoesophageal prosthesis. Third, the patient must be willing to subject himself to special attention from onlookers, or "on-listeners," as he begins to use the alternative voicing source in a full range of speaking situations.

In considering just these prerequisites for the acquisition, maintenance, and utilization of an alternative voicing source, it becomes apparent that there is a wide variability in terms of the demands made on the patient. Not surprisingly, patients will respond differently to these requirements.

Psychosocial Factors

The consensus among authors regarding psychosocial influences on laryngectomy rehabilitation is not easily ascertained. Gates and coworkers[2, 3] recently undertook an extensive investigation of a number of variables influencing laryngectomy rehabilitation. "Successful outcome" in this study was determined by extent of return to pre-morbid lifestyle, effective communication, and psychologic adjustment. The authors reported that successfully rehabilitated laryngectomees were relatively more flexible and imaginative, independent, and self-assured. In contrast, patients with failed rehabilitation showed greater denial, poorer self-images, and a decrease in socializing activities. In addition, Gates et al described a lack of desire, not associated with depression, as a factor that contributed adversely to laryngectomy rehabilitation.

Using a very different methodology, Amster et al[4] reported only low positive correlations between postsurgical speech intelligibility and variables related to motivation and aspiration level. Beamer,[5] using the Minnesota Multiphasic Personality inventory, reported that laryngectomees could not be

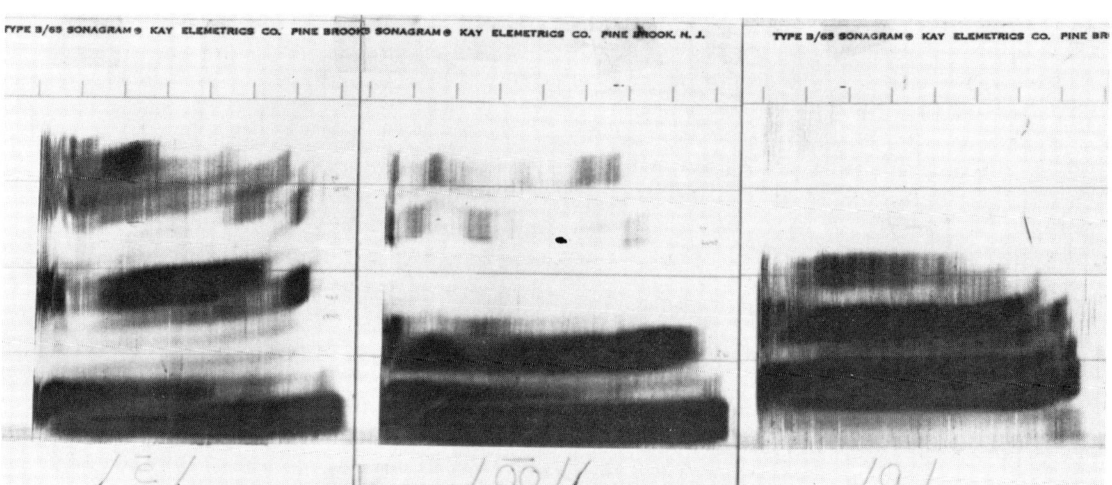

Figure 17–1. Spectrograms of a speaker saying three vowels. Frequency is represented on the vertical axis; time on the horizontal. Degree of darkness indicates relative amount of amplitude. Dark horizontal bands at different frequency locations for each vowel are called formants, and correspond to natural resonances of the vocal tract.

characterized as demonstrating a "typical profile," while Shames et al,[6] administering the Edwards Personal Preference Schedule, noted positive correlations between speech intelligibility and variables related to attention seeking and achievement. Several authors, in fact, have supported the notion that motivation, high achievement levels, and extroversion are positive factors in acquiring speech after laryngectomy, while poor self and body images, anxiety, and depression are negative factors.[7–9]

Gates et al[2, 3] did not observe age differences in laryngectomees with good or poor rehabilitation outcomes. These authors did note, however, that some effects of advanced age, including decreased strength, hearing loss, and senility, could adversely influence rehabilitation. The findings of Gates and coworkers would seem to be supported by several other authors who likewise found no significant relationship between age and speech intelligibility (Diedrich and Youngstrom,[10] Snidecor[11]). Opposition to this view is offered by Gardner,[12, 13] Shames et al,[6] and Hudson,[14] all of whom have reported an adverse influence of advanced age on speech intelligibility in laryngectomees, and by Kahane and Irwin,[15] who reported greater difficulty in learning postlaryngectomy speech with advanced age.

In contrast to the large number of studies on the relationship between age and laryngectomy rehabilitation, there is very little information available regarding possible differences between men and women in the alaryngeal population with regard to speech rehabilitation. Gates et al[2, 3] reported that sex of the speaker was not a factor either in rehabilitation outcome or in whether or not a patient acquired esophageal speech. These data appear to receive support from the results of a survey among female laryngectomees conducted by Stack.[16] Unique problems of the female laryngectomee, in terms of speech and a variety of psychosocial factors, have been reviewed by Shanks[17] and by Gardner.[12]

Interestingly, in the study by Gates et al[2, 3] education and intelligence variables were not found to influence laryngectomee rehabilitation or the acquisition of esophageal speech. Similar findings regarding educational level and quality of postsurgical speech have been supported by Hudson[14] but contradicted by Shames et al.[6] Other authors have suggested that pre-morbid verbal ability and at least average intelligence may be positively related to acquiring speech after laryngectomy.[12, 18, 19]

From even this brief review of the literature, it is apparent that the role of various psychosocial factors in laryngectomy rehabilitation is not straightforward. This lack of clarity may, in part, be related to the variable methodologies used in the studies undertaken to resolve just these issues. Obviously, it is also difficult to elucidate any one variable (age, for example) when related variables, such as hearing loss or senility, interact and confound the matter. In general, we may conclude that motivation and attitude are critical variables, while sex and levels of intelligence and education typically are not. The influence of other variables, including age, is probably best viewed as obscure.

Our own clinical experience would further suggest that the single most important factor influencing the acquisition of effective communication skills following laryngectomy is the patient's degree of communicative need and/or desire. Though many factors may intervene to prevent a given patient from developing a particular form of alaryngeal speech, if his need or desire to communicate is sufficiently strong, it is probable that this patient, by whatever means, will be a viable communicator.

Medical/Surgical Variables

Certain generalizations regarding the influence of various medical/surgical factors on patients' postlaryngectomy potential for speech are apparent. One would predict, for example, that the patient who experiences both source and transfer function deficits is a poorer candidate for any form of postsurgical speech than the patient with only one deficit. Similarly, a patient with numerous medical problems, in addition to a laryngectomy, has a poorer prognosis for alaryngeal speech than a patient who is in otherwise good health. However, beyond these rather commonsense kinds of generalizations, medical/surgical problems are more often unique to the particular form of alaryngeal voicing source being considered. Thus, problems that medical or surgical factors pose for esophageal voice may differ from those affecting electronic or pneumatic instrument voicing. For this reason, and in keeping with the "special problems" theme of this text, medical/surgical factors will be considered as they affect four major categories of alternative voicing sources: esophageal voice; voice achieved with electronic or pneumatic instruments; voice achieved primarily by prosthetic/surgical approaches; and voice achieved by surgical reconstruction alone.

Special Medical/Surgical Problems in Esophageal Voice

Esophageal voice refers to speech in which some portion of the esophagus functions as a vibrating sound source. This method of voicing is widely considered to be the ideal alternative for the alaryngeal speaker. However, Goode[20] cited studies reporting that from 17 to 50 per cent of alaryngeal speakers fail to develop esophageal speech. Gates et al[2, 3] noted that of 35 patients who attempted to learn esophageal speech, only 12, or 34 per cent, were actually using it in daily communication 6 months after surgery.

In order to produce esophageal voice, the speaker must first inject or inhale air into the esophagus. (See References 21 to 24 for descriptions of esophageal speech, air intake methods, and acoustic characteristics.) With either injection or inhalation, the initial objective is to create a pressure difference across the superior esophageal sphincter, which causes this segment to open and allows air to enter the esophagus. Then, with the esophagus functioning as an air reservoir, air is forced back across the constricted sphincter, referred to as the pharyngoesophageal (P-E) segment. To drive the P-E segment into oscillation, thereby producing voice, the speaker must develop a positive esophageal pressure sufficient to overcome the resistance of the closed P-E segment.

The P-E segment in normal individuals is most often made up of fibers of the cricopharyngeus, inferior pharyngeal constrictor, and superior esophageal muscles.[25, 26] The sound produced is low in frequency, reflecting the massive nature of the sphincter as compared with vocal folds. In addition, the sound produced is of short duration, owing to the limited amount of air that can be insufflated.

Characteristics of the P-E Segment

Morphology and Length. The structure of the segment varies among laryngectomees, and even within the same laryngectomee as he performs different tasks, but it is typically located between the fourth and sixth cervical vertebrae.[10] Cinefluoroscopic evidence has shown that in some esophageal speakers a single segment is present on voicing.[10, 27] In other patients, more than one segment may be observed, while a small number of patients exhibit no clearly defined segment. Brewer et al[28] reported wide variation in the number of segments and in the contour of the hypopharynx and cervical esophagus among 8 patients described as "good" esophageal speakers. In general, these studies appear to agree that particular size and shape characteristics of the P-E segment, as viewed radiologically, are subject to great variation among laryngectomy patients but do not influence the acquisition or quality of esophageal speech.

Some opposition to this view is offered by Damste.[29] Both Kirchner et al[27] and Damste have reported variations in appearance of the P-E segment, that is, whether it is thin or broadly based, long or short, flat or round. However, Damste has noted that patients who demonstrate extreme divergence from other laryngectomees in terms of either P-E shape or length may have difficulty achieving esophageal speech. Blom[30] has also reported that patients who demonstrate extreme divergence from other laryngectomees in terms of either the shape or length of the P-E segment may have difficulty achieving esophageal voice.

Innervation and Muscular Control. Several authors have reported that impaired innervation of the P-E segment, leading to reduced, asynchronous, or poorly coordinated activity, can interfere with esophageal speech development.[10, 31] Zwitman,[32] reviewing the course of the recurrent and superior laryngeal nerves, and the pharyngeal plexus contributions to the cricopharyngeus muscle, suggested that innervation to the P-E segment is generally spared in laryngectomy surgery. This is important, noted Zwitman, since the perfectly timed opening and closing of the cricopharyngeus and its adjacent fibers is critical to the quality of esophageal speech. Other researchers have described cricopharyngeal "spasm," in which attempts by the patient to inject or inhale air into the esophagus appear to produce a spastic tightening of the segment that precludes esophageal voicing.[33–37]

Brunner[38] observed that spasm of the cricopharyngeus muscle forms a "cross-roll" on the posterior pharyngeal wall. Brunner referred to this muscle bulk as a hypopharyngeal bar, and suggested it was analogous to Passavant's pad, which is formed higher in the pharynx by the superior pharyngeal constrictor muscle. Singer et al[35] reported that such a retropharyngeal mass was consistently observed radiographically in patients who failed to develop esophageal speech following tracheoesophageal shunts. Selective pharyngeal constrictor myotomy enabled all patients to produce esophageal voice. Singer concluded that at least partial denervation of the posterior pharynx may greatly facilitate patients' ability to tolerate pharyngoesophageal airflow for alaryngeal speech. Interestingly, Weinberg has recently suggested that a somewhat flaccid P-E segment may be a usual consequence of total laryngectomy. Weinberg's hypothesis is based on evidence that normal speakers often fail to produce esophageal voice when the esophagus is insufflated. (Weinberg B: Personal communication, 1982).

Shipp[39] reported EMG findings showing that "adequate" esophageal speakers demonstrated differential control of inferior constrictor and cricopharyngeus muscle activity across the air intake and injection phases of esophageal voicing. In contrast, speakers judged as "poor" in Shipp's study exhibited relatively more gross, undifferentiated muscle activity across preinjection, injection, prephonation, phonation, and postphonation activities.

Cricopharyngeal Sphincter Pressure. Though several authors[40, 41] have noted reduced cricopharyngeal sphincter pressures in laryngectomy patients, as compared with normal subjects, the relationship of cricopharyngeus pressure to esophageal speech proficiency is unclear and in need of further research. Winans et al[42] reported that patients judged as good esophageal speakers had lower resting cricopharyngeal sphincter pressures ($\overline{13.1}$ mm Hg) and higher gastric pressures ($\overline{18}$ mm Hg) than patients who were unable to acquire esophageal speech (cricopharyngeal sphincter pressure = $\overline{29.6}$ mm Hg; gastric pressure = $\overline{11}$ mm Hg). A criticism of Winans' study regards the validity of the assumption that findings for rest (or nonspeech activities) will hold for speech.[43] In addition, it is not clear whether cricopharyngeus sphincter pressures differ according to quality of speech, since only "good" and "non"-esophageal speakers were considered.

The data of Winans et al[42] have been contradicted by Salmon,[44] who reported no relationship between pharyngeal pressure, esophageal sphincter, and quality of esophageal voice. Salmon[45] later noted that reports of an inverse relationship between pressure measurements and proficiency of esophageal speech[46–48] must be viewed with caution. According to Salmon, extreme pressure variations observed for the same speaker repeating the same task suggest that the relationship between pressure and speech proficiency is not easily predicted.

In a recent study, Welch et al[49] observed that all prior manometric studies suffered from invalid instrumentation and indicated that future research efforts should utilize a transducer that is radially sensitive and capable of detecting pressure changes around its entire circumference. Welch's data confirmed previous reports of lowered upper esophageal sphincter pressures in laryngectomy patients as compared with normal controls. In addition, the authors reported no differences in resting pressure measurements between postlaryngectomy patients who achieved and those who failed to achieve esophageal speech.

Preservation of the Cricopharyngeus. Simpson et al,[50] examining four types of reconstruction in laryngectomy, concluded that approximating the cut ends of the cricopharyngeus muscle and anchoring it to the posterior wall of the trachea were critical to later esophageal speech development. These authors thus add their support to proponents of cricopharyngeal preservation at laryngectomy. In contrast to this view, and representing what currently appears to be a distinct minority viewpoint, Dey and Kirchner[40] have suggested that the cricopharyngeus muscle is not central to esophageal speech.

Zwitman[32] described a procedure by Calcaterra in which, when tumor margins permit, most anterior fibers of the criopharyngeus muscle are transected at their point of insertion into the cricoid cartilage. Remaining muscle is then bluntly dissected away from the posterior cricoid cartilage. According to Zwitman, this procedure assures retention of anterior mucosa and, therefore, the structural integrity of the cricopharyngeus muscle. Zwitman's impressions of patients in whom the anterior mucosal segment is intact, as compared with those in whom the cricopharyngeus muscle has been separated and the two ends then approximated, suggest an advantage of the former procedure in terms of developing very proficient esophageal speech.

Type and Extent of Surgery

Diedrich and Youngstrom[10] reported no difference in postlaryngectomy speech skill among four groups of patients, which included those who had (a) total laryngectomy only; (b) total laryngectomy and radiation; (c) total laryngectomy and radical neck dissection; and (d) total laryngectomy, radical neck dissection, and radiation treatment. Their findings have generally been supported by others,[6, 51-53] although Sako et al[54] reported, oddly enough, better results of esophageal speech development in patients with total laryngectomy and radical neck dissection than in patients with total laryngectomy only. Putney[55] observed no relationship between the degree of success of postsurgical speech and the type of neck incision, method of pharyngeal closure, or extent of adjacent cervical tissue excision in laryngectomy surgery. Robe et al[53] noted that whether the surgery field was wide or narrow did not appear to influence either the acquisition or quality of postsurgical speech.

The above reports would appear to be in some conflict with the more recent findings of Richardson,[56] who compared speech development in patients in four surgical categories: (a) laryngectomy; (b) laryngectomy and unilateral radical neck dissection; (c) laryngectomy and bilateral radical neck dissection; and (d) laryngectomy and multiple surgeries (including, for example, radical neck dissection, pharyngectomy, and fistula repair). According to Richardson, 70 per cent of patients in the "a" group had learned esophageal speech, whereas only 44 and 50 per cent of patients in the "b" and "c" groups respectively, and no patients in the "d" group, developed esophageal speech.

Simpson et al[50] compared four types of reconstruction of the hypopharynx with regard to subsequent development and proficiency of esophageal speech. The essential features of the four procedures were as follows:

A. The anterior edges of the inferior pharyngeal constrictor muscle were approximated throughout their entire length, with careful attention to an upper anchor suture to the suprahyoid musculature in the space left by the excised body of the hyoid. In addition, a lower body anchor suture was placed in which the last suture through the cricopharyngeus muscle was brought through the anterior, longitudinal esophagus and posterior wall of the trachea, thus stabilizing the P-E segment.

B. Similar to (A), but with no upper and lower anchor points, so that muscular control of the hypopharynx was somewhat impaired in these areas.

C. Inferior constrictor ends were not approximated anteriorly; rather, mucosal sutures were buttressed by stitches to deep layers of the overlapping sternohyoid muscles.

D. No attempt was made to reproduce muscular control of the hypopharynx with the inferior constrictor muscle; the pharyngeal mucosal sutures were buttressed by any readily available muscle tissue.

The authors reported that procedures (A) and (B) were associated with significantly greater numbers of patients who were able to achieve esophageal speech. In addition, the quality and proficiency of speech of the patients in Group A were judged to be better than those of patients who received procedures B, C, and D. The authors concluded that postlaryngectomy reconstruction that results in an active muscular pharyngeal wall and a controlled P-E segment allows the best results in terms of esophageal speech development.

Vrticka and Svoboda[57] and Robe et al[53] reported that the presence of the hyoid bone and intact strap muscles resulted in better esophageal speech in laryngectomy patients. This finding, however, was not supported by data presented by Diedrich and Youngstrom.[10] Duguay[58] has further hypothesized that an extensive radical neck dissection involving cranial nerves X, XII, and even the lingual branch of V, may impede oral sensations and tongue movements, and perhaps interfere with air injection in esophageal speech.

Damste[29] has noted that in cases of postcricoid carcinoma in which extensive amounts of the hypopharynx and a portion of the esophagus must be reconstructed, the ability to develop "esophageal" speech will be impaired. However, he observed "fair" voice when colon was inserted between pharynx and esophagus, and when the stomach was pulled up from under the diaphragm into the thoracic cavity. Conversely, when the hypopharynx was reconstructed with a deltopectoral flap, voice was either extremely poor or nonexistent. Duguay[58] presented an even gloomier picture, noting that he has seen only one patient with a resected esophagus develop serviceable esophageal voice. In this case, the patient's colon was used for the reconstruction. Shedd[59] observed that while Bakmajian's deltopectoral flap simplified reconstruction of the hypopharynx, as compared with the earlier Wookey method, patients undergoing complete resection of the pharynx and larynx continue to be extremely poor candidates to develop esophageal speech. Vise[60] reported a 90 per cent failure to develop esophageal speech in pharyngolaryngectomy patients. Again, this difficulty was attributed to the loss of a portion of the esophagus and the cricopharyngeus muscle.

Our clinical experience supports the observation of poor prognosis for esophageal speech in pharyngolaryngectomy patients. When sound has been produced, it has generally been weak and of poor quality. An additional concern is the long time period often required for healing to take place, a course that may be tortuous both medically and psychologically. Our emphasis has been to restore communication in these patients as quickly as possible, usually with an appropriate electronic instrument. Potential for developing esophageal speech can be explored when recuperation is complete.

Strictures, Pouches, and Fistulae

Strictures. It appears to be generally accepted that conditions causing constriction of the P-E segment, such as cicatrix or esophageal stenosis, may interfere with esophageal speech development.[10] Based on radiologic evidence, Simpson et al[50] reported three further types of postlaryngectomy constrictions that were associated with poor esophageal voice:

Type A. Described as a *permanent organic stricture* located just below the P-E juncture, this narrowed area was not observed to distend even during swallow. The authors suggested it might be related to the extent of mucosa excised, or to the degree of fibrosis.

Type B. Referred to as *pseudostrictures*, these constrictions were caused by a consistent bulging of the posterior pharyngeal wall into the hypopharynx, perhaps due to the posterior retraction of unsutured bundles of inferior constrictor muscle fibers.

Type C. In a small number of patients, x-ray data were normal at rest, and during air injection and swallow. However, during phonation the hyoid appeared to be displaced posteriorly, causing a second area of constriction. Simpson referred to these strictures as *voluntary contractions.*

In contrast to these radiologic findings in poor esophageal speakers, proficient speakers generally demonstrated a smooth, cone-shaped hypopharynx with narrowing present on voicing only at the P-E segment.

Pouches. The significance of hypopharyngeal "pouches" for esophageal speech development is not clear. Kirchner et al[27] reported that pouches located on the anterior wall of the pharynx, at its junction with the base of the tongue, were not factors in esophageal speech acquisition (pouches varied in volume from 1 to 30 cc).

In contrast to these findings, pouches of the anterior pharyngeal wall that occurred at the hyoid level just below the base of the tongue, and lower pouches, between the P-E segment and the hyoid, were found by Simpson et al[50] to occur more often in patients judged as poor esophageal speakers than in patients judged as proficient speakers. Damste[29] has further suggested that pouches in the area of the P-E segment that contain secretions from a fistula may interfere with the quality of esophageal speech.

Fistulae. The presence of fistulae in a postlaryngectomy patient is generally regarded as an indication for delaying esophageal speech therapy.[12] In fact, therapy does not typically begin until the surgeon has decided that sufficient wound-healing has taken place. The rigors of esophageal sound production, particularly in the early stages of therapy, may cause a fistula, or aggravate an existing one. Richardson,[56] however, has suggested that nonclosing fistulae in themselves do not appear to prevent esophageal speech.

An additional way in which fistulae may interfere with esophageal speech was reported by Damste.[48] This author described a pouch, or diverticulum, in the anterior wall of the P-E segment that could be traced to a fistula, that is, to the site of a suture breakdown. This sac contained secretions, which caused the speaker's voice to sound "wet and gurgling." In some cases, according to Damste, effects of such fistulae are not lasting, while in others a permanent pouch may result that significantly alters the morphology of the hypopharynx and interferes with the quality of esophageal speech.

Radiation Effects

Though our intuition and clinical experience suggest that radiation can influence esophageal speech development, supportive evidence for this view in the literature is not extensive. Several early studies suggested that radiation did not appear to be a factor in acquiring esophageal speech.[6, 10, 53] Similarly, Richardson[56] has reported that there appears to be no correlation between presurgical radiation, postsurgical radiation, or no radiation, and development of alaryngeal speech.

However, Masters et al[61] have described physiologic changes in the esophagus subsequent to radiation therapy that they believe may significantly interfere with the ability of postlaryngectomy patients to achieve esophageal speech. Gates and coworkers[2,3] reported that a considerably smaller percentage (33 per cent) of their esophageal speakers had received postoperative radiation, as compared with 66 per cent of patients using some other form of alaryngeal speech. Certainly clinical experience suggests that the effects of postoperative radiotherapy may include, at least temporarily, swelling and fibrosis, as well as mucositis and subsequent dryness, which interfere with both swallowing and speech. Other problems related to radiotherapy, such as breakdown of wounds, retarded healing, and fistula formation, may also be significant obstacles to acquiring esophageal speech.[62]

Hearing Loss

In contrast to the scant data regarding the prognostic implications of radiotherapy, there is considerable evidence to suggest that loss of hearing acuity and/or auditory discrimination ability may significantly interfere with esophageal speech acquisition.[10, 15, 19, 63–66] Diminished auditory acuity may interfere with a patient's ability to receive adequate instruction, or to monitor and differentiate various acoustic features of esophageal speech production.

In an extensive study of 90 per cent esophageal speakers, Kahane and Irwin[15] investigated the variables of auditory sensitivity for high frequencies and speech frequencies, ratings of stoma noise and speech proficiency, and time spent in therapy. The authors reported high positive correlations between high-frequency hearing loss, presence of stoma noise, and poorer speech proficiency ratings. Kahane and Irwin recommended hearing assessment in all postlaryngectomy patients. This suggestion is particularly appropriate in view of evidence that hearing loss may be a sequel to various head/neck carcinomas and their treatment regimens.[67]

Other Medical Problems

Hernia, Gastroesophageal Reflux, Esophagitis. Wolf et al[68] reported that hiatal hernia and/or gastroesophageal reflux with varying degrees of esophagitis were implicated in several cases of poor or failed esophageal speech development. These findings, which appear to be supported by the cinefluoroscopic data of Doubravsky and Prasil,[69] caused Wolf to recommend that alternatives to esophageal speech be found for postlaryngectomy patients with hiatal hernias that might be aggravated by attempts to learn this method of alaryngeal voice.

Pulmonary Factors. The presence of pulmonary disease has often been mentioned as an adverse factor in the development of esophageal speech,[17, 62] although there appears to be little statistical evidence available to support this contention. Greene[19] also reported that clavicular breathing, involving excessive tension of the strap muscles, may significantly interfere with esophageal speech development.

Samuel and Adams[70] have described the importance of coordinated esophageal and diphragmatic movements to quality of esophageal speech. From videocinefluoroscopic recordings, these authors observed the following sequence of events during air injection and phonation in esophageal speakers: (1) relaxation of the neoglottis occurring just as the diaphragm begins its descent; (2) sudden dilation of the esophagus as the diaphragm nears the end of its descent; (3) almost complete dilation of the esophagus (except for a variable lower section of the hiatus) coinciding with the point of maximum diaphragmatic descent; and (4) neoglottic closure in preparation for voicing with the beginning of diaphragmatic ascent.

According to Samuel and Adams, in good speakers only the lowermost portion of the esophagus collapses during voicing, while the remainder increases slightly in diameter. This process repeatedly continues in the manner of an inflated balloon being squeezed at the end away from its orifice, until phonation ceases. If neoglottic opening is premature or delayed, and the esophagus fails to dilate, the voice will be very quiet, or effortful, and of poor quality.

In our clinic, experience indicates that patients for whom "rest" breathing is noisy and effortful are not likely to be good candidates to develop esophageal speech. Even those patients with less severe pulmonary difficulty may be unable to avoid excessive stoma noise during speech attempts.

Special Medical/Surgical Problems in Voice Achieved with Electronic or Pneumatic Instruments

A second alternative for the alaryngeal speaker is an "artificial larynx." In the case of an electronic instrument (electrolarynx), sound is produced electronically and then transmitted through the tissues of the skin or directly into the oral cavity. Introduction of sound into the vocal tract, and the excitation of this column of air, permits the speaker to

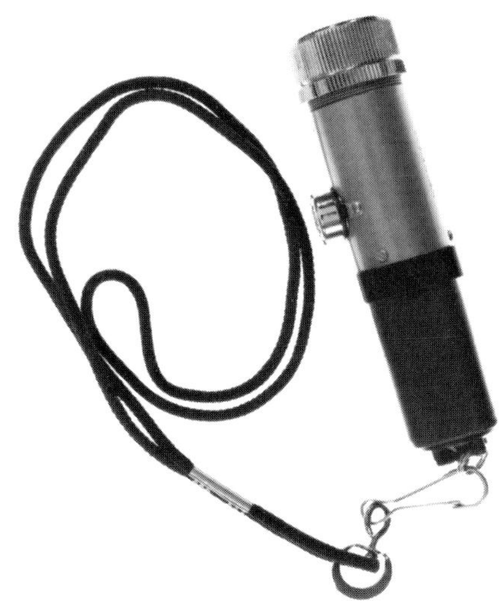

Figure 17–2. Throat-type electrolarynx (Aurex "Neovox").

articulate the voiced sounds of speech. There are two major types of electronic instruments, throat (Fig. 17–2) and intraoral (Fig. 17–3). With a throat- or neck-type device, the electrolarynx is placed on the side of the neck (or cheek) and sound is transmitted through transcervical tissues of the body into the airway. An intraoral device transmits sound directly from the electronic source into the oral cavity through a plastic tube that the speaker holds in his mouth. In other cases, the electronic sound source may be encased in a dental prosthesis and affixed inside the oral cavity.[71] Recently, electronic sound sources that can be implanted have been described.[72, 73] These latter devices are still in the developmental stages; problems of tissue rejection and infection, migration of the implant, and instrument malfunction while implanted must be resolved if these devices are to become viable alternatives for the alaryngeal speaker.

Throat and intraoral type electrolarynges, on the other hand, may rank second to esophageal speech in terms of most frequently used form of alaryngeal voicing. Putney[55] and McComb and Fletcher[74] have estimated that approximately 20 per cent of alaryngeal speakers use an electrolarynx as their primary means of communication. These instruments have the advantage of being easier to learn and more quickly mastered than esophageal speech, and may be an especially appropriate means of communication in the immediate postlaryngectomy period. In addition, even the most inexpensive model has good volume and is likely to be serviceable in most speaking situations. Electrolarynges may represent the method of choice for patients who are very elderly or in poor health, or who for other reasons are not good candidates for other alaryngeal alternatives.

Criticism of electrolarynges is usually related to the quality of speech they enable. In general, electronic instruments produce voicing that is very limited in terms of frequency and intensity variability, with resulting monopitch and monoloudness features that some speakers, and listeners, may find unsatisfactory. Another frequent objection (one typically rendered by professionals involved in a patient's rehabilitation, if not the patient himself) is that use of an electrolarynx will interfere with a patient's motivation to learn esophageal speech, which is viewed by some as a more "desirable" alternative. However, the data of Gates et al[2] do not support this observation; indeed, these authors reported that previous instrument use was not a factor in whether a patient developed esophageal speech.

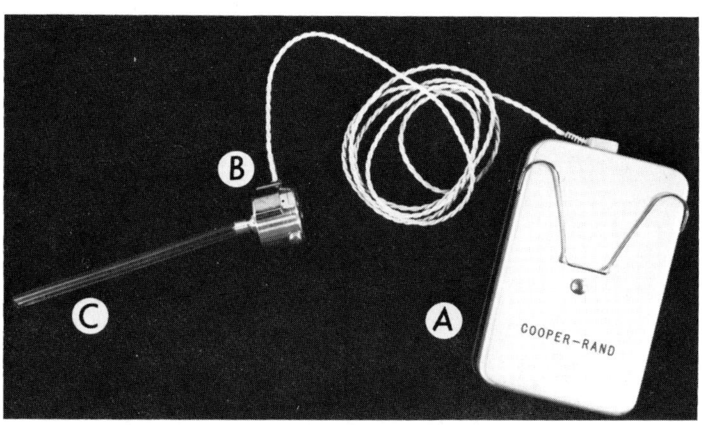

Figure 17–3. Intraoral-type electrolarynx (Cooper-Rand). *A,* Battery case and pulse generator. *B,* Tone generator. *C,* Mouth tube.

Pneumatic instruments (Fig. 17–4) are similar to electrolarynges in that the sound source is external. In this case, however, power to set the source into vibration is supplied by the patient's pulmonary air. Though there are several types of pneumatic instruments available, each with its own variations, in general they function in the following way. When preparing to speak, the speaker places the small rubber or steel cup over his stoma. As he exhales, air is directed into the cup and through a small pipe leading to a chamber over which a rubber membrane has been stretched. When air passes over this diaphragm, it vibrates and produces sound. This sound is then transmitted through a plastic tube from the vibration chamber into the speaker's mouth. (See the article by Weinberg and Riekena[75] for a description of speech with the Tokyo artificial larynx.)

Perhaps the primary advantage of the pneumatic instrument, as compared with an electrolarynx, is that speech may be much more natural. With the inclusion of the speaker's own pulmonary supply into the speech production process, quality, phrasing, and pitch and loudness variation may all be improved. However, compared with electrolarynges, pneumatic instruments may be more cumbersome to use, and require more time and effort in order to achieve a high level of proficiency. (The reader is referred to Salmon and Goldstein[76] for an excellent detailed description and analysis—with accompanying tape recordings—of most currently available electronic and pneumatic instruments.)

Medical/surgical problems that may interfere with a laryngectomy speaker's ability to use an electronic or pneumatic instrument include the following:

*1. **Condition of Superficial Tissues.*** In patients with large, thick necks, neck-type electrolarynges may not be appropriate unless a more powerful (and usually more expensive) model is available. Similarly, the presence of necrosed or scarred tissues, pain, or a wound site may preclude the use of neck-type devices, or require placement on the patient's cheek. In such cases, an intraoral type electolarynx, or a pneumatic instrument, may be more successful.

*2. **Fistulae.*** A neck-type electrolarynx may not be appropriate in a patient with a postoperative fistula that might be aggravated by the vibration of neck tissues. Again, an intraoral or pneumatic instrument that bypasses the neck may be indicated.

*3. **Radiation Effects.*** Richardson[56] has suggested that radiation, received either pre- or postoperatively, appears not to be a factor in patients' ability to achieve speech with an electrolarynx. However, in our own clinical experience, swelling and fibrosis caused by radiation has sometimes made it necessary to use a more powerful throat-type electrolarynx, or an intraoral device, on either a temporary or permanent basis.

*4. **Type and Extent of Surgery.*** Richardson's data[56] offer some insight into this variable. She investigated laryngectomy patients who were using a variety of alaryngeal speech alternatives, including esophageal speech, electrolarynges, and handwriting. In one instance, the author considered the number of speakers using each alternative according to how extensive their surgeries had been. Of interest is her finding that, while only 26 per cent of speakers who had received a total laryngectomy alone were using electrolarynges, 50 per cent of all speakers who had undergone a laryngectomy in addition to other, multiple surgeries (such as pharyngectomy) were using electrolarynges.

The report of an increase in the number of electrolarynx users with increasing severity of surgery, or multiple surgeries, would appear to provide support for the clinical observation that an electrolarynx makes fewer demands on a patient, at least in terms of physiologic

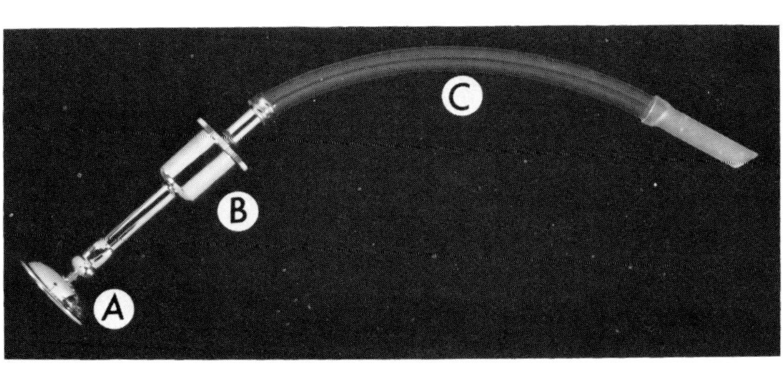

Figure 17–4. Pneumatic instrument (Tokyo artificial larynx). *A,* Stoma cover. *B,* Housing for rubber membrane sound source. *C,* Tube held in mouth.

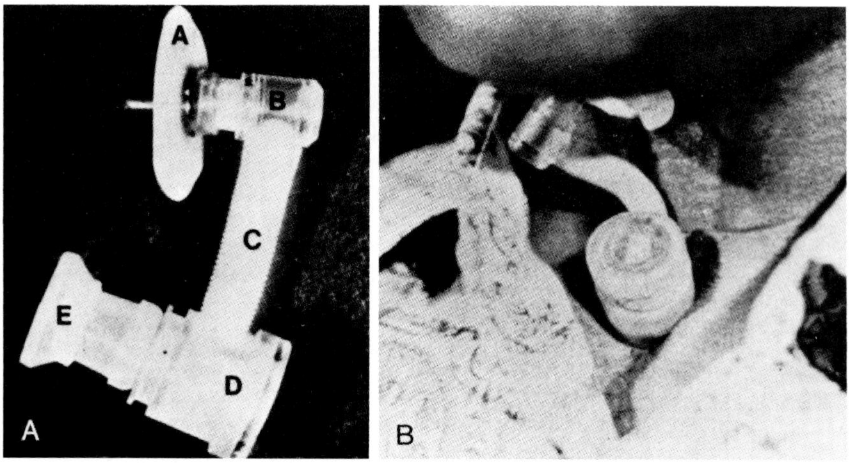

Figure 17–5. *A,* Northwestern voice prosthesis. *A,* Fistula fitting. *B,* Saliva valve. *C,* Conduit. *D,* Respiratory valve. *E,* Tracheostoma fitting. (Reprinted with permission from McConnel FMS, Sisson GA, Logemann JA: Three years' experience with a hypopharyngeal pseudoglottis for vocal rehabilitation after total laryngectomy. Trans Am Acad Ophthalmol Otolaryngol 84:64, 1977. *B,* Northwestern voice prosthesis in position. (Reprinted with permission from Keith RL, Darley FL (eds): Laryngectomee Rehabilitation. San Diego, College Hill Press, 1979).

integrity, than does esophageal speech, and thus may be a method of choice for patients who have undergone more extensive surgery. The same observation cannot be made for pneumatic instruments, since these alternatives generally require greater effort in terms of learning and use.

5. Hearing Loss. Berry[77] reported that significant hearing impairment is a serious obstacle for electronic instrument users. He suggested that the vibration of throat-type electrolarynges, in particular, may prevent the patient from adequately monitoring auditory feedback of his own speech. In addition, placement of throat-type devices on the cheek can impede auditory feedback of speech by conducting extraneous sound via bones of the face and skull directly into the cochlea.

Special Problems in Surgical-Prosthetic Reconstructions

The concept of a combined surgical-prosthetic approach to voice restoration is not new. In fact, very early laryngectomy procedures typically left a pharyngeal opening to accommodate the introduction of sound into the hypopharynx.[59] In this section, some of the major problems of recent surgical prosthetic approaches will be reviewed. In general, these strategies can be conceptualized as bypass procedures that direct air either externally or internally into the esophagus or pharynx.

External Bypass Procedures

Tracheopharyngeal Approaches. Sisson et al,[78] and Malone and Komorn[79] have described a voice prosthesis, referred to as the Northwestern prosthesis, that shunts air from the trachea into the hypopharynx through a fistula created in the lateral neck. This device, shown in Fig.17–5, includes a variable pressure-sensitive respiratory valve that automatically closes when pulmonary pressures increase prior to speech. With this valve closed, air is directed through the prosthesis conduit to a one-way saliva valve in the pharyngeal opening. This valve is intended to open only in response to respiratory air pressures and thus should not permit leakage back into the trachea.

Edwards[80] demonstrated a procedure in which a posterior tongue flap is elevated and then drawn through the former site of the hyoid corpus and tubed along its lower third. The end of the tube is sewn to the edge of an incision in the neck. A prosthesis, pictured in Figure 17–6, then serves to direct pulmonary air into the hypopharynx. The prosthesis is typically held in place in the trachea by a self-retaining flange. The pharyngeal end of the prosthesis is valved to prevent leakage.

Neither the Sisson nor Edwards prostheses include a vibratory mechanism; rather, they are simply shunts that direct pulmonary air into the pharynx. Exactly what vibrates in response to pulmonary air, thus providing a voicing "source," is open to some speculation. Fluoroscopic studies by Logemann (re-

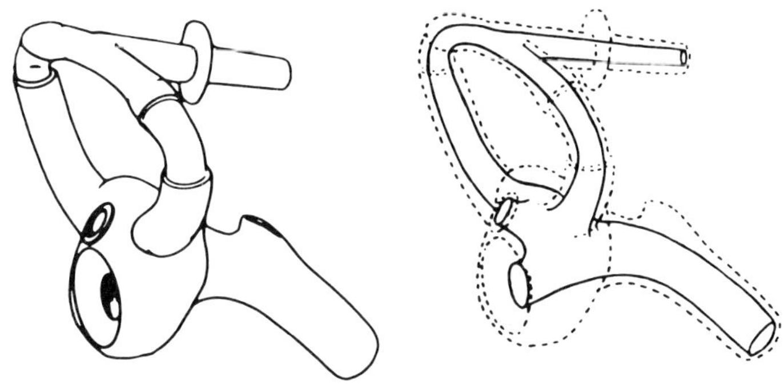

Figure 17–6. Edwards' voice prosthesis. (Reprinted with permission from Edwards N: Postlaryngectomy vocal rehabilitation using expired air and an external fistula method. Laryngoscope 85:694, 1975.)

ported in McConnel et al[81]) of patients using the Sisson device indicate that the base of the tongue, the pharyngeal walls, or the fistula itself may serve this purpose. Edwards has suggested that the fistula tract formed by the tubed tongue flap constitutes the vibratory source in this procedure.

The vibratory source is more specifically accounted for in a further surgical-prosthetic approach described by Shedd et al[82] and Weinberg et al[83] for use in patients who have had laryngectomy-pharyngectomies. These patients typically undergo deltopectoral flap reconstructions and are left with a hypopharyngeal fistula at the jaw-neck angle that can be used to accommodate a "reed-fistula" prosthesis (Fig. 17–7).

In this procedure, both an external air bypass and a "pseudolarynx" are incorporated in the prosthetic appliance. Pulmonary air directed from the tracheal stoma passes over a taut rubber or Silastic reed that is housed in the central, horizontal portion of the "H"-shaped prosthesis. When set into vibration, the reed produces sound that is then conducted into the pharynx. (See the article by Weinberg et al[83] for a description and analysis of speech characteristics with reed-fistula prostheses.)

Perhaps the major difficulty of the external tracheopharyngeal prostheses is the salivary fistula, which, in spite of efforts to create a watertight, one-way valve, still permits leakage. Other reported problems include tracheal irritation, infection, and stenosis of the fistula. Problems related to voice production include achievement of a tight seal in the trachea. In addition, in the case of bypass techniques without a built-in vibrating source, placement of the pharyngeal stoma is critical; if it is too high, speech may be breathy or whispered. With the reed-fistula prosthesis, experimentation with the vibratory mechanism may be required to produce satisfactory "voice."

Tracheoesophageal Approaches. In 1972, Taub and Spiro[84] reported a combined surgical-prosthetic method of voice restoration in which a bypass from the trachea to the esophagus was created. In this procedure, a cervical esophagostomy is performed at a point previously determined to assure maximum phonatory vibration of the pharyngoesophageal segment, as well as to prevent diverted air from entering the stomach. The esophagus is exposed posteriorly and laterally and a rectangular skin flap (including platysma) that parallels the anterior border of the sternocleidomastoid muscle is elevated. The sternal head of this muscle may be used to protect the great vessels if the carotid sheath is exposed during the procedure.

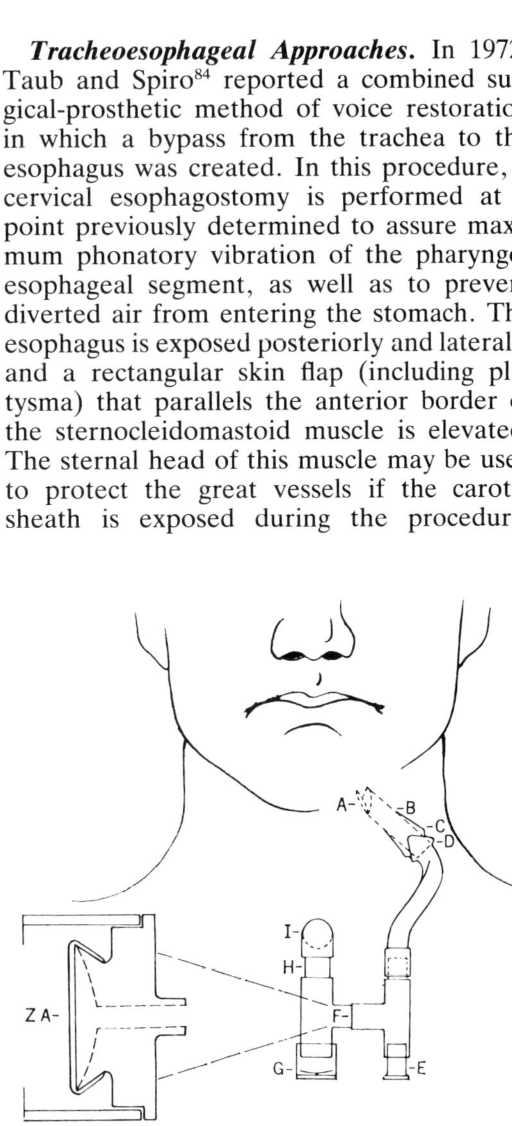

Figure 17–7. Reed-fistula appliance. *A,* Secretory valve. *B,* Fistula tube. *C,* Secretory collar. *D,* Fistula opening. *E,* Secretory collector. *F,* Voicing (reed) mechanism. *G,* Respiratory valve. *H,* Tracheal connector. *I,* Stomal opening. Insert *F* portrays voicing mechanism. Reed membrane. (Reprinted with permission from Weinberg B, Shedd DP, Horii V: Reed-fistula speech following pharyngolaryngectomy. J. Speech Hear Disord 43:402, 1978.)

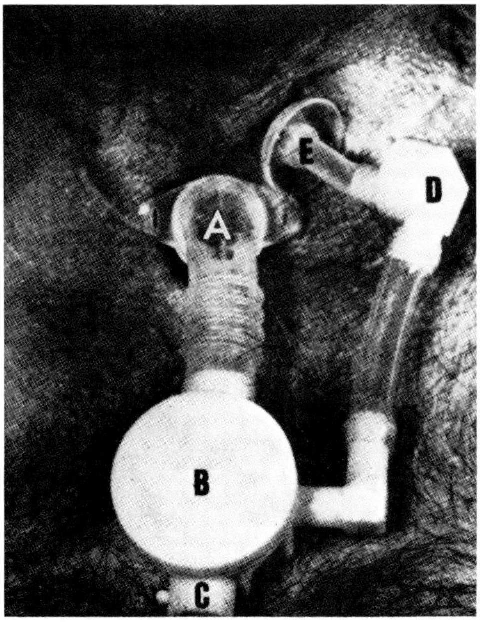

Figure 17–8. La Barge Voicebak prosthesis. *A,* Tracheal interconnector. *B,* Air-bypass flapper valve mechanism. *C,* Adjustable breathing port. *D,* One-way fistula valve. *E,* Flanged Silastic fistula tube with tension. (Courtesy of La Barge Inc, St. Louis, Missouri.)

(Note: if Eberle's recommended esophagostomy is utilized, Taub suggests this should not be necessary.[85]) The superiorly based flap is then raised from the lateral side of the original incision, tubed with the skin surface turned in, and directed retrograde to the esophageal incision. The end of the tube is anastomosed to the esophageal incision

The prosthesis, called Voicebak (Fig. 17–8), can then be interposed between the tracheostoma and the neck fistula. The prosthesis allows air to pass in and out of the trachea until a pressure increase consistent with speaking is detected. At that point, the breathing valve is closed and air passes through a side port into the neck fistula and on into the esophagus. Voice is produced when pulmonary air is driven across the P-E segment. (See the article by Blom[86] for a description of speech characteristics with Voicebak.) If the patient has undergone presurgical evaluation methods as recommended by Taub, the resulting phonatory characteristics should be optimal.

Medical/surgical complications that have been reported with Voicebak include fistula irritation and erosion, and even carotid artery rupture. Taub[87] reported that modifications in esophagostomy technique and fistula tubes have minimized both these possibilities. Additional problems include granulation tissue in the fistula and leakage problems. The procedure is only occasionally appropriate for patients who have been irradiated.

Internal Bypass Procedures

Based on their experience with the mucosal tracheoesophageal anastomosis described by Amatsu,[88] Singer and Blom[89] have recently developed a small silicone valve designed to maintain a communication between tracheal and esophageal lumens. The valve is accommodated surgically by a midline tracheoesophageal puncture through the back wall of the trachea into the anterior wall of the esophagus (see Chapter 4). As shown in Figure 17–9, the proximal end of the prosthetic valve is a narrow slit that permits airflow into the esophagus while minimizing reflux of liquids into the airway. The distal end includes an inferior opening positioned perpendicular to the airway. Flanges are used to retain the valve against the skin of the neck.

With the valve in place, the patient can speak by occluding the permanent tracheostoma. Exhaled air is then diverted into the inferior port of the valve and through the duckbill slit into the esophagus. Voice is produced when pulmonary air forced through the valve sets the P-E segment (and perhaps the tube itself, and/or surrounding tissues) into vibration. Thus, the result is esophageal speech powered by pulmonary air. Since the speaker can introduce a much greater volume

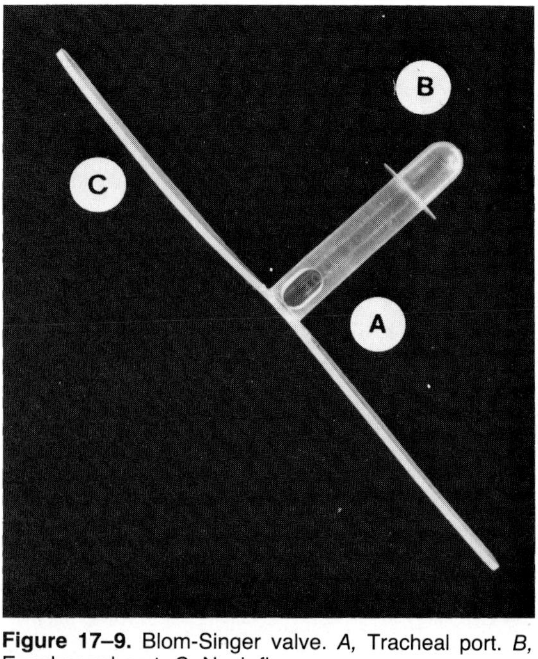

Figure 17–9. Blom-Singer valve. *A,* Tracheal port. *B,* Esophageal port. *C,* Neck flanges.

of air into the esophagus in this manner than is possible with the traditional esophageal method, in which the speaker must inject air into the esophagus, the ease and naturalness of speech are enhanced.

Problems with the valve in terms of voice production can be minimized with attention to the following: (1) establishment of viability of the P-E segment as a sound source prior to the procedure, by means of the insufflation test described by Taub,[90] and (2) rigorous case selection with respect to a number of anatomic and personal characteristics, as detailed in the article by Blom and Singer.[91] Medical/surgical problems associated with the technique appear minimal. The major liabilities observed include stenosis of the fistula if the valve is dislodged, as by poor fit of the tube, and vigorous coughing during sleep. In addition, slight leakage on swallowing liquids may occur, particularly if the valve becomes worn.

An additional surgical-prosthetic approach, similar to the Blom-Singer procedure, has been described by Panje.[92] Variations in both the design of the Panje prosthesis (Fig. 17–10) and placement of the tracheoesophageal puncture have minimized the problems with fitting and retention to the neck that have been associated with the Blom-Singer prosthesis. However, recent work by Weinberg[24] indicates that certain physical properties of the Panje button may make it more resistant to airflow, thus increasing the effort required by the speaker to produce voice.

Special Problems in Surgical Reconstruction

Subtotal Laryngectomies to Preserve Voice and Airway Function

Several authors have described procedures designed to restore both voice and respiratory functions using cartilaginous tissues remaining in subtotal laryngectomies. In general, these procedures are done at the time of laryngectomy and require elevation of the trachea, lowering of the hyoid, or both, to establish continuity between the trachea and hypopharynx. Labayle,[93] for example, preserves the hyoid along with the lower half of the cricoid ring, the cricoid plate, and one arytenoid to establish glossopharyngotracheal continuity and a so-called "neolarynx." A somewhat similar strategy by Mozolewski[94] incorporates the cricoid and one arytenoid in the reconstruction effort. A procedure by Piquet[95] requires preservation of the hyoid, the cricoid, one arytenoid, and, if possible, the epiglottis for restoration of the airway and voicing functions. Serafini has described one- and two-stage reconstructions in which the inferior posterior cricoid is preserved, as well as the extralaryngeal epiglottis.[96 97] The trachea is then elevated and sutured to the

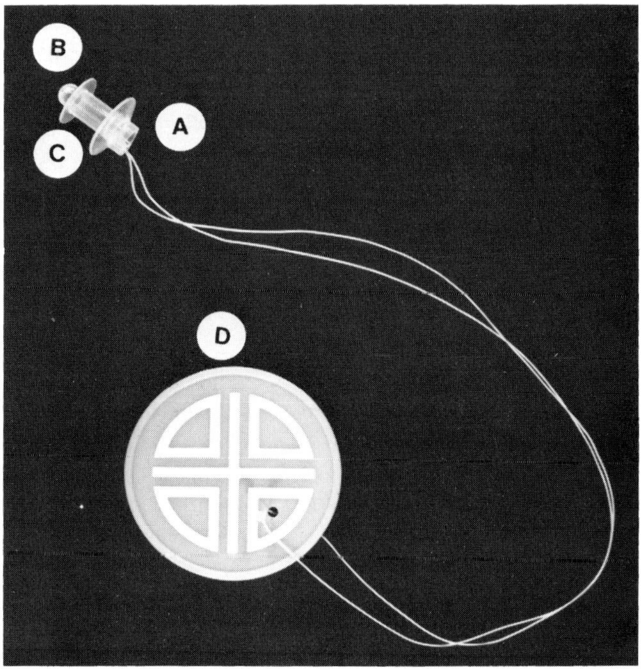

Figure 17–10. Panje voice prosthesis. *A,* Tracheal port. *B,* Esophageal port. *C,* Retention collars. *D,* Safety button.

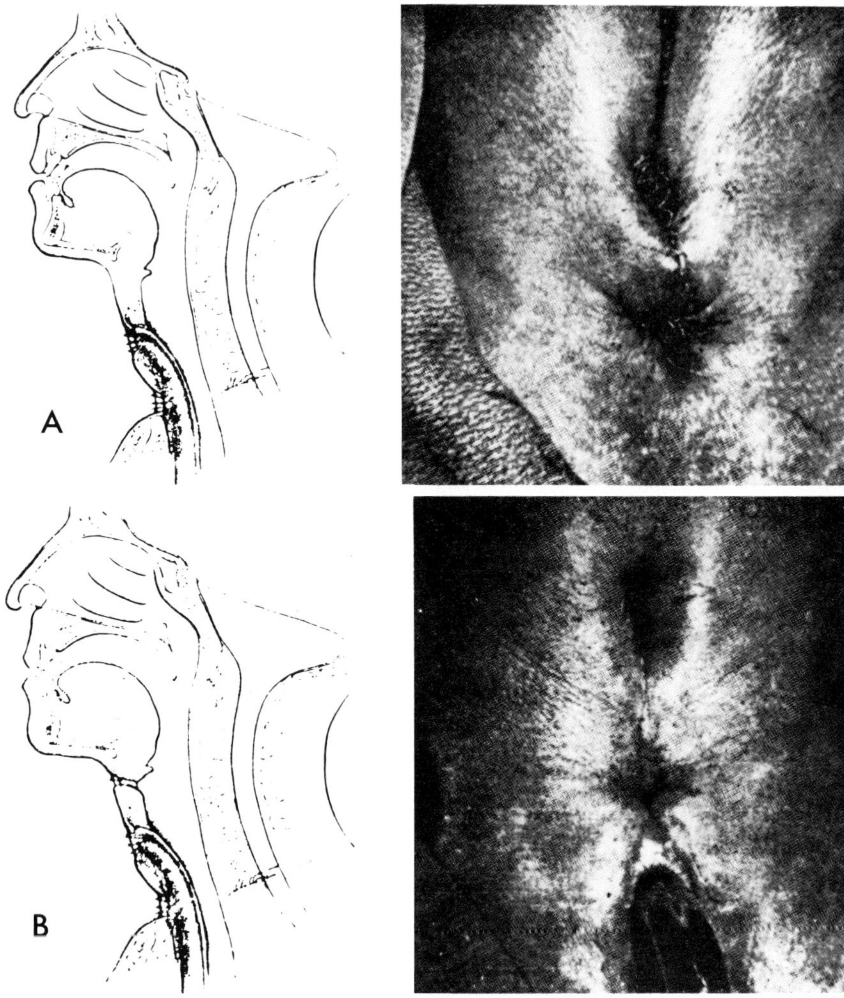

Figure 17–11. Asai procedure. *A,* End of first stage. *B,* End of second stage.

Illustration continued on opposite page

hyoid to establish tracheopharyngeal anastomosis. Vega and Siola subsequently demonstrated a modification of Serafini's procedure that allows greater excision of tissue, including the entire cricoid.[98, 99]

From the point of view of voice restoration, one of the concerns with the design of subtotal laryngectomies is that the voicing "source" is not defined and accounted for in the reconstruction. While all of the procedures appear to allow for tracheopharyngeal anastomosis and airflow into the hypopharynx, the structure or structures that actually vibrate in response to pulmonary air may not be specified. Therefore the capabilities of, and the requirements for, these structures to produce "quasiperiodic" sound, thus simulating the larynx, are unresolved. Clearly, voice *may* sometimes be produced by driving air through the hypopharynx and setting one or more structures into vibration. These may include the pharyngeal walls, the base of the tongue, or tissues involved in the reconstruction effort. However, there is an element of chance in having only a vague notion of what will become the actual vibratory source. As a result, neither success nor failure of the procedure to produce voice can be fully understood.

In contrast to these procedures are those surgical prosthetic methods previously described that incorporate the P-E segment into the reconstruction effort. Proponents of these techniques (Taub, Blom and Singer, Panje) stress the importance of placing the esophageal fistula just under the segment in a manner that maximizes and facilitates esophageal sound production. In addition, these authors emphasize the need to determine, on an "a priori" basis, the viability of the segment as a voicing source. From a theoretical view, and from a retrospective comparison of "success" of the various techniques, it would seem that those approaches that initially specify a sound source are to be preferred.

Perhaps a more general concern among surgeons is that such subtotal laryngectomies jeopardize the eradication of disease. Beyond this, major complications of subtotal procedures include problems with deglutition and aspiration. Other sequelae reported are prolapse of the neolarynx, stenosis of the neolarynx, and cartilage necrosis. In addition, the need for a permanent tracheostoma has apparently persisted in many cases.

Total Laryngectomies with Shunt Reconstruction to Preserve Voice

In contrast to subtotal laryngectomies, surgically created shunts following or accompanying total laryngectomy are intended only to restore voice—that is, no attempt is made to eliminate the need for a permanent tracheostoma or to restore airway functions. These procedures differ from shunts described in the surgical-prosthetic approaches section in that they require no prosthesis.

Tracheopharyngeal Anastomoses. Asai described a multi-stage surgery (Fig. 17–11) for shunting air from the trachea into the hypopharynx.[100, 101] At the end of a wide-field

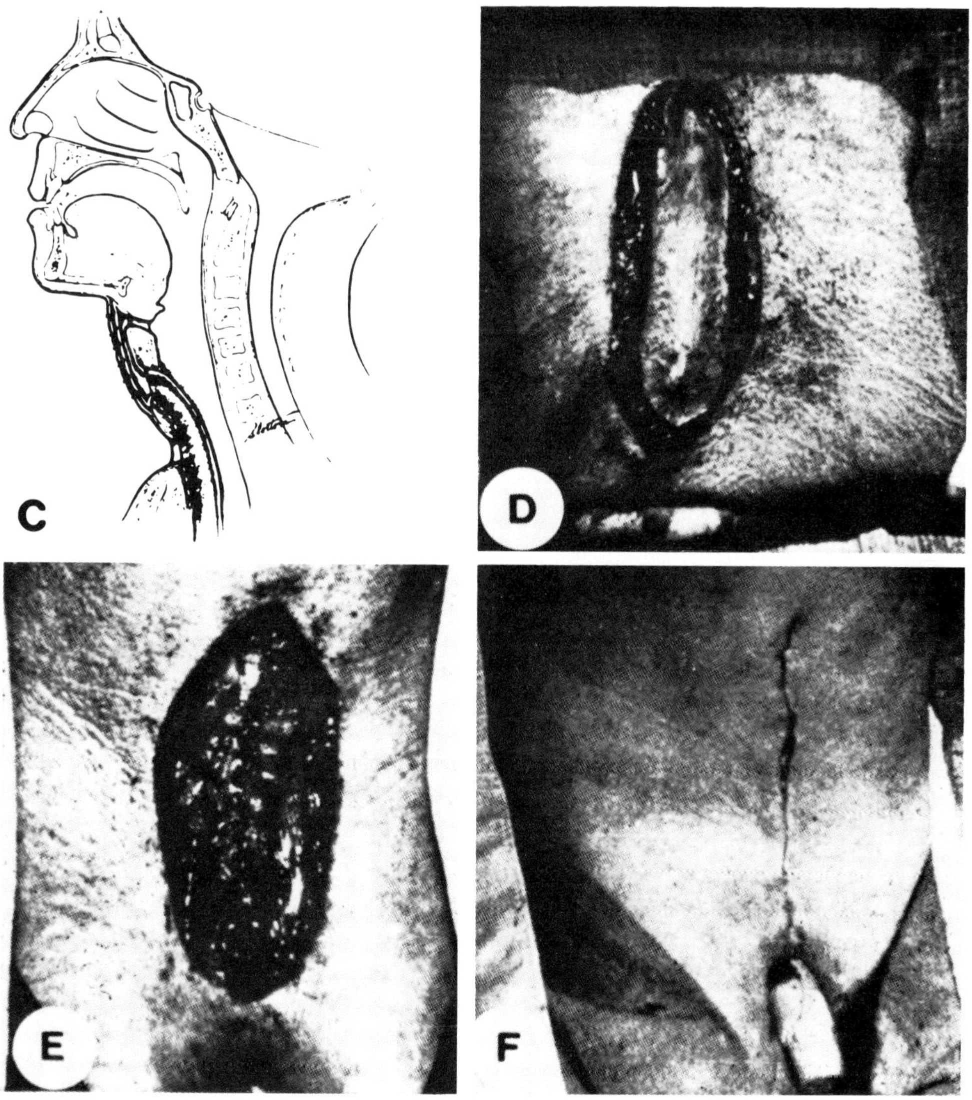

Figure 17–11 *Continued. C,* End of third stage. *D,* First step of third stage. *E,* Second step of third stage. *F,* Third step of third stage. (Reprinted with permission from Miller AH: First experiences with the Asai technique for vocal rehabilitation after total laryngectomy. Ann Otol Rhinol Laryngol 76:829, 1962.)

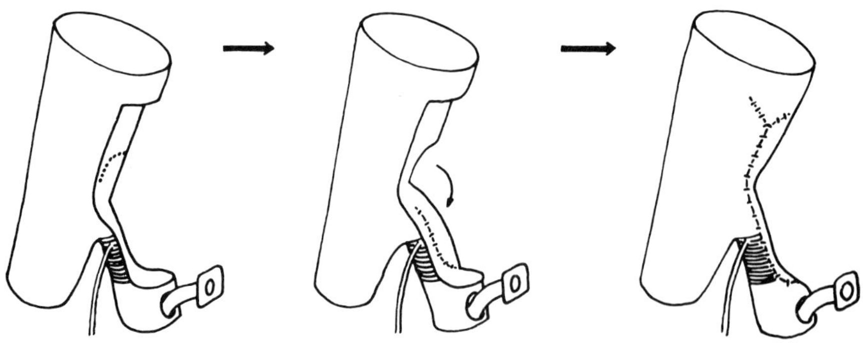

Figure 17–12. Concept of composite shunt. The endolaryngeal bridge between the trachea and pharynx, preserved by subtotal laryngectomy, is too narrow to tube into an adequate speaking shunt. Its width can be slightly increased by the addition of a pharyngeal flap. The speaking shunt is thus a composite of laryngeal and pharyngeal elements. (Reprinted with permission from Pearson BW: Subtotal laryngectomy. Laryngoscope 91:1904, 1981.)

laryngectomy, a tracheostoma is created above the larger, permanent stoma located at the fourth or fifth tracheal ring. In a second procedure, an additional fistula into the patient's hypopharynx is placed at the jaw-neck angle. Finally, a dermal tube is created from a flap of neck tissue. The upper end of the tube opens into the pharynx, the lower into the upper tracheal stoma. When the patient wants to speak, he occludes the permanent stoma and exhaled air is then diverted through the dermal tube into the hypopharynx. Typically, the speaker must also apply digital compression to the tube itself in order to produce sound.

An additional hypopharyngeal fistula procedure, similar in concept to Asai's but much different in terms of required surgery, has recently been described by Pearson.[102, 103] He suggests that, following a total laryngectomy, there is often uninvolved endolaryngeal tissue remaining that is generally sacrificed not to eliminate cancer but to separate airway from foodway. This myomucosal strip (Fig. 17–12), connecting the upper trachea to the pharynx, may include normal tracheal wall, a portion of the subglottis, and a small remnant of the true cord and its arytenoid, as well as false and aryepiglottic folds on the uninvolved side. These tissues are dissected away from the thyroid and cricoid cartilages (which are discarded) and formed into a soft tissue tube. Supplemented by a pharyngeal flap, this tube is connected to the cut ends of the trachea and hypopharynx (see Chapter 4). According to Pearson, the soft-walled tube will contract on swallowing and thereby prevent aspiration, because it contains endolaryngeal muscle innervated principally by the recurrent laryngeal nerve. Resistance to stenosis is afforded by the undisturbed mucosal pathway from trachea to pharynx. The patient may speak by occluding the permanent tracheostoma and diverting exhaled air through the flaccid phonatory shunt into the pharynx.

Staffieri has described a tracheohypopharyngeal shunt (Fig. 17–13) that results in a "phonatory neoglottis."[104–107] According to Staffieri, the neoglottis, which is best constructed at the time of total laryngectomy, is created by making a small vertical incision in the exterior muscle layer of the anterior cervical esophagus. Submucosa, connective mucosa, and internal epithelium are, in turn, pulled through the incision and sutured to pharyngeal wall muscle. The anterior hypopharyngeal wall is then sutured to the first or second tracheal ring in such a manner that the small slit is centered over the tracheal opening. The remaining anterior hypopharyngeal wall is sutured to the base of the tongue, and a permanent stoma is created at the third or fourth tracheal ring.

The exact nature of the vibratory source in hypopharyngeal shunts is not clear. Asai[100] and Kitamura et al[108] reported that in the Asai procedure, the dermal tube itself is the vibratory source, and suggested that the diameter and shape of the tube are critical variables with regard to the quality of voice produced. These observations are supported by the fact that the speaker must manually constrict the tube in order to produce voice. In the procedures described by Pearson and Staffieri, it would seem that the edges of the fistula, or perhaps other tissues in the pharynx, must serve as the vibratory source. The difficulty with Staffieri's procedure is that exceedingly high intrathoracic pressure may be required to produce phonation. As noted earlier, properties of the vibratory source should be understood if patients are to receive the fullest benefit from procedures undertaken for voice restoration. Such information is critical both to the design of these procedures and to the evaluation of their success or failure.

From a medical/surgical perspective, the chief difficulties reported for surgically-created hypopharyngeal shunts have included (1) aspiration; (2) problems with deglutition; (3) fistula; (4) stenosis and scarring of the tunnel with the Asai procedure; and (5) hair growth in the Asai dermal tube. The need for multiple surgeries in the Asai reconstruction is an additional concern. The Staffieri procedure may be done at a second stage, but this method is less successful. The need to preserve some tissue normally excised during total laryngectomy may render both the Pearson and Staffieri procedures inappropriate in some cases. All of these procedures may be restricted by the patient's history of irradiation.

Tracheoesophageal Anastomoses. In 1958, Conley[109] described a mucosal tunnel (later he used a vein graft), angling down from the trachea to the esophagus, that could be used to divert air into the esophagus. Animal

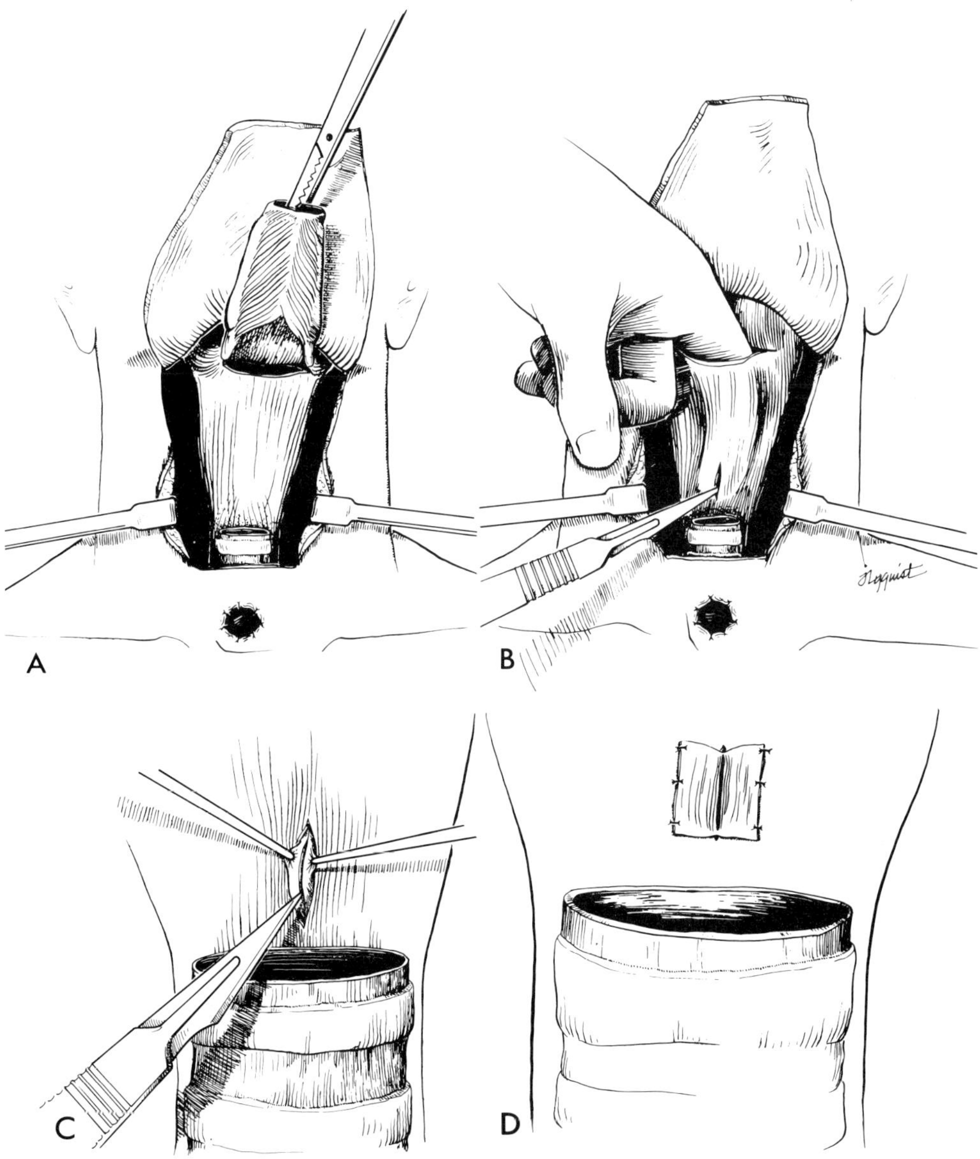

Figure 17–13. Staffieri procedure for neoglottic reconstruction. *A,* Detachment of larynx from esophagus. *B,* Manner of incision of muscular layer in forming the phonatory neoglottis. *C,* Incision of the submucosal layer. *D,* Completion of the suturing of mucosa.

Illustration continued on following page

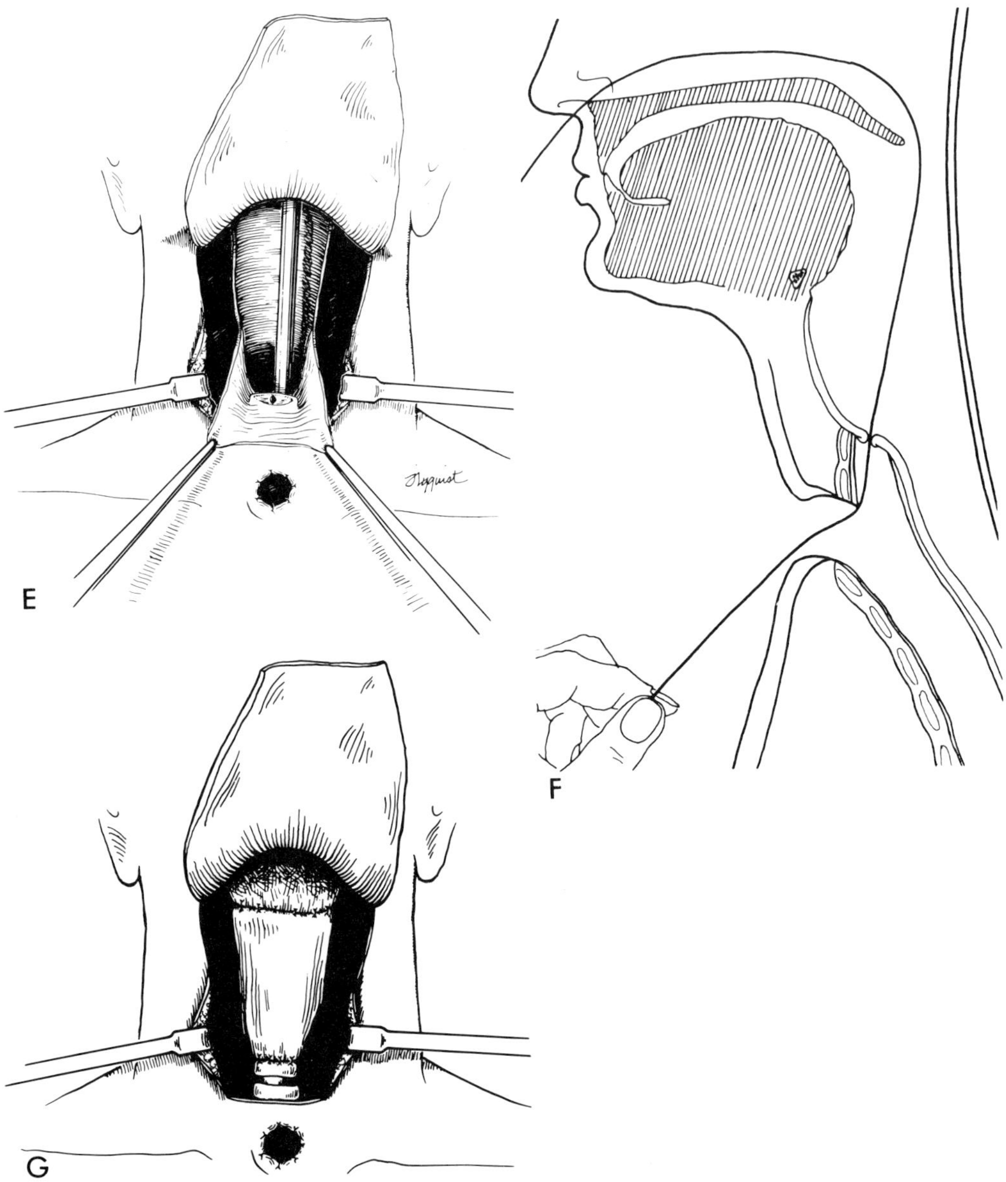

Figure 17–13 *Continued E,* Deflection of esophageal wall over the tracheal opening. *F,* A heavy thread passed through the neoglottis as a guide for dilatation or revision. *G,* Completion of closure of pharyngostomy. (Reprinted with permission from Shedd DP, Weinberg B: Surgical and Prosthetic Approaches to Speech Rehabilitation. Boston, GK Hall & Co, 1980.)

research by Calcaterra and Jafek[110] demonstrated that use of a full-thickness cervical esophageal wall tunnel could improve the tunnel technique. Subsequently, Komorn[111] described a tracheoesophageal shunt that can be constructed at or following total laryngectomy (Fig. 17–14). In this procedure, an inferiorly based full-thickness flap is raised from the anterior cervical esophagus. The posterior wall of the trachea is also incised and a mucosal tube is formed with one end in the trachea and the other in the esophagus. In a slight variation of T-E "tunnels," Amatsu[88] described an inferiorly based membranous tracheal flap used to create a side-to-side anastomosis between the incised margins of the tracheal flap and the esophagus.

With a completed tracheoesophageal shunt, the patient can produce voice by occluding the tracheostoma and diverting pulmonary air into the esophagus. Since the primary vibratory source is likely to be the P-E segment, it is critical that the shunt enter the esophagus below the cricopharyngeus

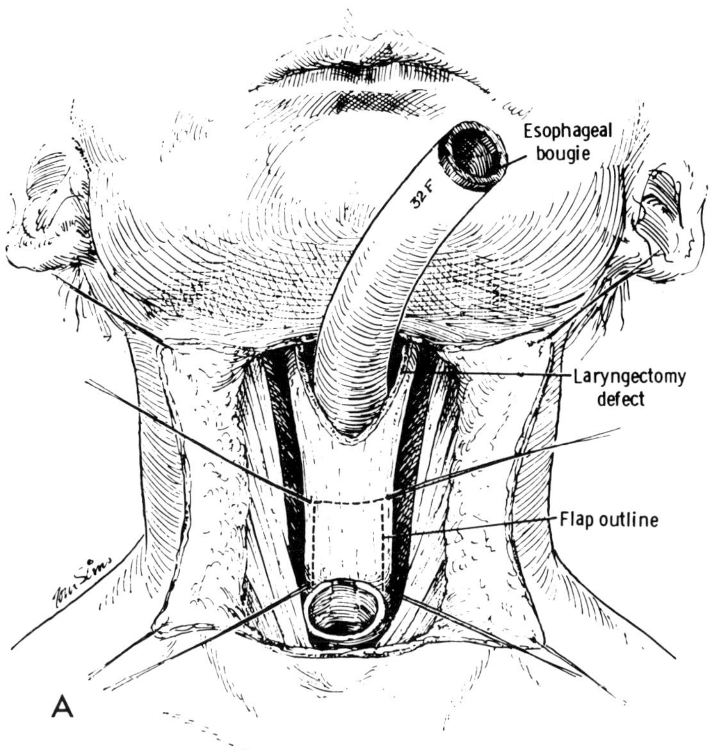

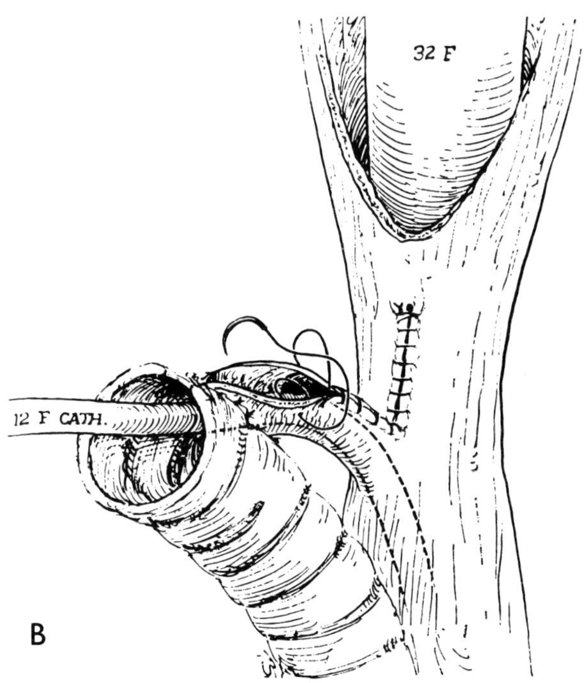

Figure 17–14. Komorn tracheoesophageal shunt. *A,* Methylene blue and silk stay sutures outlining a 2½ × 5 cm full-thickness inferiorly based flap. A bougie inserted through either the mouth or the hypopharyngeal defect present at the time of surgery stabilizes the esophagus. *B,* After the flap to the tracheal anastomosis is completed, a catheter is placed through the meatus into the esophagus and the flap tubed around this catheter. A continuous Connell suture is used to both close the esophageal defect and tube the flap. (Reprinted with permission from Komorn RM: Vocal rehabilitation in the laryngectomized patient with a tracheoesophageal shunt. Ann Otol Rhinol Laryngol 83:445, 1974.)

muscle. One of the strengths of T-E shunts, from the perspective of voice restoration, is that there is at least one vibratory source, the P-E segment, specified and incorporated in their design. (There may be additional sources—such as the shunt itself, which vibrates to produce sound—although this has not yet been adequately determined.) Since the vibratory source is specified, evaluation of patients as candidates on an a priori basis is enhanced. For example, the viability of a patient's P-E segment as a voicing source can be ascertained by insufflating the esophagus in accordance with the air-blowing test described by Taub (1980). Similarly, the patient can preview the quality and nature of sound produced prior to undergoing the procedure.

Major and persistent medical/surgical problems reported for surgically created T-E shunts include stenosis and scarring of the tunnel, aspiration, and fistula. In addition, many patients have complained of discomfort arising from air entering the stomach following the T-E shunt procedures.

In concluding this review of alternatives for the alaryngeal speaker, a word of caution is urged. The regular appearance of new, often promising techniques for voice restoration has certainly brightened the rehabilitative outlook for laryngectomy patients. However, it should be noted that literature reports of these procedures may showcase successes and minimize failures. That is, success may not be an assured, or even a usual, result. In fact, failures associated with new techniques have often provided the stimulus for further innovation and inquiry and, subsequently, other new procedures. Each of the alternatives described here has definite indications that limit its applicability. As noted earlier, the selection of an appropriate alternative for the alaryngeal speaker is more complicated than the simple expression of a preference by the patient or by the professionals involved.

REHABILITATION PROBLEMS IN PATIENTS WITH UPPER VOCAL TRACT (TRANSFER FUNCTION) DEFICITS

Effects of Orofacial Surgery on Speech

Speakers with the larynx (voicing source) intact, but with anomalies of the upper vocal tract, may experience two types of alteration. Articulation problems may result if the speaker's ability to appropriately constrict and occlude the vocal tract is impaired. That is, the speaker may be unable to effect normal resonance changes of the vocal tract, or to generate noise sources required for some consonant sounds, or to manipulate airflows and air pressures in accordance with normal speech requirements. In addition, changes in the overall size and shape of the vocal tract may alter those properties of speech that allow listeners to identify the speaker, to differentiate him or her from every other speaker, and to make accurate judgments about the speaker's age, sex, and other personal characteristics.

The more serious problem, from the standpoint of communication, is that of articulation skill and resulting intelligibility. Certainly the thrust of restorative therapy with these patients is articulation skill that affords intelligible speech. But it should be remembered that our voice and speech characteristics are unique, and reflect our individuality as much as facial and bodily characteristics do. The patient who undergoes surgical excision of highly visible structures experiences orofacial deformity in a society where facial appearance is highly prized. (See the article by Gillis[112] for an excellent discussion of psychologic factors in patients with orofacial deformities.) Voice and appearance constitute important components of our identity. Both may be altered, sometimes radically, by orofacial cancer and its treatment. Strategies for improving communication skills in such patients must be individualized to reflect the treatment of the speaker and should attempt to permit the patient a unique speaking "identity" that is acceptable to him.

This section will attempt to review some specific surgical obstacles to speech in patients with upper airway deficits. In contrast to the extensive literature in alaryngeal speech, there has been little experimental inquiry into the nature of speech in patients with acquired orofacial anomalies. For our purposes, general categories of surgical procedures will be considered in terms of their effects on speech. No attempt will be made to relate speech characteristics to specific types of surgeries within a general category, other than as allowed by clinical observation. It is also recognized that eradication of cancer often requires crossing anatomic boundaries, and perhaps seldom permits a singular procedure. It would be unwise to speculate that for a particular surgery, the greater the amount of excision and required reconstruction, the greater the likelihood for speech impairment. Similarly, it cannot be assumed that crossing anatomic boundaries will produce greater effects than if only one structure is a surgical focus. Rather, severity of speech impairment is dependent on the specific structure or structures involved and, further, on the particular portion of the structure affected.

Specific Surgical Obstacles to Speech

Glossectomy

The tongue plays a role in producing all the sounds of speech except */w, h, p, b* and *m/*. It is considered the major, premier articulatory structure of the vocal tract. The muscular complexity of the tongue is such that, during speech, the anterior and posterior portions of it appear to act almost independently. When some or all of the tongue is removed, a speaker may learn compensatory movements in an attempt to minimize the loss of function. (See References 113 to 116 for discussions of articulation errors and articulatory compensations in glossectomy speech.) In fact, partial glossectomy patients with extensive amounts of missing tissue may retain a high degree of intelligible speech.[113, 117] A remarkable capacity for compensation notwithstanding, an inability to constrict or occlude the vocal tract with the tongue can cause serious problems for a glossectomy speaker.

Presented in Figure 17–15 are formant values, measured from spectrograms as normal speakers and two glossectomy speakers produced vowel sounds. It will be recalled from earlier in this chapter that formants correspond to the natural resonance locations of the vocal tract. The concentrations of sound energy at these frequency locations are powerful perceptual cues; that is, listeners rely on this information to make judgments about what sounds they are hearing. If the glossectomy speakers' first and second formant values (F1 and F2) are compared with those of the normal speakers, it is apparent that F1 locations for the normal speakers are quite similar to those of the total glossectomy speaker. This is not surprising, since F1 is generally thought to be more related to constriction at the lips and mouth opening than it is to tongue dynamics.

Of interest in Figure 17–15 is the observation that F1 values of the partial glossectomy speaker are relatively more disparate from

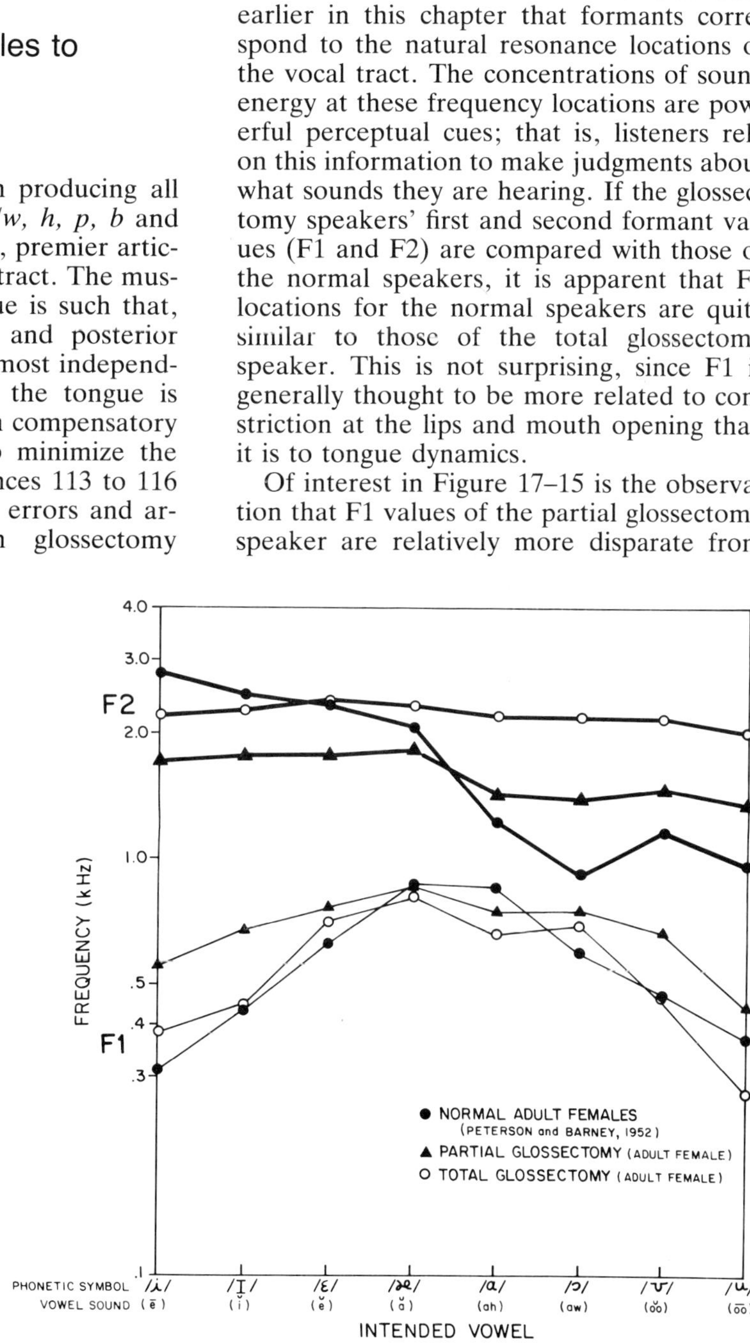

Figure 17–15. Comparison of vowel formant characteristics for normal adult females, an adult female with partial glossectomy, and an adult female with total glossectomy.

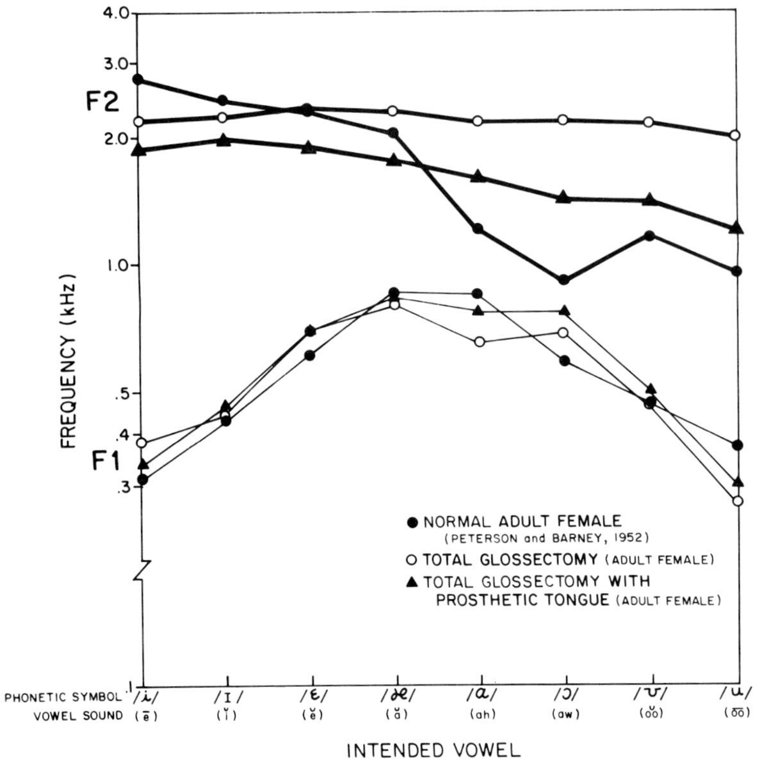

Figure 17–16. Comparison of vowel formant characteristics for normal adult females, an adult female with total glossectomy, and the same adult female using a prosthetic tongue.

normal than are F1 values of the total glossectomy speaker. This finding reflects impaired anterior tongue mobility with an accompanying restriction of mandibular movement experienced by the partial glossectomy speaker. The fact that mandibular mobility is unimpaired in the total glossectomy speaker accounts for F1 values that more closely approximate normal than do the values of the partial glossectomy speaker.

In contrast to the F1 data, F2 values are markedly altered by both glossectomy procedures. Most notably, the differentiation of F2 across vowels, encompassing a range of over 1800 Hz for the normal speaker, is seriously diminished in the glossectomy speakers. For the patient with total glossectomy, the F2 curve approximates a straight line. This tendency toward compression of the F2 range, and resulting neutralization of vowel acoustics, is also apparent in data obtained for the partial glossectomy patient. The unique location of F2 is a major cue to the accurate perception of vowels; obviously, if it is undifferentiated across vowels, listeners are likely to have difficulty discriminating these sounds. In fact, data indicate that vowels spoken by this partial glossectomy patient were perceived correctly 55 per cent of the time, while vowels spoken by the patient with total glossectomy were perceived correctly on only 48 per cent of trials.

In Figure 17–16, formant data for the total glossectomy patient and normal adult female speakers are again displayed, along with formant values obtained for the total glossectomy patient while wearing a prosthetic tongue. The prosthesis was designed to improve speech (and swallowing) in this patient.[118, 119] The data shown in Figure 17–16 demonstrate that the prosthesis did, in fact, improve differentiation of F2 across vowels. These acoustic findings were supported by perceptual data indicating improved intelligibility with the prosthetic tongue (from 48 to 64 per cent). Currently, we are investigating the nature of speech problems in patients who demonstrate considerable variety in terms of how much tongue tissue is removed, and from what area of the tongue it is excised. Initial results suggest that, in general, patients with right or left hemiglossectomies may have fewer problems with speech than patients with anterior or posterior excisions, while patients with extensive anterior excisions may be rendered most impaired in terms of speech. Substantiation of this observation with acoustic and perceptual data, however, is not complete. It is hoped that our analyses will enable us to approach rehabilitation—be it surgical, prosthetic, or speech therapy—with greater insight, allowing us to maximize communicative potential in these patients.

Mandibulectomy and Floor of Mouth Procedures

Mandibular movements during speech typically encompass less than a centimeter. Thus, mandibular excisions that permit some mobility of the mandible at normal velocities may not interfere significantly with speech intelligibility, provided that other structures (tongue and lips) are unimpaired and free to compensate for any mandibular restrictions. Bloomer and Hawk[120] report that speech dysfunction may not occur even in hemimandibulectomy unless bone resection is done across the midline symphysis. Unfortunately, many mandibular carcinomas also involve tongue tissue. In such cases, the effects of resection on speech are likely to be much more pronounced.

In a discussion of prosthetic approaches to the mandibulectomy patient, Cantor and Curtis[121] described residual problems of each major type of postsurgical condition. With respect to speech and each of these surgical categories, these authors noted the following:

Class I: Radical Alveolectomy with Preservation of Mandibular Continuity. Speech remains essentially normal with these procedures, although scarring in the area of resected mylohyoid muscle may restrict elevation of the floor of the mouth, and thus tongue mobility. Loss of the hypoglossal nerve and sensation in the oral cavity can also alter speech.

Class II: Lateral Resection of the Mandible Distal to the Cuspid. Defects in this group are more extensive than those in Class I, but involve similar sensory and motor losses. The posterior tongue may be sutured to buccal mucosa on the affected side, further restricting lingual movement. Speech is more impaired than in Class I.

Class III: Lateral Resection of the Mandible to the Midline. Speech may be severely restricted, primarily as a function of missing tongue tip and genioglossus muscle. In addition, the tongue's position in the oral cavity is lowered, further restricting its mobility.

Class IV: Lateral Bone Graft Surgical Reconstructions. If radical alveolectomy and subsequent bone augmentation are performed, problems in this category are similar to those associated with Class I excisions. However, if bone grafts connect condylar fragments with remaining mandible, the reduced condylar mobility, scar contractions, and loss of sensory-muscular functions may produce greater impairment.

Class V: Anterior Bone Graft Surgical Reconstruction. Extensive bilateral resections of the anterior floor of the mouth and the ventral surface of the tongue will have serious effects on speech, even though facial contour and bilateral mandibular function may be restored. Effects are worse if the hypoglossal nerve is lost bilaterally.

Maxillectomy and Palatectomy

Next to glossectomy, surgical excision of some portion of the palate presents perhaps the greatest deterrent to normal speech. Effective separation of oral and nasal cavities during speech is critical to the production of all sounds except the nasals /*m, n,* and *ng*/. If this separation is not maintained, the vocal tract becomes larger, and resonances change. Speech sounds are affected differentially, with those requiring the greatest amounts of intraoral pressure and flow (fricatives /*f, v, s, z, sh, zh, th*/, stop consonants /*p, b, t, d, k, g*/, and affricates /*ch, j*/) being most vulnerable to the effects of nasalization.

Major perceptual consequences of a palatectomy on speech may include a hypernasal quality perceived on some or all sounds, nasal emission of sound and air, and loss of appropriate pressures and flows for, in particular, high-pressure consonants. From a rehabilitative point of view, a prosthetic device is often satisfactory, allowing obturation of the defect and, at the same time, providing no interference to examination of the site for recurrence. Speech rehabilitation is perhaps facilitated when the defect is of the hard palate as opposed to a similar-sized defect of the soft palate. A prosthesis that must simply close a defect is much easier to design than one that must interact with muscular structures to restore velopharyngeal competence for speech.

Larger lesions, extending from the palate into other portions of the maxillae and perhaps involving sinuses, can produce marked deleterious effects on speech. Clinically, patients with such defects may demonstrate diminished intelligibility that goes beyond the effects of hypernasality. Speech may be labored as a patient struggles to generate air pressures and flows appropriate for speech. Changes in articulation, timing, and phrasing characteristics are likely sequelae. Majid et al[122] reported speech intelligibility characteristics of a group of six patients who had undergone extensive partial maxillectomy and were subsequently obturated with a variety of maxillary prostheses. Without their prostheses, these patients demonstrated average intelligibility scores of 62 per cent for consonant sounds and 58 per cent for vowel sounds on the Consonant and Vowel Rhyme Tests, respectively.[123, 124] With prosthetic treatment, articulation scores were improved to 96 per cent for consonants and 94 per cent for vowels.

Fletcher et al[125] investigated the extent of nasality in patients who had experienced a variety of surgically created maxillary defects, including procedures described as either hemi-, subtotal, or partial maxillectomy, or resections of the soft palate. In an unobturated condition, measures of nasality on speech were found to be elevated, ranging from 10 to 55 per cent higher than data obtained for normal speakers. With obturation, 6 of 12 patients studied by Fletcher reduced nasality to within normal limits.

The beneficial effects on speech of prosthetic reconstruction in maxillary defects are well documented. It should also be noted that intelligibility scores may reflect the ability of both speaker and listener to compensate for limitations or alterations in the speech signal. Insight into the nature of such compensations may afford additional power to rehabilitative strategies with these patients.

Pharyngectomy (and Laryngectomy)

Patients who have undergone pharyngectomy procedures involving primarily the hypopharynx may experience alterations of the airway that lead to subtle changes in resonance characteristics. Reconstruction of the hypopharynx following complete laryngectomy typically results in a narrowed hypopharynx, with a shorter effective vocal tract length,[10] and a resulting increase in resonance frequencies.[126] Such changes may not interfere with a speaker's ability to occlude or constrict the vocal tract, and therefore may not result in an articulation problem. Rather, the changes wrought are those related to properties of the speech signal that provide information about the speaker's identity and unique personal characteristics.

Resections involving certain structures of the oropharynx, on the other hand, may be a source of articulation difficulty. If pharyngeal contributions to the base of the tongue, soft palate, palatine arch, or velopharyngeal port are affected, speech characteristics described earlier for tongue and palatal resections may also be present.

Orofacial (Soft Tissue) Procedures

If lip or cheek tissues are unable to effectively constrict or occlude the mouth opening as a result of orofacial procedures, articulation may be impaired. The lower lip, in particular, is directly involved in the production of */f/* and */v/*, while both lips participate in */p, b, m, w, wh/* and vowels that require lip rounding, including */o͞o, o͝o, ō* and *ăw/*. In addition, changes in the overall size and shape of the vocal tract may lead to changes in those characteristics of the speech signal that provide information about the unique personal characteristics of the speaker.

As reported for other orofacial anomalies, the contribution of particular surgical variables to speech impairment in patients with facial deformity is not well understood. A comparison of surgical and prosthetic approaches to reconstruction, and their accompanying effects on certain acoustic characteristics of speech, may prove especially fruitful. Similarly, an investigation of prosthetic variables, including the type of material used, whether it is more or less porous, or hollow, may be worthwhile. An initial study by Oral et al,[127] for example, suggests that a buccal flange obturator that is used to cover a palatal defect, but does not extend into or fill the defect, may produce better speech results than hollow obturators that fill the defect. In general, however, little has been done to investigate ways to improve prosthesis design for speech.

An Additional Concern for Speech-Sensory Deprivation and Alterations

The preceding section has been generally based on two principles. The first is that ablative procedures that interfere with the typical dynamics of structures involved in speech production may produce articulation impairments. Second, changes in the size and shape of the vocal tract, unrelated to mobility, may alter those aspects of the speech signal that convey information about the speaker, i.e., identity, age, and gender characteristics.

An additional note should be included regarding possible alterations in the sensory integrity of the speech mechanism occasioned by orofacial resections. An extensive, if controversial, literature is available regarding the role of various sensory feedback mechanisms in normal speech production.[128] There is perhaps general agreement that at least certain aspects of speech production are influenced or regulated by sensory capabilities of receptors in the skin, muscles, and joints of pertinent structures. Certainly, touch-pressure, kinesthetic, and proprioceptive sensory receptors in orofacial structures may undergo temporary or permanent alteration as a consequence of ablative and reconstructive surgical procedures done to eliminate cancer. Exactly what these changes might be, and how they might contribute to the degree of speech impairment, is not known.

Similarly, the effects of radiation therapy on sensory capabilities of orofacial structures are unresolved. Mirza and Dikshit[129] have described short- and long-term effects of radiation therapy on oral tissues. Short-term effects are described as mucositis and mucosal soreness, and lost or diminished sensations of taste or smell. Among the long-term effects noted by these authors are dryness of the mouth, reduced blood supply to tissues, and increased connective tissue fibrosis.

Tissue changes and, particularly, the well-known evidence of diminished taste and smell, may be associated with alterations in sensory receptors that are utilized in speech production. Speculation regarding the relative contributions of sensory and motor aspects of speech impairment related to surgically or radiation-induced deficits is extremely difficult. Precise differentiation is further clouded by the speaker's ability to compensate—to reorganize—in the face of alterations to structure and function. Nevertheless, this aspect of the normal control of speech is sufficiently important that it should be included in discussions concerning effects on speech of surgical and radiation treatments of head and neck cancer.

Relatively more information is available regarding the influence of head/neck cancer and its treatment on auditory sensitivity. Our clinical experience indicates that conductive hearing loss related to serous otitis media may follow treatment for head and neck carcinomas. This is especially true with patients who have maxillary, palatal, or mandibular involvement, though hearing loss may also occur in patients with laryngectomy and pharyngectomy. Most often, the cause of difficulty appears to be eustachian tube malfunction as a consequence of tissue changes associated with surgery or radiation. Myringotomy and tubes, and sometimes temporary amplification, are generally successful in the treatment of these cases. Glazer[67] has noted that while serous otitis media is the most common otologic diagnosis in this population, sensorineural loss due to radiation damage of the inner ear is an additional possibility. Moretti[130] has indicated that when sensorineural loss does occur in an irradiated patient, it is typically progressive and nonreversible.

Speech Therapy Objectives for Patients with Transfer Function Deficits

Restoration of Intelligibility

Efforts to rehabilitate speech in patients with upper vocal tract deficits are twofold. First, intelligibility must be restored to the extent that the speaker is an effective communicator in at least most situations. Interestingly, our patients who estimate their own intelligibility in everyday speaking as greater than 80 per cent, improving to 90 per cent and higher if repeated efforts are considered, appear to function very well in a communicative sense. Though they may have difficulty in particular circumstances, such as in talking to elderly, hard-of-hearing, or non–native English speakers, or on the telephone, generally their experiences are successful. On the other hand, patients who consistently rate themselves as only 60 to 80 per cent effective are often extremely frustrated by their failure to be understood. Some of these patients—and many of those who estimate their proficiency at even lower levels—report that if they speak they do it primarily within the confines of their own home, with listeners who are most familiar with them. Otherwise they may rely on handwriting, or remain silent.

Restoration of speech intelligibility depends, of course, on the restoration of the vocal tract's structure and function. Surgical and prosthetic approaches to this task have generally emphasized cosmesis and function, but not specifically speech function. Systematic evaluation of these approaches as they affect the patient as a speaker can be expected to facilitate our understanding of speech disorders in this population. It is hoped that this needed inquiry will also help maximize communicative potential in our patients.

Restoration of intelligibility beyond surgery or a prosthetic device is in the form of "compensated speech," that is, the ability of the speaker to compensate for the articulation difficulty he experiences. The role of the speech pathologist at this stage of the rehabilitation process is to determine whether there are ways in which the speaker, utilizing available structures, can learn to achieve new speech sound targets that approximate the acoustic characteristics of the originals so closely that the listener will perceive them as the originals. Of course, these new productions must also differ sufficiently from remaining intact sounds that ambiguity does not result. Critical to this approach is knowledge of listener expectations. Listeners recognize certain auditory signals as "speech sounds." A speaker may lose the ability to produce such an acoustic event in the normal or typical manner, as in the case of a glossectomy speaker who can no longer put his tongue tip on the alveolar ridge to say /*t*/. However, if he can constrict the vocal tract in a similar manner, as by holding his teeth together, and manipulate airflows and air pressures as he did for the original /*t*/, he may be able to produce an acoustic signal that a listener perceives as /*t*/. Since no other English speech sound is produced in the new manner (and since the listener expects to hear a speech sound), ambiguity should be minimal.

Next, attempts can be made to enhance the effectiveness of those cues to speech sound perception that remain intact. For example, the vowel /*o͞o*/ is produced primarily by the action of the tongue. Again, a patient with impaired tongue mobility may be unable to shape the vocal tract for this sound in the usual manner. But the speaker's lips should also be rounded for this vowel, and mandibular opening should be minimal. By calling attention to these aspects of the sound's production, perception—and thus intelligibility—may be improved.

Sounds differ from each other not only in terms of their resonance characteristics but also in accordance with temporal/durational parameters, voicing characteristics, airflows and air pressures, and other variables. In connected speech, other cues, such as intonation and stress, can also be imposed on a phrase or sentence, and can influence the listener's perception of the intended utterance. Furthermore, in connected speech, the listener is aided by contextual cues afforded by other intact speech sounds. Obviously, the listener's familiarity with the topic of discussion can also be of tremendous value. By manipulating both articulatory and environmental factors, the speech pathologist can help to emphasize aspects of a patient's speech that increase predictability to the listener, and can thereby improve the likelihood of communicative success.

If restoration of speech intelligibility to a satisfactory level is not a possible objective, then establishment of a communication system that allows the patient the greatest ease and freedom of expression possible is a desirable alternative. Unfortunately, the typical alternative to compensated speech at this time is handwriting. Writing does allow a patient to communicate, and probably more completely than many other alternatives such as manual communication (i.e., sign language or gestures) or a variety of communication boards. Certainly our patients who are unable to write experience severe restrictions in their ability to communicate. But handwriting can be tedious and time consuming, and seldom does the patient have an opportunity (or desire) to freely elaborate on paper as he might through speaking. New computerized instruments that have been advertised largely for patients with multiple physical handicaps would seem to offer great promise for those head and neck cancer patients who are unable to achieve a satisfactory level of speech proficiency. As improvements in these devices continue, and as their cost becomes less prohibitive, they will no doubt fill a very serious need for patients with a variety of communication handicaps.

Restoration of Identity

A second objective of speech rehabilitation, essential for *all* patients with speech problems related to head/neck cancer, concerns the restoration of a speaking, or communicating "identity." As noted earlier, head and neck cancer patients are often subjected to dramatic alteration of features that for all of us signal our unique identities as individuals. Appearance and speech are essential components of this identity. One of our patients, a young woman who had been a university professor, elaborated this point rather eloquently. She said, in essence,

I can manage the loss of function, the difficulties I have eating and swallowing, or just trying to clean out my mouth, or even trying to make some speech sounds. But the really devastating thing is to talk with someone, or to try to do the kind of work I have always done, and to watch myself fail. The feeling I have is that I'm failing to meet my own expectations, as well as theirs—that I'm not realizing my competencies, as if I'm not who I was before.

Feelings of failure and incompetence are surely not far removed from loss of confidence and self-esteem. Our attempts to rehabilitate speech are negligent if we fail to consider not only that a speaker's intelligibility may be impaired by the effects of head and neck cancer but that his self-identity may be threatened as well. Restoration of effective, efficient communicative skills that allow the fullest possible range of expression, and that provide the speaker with a unique speaking identity that he finds acceptable, may serve to accomplish, or at least to approximate, both objectives.

References

1. Fant G: Acoustic Theory of Speech Production. The Hague, Mouton & Co, 1970.
2. Gates G, Ryan W, Cooper J, et al: Current states of laryngectomee rehabilitation. I. Results of therapy. Am J Otolaryngol 3:1, 1982.
3. Gates G, Ryan W, Cantu E, et al: Current states of laryngectomee rehabilitation. II. Causes of failure. Am J Otolaryngol 3:8, 1982.
4. Amster W, Love R, Menzel O, et al: Psychosocial factors and speech after laryngectomy. J Commun Disord 5:1, 1972.
5. Beamer M: A qualitative study of the personality adjustment of laryngectomized subjects. Unpublished Master's Thesis, Texas State College for Women, 1954.
6. Shames G, Font J, Matthews J: Factors related to speech proficiency of the laryngectomized. J Speech Hear Disord 28:273, 1963.
7. DiBartolo R: Psychological considerations in the attainment of esophageal speech. J Surg Oncol 3:451, 1971.
8. Levin N: Total laryngectomy and speech rehabilitation. Eye Ear Nose Throat Monthly 34:585, 1955.
9. Stoll B: Psychological factors determining the success or failure of the rehabilitation program of laryngectomized patients. Ann Otol Rhinol Laryngol 67:550, 1958.
10. Diedrich W, Youngstrom K: Alaryngeal Speech. Springfield, IL, Charles C Thomas, 1971.
11. Snidecor J: Speech rehabilitation of the laryngectomized. Springfield, IL, Charles C Thomas, 1974.
12. Gardner W: Laryngectomee speech and rehabilitation. Springfield, IL, Charles C Thomas, 1971.
13. Gardner W: Adjustment problems of laryngectomized women. Arch Otolaryngol 83:57, 1966.
14. Hudson A: Influences on the acquisition of esophageal voice in a group of laryngectomized veterans. Proc 13th Soc Logopedics & Phonetics, Vienna Academy of Medicine, 2:183, 1965.
15. Kahane J, Irwin J: Comparison of hearing sensitivity and stoma noise in 90 esophageal speakers. Paper presented at Annual Convention of American Speech and Hearing Association, Washington DC, 1975.
16. Stack M: The feminine viewpoint on being a laryngectomee. *In* Keith R, Darley F (eds): Laryngectomee Rehabilitation. Houston, College Hill Press, 1979.
17. Shanks J: Essentials for alaryngeal speech—psychology and physiology. *In* Keith R, Darley F (eds): Laryngectomee Rehabilitation. Houston, College Hill Press, 1979.
18. DiCarlo L, Amster W, Herer G: Speech After Laryngectomy. Syracuse, NY, Syracuse University Press, 1955.
19. Greene M: The Voice and Its Disorders. Philadelphia, JB Lippincott, 1964.
20. Goode R: Artificial laryngeal devices in postlaryngectomy rehabilitation. Laryngoscope 85:677, 1969.
21. Diedrich W: The mechanism of esophageal speech. Ann NY Acad Sci 155:559, 1965.
22. Isshiki N, Snidecor J: Air intake and usage in esophageal speech. Acta Otolaryngol 59:559, 1965.
23. Moolenar-Bilj A: Connection between consonant articulation and intake of air in aesophageal speech. Folia Phoniatr 5:212, 1953.
24. Weinberg B: Speech alternatives following total laryngectomy. *In* Darby J (ed): Speech Evaluation in Medicine. New York, Grune & Stratton, 1980.
25. Ellis F: Upper esophageal sphincter in health and disease. Surg Clin North Am 51:553, 1971.
26. Zainow D, Jacobson H, Lepow H, et al: The pharyngo-esophageal sphincter. Springfield, IL, Charles C Thomas, 1970.
27. Kirchner J, Scatliff F, Dey F, et al: The pharynx after laryngectomy. Laryngoscope 73:18, 1963.
28. Brewer D, Gould L, Casper J: Fiberoptic video study of the postlaryngectomized voice. Laryngoscope 85:666, 1975.
29. Damste P: Some obstacles in learning esophageal speech. *In* Keith R, Darley F (eds): Laryngectomee Rehabilitation. Houston, College Hill Press, 1979.
30. Blom E: Radiographic and manometric assessment of the patient who fails to acquire esophageal voice. *In* Keith R, Darley F (eds): Laryngectomee Rehabilitation. Houston, College Hill Press, 1979.
31. Ingelfinger F: Esophageal motility. Physiol Rev 38:533, 1975.
32. Zwitman D: The function of the pharyngo-esophageal segment during speech. *In* Keith R, Darley F (eds): Laryngectomee Rehabilitation. Houston, College Hill Press, 1979.
33. Hurst A: Nervous disorders of swallowing. J Laryngol Otol 58:60, 1943.
34. Van den Berg J, Moolenar-Bijl AJ: Crico-pharyngeal sphincter, pitch, intensity and fluency in oesophageal speech. Pract Otorhinolaryngol (Basel) 21:298, 1959.
35. Singer M, Blom E, Hamaker R: Further experience with voice restoration after total laryngectomy. Ann Otol Rhinol Laryngol 90:498, 1981.

36. Faulkner W, Rodinbaugh F, O'Neill J: Influence of emotions upon esophageal function: comparison of esophagoscopic and roentgenologic findings. Radiology 37:443, 1941.
37. Clerf L, Putney F: Cricopharyngeal spasm. Laryngoscope 52:944, 1943.
38. Brunner H: X-ray examination of the cricopharyngeal sphincter "hypopharyngeal bar." J Laryngol Otol 66:276, 1952.
39. Shipp T: EMG of pharyngo-esophageal musculature during alaryngeal voice production. J Speech Hear Res 13:184, 1970.
40. Dey F, Kirchner J: The upper esophageal sphincter after laryngectomy. Laryngoscope 71:99, 1061.
41. Collo D, Weihrauch I, Förster C: Course of the intraluminal esophageal pressure after laryngectomy. Laryngol Rhinol Otol 57:1003, 1977.
42. Winans C, Reichbach E, Waldrop W: Esophageal determinants of alaryngeal speech. Arch Otolaryngol 99:10, 1974.
43. Zinner E, Fleshler B: Intraesophageal pressures during phonation in laryngectomized patients. J Laryngol Otol 86:129, 1972.
44. Salmon S: Pressure Variation in the Esophagus, Pharyngeal-Esophageal Constriction and Pharynx Associated with Esophageal Speech Production. Unpublished Doctoral Dissertation, State University of Iowa, Iowa City, 1965.
45. Salmon S: Factors that may interfere with acquiring esophageal speech. *In* Keith R, Darley F (eds): Laryngectomee Rehabilitation. Houston, College Hill Press, 1979.
46. Crouch Z: The relationship of intraluminal swallowing, resting, and phonation pressures to esophageal phonation "goodness" and maximal durational phonation. Unpublished Doctoral Dissertation, University of Kansas, 1974.
47. Bozynski R, Pharr S: Esophageal manometry and speech proficiency in post laryngectomy patients. Abstracted in Gastroenterology 62:622, 1972.
48. Damste P: Oesophageal Speech. Gebr Hoitsema, University of Groningen, The Netherlands, 1958.
49. Welch R, Gates G, Ricks P, et al: Change in the force-summed measurements of the upper esophageal sphincter prelaryngectomy and postlaryngectomy. Ann Otol 88:804, 1979.
50. Simpson I, Smith J, Gordon M: Laryngectomy: The influence of muscle reconstruction on the mechanism of oesophageal voice production. J Laryngol Otol 86:961, 1972.
51. Gilchrist A: Rehabilitation after laryngectomy. Acta Otolaryngol 75:511, 1973.
52. Smith J, Rise E, Gralnek D: Speech recovery in laryngectomized patients. Laryngoscope 76:1540, 1966.
53. Robe E, Moore P, Andrews A, et al: A study of the role of certain factors in the development of speech after laryngectomy: 1. Type of operation. 2. Site of pseudoglottis. 3. Coordination of speech with respiration. Laryngoscope 66:173 (Part 1); 382 (Part 2); 418 (Part 3), 1956.
54. Sako K, Cardinal S, Marchetta F, et al: Speech and vocational rehabilitation of the laryngectomized patient. J Surg Oncol 6:197, 1974.
55. Putney F: Rehabilitation of the post laryngectomized patient. Ann Otol Rhinol Laryngol 67:544, 1958.
56. Richardson J: Surgical and radiological effects upon the development of speech after total laryngectomy. Ann Otol Rhinol Laryngol 90:294, 1981.
57. Vrticka K, Svoboda M: A clinical and x-ray study of 100 laryngectomized speakers. Folia Phoniatr 13:174, 1961.
58. Duguay M: Special problems of the alaryngeal speaker. *In* Keith R, Darley F (eds): Laryngectomee rehabilitation. Houston, College Hill Press, 1979.
59. Shedd D: Speech rehabilitation with external vibrators. Ear Nose Throat J 60:268, 1981.
60. Vise C: Rehabilitation of the voice after pharyngolaryngectomy and skin repair. I. Cineradiography. Clin Otolaryngol 1:107, 1976.
61. Masters J, Berry R, Pepa L: The effect of radiation therapy on the acquisition of esophageal speech. Paper presented at Annual Convention of American Speech and Hearing Association, Las Vagas, Nevada, 1974.
62. Martin D: Pre- and postoperative anatomic/physiologic observation in laryngectomy. *In* Keith R, Darley F (eds): Laryngectomee Rehabilitation. Houston, College Hill Press, 1979.
63. Martin D, Hoops H, Shanks J: The relationship between esophageal speech proficiency and selected measures of auditory function. J Speech Hear Res 74:80, 1974.
64. Berlin C: Hearing loss, palatal function and other factors in postlaryngectomy rehabilitation. J Chronic Dis 17:677, 1964.
65. Svane-Knudson V: The substitute voice of the laryngectomized patient. Acta Otolaryngol 52:85, 1959.
66. Hoopla G, Brewer D: Voice production in the laryngectomized patient. Ann Otol Rhinol Laryngol 63:640, 1954.
67. Glazer D: Audiologic management of head and neck carcinoma patients. J Speech Hear Disord 45:216, 1980.
68. Wolf R, Olson J, Goldenberg D: Rehabilitation of the laryngectomee: the role of the distal esophageal sphincter. Laryngoscope 81:1971, 1971.
69. Doubravsky J, Prasil J: X-ray picture of the esophagus and the esophagogastric junction in laryngectomized patients. Cesk Radiol 23:111, 1969.
70. Samuel P, Adams F: The role of esophageal and diaphragmatic movement in alaryngeal speech. J Laryngol Otol 90:1105, 1976.
71. Lowry Z: Artificial larynges: a review and development of a prototype self-contained intraoral artificial larynx. Laryngoscope 91:1322, 1981.
72. Young K, Bailey B, Everett R, et al: Electronic laryngeal prosthesis for implantation: a progress report. *In* Shedd D, Weinberg B (eds): Surgical and Prosthetic Approaches to Speech Rehabilitation. Boston, GK Hall Medical Publishers, 1980.
73. Charles D, Fredrickson J, Bryce D: An implantable electromagnetic sound source: preliminary results of human implantation. *In* Shedd D, Weinberg B (eds): Surgical and Prosthetic Approaches to Speech Rehabilitation. Boston, GH Hall Medical Publishers, 1980.
74. McComb W, Fletcher G: Larynx: Cancer of the Head and Neck. Baltimore, Williams & Wilkins, 1967.
75. Weinberg B, Riekena A: Speech produced with a Tokyo artificial larynx. J Speech Hear Disord 38:383, 1973.
76. Salmon S, Goldstein L (eds): The Artificial Larynx Handbook. New York, Grune & Stratton, 1978.
77. Berry W: Indications for the use of artificial larynx devices. *In* Salmon S, Goldstein L (eds): The

artificial Larynx Handbook. New York, Grune & Stratton, 1978.

78. Sisson G, McConnel F, Logemann J, et al: Vocal rehabilitation after laryngectomy: Results with the use of hypopharyngeal prosthesis. Arch Otolaryngol 101:178, 1975.
79. Malone P, Komorn R: Speech rehabilitation following laryngectomy and construction of a T-E shunt. Paper presented at the Annual Convention of American Speech and Hearing Association, Detroit, Michigan, 1973.
80. Edwards N: Vocal rehabilitation by external vocal fistula and valved prosthesis: Edwards method. *In* Shedd D, Weinberg B (eds): Surgical and Prosthetic Approaches to Speech Rehabilitation. Boston, GK Hall Medical Publishers, 1980.
81. McConnel F, Sisson G, Logemann J: Three years' experience with a hypopharyngeal pseudoglottis after total laryngectomy. Trans Am Acad Ophthalmol Otolaryngol 84:63, 1977.
82. Shedd D, Bakamjian V, Sako K, et al: Reed fistula method of speech rehabilitation after laryngectomy. Am J Surg 124:510, 1972.
83. Weinberg B, Shedd D, Horii Y: Reed-fistula speech following pharyngolaryngectomy. J Speech Hear Disord 43:401, 1978.
84. Taub S, Spiro R: Vocal rehabilitation of laryngectomees. Am J Surg 124:87, 1972.
85. Eberle R, Taub S: Air-bypass voice prosthesis for vocal rehabilitation of laryngectomees. Ear Nose Throat J 60:273, 1976.
86. Blom E: A comparative investigation of acoustical and perceptual features of esophageal speech and speech with the Taub voice prosthesis. Unpublished Doctoral Dissertation, University of Maryland, 1972.
87. Taub S: Air-bypass voice prosthesis for vocal rehabilitation of laryngectomees. Ear Nose Throat J 60:42, 1981.
88. Amatsu M: A new one-stage surgical technique for postlaryngectomy speech. Arch Otorhinolaryngol 220:149, 1977.
89. Singer M, Blom E: An endoscopic technique for restoration of voice after laryngectomy. Ann Otol Rhinol Laryngol 89:529, 1980.
90. Taub S: Air-bypass voice prosthesis: an 8-year experience. *In* Shedd D, Weinberg B: Surgical and Prosthetic Approaches to Speech Rehabilitation. Boston, GK Hall Medical Publishers, 1980.
91. Blom E, Singer M: Surgical prosthetic approaches for postlaryngectomy voice restoration. *In* Keith R, Darby F (eds): Laryngectomee Rehabilitation. Houston, College Hill Press, 1979.
92. Panje W: Prosthetic vocal rehabilitation following laryngectomy: the voice button. Ann Otol Rhinol Laryngol 90:116, 1981.
93. Labayle J: Restorative total laryngectomy. *In* Shedd D, Weinberg B (eds.): Surgical and Prosthetic Approaches to Speech Rehabilitation. Boston, GK Hall Medical Publishers, 1979.
94. Mozolewski E: Arytenoid vocal shunt in laryngectomized patients. Laryngoscope 85:853, 1975.
95. Pique J: Functional laryngectomy (cricohyoidopexy). *In* Shedd D, Weinberg B (eds): Surgical and Prosthetic Approaches to Speech Rehabilitation. Boston, GK Hall Medical Publishers, 1980.
96. Serafini I: Reconstructive laryngectomy. *In* Shedd D, Weinberg B (eds): Surgical and Prosthetic Approaches to Speech Rehabilitation. Boston, GK Hall Medical Publishers, 1980.
97. Arslan M, Serafini I: Reconstructive laryngectomy: report of the first 35 cases. Ann Otol Rhinol Laryngol 81:479, 1972.
98. Vega M, Siola B: Surgery for laryngeal cancer with preservation of voice. *In* Shedd D, Weinberg B (eds): Surgical and Prosthetic Approaches to Speech Rehabilitation. Boston, GK Hall Medical Publishers, 1979.
99. Vega M: Larynx reconstructive surgery—a study of three-year findings—a modified surgical technique. Laryngoscope 85:866, 1975.
100. Asai R: Laryngoplasty after total laryngectomy. Arch Otolaryngol 95:114, 1972.
101. Miller A: First experiences with the Asai technique for vocal rehabilitation after total laryngectomy. Ann Otol Rhinol Laryngol 76:829, 1967.
102. Pearson B: Subtotal laryngectomy. Laryngoscope 91:1904, 1981.
103 Pearson B, Woods R, Hartman D: Extended hemilaryngectomy for T_3 glottic carcinoma with preservation of speech and swallowing. Laryngoscope 90:1950, 1979.
104. Staffieri M: Phonatory neoglottis surgery. Ear Nose Throat J 60:254, 1981.
105. Griffiths C: Reconstruction of the glottis after total laryngectomy. Ear Nose Throat J 60:259, 1981.
106. Sisson G, Hurst P, Goldman M, et al: Prosthetic devices in neoglottis surgery. Ear Nose Throat J 60:282, 1981.
107. Leipzig B, Griffiths C, Shea J: Neoglottic reconstruction following total laryngectomy: the Galveston experience. Ann Otol Rhinol Laryngol 89:204, 1981.
108. Kitamura T, Kaneko T, Togawa K, et al: Supracricoid laryngectomy: a new technique for vocal rehabilitation. Laryngoscope 80:300, 1970.
109. Conley J, De Amesti F, Pierce M: A new surgical technique for the vocal rehabilitation of the laryngectomized patient. Ann Otol Rhinol Laryngol 67:655, 1958.
110. Calcaterra T, Jafek B: Tracheoesophageal shunt for speech rehabilitation after total laryngectomy. Arch Otolaryngol 94:124, 1971.
111. Komorn R: Vocal rehabilitation in the laryngectomized patient with a tracheoesophageal shunt. Ann Otol Rhinol Laryngol 83:445, 1974.
112. Gillis R: Psychologic implications of patient care. *In* Laney W, Gardner A (eds): Maxillofacial prosthetics. Postgraduate Dental Handbook Series, Vol 4, 1980.
113. La Riviere C, Seilo M, Dimmick K: Report on the speech intelligibility of a glossectomee: perceptual and acoustic observations. Folia Phoniatr 27:201, 1975.
114. Amerman J, Laminack C: Evaluation and rehabilitation of glossectomy speech behavior. J Comm Dis 7:365, 1974.
115. Skelly M, Spector D, Donaldson R, et al: Compensatory physiologic phonetics for the glossectomee. J Speech Hear Disord 36:101, 1971.
116. Massengill R, Maxwell S, Pickrell K: An analysis of articulation following partial and total glossectomy. J Speech Hear Disord 35:170, 1970.
117. Duguay M: Speech after glossectomy. NY State J Med 64:1836, 1964.
118. Leonard R, Gillis R: Effects of a prosthetic tongue on vowel intelligibility and food management in a patient with total glossectomy. J Speech Hear Disord 47:25, 1982.
119. Gillis R, Leonard R: Approach to prosthetic treat-

ment in a patient with total glossectomy. J Prosthet Dent 50:808, 1983.
120. Bloomer H, Hawk A: Speech considerations; speech disorders associated with ablative surgery of the face, mouth, and pharynx—ablative approaches to learning. ASHA Rep 8:42, 1972.
121. Cantor R, Curtis T: Prosthetic management of edentulous mandibulectomy patients. Part 1. Anatomic, physiologic and psychologic considerations. J Prosthet Dent 25:446, 1971.
122. Majid A, Weinberg B, Chalian V: Speech intelligibility following prosthetic obturation of surgically acquired maxillary defects. J Prosthet Dent 32:87, 1974.
123. House A, Williams C, Hecker M, et al: Articulation testing methods: consonantal differentiation with a closed response set. J Acoust Soc Am 37:158, 1965.
124. Horii Y: Specifying the speech-to-noise ratio: development and evaluation of a noise with speech-envelope characteristics. Doctoral Dissertation, Purdue University, 1969.
125. Fletcher S, Iradq S, Frost S: Quantitative and graphic analysis of prosthetic treatment for "nasalance" in speech. J Prosthet Dent 32:284, 1974.
126. Sisty N, Weinberg B: Formant frequency characteristics of esophageal speech. J Speech Hear Disord 15:439, 1972.
127. Oral K, Aramany M, McWilliams B: Speech intelligibility with the buccal flange obturator. J Prosthet Dent 41:323, 1979.
128. Putnam A, Ringel R: Oral sensation and perception. *In* Wolfe F, Goulding D (eds): Articulation and Learning. Springfield, IL, Charles C Thomas, 1980.
129. Mirza F, Dikshit J: Use of implant prostheses following radiation therapy. J Prosthet Dent 40:663, 1978.
130. Moretti J: Sensorineural hearing loss following radiotherapy to the nasopharynx. Laryngoscope 86:598, 1976.

INDEX

Note: Page numbers in *italics* refer to illustrations; page numbers followed by the letter t refer to tables.